UNDERSTANDING Y

UNDERSTANDING YOUR BODY

❖

Every Woman's Guide to a Lifetime of Health

Felicia H. Stewart, M.D.

Practicing in Gynecology
Clinical Instructor in Obstetrics
and Gynecology
University of California, Davis
School of Medicine
Sacramento, California

Gary K. Stewart, M.D., M.P.H., F.A.C.O.G.

Practicing in Obstetrics and
Gynecology
Medical Director
Planned Parenthood of
Sacramento Valley
Assistant Clinical Professor in
Obstetrics and Gynecology
University of California, Davis
School of Medicine
Sacramento, California

Felicia Guest

Health Educator,
Medical Sciences Writer
Training Specialist for Patient
Education and Counseling
Regional Training Center for
Family Planning
Emory University School of Medicine
Department of Gynecology and
Obstetrics
Atlanta, Georgia

Robert A. Hatcher, M.D., M.P.H., F.A.A.P.

Director of Family Planning Program
Emory University—Grady Memorial
Hospital Family Planning Program
Professor of Gynecology and Obstetrics
Emory University School of Medicine
Atlanta, Georgia

With Illustrations by Nelva B. Richardson
Medical and Dental Illustrator

BANTAM BOOKS
NEW YORK • TORONTO • LONDON • SYDNEY • AUCKLAND

This book is dedicated to
our mothers, with gratitude

Lena Johnson Hance
Janie C. Guest
Della Jensen Stewart
Meta Lieber Hatcher, 1899–1975

AUTHORS' NOTE

The information contained in this book is intended to complement, not replace, the advice of your own clinician, with whom you should always consult before starting any medical treatment, diet, or exercise program. Readers should keep in mind that there are references to drug or vitamin dosages in this book which are generally recommended dosages only, not individual prescriptions. Only your personal clinician can give you the individual prescription and medical counseling that you need.

UNDERSTANDING YOUR BODY
A Bantam Book / December 1987

Illustrations by Nelva B. Richardson.

Library of Congress Cataloging-in-Publication Data

Understanding your body.

Includes bibliographies and index.
1. Gynecology—Popular works. I. Stewart, Felicia Hance, 1943-   . [DNLM: 1. Gynecology—popular works. WP 120 U19]
RG121.U53   1987   618.1   87-47577
ISBN 0-553-34451-X

Published simultaneously in the United States and Canada

PRINTED IN THE UNITED STATES OF AMERICA

BOMC offers recordings and compact discs, cassettes and records. For information and catalog write to BOMR, Camp Hill, PA 17012.

A C K N O W L E D G M E N T S

Most of all, we are indebted to our patients. Their questions and their experiences are the backbone of this book.

We also want to acknowledge the support we have had from colleagues and friends and from our families; their help and encouragement made this book possible. Our reviewers have given invaluable help, with more generosity, conscientiousness, and insight than we would have dared to hope for when we began. Gary and Felicia Stewart particularly want to thank their partners in medical practice, who gave their support and encouragement and shouldered extra burdens so there would be time for writing.

Without Roxanne Delano, Cathy Vincent, and Diana Pursglove, this book would still be a 5-foot stack of handwritten yellow pages. Roxanne Delano, especially, was the patient and tireless person who transformed our drafts into a triple-checked batch of ten computer discs, and coordinated the review process as well. We appreciate too the contributions of Cynthia Ellis and Julia Barry, who helped us find source materials and references.

This work has also benefited from the many colleagues and friends who helped with the first and second editions of *My Body, My Health*. For their generous time, effort, and insight we continue to thank Geraldine Oliva, Mina Robbins, Susan Worth, Ann Reed, Rita R. Harris, Ward Cates, Michael Castleman, Matelle Goldstein, Lorrie Morris, Robin Bernard, Marsha Ross, Jane Sugarman, Judy Wolen, Elinor Hackett, Martha Kayne, Karen Shaffer, Carol Binns, Beverly Richardson, Florence Winship, Nancy Clark, Doug Cook, Mattie Baker, Sylvia Kelly, Mike Bennett, and Ed Brann.

And for special help in preparing the index, we want to thank Robin Bernard, Gene Bessent, Carol Binns, Paula E. Bunnell Robb, Beverly Daves, Nancy E. Dimick, Mary Driscoll, Sarah Freeman, Sandra Beers Garese, Charlie Godwin, Jenny Godwin, Elizabeth Hervert-Gaines, Priscilla Munson Johnson, Kathy Kallvet-Webber, Dick King, Kathey Stubbs, and Therese Techman.

Finally, we appreciate the inspiration and help of the many friends, patients, colleagues, and readers who over the years have shared new ideas, helped identify priorities, and offered us the benefit of their criticisms. We appreciate especially the readers who have written to us with their questions and concerns. This book is stronger as a result.

FOREWORD

Understanding Your Body: Every Woman's Guide to a Lifetime of Health is a book containing straightforward and comprehensive information for both women's clinicians and women, presented in a warm and positive manner. It is essential for women to know how their body functions and to have available new and up-to-date information on all aspects of health care. Understanding the anatomy of the female body, the physiology of the menstrual cycle, conception, and pregnancy gives a woman confidence and helps her make decisions in her best interest. The information contained in this book will allow a woman to participate actively in health care decisions; it will encourage her to select appropriate options for restoring health and to choose lifestyles that will help prevent disease and maintain her health and that of her family.

It is essential for clinicians to know and understand women's needs for information and to accept the varying attitudes and alternatives women choose. Authoritarian attitudes and dogmatic directives by physicians are outmoded and counterproductive.

The book is organized as a reference manual for looking up facts and information on specific problems. There is no need to approach it as a book to read from beginning to end.

Ignorance and lack of information often lead to concerns, anxiety, and fears that rob a woman of energy and confidence for everyday living and may result in her being isolated and alienated from health care. This practical information on health problems and treatment choices should go a long way in helping women understand there often are a wide range of ways to cope with common health problems. There are excellent discussions of the premenstrual syndrome, the menopause, and hysterectomy. It is important to understand that there is often no consensus among physicians and clinicians on diagnostic tests, procedures, and treatment even for serious medical problems.

Facts are essential for a woman to protect herself physically and psychologically from sexually transmitted disease, pelvic infection, and resultant infertility. Information on sexuality and pregnancy prevention allows a woman to prevent unintended pregnancy and gives her control over her own body and her life.

Self-knowledge is the most important knowledge to have; this book will help a woman know herself.

LUELLA KLEIN, M.D., CHAIRMAN
Department of Gynecology and Obstetrics
Emory University School of Medicine
Atlanta, Georgia

P R E F A C E

Some of the most momentous decisions a woman makes have a direct and immediate impact on the health of her reproductive organs. As you decide whether to have a baby or to begin a sexual partnership, health probably is not your primary consideration; nor should it always be. But health certainly is *one* factor that you will want to consider and plan for.

This book provides facts about your body and your health that you will need for making plans and decisions when your reproductive system demands your attention. You may be trying to become pregnant or trying to avoid pregnancy; you may have questions about an infection or about fibroid tumors; you may be considering whether to take hormones after menopause; or you may be worried about surgery that your clinician has recommended. Almost every woman faces one or more of these problems at some time during her life, and almost every woman has unanswered questions.

We have written about gynecology because our patients have asked so many good questions, and because we believe that each person has the right to know all the facts that are germane to personal health care decision making. As you decide about medical treatment or surgery, you have the right and the responsibility to learn about your problem, your treatment alternatives, and the possible complications. Your clinician has a legal obligation to provide the information you need, and your consent to treatment is your acknowledgment that you do understand. This book can help insure that your consent is truly informed.

No book can recommend or prescribe medical treatment specifically for you. You and your clinician are obviously in a better position to assess your needs. Also, your clinician may not agree with some of the recommendations in this book. Don't be concerned about such disagreement; it is the rule in medicine. Even the four authors of this book don't always agree. One important reason for disagreement is that there are many gaps in knowledge in the field of gynecology, just as there are in almost all areas of medical science.

You may not be familiar with the term "clinician." We have used clinician throughout the book to mean physician, nurse practitioner, or physician assistant because we enthusiastically support the expanded roles of nurses and other specially trained members of the health care field. Their skills are especially well adapted to the field of gynecology.

Reference citations in the text are intended for those who want to find the medical articles we have used as sources for statistics. Most of these sources are available only in medical libraries. If you want to read more but do not have an extensive medical background, the "Suggested Reading" lists may be of help.

We expect to keep this book current by revising it regularly. Some of the issues in reproductive health need to be reevaluated almost weekly. Nothing would be more helpful to us and to future readers than your constructive comments for improving the next edition. We would like to hear from you. Please send your comments and suggestions to Felicia Stewart, Planned Parenthood of Sacramento Valley, 501 S Street, Suite 3, Sacramento, California 95814.

FELICIA HANCE STEWART
FELICIA JANE GUEST
GARY K. STEWART
ROBERT A. HATCHER

C O N T E N T S

L I S T O F T A B L E S

R E V I E W E R S

The authors wish to express their heartfelt gratitude to the many colleagues whose inspiration and scholarly work are the foundations for this book. We also truly appreciate the invaluable help of the following reviewers, who have so generously given us the benefit of expert criticism. Their help has made this book more carefully considered than would otherwise have been possible, and we have tried to integrate each criticism honestly and accurately. Lapses and inaccuracies, however, belong to the authors, not the reviewers. Each reviewer provided comments in her/his area of expertise, but the final product is our responsibility.

John S. Abele, M.D., F.A.C.P.
Diagnostic Pathology Medical Group
Sacramento, California

Donna Armstrong, President
Printed Matter, Inc.
Atlanta, Georgia

Mary Lou Ballweg, President and Co-founder
U.S.–Canadian Endometriosis Association
Milwaukee, Wisconsin

Lonnie Barbach, Ph.D.
Clinical Faculty
University of California, San Francisco

Stephen Bearg, M.D., F.A.C.O.G.
Co-Medical Director, Women's Health Associates, Inc.
Larkspur, California

Gerald S. Bernstein, Ph.D., M.D., F.A.C.O.G.
Department of Obstetrics and Gynecology
University of Southern California School of Medicine
Los Angeles, California

N. Edward Boyce, Jr., M.D., F.A.C.O.G.
Clinical Assistant Professor of Obstetrics, Gynecology, and Reproductive Sciences
University of California, San Francisco

Medical Director, Planned Parenthood
of Marin and Sonoma Counties
San Rafael, California

J. Robert Bragonier, M.D., Ph.D., F.A.C.O.G.
Chairman, Department of Obstetrics and Gynecology
CIGNA Healthplans of California
Adjunct Professor of Obstetrics and Gynecology
University of California, Los Angeles

Ronald T. Burkman, Jr., M.D., F.A.C.O.G.
Chairman, Department of Gynecology and Obstetrics
Henry Ford Hospital
Detroit, Michigan

Michael S. Burnhill, M.D., D.M.Sc., F.A.C.O.G.
Professor of Clinical Obstetrics and Gynecology
Robert Wood Johnson Medical School
University of Medicine and Dentistry of New Jersey
New Brunswick, New Jersey

Dwana Marie Bush, M.D.
Family Physician, Private Practice
Assistant Clinical Professor of Medicine
Emory University School of Medicine
Atlanta, Georgia

Harvey W. Caplan, M.D., F.A.C.P.
Private Practice, Psychotherapy
Former Co-director of Clinical Training
Human Sexuality Program
University of California, San Francisco

Carol Cassell, Ph.D.
Past President, American Association of
   Sex Educators, Counselors and Therapists
Albuquerque, New Mexico

Willard Cates, Jr., M.D., M.P.H.
Director, Division of Sexually Transmitted Diseases
Centers for Disease Control
Atlanta, Georgia

Charles Collins, M.D., F.A.C.A.
Sacramento, California

Winnifred B. Cutler, Ph.D.
Research Director, Athena Institute
   for Women's Wellness Research
Haverford, Pennsylvania

Philip D. Darney, M.D., F.A.C.O.G.
Associate Professor of Obstetrics, Gynecology,
   and Reproductive Sciences
School of Medicine
University of California, San Francisco

Patrick Dietler, M.D., F.A.C.S.
Sacramento, California

Kemp B. Doersch, M.D., F.A.C.S.
Clinical Professor of Surgery
School of Medicine
University of California, Davis

Robert M. Faggella, Jr., M.D., F.A.C.S.
Associate Clinical Professor of Plastic and
   Reconstructive Surgery
School of Medicine
University of California, Davis

Arthur C. Feinstein, M.D., F.A.C.S.
Atlanta, Georgia

Julita A. Fong, M.D., F.C.A.P.
Fong Diagnostic Laboratory
Sacramento, California

Katherine Forrest, M.D., M.P.H.
Medical Research and Marketing Consultant
Portola Valley, California

Lise Fortier, M.D., F.A.C.O.G.
Medical Director, Planned Parenthood World
   Population
Los Angeles, California

Malcolm G. Freeman, M.D., F.A.C.O.G.
Professor of Gynecology and Obstetrics
Emory University School of Medicine
Atlanta, Georgia

Celso-Ramón García, M.D., F.A.C.O.G.
Professor of Obstetrics and Gynecology
Hospital of the University of Pennsylvania
Philadelphia, Pennsylvania

Mitchell S. Golbus, M.D., F.A.C.O.G.
Professor of Obstetrics, Gynecology, and
   Reproductive Sciences
School of Medicine
University of California, San Francisco

Matelle Goldstein, R.N., N.P.
Valley Center for Women's Health
Sacramento, California

William M. Green, M.D.
Associate Clinical Professor of Internal Medicine
Division of Critical Care/Emergency Medicine and
   Clinical Toxicology
School of Medicine
University of California, Davis

Sheldon Greenfield, M.D., F.A.C.M.
Professor of Medicine and Public Health
School of Medicine and School of Public Health
University of California, Los Angeles

Sadja A. Greenwood, M.D., M.P.H.
Assistant Clinical Professor of Obstetrics,
Gynecology, and Reproductive Sciences
School of Medicine
University of California, San Francisco

David Grimes, M.D., F.A.C.O.G.
Professor of Obstetrics and Gynecology
School of Medicine
University of Southern California
Los Angeles, California

Jean Guenza, L.V.N.
Valley Center for Women's Health
Sacramento, California

Janie C. Guest
Fort Payne, Alabama

Lena Hance
Palo Alto, California

Elizabeth Harrison, M.D.
Clinical Consultant, Sacramento AIDS Foundation
Sacramento, California

James K. Hepler, M.D., F.A.C.O.G.
Associate Clinical Professor of Obstetrics and
    Gynecology
School of Medicine
University of California, Davis

Warren M. Hern, M.D., M.P.H.
Director, Boulder Abortion Clinic, P.C.
Boulder, Colorado

Howard H. Hiatt, M.D., F.A.C.M.
Professor of Medicine
Harvard Medical School and School of Public
    Health
Boston, Massachusetts

Edward C. Hill, M.D., F.A.C.O.G.
Professor of Obstetrics, Gynecology, and
    Reproductive Sciences
School of Medicine
University of California, San Francisco

Carol J. Rowland Hogue, M.P.H., Ph.D.
Chief, Pregnancy Epidemiology Branch
Division of Reproductive Health
Centers for Disease Control
Atlanta, Georgia

T. Warner Hudson, M.D., F.A.C.F.P.
Assistant Clinical Professor and Associate
    Residency Director
Department of Family Practice
School of Medicine
University of California, Davis

Patricia Lawver Humphries, M.Ed.
Atlanta, Georgia

Richard M. Hutchinson, M.D., F.A.C.O.G.
Santa Rosa, California

Kathleen L. Irwin, M.D.
Division of Reproductive Health
Centers for Disease Control
Atlanta, Georgia

Henry S. Kahn, M.D., F.A.C.P.
Department of Community Health
Emory University School of Medicine
Division of Reproductive Health
Centers for Disease Control
Atlanta, Georgia

Barbara Kass-Annese, R.N., C.N.P.
Los Angeles Regional Family Planning Council,
    Inc.
Los Angeles, California

Maxine M. Keel
Emory University Family Planning Program
Atlanta, Georgia

Robert E. Keller, P.A.-C.
Lifestyle Health Services
Nashville, Tennessee

Juliette S. Kendrick, M.D.
Division of Reproductive Health
Centers for Disease Control
Atlanta, Georgia

Annabelle Kenward, Coordinator
Religious Coalition for Abortion Rights of
    Northern California
Sacramento, California

Joyce King, R.N.
Assistant Professor Emory University School of
    Nursing
Atlanta, Georgia

Mary E. Lane, M.D.
Director, Women & Youth Services
Westchester County Department of Health
White Plains, New York

Nancy C. Lee, M.D., Medical Epidemiologist
Division of Reproductive Health
Centers for Disease Control
Atlanta, Georgia

James A. McGregor, M.D.C.M., F.A.C.O.G.
Associate Professor of Obstetrics and Gynecology
School of Medicine
University of Colorado Health Sciences Center
Denver, Colorado

H. Trent MacKay, M.D., M.P.H., F.A.C.O.G.
Clinical Professor of Obstetrics and Gynecology
School of Medicine
University of California, Davis

David Magnus, M.D., F.A.C.S.
Urologist
Sacramento, California

Byrne R. Marshall, M.D., F.A.C.O.G.
Obstetrician/Gynecologist
Carmichael, California

Arthur M. McCausland, M.D., F.A.C.O.G.
Associate Clinical Professor of Obstetrics and
    Gynecology
School of Medicine
University of California, Davis

Suellen Miller, R.N., C.N.M.
Marin Maternity Services, Inc.
Greenbrae, California

Daniel R. Mishell, Jr., M.D., F.A.C.O.G.
Professor and Chairman of Obstetrics and
    Gynecology
University of Southern California School of
    Medicine
Chief, Professional Services, Women's Hospital
Los Angeles, California

Dorothy Eilers Mitchell, M.D., F.A.C.O.G.
Director, Division of Reproductive Endocrinology
    & Infertility
Assistant Professor of Gynecology and Obstetrics
Emory University School of Medicine
Atlanta, Georgia

Lorrie Morris, R.N., N.P.
Ob/Gyn Nurse Practitioner
Sacramento, California

Madge E. Mulkey, R.N., C.N.M., M.S.
Valley Center for Women's Health
Sacramento, California

Morris Notelovitz, M.D., Ph.D.
Founder and President Midlife Centers of America
    and the Climacteric Clinic
Gainesville, Florida

Geraldine Oliva, M.D., M.P.H., F.A.C.P.
Director, Family Health
San Francisco County Department of Public
Health

David L. Olive, M.D., F.A.C.O.G.
University of Arkansas Medical Center
Little Rock, Arkansas

James W. Overstreet, M.D., Ph.D.
Professor of Obstetrics and Gynecology
School of Medicine
University of California, Davis

Margaret J. Oxtoby, M.D.
Meningitis and Special Pathogens Branch
Division of Bacterial Diseases
Centers for Disease Control
Atlanta, Georgia

Kirtley Parker-Jones, M.D., F.A.C.O.G.
Department of Obstetrics and Gynecology
University of Utah Medical Center
Salt Lake City, Utah

Diana B. Petitti, M.D.
Assistant Professor of Community Medicine and
    Epidemiology
Division of Family and Community Medicine
University of California, San Francisco

Harriet F. Pilpel, J.D.
Practicing Lawyer with Weil, Gotshal and Manges
General Counsel, Planned Parenthood Federation
    of America
Vice-Chair, National Advisory Committee of the
    American Civil Liberties Union
New York, New York

Virginia C. Poirier, M.D., F.A.C.R.
Director of Radiology, Kaiser Permanente Hospital
Sacramento, California

Sandy Pomerantz, M.D.
Co-Medical Director, Sacramento AIDS Foundation
Sacramento, California

Mark D. Reiss, M.D.
Radiological Associates of Sacramento Medical
    Group
Sacramento, California

Mary J. Retzer, M.D., F.A.Co.M.
Medical Oncologist
Sacramento, California

Ralph M. Richart, M.D., F.A.C.O.G.
Professor of Pathology
Columbia University College of Physicians &
  Surgeons
Director, Division of Ob/Gyn Pathology and
  Cytology
The Sloane Hospital for Women
New York, New York

Eugene D. Robin, M.D., F.A.C.M.
Professor of Medicine and Physiology
Stanford University
Palo Alto, California

Judith P. Rooks, C.N.M., M.S., M.P.H.
Portland, Oregon

George L. Rubin, M.D.
Division of Reproductive Health
Centers for Disease Control
Atlanta, Georgia

George W. Rutherford, M.D.
Medical Director, AIDS Office
San Francisco Department of Public Health
San Francisco, California

Jack M. Schneider, M.D., F.A.C.O.G.
Director and Clinical Professor of Maternal–Fetal
  Medicine
Department of Obstetrics and Gynecology
University of California, Davis School of Medicine
Director, The Perinatal Center and Department of
  Perinatology
Sutter Community Hospitals
Sacramento, California

Kay Scott, Executive Director
Planned Parenthood–Atlanta
Atlanta, Georgia

William Silen, M.D., F.A.C.S.
Johnson & Johnson Professor of Surgery
Harvard Medical School
Surgeon-in-Chief, Beth Israel Hospital
Boston, Massachusetts

Lloyd H. Smith, M.D., Ph.D.
Fellow, Section of Gynecologic Oncology
Stanford University School of Medicine
Stanford, California

Richard M. Soderstrom, M.D., F.A.C.O.G.
Reproductive Health Specialists
Seattle, Washington

Leon Speroff, M.D., F.A.C.O.G.
Professor of Obstetrics and Gynecology
Case Western Reserve University
Cleveland, Ohio

Lucinda L. Thomas, M.A., A.C.S.E.
Director, Public Health Education
Pee Dee II Public Health District
South Carolina Department of Health &
  Environmental Control
Bennettsville, South Carolina

J.D. Thompson, M.D., F.A.C.O.G.
Professor of Gynecology and Obstetrics
Emory University School of Medicine
Woodruff Medical Center
Atlanta, Georgia

Duane E. Townsend, M.D., F.A.C.O.G.
Professor and Vice-Chairman of Obstetrics and
  Gynecology
School of Medicine
University of California, Davis

James Trussell, Ph.D.
Professor of Economics and Public Affairs
Princeton University
Princeton, New Jersey

Catherine Underwood
Sacramento, California

Joyce M. Vargyas, M.D., F.A.C.O.G.
Assistant Professor of Obstetrics and Gynecology
Women's Hospital
University of Southern California School of
  Medicine
Los Angeles, California

Burnell Vassar, P.S.S. II
Planned Parenthood of Sacramento Valley
Sacramento, California

C. Phillip Weaver, M.D., F.A.C.O.G.
Sacramento, California

Wendy Lucas Wood
Davis, California

Bill Yee, M.D., F.A.C.O.G.
Director of In Vitro Fertilization
Assistant Professor of Obstetrics and Gynecology
California College of Medicine
University of California, Irvine

F O R E W O R D
to the First and Second Editions

"What do women want?" is a question ascribed to Freud that became a riddle in Victorian times. Answers are more obvious today. Among other things, women want basic tools for self-direction and growth—among these tools are knowledge of their body's rhythms, and knowledge of their inner space and how to protect it. As more is known about the reproductive sciences, the task of presenting such knowledge to the public grows more challenging. Women must be informed about their anatomy and functioning from an early age; they must learn how to prevent sexually transmitted diseases and unwanted pregnancy; they must be encouraged to become students of their own individual condition—surely an interesting quest, if occasionally an uncomfortable one.

In this book, the authors have taken on the task of such education and motivation—with wisdom, warmth, and clarity. Their book is exceedingly thorough, scientific, and understandable. The reader becomes a colleague in the quest for accurate information and its application to unique individuals. This book will please the women's movement and consumer medicine advocates with its honesty and emphasis on self-care and informed choice. Yet it will reach an even larger audience, as it has humor and balance and is never doctrinaire. Counselors, sexologists, and perusers of birth control manuals will be delighted to find—at last—a thorough discussion of the sexual aspects of various contraceptive measures and an acknowledgment of the importance of sexuality in birth control choice.

One need spend only a day in a woman's clinic or hospital emergency room to appreciate the difficulties that can visit the female reproductive system when women are not educated to be vigilant in self-protection. May this book be widely read and wisely heeded!

SADJA GREENWOOD, M.D.
University of California
San Francisco Medical Center
San Francisco, California

1

Coping with Health Care

The average woman visits a doctor's office or clinic roughly three times each year; more than 100 times in an average adult life span. Most of these visits are for routine care, or for minor problems. Nevertheless, it is safe to guess that many are less than enjoyable, and some may be downright terrifying.

It makes sense to do whatever you can to insure that your own inevitable medical experiences are positive for you. Many women are able to accomplish this. One of the nice things in life is the comfort of knowing that you are doing a good job of protecting your health, and that you have a source of medical care you feel is optimal. For this comfort you need to have confidence in your clinician's competence and in her/his ability to communicate well with you.

You also need to have confidence in yourself. You are the final judge of your clinician's competence, and you can make a good judgment. You will certainly want to consider factors such as medical training and certification and the opinion of other knowledgeable people, but your own observations are also very important. Similarly, you will be the one to make final decisions about any treatment or surgery that is proposed. Good decisions may require that you learn about the problem, take time to weigh the pros and cons, and perhaps even obtain a second or third medical opinion. When you reach a decision, though, you will have the confidence that your judgment truly is informed.

Finally, it is very helpful to understand how the medical care system works, what you can reasonably expect, what you shouldn't expect, and what you can do to make your own experiences better.

There are many important "unwritten" principles in health. (The health homilies your mother taught are probably most important of all: you'd feel better if you'd eat some vegetables, go outside and get some **exercise** . . . you know the ones.) The following concepts may help you avoid frustration, misunderstanding, or even serious medical disaster.

Health Versus Health Care.　Health care does not determine health. What you do to safeguard your own health is much more important overall than what your clinician does. In fact, except for the few minutes that you may be undergoing surgery for appendicitis or receiving emergency treatment, your clinician's main role is in **helping you learn to take care of yourself**. Your diet and lifestyle, and your own health habits, such as breast self-exam, wearing seat belts, avoiding cigarettes, having your tetanus booster, are what determine your healthiness.

A Checkup Isn't Magic.　A checkup can tell you that you don't have any evidence of the specific problems you are tested for, but cannot tell you that you are entirely well. The purpose of a routine checkup is to be sure that you do have the tests and treatments that are of demonstrated value for a person your age, and to give your clinician the chance to review your personal and family medical history and lifestyle for any additional recommendations that may be appropriate.

Some routine exams and tests are of value in detecting problems before symptoms occur, and earlier treatment in some cases does prevent more serious medical consequences later on. This is true, however, for only a small number of quite specific medical conditions (see Chapter 7 for more information about routine test recommendations).

There are many medical problems that cannot, as yet, be detected reliably in advance. Heart disease is a good example. It is entirely possible to have normal results from a complete physical exam, electrocardiogram, and extensive blood tests, and yet suffer a severe heart attack the very next day. Your clinician can assess your risk factors, high or low, for heart disease, but cannot really predict with certainty whether or when problems will occur.

Your Medical History and Current Symptoms Are Key.　When you see your clinician because of a problem, your clear and accurate description of what has happened is even more important than a physical exam or test results in arriving at a correct diagnosis. Obviously, honesty is crucial. Don't expect your clinician to guess what you are worried about. If you don't mention symptoms, your clinician can't know what areas need special attention in your exam or what tests might be needed.

You Are Responsible for Your Health Care.　Your clinician is an adviser, not a guardian angel. You will need to remember and take the initiative in scheduling your routine exams. And if special tests are ordered, you will have to see that they are done. Your clinician may have a reminder system for follow-up of truly serious problems, but most clinicians do not send routine reminders.

Details and dates will be easier to remember if you have your own personal health file or record book. Then a glance will tell you whether the "recent" tetanus shot you remember was actually last year—or ten years ago. Ask your clinician for your own copy of significant medical records such as surgery reports, pathology reports, or abnormal test results. Having your own copies may save time if they are needed for a new clinician in the future. An up-to-date written record of menstrual period dates also belongs in your health file if you are having menstrual cycles.

Choose Your Clinician While You Are Well.   Finding your ideal clinician will take research, time, and energy. The best time for this search is when you are well and strong. If you wait until illness strikes, you may have no alternative but a visit to the hospital emergency room or an urgent problem appointment with a physician whom you don't know, and who doesn't know you. Neither of these alternatives can give you the benefit of thorough, ongoing health care by someone familiar with your personal and family health history.

Nothing in This World Is 100%.   Medical exams and tests, like everything else, are not infallible. Some tests are quite accurate, with very low error rates; some are not so accurate.

A test result that is normal for a patient whose result should have been abnormal is called **false-negative**. This error can lead to false reassurance: the clinician and patient believe that there is no problem when a problem really does exist.

False-positive results can also occur. An abnormal test result that really should have been normal can lead to unnecessary worry. Because error or inaccuracy is always a possibility, your clinician may ask you to repeat tests if the results don't fit the symptoms you are having.

A Stitch in Time Saves Nine.   The old adage about the value of prevention definitely applies to health. When medical problems are identified and treated early, the chance that treatment will be successful is almost always higher. Also, recovery is likely to be quicker, and the risk of permanent damage lower. This is true whether the problem is early IUD infection or early high blood pressure. So when symptoms do occur, make health your first priority. Don't delay your visit because of a hectic work schedule. If your illness becomes severe, you won't be able to work at all.

Your Body and Soul Live in the Same Container.   What happens to your body cannot help but affect your soul, and disturbances in your emotional, social, and spiritual life are quite likely to affect your body as well. Whenever stress is high, with loss of a partner, change in job, or geographic move, for example, the risk of significant medical illness is also high. So don't be surprised when your clinician asks about nonmedical aspects of your life. They may be of great importance in understanding medical events. Also, whenever you are facing stress, take any extra precautions you can to fortify your physical self. Extra rest, the best possible diet, faithful exercise, and time for unwinding may help prevent a serious health problem that would add to your stress list.

Insuring a Successful Working Relationship with Your Clinician

I used to get frustrated and angry with my doctor. I felt invisible and misunderstood, never relieved or comforted. I realized, finally, I was expecting him to read my mind. I feel much better about my visits now, and it's simply because I've learned to be more candid.

—WOMAN, 44

WHAT YOU CAN DO

Both you and your clinician have essential responsibilities in building an optimal clinician-patient working relationship. Like any human relationship, it is a two-way interaction, so what you do and say does count.

Be Clear About What You Want.   Before each visit, try to clarify in your own mind exactly why you are going. Then let your clinician know at the beginning of your visit what you are expecting. If you have no problems and want only a routine exam, say so. If you want to discuss a specific question, raise it early. Your clinician will want to use the limited time available for your most important issues. If you wait until the end of your visit to raise a concern such as a sexual problem, then both you and your clinician are likely to be frustrated. There will not be sufficient time to deal effectively with your problem.

Sometimes a list is helpful. If you have specific questions or need medication refills, a list may help insure that they are not forgotten. If your list is long, though, your clinician may ask you to pick out your two or three most important issues. It makes more sense to focus on significant problems, and deal effectively with them, than to spend a couple of inadequate minutes on each of a dozen miscellaneous issues.

Be Ready to Be Honest.   If you think of your clinician as a detective, you are likely to be stuck with unsolved medical mysteries. Your clinician needs to know about any problems you may have with alcohol and drugs, for example, and needs a straightforward accounting of your past medical history. It is not safe to assume that your current symptoms are unrelated to the past or to your personal health habits. Also, you will need to answer questions about your psychic and social life honestly. They may be quite relevant in assessing the role of stress in your life, and essential in identifying possible risk factors for problems such as hepatitis, cervical cancer, AIDS, and other sexually transmitted diseases.

Be honest also about your reaction to the medical plans your clinician recommends. **If you do not feel comfortable about your evaluation or don't plan to follow the advice you have received, then by all means say so.** If you express your reservations directly, there is at least some chance that the two of you can reach a satisfactory plan together. If you say nothing, your clinician will assume that you agree, and your time and money will have been entirely wasted.

Also, serious medical risks may be involved. You need to understand exactly what medical problems your clinician is concerned about and why she/he is recommending the tests or treatment in question. And you need to understand what risks, if any, may result if evaluation or treatment is delayed. You may need time to think or to learn more before you make a decision. Ask your clinician for a time-line. How much thinking time is reasonable and safe? Also, you may want to have a second medical opinion. If time is limited, your clinician can (and should) help expedite arrangements for your second opinion.

Do Whatever Is Necessary to Get Your Questions Answered.   It is entirely normal to have questions, and quite essential that they be answered. It is also possible that your most important questions won't come to mind until after your visit, as you reflect on your visit or discuss it later with friends or family. And you may find that all questions vanish from your mind as soon as you walk into the office for your *next* visit. You may need to use a list or even rehearse with a friend to help overcome this problem. Or you could take a friend with you for moral support. **Don't be afraid to ask the same question twice** (or more often) if necessary. The goal is to get answers and information you need, so keep trying even if you don't feel successful at first. No one expects that you can learn all about a complex problem with just one explanation.

Remember, though, that **not all questions have answers**. Many areas of medicine are not fully understood, so you may have to be content with a discussion that clarifies what is known and what is not known. Also, there may be several different medical management schemes that are all acceptable for a specific problem or symptom. The tests or medications your clinician suggests may or may not be identical to the ones your friend had for a similar problem. If you are concerned, ask your clinician to explain the differences. You may find that your clinician prefers a different approach in your case for a specific reason, or that the apparent difference is just a matter of different brand names for the same kind of treatment.

Be Prepared to Hear Something You Weren't Expecting.   Your clinician's assessment may be a surprise, or may be something you don't want to hear. Nevertheless, she/he may be right. Many people find it particularly difficult to recognize the connection between physical symptoms such as pain or fatigue and their overall life stresses. We all tend to assume that our bodies should keep on functioning fine no matter what we are doing, or no matter how badly we abuse them with inadequate rest or a marginal diet. So if your clinician suggests that your alcohol intake needs to be reduced, or a hectic work schedule revised, try to listen.

Find Out About Practical Issues Ahead of Time.   It is entirely appropriate to ask practical or financial questions when you call for an appointment. The receptionist should be able to give you an approximate cost range for your visit, and you will be prepared if payment is expected at the time of your appointment. Also, you may want to ask about typical waiting times and the length of time you are likely to be there. If your schedule is demanding, it may pay to call the office an hour or so before your appointment time to see whether the office is running on time. If an emergency has interrupted their schedule you will be forewarned. You may prefer to reschedule your appointment to another time, or another day.

Once you are in the office, don't wait patiently and endlessly. Check with the receptionist if the delay seems long. Errors are possible. Perhaps your chart was not pulled when you initially checked in, or somehow no one realizes you are waiting. If an emergency has arisen and the delay will be long, you may prefer to reschedule rather than wait. If so, say so.

Don't Say Yes (or No) Until You Are Ready for the Decision.   You are entitled to the time you need for medical decision making. For serious decisions or complex problems, your clinician is likely to suggest that you take time to think and discuss options with your friends or family. You are also entitled to time for more minor decisions if you are unsure. **If you want time to think, say so.** Ask your clinician whether a slight delay is risky, and how soon a decision is needed. You can always come back to the office later, for example, for an injection or medication. Except in very unusual emergencies, medical care is not a "now or never" undertaking.

Reading may help you gather the information you need to be clear about a decision. Your clinician may be able to provide written materials or you can check in the library for health books or articles in recent magazines. As you read, though, **remember to pay close attention to the authors and the dates of your sources.** A medical textbook or health encyclopedia is a reasonable starting point for an explanation of your disorder, but specific testing and treatment recommendations may not be up-to-date if the book is more than one or two years old. Current medical research is reported in medical journals, most of which are published monthly and contain articles on a range of topics. Each author presents her or his results and opinions, along with a brief summary of previous work by others in that specific area, so each article is just one opinion or viewpoint. There may be other experts who disagree strongly, or other research studies with opposite conclusions. This may not be evident if you read just a few articles, or read a lay summary that selectively emphasizes one viewpoint.

Be Sure You Understand What Is Next. Before you leave your clinician's office, be sure you know what you need to do next and what to expect. If tests are ordered, you will want to know when and where to have them done, and when and from whom to expect the results. If another visit is needed, find out when it should be scheduled. Double-check to be sure you understand how to take any medications prescribed, and what they are, as well as adverse side effects you need to watch for. Ask your clinician whether there are any danger signs of problems she/he would want to hear about before your next visit.

WHAT YOU CAN EXPECT FROM YOUR CLINICIAN

You cannot reasonably expect your clinician to be perfect; she/he is a human being too. But there are some things you can and **should** expect. For most women, professional competence is at the top of the list. Communication skills and personality are important too, but competence is essential. The following are additional expectations that are reasonable.

Expect Your Clinician to Be Honest. You need to hear what your clinician actually thinks about your health problems, with neither false reassurance nor exaggerated warnings. The days when a serious diagnosis might be kept secret to spare the patient's delicate feelings are over. You should also expect your clinician to be honest about what is not known, and about her or his specific skills and competence. Your clinician should be willing and ready to refer you elsewhere for specialized evaluation or treatment that exceeds her/his training or experience. Similarly, you should expect a thoughtful referral if your clinician chooses not to perform certain services, such as sterilization surgery or abortion.

Expect Your Clinician to Be Clear About Her/His Goals. Your goals and your clinician's goals may not precisely coincide. Your primary goal may be to discover the cause of a troublesome pain, and to stop it. Your clinician, on the other hand, will want to make sure that the pain is not the first telltale sign of a serious medical problem. Once the possibility of infection, cancer, or some other serious illness is excluded, then finding the actual cause of the pain may not be so urgent. It may not even be possible. Understanding your clinician's goals can help to prevent frustration.

Making sure that you are up-to-date with routine exams and tests is also likely to be part of your clinician's agenda. Your clinician would be medically negligent to provide prescription refills or similar minor services without current routine care. So don't be surprised if you are asked to schedule your annual Pap test when your main goal is medication for cramps.

Expect Your Clinician to Explain Clearly.   You are entitled to a lucid and detailed explanation, more than once if necessary, of your medical problems. This might include their cause or causes, the symptoms your problem may produce now and in the future, options for evaluation and/or treatment, and expectations for the future. Your questions should be answered, and you should be told about danger signs, if any, that you need to watch for or report to your clinician.

Expect Your Clinician to Be Comfortable with Consultation or a Second Opinion.   Obtaining a second opinion about surgery or management of a serious or complex medical problem is entirely acceptable and very common. Your clinician should not be reluctant about it, and should cooperate fully in forwarding necessary medical information to the consulting physician.

Expect Your Clinician to Care About You.   You and your needs are the appropriate focus of your clinician–patient relationship. Your clinician should have genuine concern about you and about your well-being. This is not the same, however, as mutual love. Even though you may have strong positive feelings about each other, personal and sexual needs have no place whatsoever in the relationship.

Expect Your Clinician to Share the Decision-Making Process.   You, yourself, are the final decision maker, and you have the right to decide against even the strongest medical recommendations. The process of decision making works best, however, if you are involved from the beginning so that you understand the step-by-step logic your clinician has followed in arriving at her or his recommendations. This process, called informed consent, is described in detail in the next section.

Informed Consent

The principles of informed consent apply to all medical decisions. Historically, informed consent is a legal concept. Its real importance in medical care, however, is that this legal concept provides motivation and guidelines for essential patient education. Legally speaking, the clinician must teach and the patient must learn. And it is the patient who must make the final decision.

GUIDELINES FOR CONSENT INFORMATION

Despite the general guidelines provided by court decisions, it is not easy to decide what information is necessary for informed consent. Information must be comprehensive enough to allow the individual to make a reasonable decision; on the other hand, the law recognizes that this does not mean a miniature medical school course. A concise summary that may be of help is the seven-point requirement for informed consent included in legislative guidelines for federally funded sterilization procedures (1). The seven requirements can conveniently be remembered with the acronym BRAIDED.

- *B*enefits
- *R*isks; all discomforts and common risks, and all major risks, no matter how rare
- *A*lternatives; description of possible alternatives with enough information about each to permit a rational decision. **Informed choice** is an essential part of informed consent. In order to give consent, the patient must understand not only the potential risks and benefits of the proposed treatment, but also those for alternative treatments.
- *I*nquiries; an opportunity for discussion of questions the patient may have
- *D*ecline; the patient is free to decline or withdraw consent without prejudicing any other benefits (federal, state, or other) to which she/he may be entitled
- *E*xplanation; an explanation of the proposed treatment or procedure in lay terms
- *D*ocumentation; written record that all six aspects of informed consent have been discussed with the patient

CONSENT PRINCIPLES IN PRACTICE

My first experience with consent forms was when I was 19 and started taking birth control Pills. My first thought was, "What is this guy, a doctor or a lawyer?" It was one forbidding document! After I read it, I was glad to know all that stuff. Although it scared me to read that list of what could happen to me, I appreciated the honesty. I felt like I had a genuine *choice* to make about the Pills, and that form really made me think.

—WOMAN, 26

When the medical decision is a minor one, for example, whether or not to take antibiotic tablets for a sexually transmitted infection, little or no specific consent discussion will be needed unless you want more information. Your clinician can reasonably assume you are already aware of the benefit of treatment, as well as the common risks (adverse medication reaction). There are no real medical alternatives to antibiotic treatment, and treatment is definitely needed.

For more serious decisions such as surgery, or whenever **elective** treatment is considered, you are likely to encounter a more formal and lengthy informed consent procedure. (See Chapter 45 for more information on surgery decision making.) **Elective treatment means there is no pressing medical necessity involved.** Your decision to take birth control Pills or have sterilization surgery is in this category. Your clinician will want to be sure you understand all the possible risks of treatment before you decide. The risks may be low, but the benefits are personal rather than medical. And in the case of birth control Pills, other options are available. So don't be surprised if your clinician seems to emphasize possible problems or asks you to sign a consent form. A detailed consent form required for birth control Pills but not for antibiotic treatment does not mean that birth control is more risky. It simply means that a birth control decision is elective, while antibiotic treatment is medically necessary.

Consent forms are often used for education as well. By summarizing all the essential risk information concisely, **a consent form can help insure that you have had the opportunity to review your decision and ask questions.** If you are already well informed, your quick review is sufficient; if not, then you will be able to identify unfamiliar issues for further discussion.

Your clinician should be serious about informed consent and you should be also. When you give your consent, you are acknowledging that you have received the information you need and want, and that you agree. **Don't say yes until you really mean yes.** On the other hand, you always have the right to change your mind. Informed consent is not like a contract. If you feel worried or uncertain later on, or have more questions, let your clinician know. You can decide to stop your treatment or cancel your surgery, and your clinician should not be angry or offended.

Choosing a Clinician

Your search for a clinician might logically begin with a decision about what kind of care you need and what kind of clinician would therefore be most appropriate. (We limit our discussion in this chapter to traditional sources of care because that is our métier. No slight to nontraditional providers is intended.)

In order to be licensed, a physician must have an M.D. degree and at least one year of additional internship training. Such physicians are called general practitioners, and are qualified to provide most routine health care and to perform minor surgical procedures. Additional training, called specialty training, usually involves three or four years of full-time, supervised experience in one of the medical specialties. When training is completed, the physician is "board eligible" in that specialty and can become "board certified" after completing one or more additional years of experience in practice and passing examinations for the specialty. Board-certified physicians are entitled to use initials signifying board membership after the M.D. in their name. Board initials are F.A.C. followed by the specialty, meaning "Fellow of the American College of." For example, a board-certified obstetrician/gynecologist will have M.D.,

F.A.C.O.G. after her/his name. After specialty training some physicians continue their education for two or more years to complete a subspecialty fellowship. Within the specialty of internal medicine, for example, are subspecialties of endocrinology (hormones), cardiology (heart), and others. Surgery includes subspecialties such as orthopedics and pediatric surgery, and obstetrics/gynecology subspecialties include reproductive endocrinology, perinatology (high-risk pregnancy and delivery), and oncology (cancer).

If what you want is someone to provide routine health care, and to help you with referral if more specialized services are needed, then **primary care** is what you need. Primary care can be provided by:

- A general practitioner (no specialty training)
- A family practice specialist (specialty training in the field of family practice)
- An internist (internal medicine specialist)
- A pediatrician (specialist in children's nonsurgical medicine)
- An obstetrician/gynecologist (specialist in pregnancy and reproductive health care for women)

Specific medical needs may influence your choice. If you have medical problems such as arthritis or high blood pressure, an internist who can manage your problems is a reasonable choice for primary care as well. If you have children and want one source of care for all the members of your family, a family practice specialist or general practitioner would be a good choice. If your primary medical needs are family planning or pregnancy care, then you may wish to see a specialist in obstetrics and gynecology who also can provide primary care.

Finding a physician in general practice or family practice may not be easy. Approximately 90% of physicians completing education now pursue specialty training, and only a small portion choose family practice.

Nurse practitioners, physician assistants, and certified nurse-midwives may also be resources for your care. **Their special training allows them to provide fully competent services within a specific area.** State licensure requires that these mid-level professionals have physician backup available, and in many cases they function within a physician's office, clinic, or hospital, working side by side with their supervising physicians.

Your choice may also be influenced by your health insurance, and by the health facilities in your specific geographic area. In one city, a huge, excellent private clinic may prove to be the best alternative; in another, a university-run program or clinicians in private practice may be best. Your health insurance program may specify a panel of preferred providers, or, in the case of prepaid health programs, cover health services only when they are provided by clinicians within the health plan.

When you have decided what kind of clinician you need, it is time to begin finding specific recommendations. If you already have a relationship with a clinician, this is a good place to begin. Your eye doctor or children's pediatrician should be able to identify one or more appropriate possibilities for the care you need.

Try to gather information from several sources, and keep notes. Ask what each recommendation is based on: personal experience, experience of other friends, a general community reputation, credentials, etc. If your source is a list, ask how the list was constructed and whether there is any mechanism for evaluation or review. How does a clinician get onto the list; under what circumstances would a name be removed? Table 1-1 shows possible sources of information and the kind of information each is likely to provide.

Remember that a list is likely to include all clinicians who meet the criteria (all the members of the medical society, for example), and referrals are made on a rotation basis, or the entire list is provided. For personal information, discussion with friends or acquaintances who work in the health field is a more likely resource.

Checking credentials is a reasonable step once you have identified several possibilities. Contacting the hospital is the simplest way to verify credentials. Find out where your prospective clinician has hospital affiliations. Then call or write to the hospital medical staff office to verify that she/he is a member of the staff in good standing. When a clinician applies for hospital staff membership, a hospital committee reviews all relevant credentials to verify medical school attendance, state licensure, and specialty training. **Almost all reputable clinicians hold staff membership at one or more hospitals.** Hospital affiliation is necessary in order to provide in-hospital care, and also means that the clinician is participating in the continuous peer review required for all accredited hospitals.

For your final assessment, you will need an appointment. You may be able to schedule an appointment specifically for an interview or consultation. Alternatively, you may want to use your next routine exam for your test visit. **Once inside the office, look around carefully.** Do the facilities appear to be appropriate, up-to-date, clean, and well supervised? Does the staff convey a competent and caring attitude? What kind of literature is provided? Is patient education and health promotion stressed? Is medical equipment clean, well maintained, and modern? Does the office seem to function smoothly?

If your appointment is for consultation only, your meeting with the clinician will provide an opportunity to assess her/his overall philosophy, communication skills, and any obvious biases. **Don't expect specific medical recommendations about problems you may be having.** Even if you are able to provide a clear and detailed medical history, it would be negligent for anyone to make medical recommendations without examining you and having an opportunity to review your past medical records. You may find it helpful to think about specific questions before your visit. For example, you could ask what routine exams and lab tests would be recommended for a healthy woman your age over the next two to five years. If you are trying to arrange primary care, then ask what minor problems could be handled here, and what sort of problems would require referral to another physician.

If you are also having an initial routine exam, you will have the chance to assess medical competence as well. The visit should begin with a discussion of the purpose for

TABLE 1-1
INFORMATION SOURCES: FINDING A CLINICIAN

SOURCE	INFORMATION AVAILABLE
Medical School—Department of Family Practice, Internal Medicine, Obstetrics/Gynecology, etc.	A list of clinicians on the faculty who also see private patients; a list of clinical faculty members— community clinicians who donate time to the medical school.
Medical society	A list of clinicians who are members of the society; a list of members in a specific category (woman pediatricians, for example).
Planned Parenthood	A list of clinicians who choose to be included as Planned Parenthood resources; information on services and fees as well as evaluation may be available.
Women's Center, Rape Crisis Center	A list of clinicians who are willing to accept referrals, or a list constructed by women members of the group.
Hospital or health plan	A list of clinicians who are members of the staff.
Nurses or acquaintances who work in health care	Personal or community reputation information about clinicians who work in the same facility. A nurse who works in surgery, for example, is quite likely to have good information about the skills and experience of the surgeons who work there.
Knowledgeable friends	Personal or community reputation information; this source is especially important for assessing communication skills.
Specialty societies such as American Cancer Society, American Fertility Society, Resolve, DES Action	A list of specialists in your geographic area who are members of the national society or have registered with the society because of their interest in the field.

your appointment (a problem, a checkup) and review of your recent and past medical history. Any symptoms you may be having should also be discussed. Your exam may focus on your problem, if any, but should also include blood pressure and weight, and each of the exam steps recommended for someone your age (see Chapter 7). Routine preventive health measures such as a Pap smear should be done, or at least discussed to determine if they are needed at this visit.

With luck, you will have succeeded in finding someone who is humane, thorough, competent, and able to answer your questions in a way that makes sense to you.

How to Leave

You have the absolute right to leave anytime you wish. If you are frightened by what is happening or by the situation in the office, then you can simply walk out. You don't have to explain your feelings or decision to anyone unless you want to. You can write later to transfer your medical records to another clinician. If you wish, you can also phone or write to explain your reasons for leaving. You may also want to write to the local medical society or state medical license board if your decision was based on a serious problem like alcohol abuse or sexual advances. These problems are rare, but certainly could jeopardize other patients in the future.

Because my dad was a physician I never thought about "picking" a doctor when I was younger. As a grown-up I first went to an internist—a fancy, Harvard-trained, locally famous specialist with a huge practice. He was more doctor than I needed as a healthy 23-year-old, but more important, I couldn't talk to him. He seemed very distant and emotionally he was a blank—a pure technician. I remember telling him proudly that I had stopped smoking, and instead of praise, I got a lecture about gaining 10 pounds.

Then for 12 years I was antimedicine. Once a year I went to the health department for a Pap smear! When I developed mild hypertension I realized I needed a source of ongoing care, and I chose a family practice doc I'd heard good things about from my friends. It was gratifying to have a "full service" doctor I could depend on, and I could talk to him. Sometimes, though, I felt we were out of sync—as though he was too casual when I was feeling worried about a health issue.

Now I see another family practice doctor, and I can't imagine a better situation. I trust her competence, and she doesn't hesitate to make a referral to a specialist when she thinks I need it. (I've liked the referral physicians too.) I'm regarded as a total human being. She listens, takes my concerns seriously, and is a wonderful explainer and comforter. I hope she will be my health ally for the rest of my life.

—WOMAN, 40

REFERENCE

1. November 8, 1978, Federal Register 43:52146–52175. Regulations are summarized in Hatcher RA, Guest FJ, Stewart FH, et al: *Contraceptive Technology, 1986–1987* (ed 13). New York: Irvington Publishers, 1986.

2

How a Woman's Reproductive System Works

Components of a Woman's Reproductive System

UTERUS

The uterus is a rosy, glistening mass of muscle deep inside the lower middle abdomen (see Illustration 2-1). It is pear-shaped, domed at the top and narrowing to a neck at the bottom. It can be as small as a lime or as large as a good-sized pear. It feels firm and rubbery and becomes very tense and hard when it is touched or stimulated in any way.

Muscle layers about 1/2 inch thick cover a central cavity shaped like a flattened funnel. Colors deepen from pink to raspberry to vivid bloodred between the outer muscle layers and the soft, velvety endometrium, the lining of the inner cavity. The endometrium is sloughed away and renewed during each menstrual cycle. Menstrual discharge is nothing more than shreds of endometrial tissue, fluid from sloughing endometrium, and blood from endometrial vessels.

The uterus has three openings. Near the domed top (the fundus), two fallopian tubes open into the central cavity, one on each side. At the narrow neck (the cervix), an inch-long canal opens into the vagina.

The uterus is supported by strong, supple ligaments and can be moved easily in several directions. A rich network of uterine blood vessels lies within folds of the

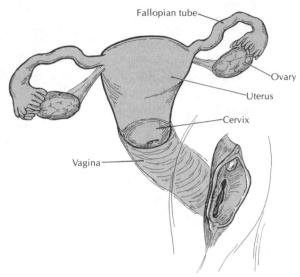

Fallopian tube

Ovary

Uterus

Cervix

Vagina

ILLUSTRATION 2-1   Internal reproductive organs include the uterus, fallopian tubes, ovaries, cervix, and vagina.

supporting ligaments, and, especially after pregnancy, blood vessels may crisscross the outer muscle layer of the uterus.

The primary function of the uterus is to house and protect a fetus for 40 or so weeks. In late pregnancy, the formerly pear-sized uterus looks more like a medium-sized watermelon as muscle fibers stretch to accommodate a growing fetus (or two). The uterus feels hard, and the pregnant woman may notice waves of slow, tightening sensations long before true labor contractions begin. No one knows what signals the uterus to begin the powerful, rhythmic contractions of labor. The uterus may be responding to hormonal messages or perhaps to something the fetus itself does.

Almost any pain message from the uterus, during menstruation or during an IUD insertion, for example, will be felt as a cramp. Sometimes uterine cramping is perceived as back pain, or even leg pain, because uterine nerves enter the spinal cord in the lower back very near nerves from the upper thighs, and the brain may have trouble sorting out the exact source of the pain message.

Uterine pain often arises as a result of firm contraction of the uterine muscle layer. If muscle contraction is prolonged or intense, blood flow to uterine muscle cells may be temporarily diminished. Like a spasm or cramp in any muscle, insufficient blood supply means insufficient oxygen supply, and that leads to pain in the muscle tissue.

Pain during a menstrual period, too, is related to intensified uterine muscle activity. As uterine lining cells are shed, they release prostaglandin hormone (described later in this chapter), which stimulates uterine muscle. Women with severe cramps have stronger, more prolonged uterine muscle contractions than do women with minimal or no menstrual cramps.

CERVIX

The cervix is the narrow neck of the uterus, and it connects the main body of the uterus with the vagina. You can feel its firm, smooth, rubbery surface (much like the tip of your nose) by using your finger to explore the inside of your vagina. When your vaginal walls are held apart with a speculum (see Chapter 3 for details on pelvic examination), your cervix is plainly visible; it looks like a small, pink, glazed doughnut, an inch or so in diameter.

Right in the middle of your cervix is the opening (os) of the inch-long canal that connects the vagina with the uterine cavity. The os is a tiny round hole. Once you have delivered a baby, the os looks more like a 1/4-inch-long horizontal slit. Sperm traverse the cervical canal to reach the uterus, and menstrual discharge and babies leave the uterus through this same passageway.

Powerful fibers in the cervix hold the fetus inside the uterus until labor begins, and then they stretch dramatically so that the cervical canal is fifty or more times its normal width at the time of delivery.

Glands line the cervical canal and produce a constant downward flow of mucus to protect the uterine cavity from bacterial invasion. Mucus characteristics are determined by cyclic hormone levels: thick and scanty mucus when estrogen levels are low; thin, slippery, abundant mucus at the time of ovulation, when estrogen levels are high. Sperm have a better opportunity to penetrate the cervical canal when mucus is slippery and abundant; they are more likely to survive the journey up the fallopian tubes and have the opportunity to fertilize an egg.

If you perceive **a pain message from your cervix,** during an IUD insertion or during delivery, for example, it **will feel like pressure, a bearing-down sensation sometimes accompanied by cramping.** Even when a portion of your cervix is frozen during cryosurgery, pricked with a needle, or pinched with a clamp, what you perceive is pressure and cramping. The cervix has a short memory for pain; for example, your clinician may leave a clamp on your cervix for five minutes to hold it steady for IUD insertion, but your perception of pain will usually subside after a minute or so.

FALLOPIAN TUBES

A limp, delicate, 5-inch-long fallopian tube droops from each side of the uterus. The soft, glistening, pale pink tubes lie beneath folds of translucent membrane (peritoneum). Each tube is about an inch thick where it joins the uterus, narrow as a telephone cord in the middle, and flared at the open end. The trumpet-shaped ends (infundibula) are lined with white, ruffled *fimbria*, millions of tiny feathery fingers that are constantly in motion to draw an egg into a tube once it has left an ovary. The passageway that runs the length of the tube is no wider than a single strand of spaghetti.

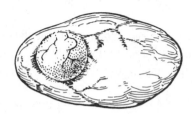

ILLUSTRATION 2-2   Ovary—actual size.

Fertilization occurs when the egg has completed about one third of the distance down the tube toward the uterus. The fertilized egg completes the journey in four to five more days, with cell multiplication and growth well under way. If you are having twins, they are separate entities before they reach your uterus. Muscular contractions in the tube nudge the fertilized egg (blastocyst) along the way to the uterus, where it implants in the blood-rich endometrium.

When fertilization does not occur, the egg simply passes out of the uterus through the cervical canal completely unnoticed. It is no bigger than the period at the end of this sentence.

The functions of the fallopian tubes are to provide a pathway between the ovary and the uterus, and a favorable milieu for conception. Also, continuous waves of contractions in the delicate tube walls may help move the fertilized egg down the tube toward the uterus and, along with gently undulating tube lining cells, provide a fluid current to orient sperm so that they will swim in the right direction as they move out of the uterus into the tube.

OVARIES

Ovaries look like miniature, firm, slightly flattened hard-boiled eggs, appropriately enough. There are two ovaries, one on each side of the uterus near the open end of each fallopian tube. The ovaries are covered with a tough, almost gristly white membrane and usually measure about 1 by 1 1/2 inches (see Illustration 2-2). They may be quite smooth, or there may be rounded lumps on the surface where egg follicles, clusters of cells that enclose a developing egg, have enlarged. Each ovary lies in a shapeless fold of uterine suspensory ligament. Ligaments also supply blood to the ovaries.

Ovaries produce eggs and reproductive hormones, including estrogen and progesterone. Each cycle about 20 of the roughly 300,000 egg follicles in your ovaries enlarge, secrete estrogen, and begin to ripen an egg in response to hormone signals from your pituitary gland. As development progresses, one follicle predominates while the others stop growing, shrink, and disappear into the ovarian tissue. (If two follicles predominate, fraternal twins may be conceived from two different eggs.) The dominant egg follicle continues to enlarge until the ovary's outer membrane gives way and the ripe egg spills out inside a transparent, gelatinous cloud (zona pellucida). This process is called ovulation.

While the fimbria draw the egg into the fallopian tube passageway, the empty follicle undergoes a dramatic transformation. Follicle cells reassemble into a small, yellow, hormone-producing lump right on the surface of the ovary called the corpus luteum. The corpus luteum produces progesterone on a hormone signal from the pituitary gland. After about 14 days it stops releasing progesterone and regresses, leaving only a smooth bump on the surface of the ovary. The 14-day life span of the corpus luteum is the most consistent, predictable interval in the entire hormone cycle.

When your clinician manipulates an ovary during your pelvic exam, you may notice a unique twinge, somewhere between pain and a tickle. You may also feel ovarian pain at the time of ovulation or if you develop an ovarian cyst. You will be able to pinpoint pain very low in your abdomen, slightly to one side or the other of your uterus.

VAGINA

The vagina is a muscular tube 4 to 5 inches long that connects the uterus with the outside of the body. When it is empty, it has no inner space at all, like an empty shirt sleeve. The pale pink vaginal lining is slippery and rippled. Glands in the lining continuously produce a small amount of thin mucus to keep the area moist. During sexual arousal these mucus-secreting glands increase their output somewhat, and quite copious amounts of additional lubricating fluid are released (''sweated'') from the vaginal lining cells. You may notice a distinctly wet sensation.

Except for the tiny cervical canal opening, your vagina is a dead-end passageway. There is absolutely no way tampons or a contraceptive sponge can get lost, for example. The opening to the outside of your body (introitus) is ringed with strong, elastic muscles that are capable of expanding to accommodate a baby during delivery.

The vagina is an exit passageway for menstrual discharge and babies, and half the equipment necessary for penis–vagina intercourse.

The vagina has few nerve endings. An ice water douche probably wouldn't feel cold, for example, and you can't feel a tampon once it is in place. Most sensations deep in the vagina feel like pressure. Nerve endings are concentrated near the introitus where skin begins, and that is where you perceive sensations of heat, cold, irritation, pain, or itching.

During sexual arousal the vagina lengthens, and because the tissue is so elastic, it accommodates easily to a penis of any size. If a woman's arousal and lubrication responses have had a chance to occur, intercourse should not cause uncomfortable or painful physical sensations.

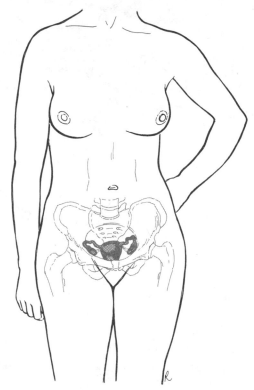

ILLUSTRATION 2-3   The internal reproductive organs are surrounded and protected by pelvic bones.

NEIGHBORS

All the internal reproductive organs lie within the abdominal cavity, closed off from air and surrounded by the large and small intestines, the tough, pink, glistening bladder, two ureters, and many blood vessels and nerves. All the organs in the pelvis are enclosed and protected by the large bones of the pelvic girdle (see Illustration 2-3). To reach your pelvic organs, a surgeon must penetrate a 1/16-inch-thick layer of abdominal skin, an ivory-colored layer of fat, a tough white layer of connective tissue (fascia), red, fibrous muscle, another layer of fascia, and the peritoneum, a thin, strong, translucent membrane that lines the entire abdominal cavity.

EXTERNAL STRUCTURES

All the external structures of the reproductive system together are called the **perineum** or **vulva** (see Illustration 2-4). The skin-colored outer lips (labia majora) and brown or pink inner lips (labia minora) shield and protect the vaginal introitus, urinary

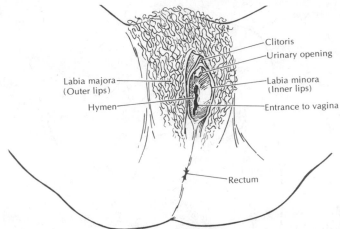

Clitoris
Urinary opening
Labia majora
(Outer lips)
Labia minora
(Inner lips)
Hymen
Entrance to vagina
Rectum

ILLUSTRATION 2-4   All the external reproductive structures together are called the vulva or perineum.

opening (urethral meatus), and clitoris. Both the inner and outer lips are responsive to pleasurable and painful tactile sensations. **Pubic hair**, much like eyebrows and underarm hair, serves to absorb and divert moisture. Pubic hair can be thick or scant; it can be confined to the skin areas covered by the briefest bikini, or spread up the abdomen toward the navel and down the inner thighs. The **mons pubis** is a fatty cushion over the frontal pelvic bones. It is the soft, hairy triangle you see when you are standing up.

The **clitoris** is a 1/4- to 1-inch-long, somewhat cylindrical mass of pink or brown erectile tissue. It lies protected beneath the clitoral hood (prepuce) just above the urinary opening. The clitoris is richly innervated and highly responsive to tactile sensations. It swells with blood during sexual arousal and is a woman's primary orgasmic focus. The sole function of the clitoris is sexual responsiveness.

Two **Skene's glands** are located near the urinary opening, one on either side (see Illustration 2-5). They serve no known function and may be vestigial glands originally intended to lubricate the urinary opening and protect it from bacterial invasion.

Two **Bartholin's glands** open into the vagina near the introitus, one on either side. They produce a thin mucus that lubricates the vagina and vulva to some degree. Most women aren't even aware of the Bartholin's glands unless they become infected. Infection can cause swelling and redness and can be extremely painful.

BREASTS

A woman's two breasts are outposts of the reproductive system that develop at puberty. Fatty tissue protects the myriad milk-producing glands, and an intricate duct system channels milk into the nipple (see Illustration 2-6). Ligaments on the chest wall support the breast; the breast itself contains no muscles.

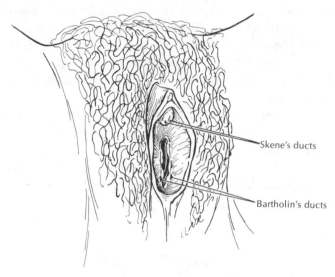

ILLUSTRATION 2-5   Ducts from Skene's glands and Bartholin's glands are practically impossible to see with the naked eye.

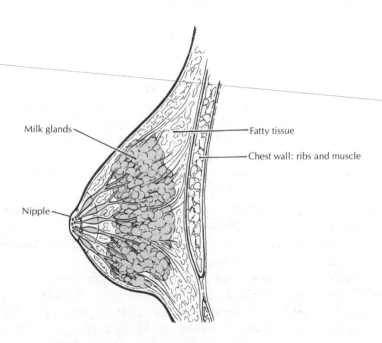

ILLUSTRATION 2-6   The breast is composed almost entirely of fatty tissue and glands.

Nipples are erectile tissue and are quite responsive to tactile sensations. Each nipple is surrounded by a pink or brown circle of skin (areola) that is also responsive to tactile sensations. The areola may be ringed with sparse hair.

Some women have erect nipples all the time; other women find that nipple erection occurs only in response to touch, cold weather, or a sneeze. Nipples are always almost erect at the moment of orgasm. In never-pregnant women, the entire breast may swell during sexual arousal.

Breasts are responsive to cyclic hormone changes. Many women have enlarged, tender breasts just before a menstrual period. Breasts also enlarge, and the nipple and areola color often darken, during pregnancy.

The two breast functions are milk production and sexual responsiveness. Breasts of any size or shape are almost certain to be fully competent in both these roles.

Hormone Coordination of the Reproductive System

• Why are my periods so light when I take birth control Pills?
• My doctor says I have a hormone imbalance, but he isn't sure exactly what kind. Why can't he tell?
• Why do I seem to run a fever the last two weeks of every cycle?
• Why did my doctor order skull x-rays when my periods stopped?

All these questions have hormone answers. Two reproductive hormones, estrogen and progesterone, are famous, but the complex hormonal coordination of your reproductive system begins three steps back and requires the participation of at least five or six other, less famous hormones, as well as input from your brain, your pituitary gland, your thyroid gland, and your adrenal glands.

Your body has two major ways to convey information from one organ or cell to another: the nervous system and the endocrine system.

The endocrine system uses hormones—chemical messengers—that are carried in the bloodstream. Hormones are produced by specialized glands such as the thyroid, the ovaries, and the adrenals. Some hormones act primarily on one specific target organ, and others have effects on a wide range of organs and cells.

A hormone's effect depends on the target organ's sensitivity to the specific hormone chemical. Target organs often have cells richly endowed with receptors for their specific hormones; the tiniest trace of hormone can cause profound changes in target cells. Hormones exert their influence by altering the chemical processes within a cell, influencing a cell to grow more rapidly or to produce a specific chemical product, for example.

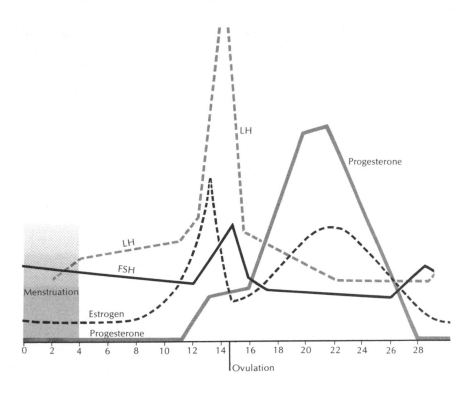

ILLUSTRATION 2-7   Hormone activity in a normal 28-day reproductive cycle.
(Speroff L, Glass RH, Kase NG: *Clinical Gynecologic Endocrinology and Infertility* (ed 3). Baltimore: Williams & Wilkins, 1983. Used with permission.)

To the endocrinologist, your reproductive system looks like Illustration 2-7. Clearly it is complex! Chances are your clinician would not be able to draw this chart from memory, and you can certainly understand the important facts about your reproductive hormones without memorizing all its details.

Notice that **the normal level for each hormone changes continuously throughout the menstrual cycle.** A normal estrogen level on cycle day 12 may be seven times higher than a normal estrogen level on cycle day 4 so **there is no one simple blood or urine test** that can determine whether your hormone levels are too high, too low, or normal.

When you read the description of hormone events in this chapter, it may be hard to believe, but this is only part of the story. This description covers only the highlights. There are still many aspects of the reproductive hormone cycle that are not fully understood; for example, no one understands the precise cause of premenstrual tension and fluid retention.

THE UNFAMOUS HORMONES

The cyclic hormone changes in the reproductive system begin in a specialized area of the brain called the hypothalamus. This organ is part of both the nervous system and the hormone system and is probably responsible for coordination between them. The hypothalamus is the only part of the hormone system that can react to messages from the outside world. The nervous system collects information from your five senses and from the rest of your body and integrates this information. The outside world can influence your hormone cycles through the hypothalamus. Nearby brain centers govern appetite and body temperature, and their proximity may explain the relationship between hormones and cyclic body temperature and weight changes.

The hypothalamus produces and secretes hormones and releasing factors that act directly on their target organ, the nearby pituitary gland.

The releasing factor responsible for reproductive hormone control is GnRH, gonadotropin-releasing hormone. The hypothalamus releases tiny pulses of GnRH approximately once each hour (60 to 90 minutes); the amount in each pulse and pulse timing probably determine exactly how the pituitary gland will respond. GnRH pulses vary in amount and frequency during each normal menstrual cycle, and disturbance in the GnRH pulse pattern is likely to disrupt normal cyclic events such as ovulation.

Alterations in GnRH pulse release may be the mechanism by which stresses such as physical exertion with athletic training and dieting can influence menstrual cycles.

GnRH may also play a role in the timing of puberty. Synthetic GnRH is used to treat young women who fail to undergo puberty because of insufficient normal GnRH production, and to treat some fertility problems as well.

The pituitary gland is part of the endocrine system and is located in the middle of the brain. It secretes many hormones, including stimulating hormones that affect the ovaries, thyroid glands, and adrenal glands. The pituitary also produces prolactin, the hormone that governs breast milk production.

Disturbances in the pituitary gland can cause changes in many hormone patterns at once. Reproductive hormone problems might be accompanied by thyroid problems or by abnormal secretion of breast milk, for example. Pituitary gland enlargement from a tumor might cause headache or vision problems because the gland is in the middle of the brain and very near the optic nerves. That is why your clinician may recommend precise measurement of your field of vision and skull x-rays if she/he suspects that a pituitary tumor is causing your menstrual irregularity.

The two pituitary gland hormones that regulate reproductive function are FSH (follicle-stimulating hormone) and LH (luteinizing hormone). The primary targets of both FSH and LH are the ovaries, which in turn produce the two famous hormones, estrogen and progesterone. Pituitary FSH and LH release is governed by GnRH from the hypothalamus and by the levels of estrogen and progesterone in the bloodstream.

FSH is responsible for development and maturation of **egg follicle**(s) in the ovary. As the follicle cells develop, they begin to release estrogen. The first half of your cycle—before ovulation—is dominated by estrogen and is called the follicular phase. As ovulation nears, estrogen production reaches a fairly high level and the pituitary is stimulated to release a burst of LH. LH triggers ovulation, the release of a ripe egg from its follicle; and LH also transforms the empty follicle into a gland called the **corpus luteum**. The corpus luteum, a regrouping of the cells that formerly lined the egg follicle, produces and releases **progesterone**, the hallmark of the last half of the cycle. The corpus luteum produces estrogen during the last half of the cycle as well. The second half of the cycle is called the luteal phase.

THE FAMOUS HORMONE: ESTROGEN

If there is a female hormone, it is estrogen. Actually, a woman's body produces several slightly different estrogens. **The primary source of estrogen is follicle cells in the ovaries.** Fatty tissue throughout the body also manufactures estrogen by converting similar hormones (including androgens, male sex hormones that are normally produced in small quantities by the adrenal glands in women as well as men) into estrogen. Even after menopause, when estrogen production by the ovaries has dropped to low levels, fatty tissue production of estrogen continues, and may provide substantial estrogen.

Your body's own estrogens are similar but not identical to the synthetic estrogens in birth control Pills and estrogen replacement therapy pills for menopausal women. Each estrogen has its own particular side effects and potency. Estrogens are carried in the bloodstream until they are deactivated by the liver and filtered by the kidneys into the urine. A woman with serious liver disease may not be able to use estrogen medication, because her estrogen may be poorly deactivated and may rise to an abnormally high level.

Estrogen can enter any body cell and has a very wide range of effects. The reproductive system is the primary target for estrogen, but alterations in other body processes do occur and may account for some of the side effects that women using estrogen may experience.

The list of known normal estrogen effects is very long and includes the following:

- Growth and development of the breasts, uterus, fallopian tubes, and vagina during fetal development and puberty
- Cyclic thickening of the lining of the uterus
- Production of thin, stringy, profuse cervical mucus at the time of ovulation
- Thickening of vaginal lining and production of vaginal mucus
- Promotion of vaginal acidity
- Promotion of feminine fat distribution patterns for body shape; increased thickness of fatty layers
- Increased water content and thickness of skin

- Decreased oil gland activity and oil secretion by skin
- Slowing and stopping of growth of long bones—especially in arms and legs
- Increased protein metabolism rate
- Protection against loss of bone density; direct effects on bone building and dismantling cells and on body calcium balance
- Increased blood level of certain plasma proteins; thyroid-binding protein, cortisone-binding protein
- Increased fluid retention
- Feedback to the brain essential for regulation of FSH and LH release

Clearly, too much or too little estrogen might cause a wide range of symptoms. The symptoms of too much estrogen are most often associated with the use of estrogen medication such as birth control Pills. Women undergoing menopause or surgical menopause may experience symptoms of too little estrogen.

THE OTHER FAMOUS HORMONE: PROGESTERONE

Progesterone is manufactured by the ovary only after ovulation. It is released in small amounts from **the adrenal glands** as well, but it does not have any other significant sources. Progesterone is produced at very high levels **during pregnancy** and was first isolated and identified in pregnant women; so its name was taken from the terms "pro" (supporting) and "gestation" (pregnancy).

Natural progesterone has a chemical structure very much like that of estrogen. Several synthetic progesterones, called **progestins**, are used in birth control Pills and for treatment of hormone disorders. Synthetic progestins often have side effects because of their structural similarity to estrogen and other hormones. A synthetic progestin may have its primary effect as a progestin, and additional effects as if it were a weak estrogen or weak androgen: a woman using a specific synthetic progestin in a birth control Pill may notice improvements (estrogen effect) or worsening (androgen effect) in her acne. Sensitivity to these effects varies from woman to woman and differs for each of the synthetic progestins. Changing to a different type of Pill may be helpful.

Deactivation of progesterone occurs at numerous sites within the body, and deactivation is not solely dependent on the liver, as is the case with estrogen. The effects of progesterone seem to be more limited than the effects of estrogen.

Known **normal** progesterone effects include the following:

- Maturation of the estrogen-primed uterine lining to promote the formation of glands, blood vessels, and distinct layers in the lining
- Decreased tendency for the uterus to contract
- Thick, sticky cervical mucus
- Maturation of the breast glands after estrogen priming

- Feedback to the ovary, pituitary gland, and hypothalamus for regulating cyclic hormone release and/or response to hormone exposure
- Increased protein formation
- Altered liver and gallbladder function
- Increased tolerance to the presence of foreign protein, such as a fetus
- Elevation of body temperature (about 0.5 to 0.8 degree Fahrenheit)

In early pregnancy, progesterone-induced maturation of the uterine lining allows the placenta to attach itself to the uterus properly and is essential for successful pregnancy. During the first three months of pregnancy, progesterone (and some estrogen) is produced by the corpus luteum. After three months, the placenta itself is able to produce both of these hormones and the corpus luteum wanes.

Maturation of the uterine lining is important for normal menstrual blood loss: the mature lining is able to shed its entire surface layer in a relatively short, predictable time period, with heaviest bleeding during the first 24 to 48 hours, followed by lighter bleeding and complete cessation of bleeding in five to seven days. Normal menstrual discharge totals about 4 to 5 tablespoons of fluid, of which one third is blood (1).

If the lining does not mature, good separation between layers and efficient shedding of the whole lining is not likely; hence, a deficiency of progesterone can account for the **prolonged or intermittent bleeding pattern** that often occurs when a woman doesn't ovulate and her uterus has been exposed to estrogen stimulation alone. Estrogen stimulates growth of lining cells. Without the maturing effect of progesterone, growth just continues. Eventually one or more areas may begin to bleed, and the amount of bleeding and pattern of bleeding may be quite unpredictable.

OTHER HORMONES

Androgen. The ovary normally produces small amounts of male hormone (androgen), in addition to estrogen and progesterone. Ordinarily the amount of androgen is not significant enough to cause noticeable effects. When a woman's normal cyclic hormone patterns are disrupted, however, excessive androgen production can cause masculine hair growth, skin problems such as acne, scalp hair loss (balding), and deepening of the voice. Such symptoms require prompt evaluation, because similar symptoms can occur with tumors of the adrenal gland or ovary.

Prolactin. Prolactin is the hormone that regulates breast milk production ("pro" means supports; "lactin" means lactation). In the normal woman who is not breastfeeding, levels of prolactin are low because its release is inhibited by the hypothalamus. Several problems including a pituitary gland tumor can cause excessive production of prolactin and may cause you to develop breast milk. High prolactin may also stop menstrual periods.

Drugs, including tranquilizers (phenothiazines), amphetamines, and blood pressure medications, can cause elevated prolactin and breast milk production. **Abnormal breast milk production demands thorough investigation to be certain that a pituitary tumor is not present.** Your clinician will probably check your prolactin levels if your menstrual periods cease inexplicably.

Prostaglandins.   The prostaglandins are a family of hormones present in semen, in the uterine lining, and in many body tissues. Each member of the prostaglandin family has its own distinct effects.

The normal role of prostaglandins is not yet fully understood. They can affect blood pressure, body temperature, kidney fluid balance, activity of the gastrointestinal tract, constriction of lung air passageways, and uterine contractions. The release of prosta-glandins as uterine lining cells shed is **the cause of ordinary menstrual cramps.** (Cramps may also be caused by gynecologic problems such as infection.) Prostaglan-dins are probably also responsible for the diarrhea, nausea, and vomiting that sometimes accompany cramps. Researchers suspect that prostaglandins may play a role in initiating labor at the end of pregnancy. The presence of prostaglandins in semen may facilitate sperm transport or in some way enable the sperm to unite with the egg.

The only approved medical use for prostaglandins so far is termination of pregnancy. The drug is most often used for abortions performed after the 15th week of pregnancy (see Chapter 18).

CHANGES IN THE OVARY AND UTERUS DURING THE HORMONE CYCLE

The menstrual cycle days are traditionally numbered **using the first day of a menstrual period as the first cycle day.** This scheme makes sense because menstrual bleeding is the most obvious external sign of internal cyclic changes. The first day of a menstrual period also turns out to be a logical starting point in relation to internal events. The menstrual bleeding phase is the time in the cycle when hormone levels are at their lowest point. As the production of estrogen and progesterone drops, the hormone support to the uterine lining is lost, the lining sloughs off, and menstrual bleeding begins.

The length of a normal cycle varies from woman to woman, and from month to month in the same woman. Ninety percent of normal cycles fall between 23 and 35 days in length. Although the total number of days in the cycle may vary, **the number of days between ovulation and the next menstrual period is very consistent—about 14 days** (plus or minus 2 days at most). The variations in normal cycles almost always occur in the first half of the cycle, **before** ovulation. Descriptions of the normal cycle traditionally assume that the cycle length is an average 28 days and that ovulation occurs on cycle day 14. You can adjust the description to fit your own cycle by mentally adding or subtracting days from the first half of your cycle.

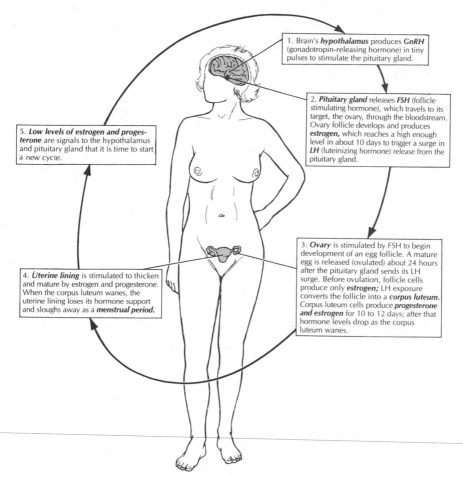

1. Brain's **hypothalamus** produces **GnRH** (gonadotropin-releasing hormone) in tiny pulses to stimulate the pituitary gland.

2. **Pituitary gland** releases **FSH** (follicle stimulating hormone), which travels to its target, the ovary, through the bloodstream. Ovary follicle develops and produces **estrogen,** which reaches a high enough level in about 10 days to trigger a surge in **LH** (luteinizing hormone) release from the pituitary gland.

5. **Low levels of estrogen and progesterone** are signals to the hypothalamus and pituitary gland that it is time to start a new cycle.

3. **Ovary** is stimulated by FSH to begin development of an egg follicle. A mature egg is released (ovulated) about 24 hours after the pituitary gland sends its LH surge. Before ovulation, follicle cells produce only **estrogen;** LH exposure converts the follicle into a **corpus luteum.** Corpus luteum cells produce **progesterone and estrogen** for 10 to 12 days; after that hormone levels drop as the corpus luteum wanes.

4. **Uterine lining** is stimulated to thicken and mature by estrogen and progesterone. When the corpus luteum wanes, the uterine lining loses its hormone support and sloughs away as a **menstrual period.**

ILLUSTRATION 2-8   Reproductive hormone cycle.

If your typical cycle length is 32 days, then the first "half" of your cycle is 17 days, and you ovulate on day 18. If your typical cycle is 22 days, you ovulate on day 8; the first "half" of your cycle is only 7 days long. In either case, the secretory phase of your cycle (the second "half") is 14 days long.

During the first few days of the cycle—the menstrual period itself—the falling level of estrogen triggers secretion of FSH to stimulate growth of ovarian follicles. Initial growth occurs in 20 or so follicles. The cells lining the follicle soon begin to produce estrogen. One or two follicles assume dominance and continue to grow and produce estrogen, while the remaining follicles subside and shrink away (see Illustration 2-8).

As the follicle cells multiply and grow, estrogen production rises dramatically toward the middle of the cycle (days 11, 12, 13); estrogen rises to a critical peak and a surge

OVARY

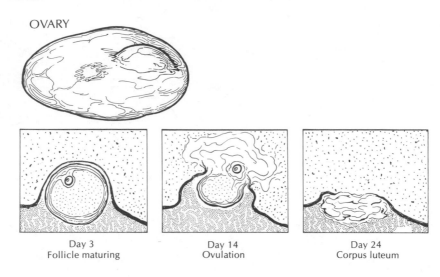

Day 3
Follicle maturing

Day 14
Ovulation

Day 24
Corpus luteum

ILLUSTRATION 2-9   Changes in the ovary during the menstrual cycle.

in the release of LH from the pituitary gland is triggered. **The sudden burst of LH is the stimulus for ovulation, the release of the mature egg** cell from inside the follicle (see Illustration 2-9).

After ovulation, the cells that line the fluid-filled egg follicle rearrange themselves into a cluster. LH changes follicular cell chemistry, and a yellow pigment called lutein accumulates within the cells (hence the name "corpus luteum"—yellow body). The cells resume production of estrogen and, under the LH influence, begin to produce progesterone as well. Both estrogen and progesterone are released during the last half of the cycle.

The LH level gradually decreases during the last half of the cycle. By cycle days 22 to 24, the LH level is so low that corpus luteum function is no longer supported and production of estrogen and progesterone declines rapidly. This drop results in menstrual bleeding and brings to an end one full cycle. The low estrogen level will soon serve as a signal to the hypothalamus and pituitary gland that more FSH is needed to begin the next cycle.

Some women notice cramping pain on one side of the lower abdomen at the time of ovulation. Fluid or blood released from the ruptured egg follicle may irritate the abdominal lining, or perhaps stretching of the surface of the ovary by follicle growth causes pain. Ovulation pain usually lasts only a few hours, but can persist as long as a day or two.

Except for ovulation pain and changes in cervical mucus, all the cyclic changes described so far are silent: they occur with few noticeable symptoms. **The external evidence of the reproductive cycle (bleeding) is the last step** in the chain of hormone

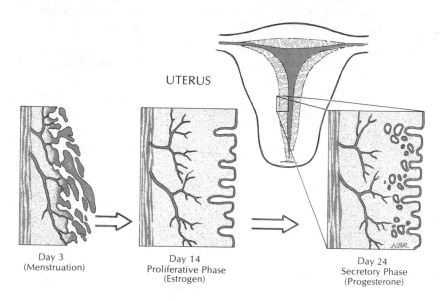

UTERUS

Day 3
(Menstruation)

Day 14
Proliferative Phase
(Estrogen)

Day 24
Secretory Phase
(Progesterone)

ILLUSTRATION 2-10   Changes in the uterine lining during the menstrual cycle.

events and involves the effects of decreased estrogen and progesterone on the uterus and cervix.

The first few days of the new cycle set the stage for changes in the uterine lining (endometrium). As the menstrual flow stops (on day 4, 5, 6, or 7), the surface layers of the endometrium have been shed to leave only the thin basal layer. At about this time (day 7 or 8), estrogen production by the ovarian follicle is beginning to rise. Estrogen stimulates growth of the uterine lining. The basal cells multiply, and gradually the lining thickens. By the middle of the cycle the lining thickness has increased five- to tenfold (see Illustration 2-10).

As ovulation occurs **there is a temporary drop in estrogen production,** followed by renewed estrogen and progesterone release. **Some women notice a brief episode of spotting at the time of ovulation** that is probably caused by the temporary lull in estrogen production.

During the last half of the cycle, after ovulation, progesterone and estrogen stimulate maturation of the uterine lining. The lining does not increase in thickness, but the cells reorganize to form mucus-producing glands and distinct layers. Small blood vessels grow into the lining to nourish it and to be available in case a fertilized egg implants. The lining cells also begin to store nutrients that would be needed for pregnancy.

At the conclusion of the cycle, estrogen and progesterone levels drop and the stimulus to the mature lining is lost. Decreasing blood flow into its tiny arteries causes shrinking and deterioration of the surface layers. **Most of the endometrium separates from the uterine wall and is shed as menstrual blood.**

Cyclic changes in estrogen and progesterone also affect mucus production by the cervix. During the initial low-estrogen days of the cycle, there is very little mucus. As estrogen rises, mucus production increases and reaches a peak that coincides with ovulation. Mucus at the time of ovulation is characteristically fluid, stringy, elastic, and abundant.

Immediately after ovulation, as estrogen drops and progesterone appears, the cervical mucus becomes thick, sticky, and much less profuse. Mucus remains scant throughout the rest of the cycle, although some women do notice a second increase in mucus a few days before menstruation that is probably the result of renewed estrogen production during the last half of the cycle.

WHEN PREGNANCY OCCURS

If fertilization occurs, the hormone patterns of the last half of the menstrual cycle are altered. Assuming that you ovulate on cycle day 14, your egg can be fertilized on day 14 or 15 and implantation of the embryo in the uterine lining will occur between day 17 and 21. Soon after implantation, the production of pregnancy hormone (HCG— human chorionic gonadotropin) by the developing placenta reaches detectable levels. HCG hormone closely resembles LH hormone and takes over its role as a continuing stimulus to the corpus luteum. The corpus luteum, in turn, continues with its production of progesterone throughout the first three months of pregnancy. After the third month, progesterone production by the placenta itself completely replaces progesterone production by the corpus luteum. **HCG interrupts the repetitive cycle of hormone changes and prevents menstrual loss** of the uterine lining by maintaining progesterone production.

Puberty

During puberty a young woman's reproductive organs mature in size and function. Puberty encompasses a whole sequence of normal changes and occurs over a period of about two years for most young women. Every female child is born with the organs and hormones described in the first sections of this chapter. During childhood, the hormone-producing thermostat of the hypothalamus is turned off, and no matter how low the level of estrogen or progesterone circulating in the child's blood, the hormonal thermostat in the brain does not switch on, as it would in a mature woman.

No one knows just why or how the reproductive hormone system begins to function at puberty. The first changes that lead to puberty are invisible. The hypothalamus becomes sensitive to the reproductive hormone levels, and the thermostat turns on. The hypothalamus gives the pituitary gland a signal to produce follicle-stimulating hormone (FSH), and FSH travels to the immature ovary and causes it to grow and to secrete estrogen.

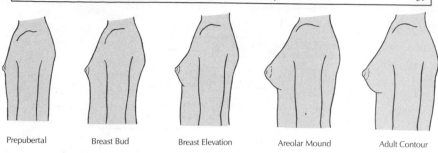

| Prepubertal | Breast Bud | Breast Elevation | Areolar Mound | Adult Contour |

ILLUSTRATION 2-11 The breast bud usually appears at about age 10; the nipple enlarges, and a firm mound of breast tissue develops under the skin. The adolescent breast often has a prominent, puffy areola.

Production of FSH by the pituitary gland begins to increase several years before puberty. Increasing LH release during sleep begins at puberty and may indicate that GnRH pulses from the hypothalamus are beginning to take on the mature pattern they have in adult women.

The timing of the changes of puberty is quite variable. Family patterns are important, but researchers suspect that external influences also play a role. The average age of puberty gradually declined over several decades in this century, and then stabilized; improvement in average nutrition and health are credited for this decline.

Puberty is also roughly linked to overall body size and weight, and researchers in the past suggested that the beginning of menstrual periods was linked to attaining a critical weight of about 100 pounds on the average. In more recent studies, body composition appears to be more significant. During childhood, fat is likely to account for a lower percentage of body weight; it increases gradually as puberty approaches, and more rapidly during the first few years after puberty. Some experts feel that it is necessary for a woman to have a body fat percentage of at least 17% for the initiation of menstrual periods, and 22% for normal ovulatory cycles to be maintained (2). The effects of athletic training on puberty events lend some support to this possibility, because young women who begin intensive physical training before menstrual periods have started may be delayed in completing their puberty changes. Studies of young ballet dancers, runners, swimmers, figure skaters, and other athletes show that menstrual periods may start as much as one to three years later than average. Nutritional deprivation related to illness, dieting, or anorexia nervosa can also cause delayed puberty.

OUTWARD SIGNS OF PUBERTY

As the body's level of estrogen rises, a young woman's sex organs grow and mature and the first signs of puberty become apparent. The first outward sign of puberty in the

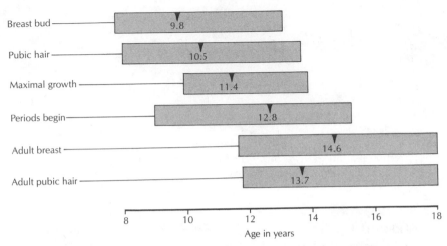

ILLUSTRATION 2-12   Normal age ranges are quite wide for each phase of pubertal development. (Adapted from Speroff L, Glass RH, Kase NG: *Clinical Gynecologic Endocrinology and Infertility* (ed 3). Baltimore: Williams & Wilkins, 1983.)

young woman is in the **breast nipple** (see Illustration 2-11). Her nipple begins to grow and stand away from the chest wall, and later the breast itself begins to grow. A **small mound of breast tissue forms just under the nipple.** In 95% of young women, breast bud development occurs between ages 8 and 13 (see Illustration 2-12). During the early part of puberty, the young woman also begins her growth spurt, a period of rapid growth that ends when adult height has been reached. Meanwhile, estrogen causes the vagina and uterus to grow, and the lining of the uterus begins to thicken. Estrogen is also responsible for fat deposits over the hips and thighs that give her body a female contour.

Next the adrenal glands start to produce male sex hormones (androgens), which play an essential role in a young woman's pubertal development. No one knows why the adrenal glands begin making more of these hormones, but we do know that it happens as the estrogen level in the blood rises. The male hormones cause the **growth of pubic hair and underarm hair and further stimulate the growth spurt.** In 95% of young women, hair appears between ages 8 and 13. The male hormones may also cause acne; for most young people the level of male hormones falls once puberty is completed, and the skin clears up.

When breast development is further along and the young woman has probably purchased her first bra, she will probably have a triangle of pubic hair and some hair under her arms, and her growth will have slowed down. She can now expect her first menstrual period.

MENSTRUATION

Menstruation usually begins between ages 9 and 15, about two years after the first signs of breast development. It is normal for periods to begin as early as six months or as late as five years after breasts begin to grow. **Often a young woman will notice some vaginal discharge six months or so before she begins to menstruate.** This discharge is clear or whitish and does not cause itching, burning, or foul odor. The young woman may simply notice a little wetness on her underclothes each day, or the discharge may be quite heavy in some cases.

The first periods occur when estrogen has thickened the lining of the uterus sufficiently that some of the lining simply falls off. **Many young women have irregular periods during the first year or two,** and they may not yet be ovulating. Periods may come twice a month or every two to three months, and may be very heavy or very light and still be normal for this stage of development.

Once ovulation begins, the young woman should have regular periods every four weeks or so. Ovulation is necessary for pregnancy to occur, and many young women think that they are safe because their periods are irregular or infrequent. **Remember that there is no way to tell when ovulation will start** and that irregular periods will not necessarily protect a young woman from pregnancy. Ovulation begins immediately after, or even before, the very first menstrual period in some cases.

PUBERTY THAT IS TOO EARLY OR TOO LATE

If a young woman has signs of puberty that begin before the age of 8, or if no signs have appeared by age 13 1/2, then evaluation for possible **precocious puberty** or **delayed puberty** will be needed. (For boys puberty is a little later; normally it begins between the ages of 9 and 14.) Treatment to counteract these problems is quite likely to be successful.

Menopause: Physical and Hormone Changes

The transition from the reproductive phase of a woman's life cycle into the postreproductive phase is called the **climacteric.** Menopause, which means cessation of menstrual periods, is the most obvious event, but many other changes occur as well. Most women are able to cope with this transition without difficulty. **Approximately 50% of women undergo menopause at or before 51 or 52 years of age,** although the normal range is fairly wide, 45 to 55. The timing of menopause is not predictable. You may follow the same pattern that your mother and sisters experienced, or your menopause may be earlier or later. Climacteric changes begin considerably before menopause. A significant decline in fertility occurs in the mid 40s. The reason for this decline is not known, but a decrease in the number of maturing ovary follicles and in ovarian estrogen production occurs at about this time.

The rate of ovarian changes varies from individual to individual. Some women seem to experience a gradual decrease in hormone production over a period of several years that is associated with irregular menstrual cycles or prolonged intervals between periods. For other women, the changes may be more abrupt, with a normal cycle one month and a complete cessation of bleeding two or three months later. **Women who undergo premature menopause because of surgical removal of the ovaries have extremely abrupt hormone changes,** and symptoms related to menopause are often quite severe.

As the climacteric nears completion, ovarian estrogen production declines to extremely low levels. The ovary is no longer responsive to the stimulating hormones produced by the brain. The pituitary FSH and LH output rises to high levels because their release is triggered by low levels of estrogen.

As estrogen production by the ovary declines, the importance of **other** sources of estrogen increases. **Fatty tissue is able to convert other hormones to estrogen;** hence, estrogen levels do not drop to zero. Ovary production of testosterone actually increases after menopause, and is maintained for at least several years. Testosterone conversion to estrogen in fat cells is one source of continuing estrogen production. The hormone precursor androstenedione can also be converted to estrogen in fat cells. It is produced mainly by the adrenal gland, but also to some extent by the postmenopausal ovary (3). Some women maintain a significant estrogen level well into old age.

The relationship between the known hormone changes and the various symptoms that occur during the climacteric is not well understood. For some women, however, the physical and hormonal changes that accompany the climacteric can be quite distressing and disabling. Physicians used to identify low estrogen levels as the cause of a host of problems, ranging from hot flashes to irrationality and decrepitude. Research in the last decade, however, has concluded that the estrogen drop can be unequivocally blamed for only a few problems: hot flashes, vaginal dryness, muscle tone loss in the urinary tract, and bone density loss caused by osteoporosis. These issues are discussed in depth in Chapter 34, along with pros and cons for estrogen replacement therapy and alternatives for nonhormonal management of menopause symptoms.

REFERENCES

1. Fraser IS, McCarron G, Markham R, et al: Blood and total fluid content of menstrual discharge. *Obstetrics and Gynecology* 65:194–198, 1985.
2. Neinstein LS: Menstrual dysfunction in pathophysiologic states. *Western Journal of Medicine* 143:476–484, 1985.
3. Speroff L, Glass RH, Kase NG: *Clinical Gynecologic Endocrinology and Infertility* (ed 3). Baltimore: Williams & Wilkins, 1983.

The Pelvic Examination

A pelvic examination provides your clinician—and you—with essential basic information about the health of your reproductive system; yet thousands of women avoid or delay pelvic exams. Some women fear that the exam will be painful, especially if they have had uncomfortable exams in the past. You probably won't ever like having a pelvic exam, but it does help to know what happens during your exam and why. It also helps to know how to prepare for an exam and what you can expect your exam to accomplish.

Most reproductive system problems can be treated successfully if they are detected early, so it is very important to be realistic about your health needs and put fear and embarrassment in perspective. "I guess I'd rather be mortified for a few minutes than put up with this itching another month," one woman said.

Preparing for a Pelvic Exam

My memory deserts me when I take off my clothes. The minute I get on an exam table—just me and that sheet—I forget *everything* I wanted to ask about. And I'm too embarrassed to call back and ask questions later!

—WOMAN, 35

Make a list of your questions at home and take them with you, right into the exam room if necessary. **Start with your most important concerns**, and be sure that your clinician is aware of them before beginning your examination. Write down the dates of your last few periods, the dates you first noticed any symptoms that concern you, and the names of any drugs you have taken recently. Be sure to tell your clinician if you took DES during pregnancy or if your mother took DES while she was pregnant with you. (See Chapter 42 for more on DES and its implications for your health.)

Avoid douching for at least 24 hours before your exam, especially if you think you have an infection. Your clinician may not be able to diagnose infection if all the evidence has been washed away. Some clinicians also recommend that you avoid intercourse for 48 hours, and tampons for 24 hours, before your exam. Your Pap smear and other lab tests will be more accurate if your normal vaginal ecosystem hasn't been tampered with.

Find out whether your clinician wants you to come in on schedule if you start your period. **Heavy menstrual flow may interfere with a Pap smear but should not be a problem for pelvic examination otherwise.** If you are a diaphragm user, take your diaphragm with you. Your clinician may want to check for proper insertion and fit. Let your clinician know if this will be your first pelvic exam and ask her/him to explain the exam along the way. Your clinician can also show you the instruments she/he will use, and provide a mirror so you can see your cervix, vagina, or other areas of interest or concern. (If you are not interested in seeing your cervix just let your clinician know. Viewing is not required!)

How a Pelvic Exam Is Done and Why

A gynecologic exam begins with a careful medical history and a general physical examination. Your clinician will probably record your weight and blood pressure, listen to your heart and lungs, examine your thyroid gland, breasts, and abdomen, and may take specimens for blood and urine lab tests. (See Chapters 4 and 7 for a full discussion of common office tests and procedures and routine checkups.)

Before your breast exam, ask about any breast changes you have noticed that puzzle or concern you. **Don't assume that your clinician will find a lump you found first yourself;** you know your breasts much better than your clinician does. Your clinician will check your breasts for lumps, tenderness, enlarged nodes, nipple discharge, and skin changes that might indicate the presence of a tumor. (See Chapter 37 for a full discussion of breast lumps.) Pay careful attention to your clinician's technique and compare it with your own technique for your monthly breast self-examination. If you are not sure how to examine your own breasts, ask your clinician to teach you (see Chapter 5).

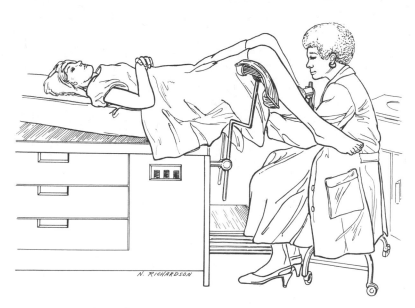

ILLUSTRATION 3-1   Speculum part of pelvic exam. Your clinician usually sits on a stool.

For your pelvic exam you will be placed in what is clinically called the dorsal lithotomy position (commonly known as the Awkward Embarrassing Position). You lie on your back with your bottom at the very end of the table and your legs supported in knee or foot stirrups. Your clinician will sit on a stool at the end of the table, between your legs (see Illustration 3-1).

Some clinicians and their patients prefer pelvic examination with the woman in a semirecumbent position. In this case you lie on your back with your upper body raised at about a 45-degree angle, much like a "reading in bed" position. This posture relaxes the thick sheath of abdominal muscle that covers the pelvis, so clinicians find the uterus and other structures much easier to feel. Women who have been examined in this position usually say the exam is quite comfortable, and that it allows good eye contact with the clinician.

EXTERNAL EXAMINATION

The first step in the pelvic examination is inspection of your vulva, the area around the entrance to your vagina (see Illustration 3-2). Your clinician will check for redness, swelling, or lesions that might indicate infection or injury. ("Lesion" simply means any tissue abnormality or loss of function: a sore or a wound or an area of irritation, for example.) Some clinicians examine the clitoris by pushing back the fold of skin (prepuce, or clitoral hood) that covers it.

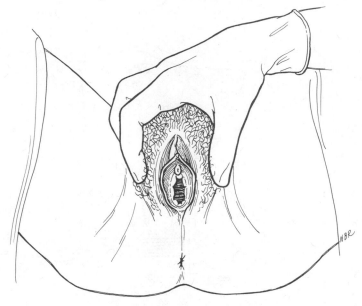

ILLUSTRATION 3-2   Your clinician examines your vulva as the first step in a pelvic exam.

SPECULUM EXAMINATION

Examination of the lining of the vagina and the cervix is the next step in a pelvic examination. **The speculum holds the vaginal walls apart so that your clinician can see your cervix and inspect the vaginal lining** (see Illustration 3-3). Specula come in several sizes, and your clinician will choose a speculum compatible with the size of the entrance to your vagina. If speculum insertion is painful, ask your clinician to stop. She/he may be able to readjust its position or switch to a smaller size.

Many clinicians begin by inserting a gloved finger into your vagina to dilate your vaginal opening and to locate your cervix. The speculum is inserted with the blades closed. Your clinician will press downward on the bottom wall of your vagina to guide the speculum in. Once inside the vagina, the speculum is rotated to the handle-downward position and the blades are opened and locked into place at the correct width. (Plastic specula make a loud crack as they snap into the locked position, so don't be surprised. Metal specula are mercifully silent, but they are cold unless they are warmed prior to insertion.) Your clinician inspects the vaginal walls and cervix for any redness, irritation, unusual discharge, or lesions. **Specimens for lab tests are collected while the speculum is in place.** A Pap smear specimen, gonorrhea and chlamydia test samples, and a wet smear preparation for diagnosing infection are often included.

Because gonorrhea and chlamydia are so common and because both men and women can have these infections without any symptoms, many clinicians believe that

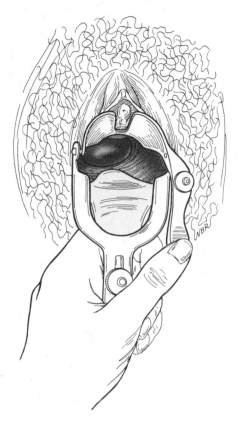

ILLUSTRATION 3-3   A speculum holds your vaginal walls apart so that the clinician can see your cervix.

the safest course is to perform routine testing on every patient. Other clinicians perform tests only when there is reason to suspect that infection may be present. Tests are essential if you have pain or an unusual discharge, if either you or your partner has been exposed or even has reason to suspect exposure, or if you are worried. It may be wise to have frequent tests if you have more than one sexual partner. Be sure to ask specifically for chlamydia and gonorrhea tests. (See Chapter 25 for a discussion of chlamydia and gonorrhea.)

It doesn't take as long to perform a speculum exam as it does to read about it here, you'll be happy to know.

BIMANUAL EXAMINATION

After laboratory specimens are collected, the speculum is removed. The next step in a pelvic exam is a bimanual (both hands) exam. Most clinicians stand up to perform a bimanual exam (see Illustration 3-4).

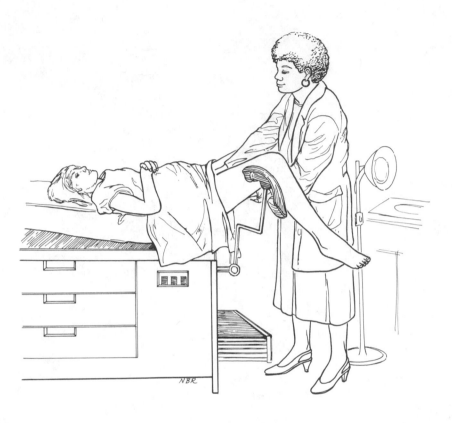

ILLUSTRATION 3-4   Bimanual part of a pelvic exam. Your clinician usually stands during this part of your examination.

Your clinician inserts two gloved fingers of one hand into your vagina and places the other hand on your abdomen. By pressing upward on your cervix and downward on your abdomen, she/he can feel the size, consistency, shape, and location of your uterus and will check for pain or tenderness (see Illustration 3-5). She/he checks both sides of your abdomen to locate your ovaries and fallopian tubes and checks your entire abdomen for masses or tender areas. At the conclusion of the bimanual exam, your clinician may insert one gloved finger into your rectum while the other remains in your vagina in order to evaluate the muscular wall that separates the rectum and vagina, to examine your uterus if it is retroflexed, or tilted toward your back, and to detect masses or tenderness deep in your pelvis (see Illustration 3-6).

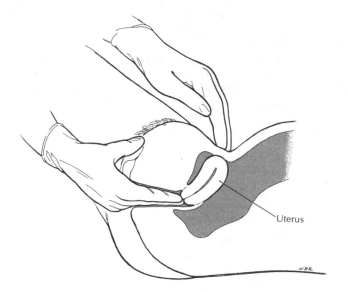

ILLUSTRATION 3-5   Bimanual exam. Your clinician can feel your uterus between her/his two hands.

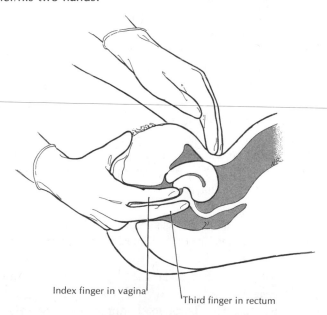

ILLUSTRATION 3-6   The rectal part of a bimanual exam permits your clinician to check your uterus even if it is retroflexed—tilted toward your back—as this uterus is.

Surviving a Pelvic Exam

I must have had about 30 pelvics by now, and I'm beginning to feel as blasé about them as my doctor does. After one child, two diaphragms, and a yeast infection I think I'll go to my grave with, it just doesn't bother me anymore. Last time, right in the middle of the exam, I caught myself wondering if Dr. Jackson dyed his hair! It proves you can get used to anything, I suppose.

—WOMAN, 33

A pelvic exam—performed on a healthy pelvis—should not be painful, but it may be uncomfortable. The speculum insertion is a strange sensation, especially if you have never had intercourse. Remember that relaxed vaginal muscles are highly flexible and elastic and that they are capable of accommodating a speculum. You can help by relaxing all your pelvic muscles completely and keeping them relaxed until the speculum is removed. When you are tense, your muscles clamp down on the speculum and increase your discomfort. If the speculum feels really awful, by all means ask your clinician to adjust it. It is almost always possible to do an adequate speculum exam without causing you significant discomfort.

A successful, informative bimanual examination is also much easier for your clinician if you are able to relax your abdominal muscles. A thick sheath of muscle completely covers your abdomen, and when muscles are tense, your clinician may find it difficult or impossible to feel your uterus underneath. **Deep breathing with your mouth open helps relax these muscles.** You may not even recognize tense muscles, especially if you are anxious or busy talking over your questions with your clinician. You might try tensing all your muscles on purpose and then relaxing them completely.

If you are having pain or tenderness, tell your clinician where it is before the exam begins; she/he will want to be especially gentle and especially thorough in examining that area.

Make sure to urinate just before your exam. Your bladder rests just above your uterus, and a full bladder can make the examination uncomfortable for you and more difficult for your clinician.

It is unlikely that your clinician will be able to tell if you have ever had intercourse. If she/he can't even insert so much as a fingertip in your vagina, she/he could reasonably conclude you haven't, but **most women are quite easy to examine, including those who have never had intercourse even once,** especially if they are tampon users.

Many clinics and private physicians now employ specially trained nurse practitioners or physician assistants who function in roles that formerly were reserved for doctors only, including routine pelvic examinations. These clinicians counsel and examine women for annual exams, family planning, prenatal care, and many other health needs. They work under a physician's supervision, and the physician assists in difficult or unusual situations. Most patients are very pleased with their nurse practitioner or physician assistant experience.

She spent *much* more time with me than my doctor ever did, and she was a very good explainer. For the *first time* I understood why I get spotting when I miss a couple of Pills!

—WOMAN, 22

When You Will Need a Pelvic Exam

Think of a pelvic exam as the starting place for all your reproductive health care needs. No one else can take the responsibility for the routine exams you need or for additional exams when problems occur. It is ideal to have your first pelvic exam before you need it, at a time when stress is low and you aren't sore or tender from infection. Under these circumstances the first exam is genuinely optional, and you can ask your clinician to terminate the exam if you are too uncomfortable to go on. Your clinician can also teach you how to dilate your vaginal opening so that future exams will be more comfortable. Most women who have gentle clinicians find that even a first pelvic exam is entirely manageable. Plan to see your clinician for a pelvic exam:

- When you think intercourse is imminent for the first time. You'll be reassured when you know your anatomy is normal and when you are prepared with good birth control.
- If you haven't begun menstruating by age 16
- At about age 20, or earlier if you begin having intercourse at an earlier age or if your mother took DES when she was pregnant with you (see Chapter 42)
- If you are having problems with severe menstrual cramps
- If your bleeding is very heavy or lasts more than 10 days
- At whatever intervals you and your clinician decide on for routine Pap smears. If you have had an abnormal Pap smear, genital warts, or more than one male sexual partner, faithfulness about Pap smears once a year is essential; more frequent smears may be needed in some cases (read about Pap smear recommendations in Chapter 7).

- Any time you are bothered by itching, redness, sores, swelling, unusual odor, or unusual discharge
- Any time you have abdominal pain or painful intercourse, especially if you also have chills or fever
- Any time you have unusual vaginal bleeding
- Any time you would like to use Pills, an IUD, or a diaphragm
- Any time you miss a period if there is any chance that you could be pregnant
- Any time you miss more than three periods (if you are not sexually active)
- Any time you have burning when you urinate, and you urinate frequently
- Any time you have had intercourse with a partner who might have an infection
- Any time you plan to become pregnant, for a thorough health assessment and prenatal advice before you conceive
- If you have been raped or suspect that you may have been injured

CHAPTER 4

Common Office
Tests and Procedures

Fifty years ago a clinician's office came equipped with a stethoscope, some bottles of pre-antibiotic-era medications, and little else. Today sophisticated lab tests and high-tech in-office diagnostic and therapeutic tools are commonplace. Labs perform assays sensitive enough to detect a teaspoonful of sugar in Lake Tahoe. Lasers stand beside tongue depressors in exam rooms. If at times we feel our medical care comes from machines, they are, at least, splendid machines.

This chapter describes some of the common office procedures that your clinician may use to help determine the cause of a specific problem. Sections here also cover office treatment procedures such as cautery, cryosurgery, and laser. The last section describes ultrasound or sonogram evaluation.

Laboratory tests are part of routine care, and are often needed to confirm the cause of a problem. If your test can be analyzed in the office, you may know the results within a few minutes. In many cases a test specimen is collected during your visit and is sent to an outside laboratory for analysis, or you may be asked to go to the laboratory yourself to have the test.

If your test is not normal, your clinician will notify you by telephone or mail and will make arrangements for any further studies or treatment you might need. Many clinicians do not routinely notify patients when test results are normal (the "no news is good news" technique).

It is likely to be at least a week before your clinician receives a report on routine test results from an outside lab. Part of that time is for the lab procedure itself, and

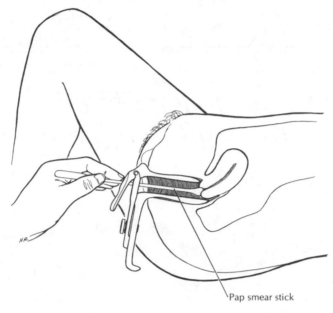

Pap smear stick

ILLUSTRATION 4-1   Your clinician scrapes surface cells from your cervix for a Pap smear.

with some tests this may require several days. Most of the time, though, it is just normal clerical and mail processing time. Urgent test results may be reported by phone, with results the next day or even sooner, and some tests may require even longer than a week. If you do not hear about your test within two weeks or so, telephone your clinician's office or clinic and ask the receptionist to verify that your test report has been received and that it is normal.

PAP SMEAR

A Pap smear specimen is collected during your speculum examination (see Chapter 3 for details on pelvic exam procedures). **Your clinician gently rotates a wooden or plastic spatula over the surface of your cervix to scrape away a thin layer of cervical cells;** she/he then spreads the cells across a glass slide (see Illustration 4-1). An additional sample of cells may be collected from your vagina or from the inside of your cervical canal in some cases. The slide is sprayed or immersed in a chemical that fixes the cells to the slide and preserves them; the slide is then sent from your clinician's office to a laboratory to be stained and examined under the microscope by a specially trained technician (cytotechnologist) or a physician specialist (pathologist). **You probably will not feel anything except the speculum during your Pap smear.** You may have light bleeding or a few spots of blood after a Pap smear.

   The purpose of a Pap smear is to detect cervical cancer or precancerous abnormalities that may be present. Vaginal infection or a low estrogen level is sometimes evident from a Pap smear as well. **The Pap smear is not reliable for detecting cancer of the uterus, ovary, or vagina.** Detailed information about abnormal Pap smears is in Chapter 35. Recommendations for timing of routine health exams, including Pap tests, are presented in Chapter 7.

Normal Pap test results provide excellent reassurance that you do not have cervical cancer or its precursors. **No test, however, is 100% accurate, and that includes Pap tests.** Pap test inaccuracies are discussed in Chapter 35. You can help insure accurate results by planning ahead for optimal Pap test conditions.

• Schedule your exam and Pap smear midway between menstrual periods if possible
• Do not put anything inside your vagina for one or two days prior to your test; don't have intercourse, don't douche, and don't use vaginal medication, lubricants, or contraceptive products

If you are having bleeding problems **you may be tempted to delay your Pap test, waiting for a blood-free time. Don't do it.** Bleeding can be a sign of serious uterine problems as well as cervical problems or even cervical cancer, so an exam and Pap test are essential. Bleeding will not bother your clinician, and at worst it may mean repeating your Pap test later if initial results are unsatisfactory because of too much blood.

WET SMEAR

If you have been bothered by itching, burning, an unusual odor, or excessive discharge, your clinician will probably recommend a wet smear (wet mount, wet prep). She/he places a small sample of your vaginal discharge on a glass slide and adds one or two drops of salt solution so that vaginal cells float in suspension, or one or two drops of mild alkaline solution to dissolve vaginal cells and make yeast infection cells appear more prominent. **Your clinician examines the slide immediately** under a microscope to look for fast-moving organisms that cause trichomonas, the branched colonies of fungus that cause yeast infection, or the stippled cells that indicate a bacterial vaginosis. All competent clinicians who treat gynecologic problems have microscopes and perform wet smears frequently. **The wet smear does not provide a conclusive diagnosis for gonorrhea or chlamydia.** Tests specifically for gonorrhea and chlamydia must be performed to detect these small, fragile bacteria (see "Infection Tests and Cultures" later in this chapter).

PH TEST

If your clinician suspects that you may have a vaginal infection, she/he may check the acidity of your vaginal secretions. Acidity (or alkalinity) is expressed as pH (potential for hydrogen), a number from 0 to 14 (zero is very acid, 7 is neutral, 14 is very alkaline). To determine vaginal pH your clinician will dip a strip of pH paper into a small sample of secretions and watch for the color change that corresponds to pH. Normal vaginal pH is 3 to 4. A high pH, 5 or more, shows that your vaginal environment is less acid than normal; high pH is a common finding with trichomonas vaginal infection and with bacterial vaginosis.

URINE TESTS

Many different kinds of tests can be performed on a urine sample. Don't be misled by thinking that the normal urine test you had two months ago proves that your entire urinary system is perfect.

Careful urine collection is important for accurate results. Blood or discharge from your vagina or bacteria from your skin may interfere with the test procedures or cause incorrect results. For a "clean catch" specimen you will be asked to wipe your vulva clean before urinating and use your fingers to spread the vaginal lips gently as you urinate. Use your other hand to hold the urine container. A sample collected in the middle of your urine stream (not the first or last few drops) is least likely to be contaminated.

Dipstick urine tests are routinely performed in many clinicians' offices. A small strip of chemically treated paper is dipped into a urine specimen, and the results immediately appear as a color change in the paper. **The dipstick test reveals the presence of blood, abnormal protein, sugar, and acids produced in diabetes in your urine.** An abnormal dipstick result may indicate kidney disease, diabetes, or infection in your bladder or kidneys; or it may simply mean that your urine specimen was contaminated by menstrual blood or vaginal discharge washed from your vulva into your specimen cup.

Urinalysis is a more complete urine evaluation that can be performed either in your clinician's office or by an outside lab. The concentration and acidity of your urine are tested, and a dipstick test is performed. A tube of urine is spun in a centrifuge for several minutes to collect the cells and particles in a sediment at the bottom of the tube. The sediment is spread on a glass slide and examined under a microscope; if infection is present, the sediment will contain white blood cells and bacteria. Abnormal microscopic crystals or clumps of cells in your urine may indicate kidney disease.

A urine sample may also be used for a pregnancy test. Two-minute slide tests for pregnancy use a urine sample, and are quite likely to be performed in your clinician's office. More sensitive pregnancy tests, also using urine, are also performed in many offices. Pregnancy tests are described in detail in Chapter 8.

Many other less common tests can be performed on a urine sample; determination of hormone levels, for example, may require analysis of your entire urine output over a 24-hour period. **Urine cultures** are described in a later section. When you have a urine test your clinician will not be checking for all possible problems. A normal urinalysis does not mean that a pregnancy check has been done, and vice versa. So if you are concerned about a specific problem such as pregnancy, be sure your clinician understands your concern and that the appropriate test is done.

BLOOD TESTS

Hundreds of tests can be performed on a blood specimen. If you want to find out whether you have syphilis, for example, you must ask specifically for a syphilis test. It is entirely possible to submit 15 different tubes of blood and learn whether you have ever had German measles, whether your liver is damaged, whether your thyroid hormone is low, and so forth, and still not find the answer to your question about syphilis.

One very common blood test, the **blood count,** can be done with a specimen drawn either from a vein in your arm or from a fingertip or earlobe prick. Your clinician may perform a blood count right in the office or clinic, or send you to an outside lab. **A blood count detects anemia.** Two slightly different techniques are widely used. The **hematocrit** method determines what percentage of your blood volume is made up of red cells. A result of 35% to 40% is normal, and a lower percentage means that you are anemic. The **hemoglobin** method measures the concentration of red pigment (hemoglobin) in your blood. Normal hemoglobin values are 12 to 14 gm per 100 cc of blood, and lower values indicate anemia. If you have a finger or earlobe prick test, most likely you are being checked for anemia. Most other blood tests require a tube of blood from an arm vein.

In some cases, **timing and special instructions may be important for meaningful blood test results.** A fasting blood sugar means just that. Results of a sugar (glucose) level obtained when you have eaten a meal in the previous six to eight hours are not meaningful. Tests for triglyceride and cholesterol should also be drawn after an overnight fast (no food), and may also be elevated if you have eaten unusually rich food during the previous day or two. Cholesterol and triglycerides are also somewhat higher during the first part of a woman's menstrual cycle than they are during the last two weeks (1). If you are having these tests repeated, plan to have the specimen drawn at about the same time in your cycle so results will be comparable.

Hormone tests also may require special planning. Prolactin hormone rises whenever breast or nipple tissue is stimulated. Ideally, a sample for prolactin should be drawn after an overnight fast, with no recent breast stimulation, and after a 15-minute rest. Don't go to the lab immediately after a routine visit and breast exam! Other hormone tests, such as progesterone, may need to be timed with your menstrual cycle. Be sure you understand your clinician's instructions.

INFECTION TESTS AND CULTURES

A culture identifies the specific bacterial agent or other organism that is causing infection. Your clinician collects a blood, urine, pus, or discharge sample from your

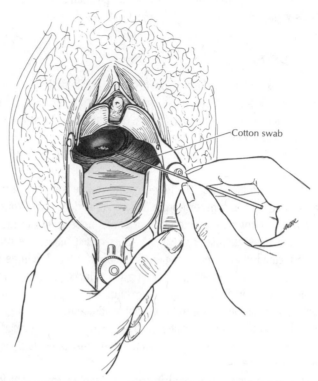
Cotton swab

ILLUSTRATION 4-2   Your clinician collects a specimen of fluid from inside your cervical canal for a bacterial culture.

infection site with a sterile cotton swab (see Illustration 4-2), transfers the sample to a jelly-like nutrient where organisms are likely to thrive, and sends the specimen to a lab, where it is incubated at roughly 98 degrees. Bacteria begin to multiply rapidly in this ideal environment. Lab specialists identify the specific bacteria and determine its sensitivity and susceptibility to various antibiotics. Incubation, identification, and sensitivity tests take several days.

Some bacteria are more difficult to culture than others and require special handling. In order to culture the fragile gonorrhea bacteria, for example, laboratories use a nutrient treated with antibiotics to reduce growth of competitive bacteria that might overshadow gonorrhea. Gonorrhea cultures must also be protected from exposure to oxygen in the air, so culture samples are immediately stored in an oxygen-free atmosphere. Culture tests for gonorrhea are not reliable if these safeguards are ignored.

As an alternative to cultures, tests are now available to **detect some infections using chemical techniques,** so it is not necessary to grow the organism in a laboratory. These techniques are especially helpful for bacteria that are difficult to grow, such as *Chlamydia trachomatis* and *Neisseria gonorrhoeae,* and may also provide quicker test results. Chemical tests for several common pathogens are in wide use, and many more new tests are anticipated. The test or culture technique your clinician chooses will depend on laboratory resources available and relative costs in your area.

If you are concerned about a sexually transmitted infection such as chlamydia or gonorrhea, be sure to ask specifically for testing so your clinician can use the proper collection and storage techniques. Separate samples will be needed for chlamydia and gonorrhea tests, and additional test samples from the rectum, urethra, and cervix may be recommended for maximum test reliability. A specimen from your throat should be tested if oral sex exposure to gonorrhea or chlamydia is a possibility.

IDENTIFICATION OF HERPES

Many laboratories have specialized equipment for culturing herpes and other viruses. Although virus culture is a fairly complex and costly procedure, it may be advisable if there is any question about whether you have herpes (see Chapter 26). Specimens for herpes cultures are collected with a cotton swab from your cervix or from a blister.

Another technique used for identifying herpes is microscopic examination of a sample of cells scraped from a suspicious sore; if herpes is present, it is often possible to identify giant cells with multiple nuclei when your cell sample is processed like a Pap smear and examined under the microscope.

SCHILLER'S STAIN

In a simple procedure often done during the speculum examination, Schiller's solution or a similar iodine mixture such as Lugol's solution is painted over the surface of your cervix and vagina. A normal cervical surface and vaginal lining absorb iodine from the solution and are stained mahogany brown; abnormal areas remain light pink. Iodine staining was often used to pinpoint an area for biopsy before colposcopy was available, and may now be used in conjunction with colposcopy.

WOOD'S LIGHT

Wood's light is an ultraviolet light bulb used to identify fungus infections of the scalp and skin. Some common fungus infections appear fluorescent under ultraviolet light.

HOME TESTS

Drugstore home test kits arrived in 1977 with the first do-it-yourself pregnancy test and are now a significant growth industry. Kits are available without prescription to test for pregnancy, ovulation timing, stool blood, menopause, urinary tract infection, and diabetes. Pregnancy, ovulation, and menopause kits test for hormone levels of HCG (human chorionic gonadotropin), LH (luteinizing hormone), and FSH (follicle-stimulating hormone), respectively; elevated levels of these hormones provide reliable

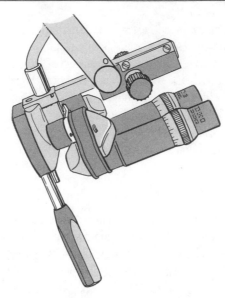

ILLUSTRATION 4-3   With the colposcope your clinician can see details on the surface of your cervix or skin magnified about 10 times.

diagnosis for the condition in question. The stool blood test detects traces of blood too small to be visible. The urinary tract infection test detects abnormal cells present in urine and the diabetes test detects abnormally high sugar levels. A do-it-yourself gonorrhea test kit for men is available in some areas, and many more tests are being developed.

Home tests have some big advantages in convenience and cost, and may help you avoid delay in identifying a pregnancy, for example. Checking your own stool samples for blood three times each year is easier and less costly than similar tests at a laboratory, and many clinicians recommend these home tests as a routine screening step for colorectal cancer.

The main disadvantage of home testing is that you could be misled by incorrect test results, and may not be able to identify possible test errors as well as your clinician could. Also, you are likely to need an exam and confirming lab work if your home test is abnormal, so your test may have to be repeated anyway.

COLPOSCOPY

A colposcope is a diagnostic instrument that looks like binoculars mounted on a tripod or suspended from a movable, mechanical arm (see Illustration 4-3). During a pelvic examination your clinician can look through the colposcope to see the surface of your cervix magnified 10 to 20 times normal size. With magnification and high-intensity colored lights, it is possible to see details of cervical structure that are not visible to the naked eye. Colposcopy is also helpful in evaluating abnormalities on the vaginal lining and on the skin of the vulva.

Colposcopy requires special training. Many clinicians did not have a chance to learn colposcopy as part of their specialty education in gynecology, and unless your clinician has been trained to interpret colposcopic findings, the procedure is not worthwhile.

Colposcopy is painless; the instrument does not even touch you, and the light source provides cool light. Your clinician will use a dilute vinegar solution (acetic acid) mopped over the cervix with a cotton swab to remove mucus and make the surface features more clearly visible. You may notice a mild stinging sensation with the vinegar, particularly if you have any vaginal or vulvar irritation at the time. Colposcopy is time-consuming and expensive, and thorough colposcopic examination requires that you lie still for 10 to 20 minutes with a speculum in place.

Colposcopy is often used to evaluate abnormal Pap smear results (see Chapter 35) or to identify an abnormal area for biopsy. Your clinician may perform a colposcopic exam if you have pain or bleeding with intercourse that may be caused by a cervical abnormality. **Colposcopic examination of both the cervix and the vaginal walls may be recommended for DES daughters** (see Chapter 42). Your clinician may use a colposcope to examine ulcers, sores, or other abnormal skin areas on your vulva.

Colposcopy can help your clinician identify areas of the cervix where cell multiplication is increased. After swabbing with vinegar solution, these areas appear white and dense compared to the normal cervical surface areas because dense, white nuclei of young cells are closely packed together. Such areas are called **white lesions** and are often the source of abnormal cells found in a Pap smear.

The distribution of tiny blood vessels near the surface of your cervix can also be seen through a colposcope. The blood vessel pattern is often altered when precancerous changes occur, and the pattern is significantly altered by cancer. These clues may help your clinician **identify the most abnormal areas for biopsy or treatment.**

Biopsies performed after careful colposcopic examination (called colposcopically directed biopsies) are especially valuable, because you and your clinician have some assurance that your biopsy specimens are from the most abnormal areas. The same principle applies when your clinician uses the colposcope to examine an abnormal area on your vulva.

If your clinician is not able to see the entire extent of the abnormal areas, she/he will recommend further tests or treatment. For example, if the abnormal area extends up inside your cervical canal out of view, your clinician may perform endocervical curettage (described later in this chapter) or recommend surgery to remove the entire surface of the cervix and the outer part of the cervical canal (called conization of the cervix).

CERVICOGRAPHY

Cervicography, analysis of a photograph of your cervix, is a new technique that may

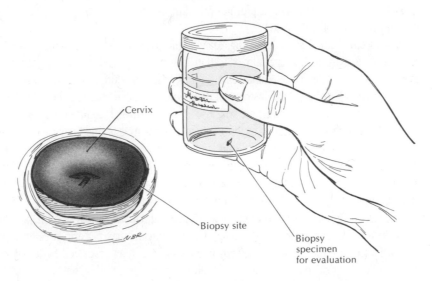

Cervix

Biopsy site

Biopsy
specimen
for evaluation

ILLUSTRATION 4-4   A cervical biopsy requires only a tiny fragment of tissue.

offer some of the advantages of colposcopy at lower cost. The camera equipment
necessary for cervicography is less expensive than colposcopy equipment, and less
training is required for the clinician. The photographic slides obtained are sent to
certified experts for interpretation and the results are reported back to the clinician.
Cervicography is used along with a Pap smear for routine screening to reduce the risk
that a significant abnormality might be overlooked with Pap smear alone.

BIOPSY

If you have a lump, a wart, or an ulcerated or abnormal-appearing area, your
clinician may recommend biopsy, the removal of a small piece of tissue for microscopic examination by a pathologist. Biopsy is a procedure that usually allows your
clinician to arrive at a precise, definite diagnosis. Almost any tissue can be subjected to
biopsy, including skin, vaginal lining, cervix, or uterine lining.

Taking the biopsy sample is usually a minor office procedure. A local anesthetic is
often used, and discomfort is likely to be minimal. The pathologist needs only enough
tissue to include several cell layers so that she/he can assess the pattern of cell changes
beneath the surface layer. Laboratory evaluation of a biopsy specimen requires several
days.

Vulvar Biopsy.   Vulvar biopsy is particularly helpful when skin cancer is a
possibility. Your clinician removes a 1/4-inch patch of anesthetized skin from the
junction of normal and abnormal-looking areas. In some cases, she/he will close your
biopsy site with a stitch, and in other cases, it can be left to heal over by itself. Keep

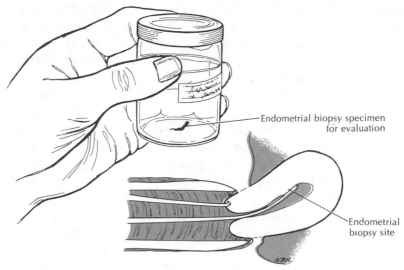

Endometrial biopsy specimen
for evaluation

Endometrial
biopsy site

ILLUSTRATION 4-5   Your clinician scrapes away a narrow strand of uterine lining for an endometrial biopsy.

the biopsy area clean and dry to prevent infection. If tenderness, swelling, or redness occurs in the biopsy area, see your clinician promptly.

Cervical Biopsy.   Your clinician may recommend biopsy of the cervix if you have an abnormal Pap smear. Colposcopy (see preceding section) may help your clinician pinpoint abnormal areas for biopsy. A local anesthetic usually is not necessary; pain nerves to your cervix are sparsely distributed, and you are likely to feel only mild cramping when a biopsy specimen is taken (see Illustration 4-4). Avoid intercourse, douching, and tampons for a week or so after biopsy so that your cervix can heal properly. It is normal to have some spotting after a biopsy, but if heavy bleeding occurs, see your clinician promptly. Symptoms of infection, such as pain, unusual vaginal discharge, or fever, require prompt evaluation as well.

Endocervical Curettage (ECC).   ("Endocervix" means the cervical canal; "curettage" means scraping.) If an abnormal area on your cervix extends up into your cervical canal, or if you are being evaluated because of an abnormal Pap test result, your clinician may recommend endocervical curettage to obtain shreds of tissue for microscopic evaluation. The scraping instrument (curet) has a tiny spoon-shaped tip that removes a shallow strand of cervical lining as it is scraped downward inside the canal. The strand is evaluated in the same way as any other biopsy sample. Endocervical scraping is likely to cause fairly intense cramping that lasts for one or two minutes. After ECC, watch for infection symptoms such as fever, pain, and unusual discharge, and call your clinician promptly if you think you have an infection.

Endometrial Biopsy. A small curet is inserted through your cervical canal into your uterine cavity and then scraped downward along the uterine lining (see Illustration 4-5) to remove shallow strands of lining (endometrium). Most women experience moderate to strong cramping with endometrial biopsy. Your clinician may use a local anesthetic or intravenous sedation to decrease pain, and may recommend a pain reliever like ibuprofen (one or two tablets of Advil or Nuprin) an hour or so before your appointment.

Endometrial biopsy may be recommended for evaluation of abnormal bleeding, especially if you are over 35 or have a family history of uterine cancer. Endometrial biopsy is often used to evaluate fertility problems. The pathologist can determine whether your uterine lining shows evidence of normal ovulation and normal progesterone-influenced changes.

Complications with endometrial biopsy are rare. Damage to the uterus or nearby pelvic structures such as the bladder, intestine, or uterine blood vessels is possible if a biopsy instrument punctures (perforates) your uterus. More significant is the risk of pelvic infection after biopsy. Any time instruments traverse the cervical canal, it is possible for bacteria present on your cervix to be carried up inside the uterus. This would be particularly dangerous if you had gonorrhea or chlamydial cervical infection at the time biopsy was performed. **During the first two weeks after endometrial biopsy you should watch for signs of possible infection** such as fever (temperature over 100.4 degrees Fahrenheit by mouth), pain, cramps, or abnormal bleeding or discharge. Contact your clinician immediately if one or more of these symptoms occur. The risk is highest if you have had pelvic infection in the past.

Endometrial biopsy can also cause temporary bacterial contamination in your bloodstream. This is not a significant health risk unless you have a heart valve problem such as rheumatic heart disease or mitral valve prolapse that increases your risk for heart valve infection (bacterial endocarditis). If so, your clinician may advise you to take antibiotics prior to endometrial biopsy, just as you would for dental work or other minor surgery procedures (2). The risk of endocarditis after biopsy is very low, however, so antibiotic treatment may not be necessary unless your heart problem is serious (3).

Uterine Vacuum Scraping. Your clinician may insert a narrow plastic tube through your cervix into the uterine cavity and connect it to a vacuum source to obtain small shreds of uterine lining tissue that can be examined microscopically by a pathologist. The vacuum scraping procedure is similar to early vacuum abortion. Antibiotic treatment before the procedure may be needed if you have rheumatic heart disease or abnormal heart valves (see discussion in the preceding section).

The purpose of vacuum scraping is to be sure that you do not have abnormal thickening of the uterine lining (endometrial hyperplasia) or uterine cancer. In some cases, uterine vacuum scraping can be a substitute for full dilation and curettage

(D&C, see Chapter 47). Some clinicians recommend vacuum scraping as a routine test for women who choose to take estrogen medication after menopause.

Your clinician will probably use a local anesthetic to block nerves in your cervix and decrease your discomfort during the procedure. You are likely, however, to have some cramping during and a few minutes after vacuum scraping. Most clinicians believe that more accurate diagnostic information is obtained with vacuum scraping than with older techniques that used a salt solution to wash cells from the uterine cavity.

Possible risks and complications for vacuum scraping are similar to those for endometrial biopsy described in the preceding section. If you have fever, pain, or unusual discharge after uterine scraping, be sure to call your clinician promptly.

CRYOSURGERY, CAUTERY, AND LASER

Cryosurgery (freezing, cold cautery) and cautery (burning, heat cautery) are commonly used to **destroy abnormal tissue such as warts on the vulva, cervix, or vaginal walls.** Laser treatment, now available in many communities, is another option for eradicating abnormal tissue. When an abnormal area of surface tissue is destroyed, the nearby normal cells have an opportunity to grow into the area and replace destroyed abnormal tissue with new, normal cells. Laser and cryosurgery are both commonly used to treat precancerous abnormalities of the cervix that have been confirmed by Pap smear, colposcopy, and biopsy. Cautery can also be used for this purpose but is less likely to be recommended if cryosurgery or laser equipment is available.

Heat cautery is the oldest of these three approaches. Cautery equipment is simple and inexpensive; electricity produces a controlled current at the tip of the cautery probe. The probe is touched to an abnormal area, and heat destroys abnormal cells. The heat current penetrates only a few cell layers, so only surface cells are killed. Cautery causes mild to moderate pain, depending on what part of the body is treated and the size of the area involved.

Cryosurgery is a newer technique and has several advantages over cautery. **It is less likely to be painful and produces a more uniform area and depth of tissue destruction.** Freezing can eradicate a more extensive surface area without as much risk of damage to underlying tissue; it causes less scarring and is less likely to cause narrowing of the cervical canal (stenosis) than cautery.

Cryosurgery equipment is fairly sophisticated and expensive. The cold source is compressed nitrous oxide or carbon dioxide gas from a tank. The tank is connected to a pressure regulator and a hand-held instrument that looks like a gun. Compressed gas is released into the gun and expands rapidly to produce intense cold, about –60 degrees Centigrade. Cold is conducted from the gun's metal tip to any tissue that it touches.

When cryosurgery is used to treat cervical problems, your clinician first selects a metal tip that fits the contour of the area to be frozen. With the speculum in place as in a routine pelvic examination, she/he touches the metal tip to your cervix and turns

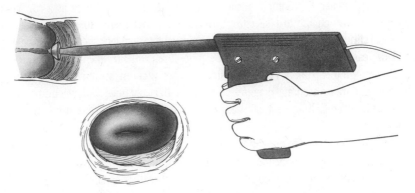

ILLUSTRATION 4-6   Only the tip of the cryosurgery instrument is cold. Your clinician can use freezing to eradicate a small area of abnormal surface tissue.

on the gas (see Illustration 4-6). Thorough freezing usually requires about two minutes. You may experience a vague sensation of coldness in your vagina and mild menstrual-like cramps, but discomfort usually subsides rapidly after the freezing is completed.

Laser, which stands for "light amplification by stimulated emission of radiation," is the high-tech newcomer in this office treatment field. **Laser treatment uses an intense, focused beam of light to evaporate one, tiny, precise area of surface tissue at a time.** For procedures described here, a CO_2 (carbon dioxide) laser would probably be used. Laser equipment is quite expensive and special training is required for its use, so laser treatment is not as widely available as cryosurgery. Some physicians have laser equipment for office use, and treatment can often be undertaken without general anesthesia; alternatively, laser treatment may require a trip to a hospital or surgery center if equipment is not available elsewhere or general anesthesia is needed. Laser equipment can also be used in conjunction with major surgery procedures for fertility problems, and techniques combining laser with laparoscopy and hysteroscopy (see Chapters 46 and 48) have been developed.

For laser treatment of cervical abnormalities you will be positioned as for a routine pelvic exam, with a special nonreflecting speculum in place. Your physician will focus and position the laser beam, and then use short pulses of laser to evaporate one area of surface cells at a time. The laser equipment does not touch you, only the light beam, but you may have a sensation of warmth and crampy pain during treatment not unlike the response of a cervix to cautery or freezing. Laser can also be used to treat abnormalities on the skin of the vulva. For this your physician is likely to use a local anesthetic, or a general anesthetic if the area involved is large, so your treatment should be painless.

Overall success rates in treating precancerous cervical abnormalities are similar for laser and cryosurgery. Laser has advantages, however, in certain situations: if the abnormal area is very extensive, laser treatment helps insure that every bit of abnormal tissue is removed. Also, with laser it may be possible to eradicate abnormal tissue that extends up inside the canal of the cervix. Cervical canal treatment is more difficult to accomplish with freezing. Laser is also preferable in treating precancerous vulvar skin problems when surgery may be the only other option.

Cryosurgery or heat cautery can cause swelling in the cervix that might temporarily narrow or obstruct your cervical canal, so these procedures are usually performed immediately after a normal menstrual period. Swelling should be resolved by the time your next period is due.

After cervical treatment with any of these procedures, you will have a profuse, watery vaginal discharge lasting as long as a week or two. You may also have spotting or bleeding, especially if your cervix is touched or bumped. While your cervix is healing, you will also be instructed to abstain from intercourse and to avoid tampons and douching, especially during the initial two weeks or so after treatment. Complete healing will require six to eight weeks. If you do resume intercourse, use condoms until your follow-up Pap smears show that your cervix is healed and your abnormalities are gone.

After treatment to eradicate vulvar problems you can expect some discomfort as the abnormal skin sloughs away leaving some areas temporarily raw and tender until new skin can grow. The amount of discomfort depends on the size of the abnormal area. In some cases, several treatment sessions will be scheduled to avoid having a large area undergoing healing at any one time. Keep the healing area clean and dry to speed healing and reduce the chance that your raw areas will become infected. Be sure you understand any special instructions your physician may have for taking care of yourself during the healing period.

Serious complications after laser, cryosurgery, or heat cautery are rare. Infection may occur and may require antibiotic treatment. Excessive tissue destruction can result in permanent narrowing of the cervical canal, and is more likely after heat cautery than cryosurgery. Accidental damage to deeper cervical tissue could cause serious hemorrhage, especially with hot cautery when tissue destruction is rapid and difficult to gauge accurately. Extensive destruction of cervical mucus glands might result in a significant decrease in cervical mucus production and might even impair fertility.

Being faithful about follow-up after cryosurgery, laser, or cautery is essential. Your treatment is likely to be effective, but you will need further evaluation and treatment if the abnormality is not entirely gone. Precancerous cervical abnormalities, for example, are eradicated in about 90% of cases by one treatment with cryosurgery or laser. In the other 10%, more than one treatment may be needed. The only way to be sure is to have the follow-up exams and tests your clinician recommends. Precancerous abnormalities are obviously serious, and following instructions to the letter could save your life.

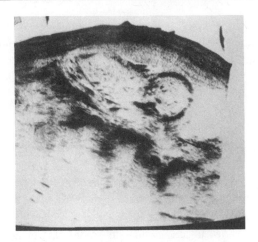

ILLUSTRATION 4-7　The head and back of this five-month fetus are visible on the sonogram. The pregnant woman's navel is the bulge on top, and her ribs are to the left, pelvis to the right.

SONOGRAM (ULTRASOUND, SONOGRAPHY)

I saw my heart beating! It's white on black, and it's fuzzy, and it's disorienting, but just the same it's very precious. An in-motion look at my insides. Wow!

—WOMAN, 28

Sonography is an adaptation of marine sonar technology. **Sound echos provide a picture of soft tissue structures inside your body.** A sonogram (see Illustration 4-7) may be recommended to determine the size of your uterus, pregnancy dates, or the position of a fetus; to confirm the presence of twins; and to help in evaluating many pregnancy problems as well. It can also be used to evaluate ovarian enlargement or a pelvic mass, or to help detect an ectopic pregnancy. Ultrasound is also used in evaluating problems such as gallbladder disease and heart problems. It is a painless procedure.

Some clinicians have ultrasound equipment in the office and others will send you to an x-ray laboratory for your sonogram. **Sonography does not use x-rays,** but it does require special equipment and special training for your clinician or for a technician who conducts the examination. You will be asked to drink several glasses of water before your test, and your bladder will be uncomfortably full. (You will be able to urinate immediately after your test!) Your full bladder provides a landmark for the sonar echos and fills the space between the surface of your lower abdomen and the uterus and ovaries so that loops of intestine stay out of the way. The ultrasound view is clearest when your fluid-filled bladder is the only structure above your pelvic organs.

During the test, you will be positioned on a flat table and your clinician or technician will move a small transmitter-receiver that looks like a microphone back and forth across your abdomen to trace the sonar echos. The surface of your abdomen will be coated with a water-soluble gel to provide good contact between the transmitter-receiver and your skin. You can wipe it off afterward, or wash it off with water. Alternatively, a sausage-shaped transmitter-receiver positioned inside your vagina may be used to provide a clearer view of your ovaries. An ultrasound evaluation may require 30 minutes or more, but you will probably be able to watch some of the echo patterns yourself on the ultrasound screen. Many women find it a fascinating experience.

Most radiologists (physicians specializing in x-ray techniques and ultrasound) believe that the risks associated with sonography are minimal. Sound waves do not have the same potential for altering molecular structure that x-rays do and are almost certainly safer. Ultrasound has been in widespread use for about 20 years and so far there is no reported evidence of harmful effects from diagnostic exposure. Ultrasound equipment emits high-frequency sound waves and records the returning echo to create a picture. The small doppler device used to count fetal heart rate during pregnancy uses a continuous sound emitter. Larger scan machines that create a picture use short pulses of sound lasting 1/1,000 of a second; exposure is lower because the pulse is "off" 99% of the time. Experts are nevertheless cautious, especially about recommendations for use of ultrasound in pregnancy. Animal research and studies of cell cultures have shown possible adverse effects with prolonged exposure at high doses. For this reason ultrasound should not be used for frivolous reasons, or to satisfy curiosity, and is not recommended as routine in every pregnancy. Overall, though, ultrasound has many medically important uses, and can provide essential answers more safely and effectively than any alternative test procedure in many situations.

REFERENCES

1. Hemer HA, de Bourges VV, Ayala JJ, et al: Variations in serum lipids and lipoproteins throughout the menstrual cycle. *Fertility and Sterility* 44:80–84, 1985.
2. Livengood CH III, Land MR, Addison WA: Endometrial biopsy, bacteremia, and endocarditis risk. *Obstetrics and Gynecology* 65:678–681, 1985.
3. Seaworth BJ, Durack DT: Infective endocarditis in obstetric and gynecologic practice. *American Journal of Obstetrics and Gynecology* 154:180–188, 1986.

Breast Self-exam and Mammography

Commitment to your own personal breast surveillance program is an important aspect of preventive medical care if you are a woman over 30. Breast cancer and lung cancer are the leading causes of cancer death for women over 40, and steps to prevent them far, far outweigh all the medical steps you can take, including blood tests, Pap tests, and even routine exams, for saving lives. One in 11 women in the U.S. develops breast cancer. If the disease hasn't touched your life at least indirectly, it will.

There are no proven steps for preventing breast cancer, but your lifestyle choices may affect risk. Women whose diet is high in fat or whose weight is above the normal range have a risk that is higher than average. In general, though, reducing breast cancer death risk means detecting and treating the disease as early as possible. Cure can be confidently expected for 90% of women with breast cancer who are treated early, before there is evidence of any cancer spread, and the treatment required is simpler, easier, and safer than for more extensive disease.

Paying attention to danger signs and avoiding delay are probably the most important steps you can take in reducing your health risks with breast cancer. If you notice a lump or one of the other danger signs shown in Illustration 5-1, don't ignore it and don't wait to see whether it goes away. Don't wait even if your recent routine exam was normal or your mammogram last month was normal. **About one third of cancers are found in between routine exams.** Delay may increase the chance that the cancer will have spread.

5:1   BREAST CANCER DANGER SIGNS

Breast lump
Lump in underarm or above collarbone
Persistent skin rash, flaking, or eruption near the nipple
Dimpling, pulling, or retraction in one area of the breast
Nipple discharge
Sudden change in nipple position (such as inversion)

See your clinician at once if you have any of these signs.

Also, be persistent. If you can feel a lump, or have other danger signs, be sure your evaluation is thorough. Your clinician may be reassuring, but if you continue to feel a lump you should go back again for a second exam, or see another clinician for a second opinion. The same is true for any other persistent danger signs you are noticing. Chances are good that your lump is not cancer, because most lumps aren't. But there is no way to be certain without thorough evaluation.

Breast self-exam, regular exams by your clinician, and periodic mammograms are the best tools now available for breast screening. During your self-exams (and at other times as well) you should be watching for the breast cancer danger signs shown in Illustration 5-1.

The following recommendations of the American Cancer Society are based on careful review of available research information by their national panel of medical experts (1). These recommendations are endorsed by many other professional health organizations, and are likely to be your own clinician's recommendations as well.

- Breast self-exam every month for life beginning at age 20
- Breast exam by your clinician every three years from age 20 to 40, and every year after that
- Initial mammography at age 35 to 40
- Mammography every one to two years from initial screening through age 50, depending on initial findings and personal risk factors
- Mammography every year beginning at age 50

(The authors of this book recommend a breast exam by your clinician each year, beginning at age 20. You'll probably be there anyway, and it adds only a few minutes to your routine exam.)

Weighing benefits against costs and possible risks for breast self-exam is fairly easy. It has no direct adverse health effects, and a benefit in reducing the likelihood of breast cancer death has been documented. Similarly, an exam by your clinician adds little if any cost to a routine checkup, and there are no direct health risks. Even an exam, however, could have indirect health risks if it failed to find a lump that was present, and the false confidence thus inspired led a woman to ignore her breasts in the subsequent weeks or months, or to delay evaluation of a lump or other sign she noticed soon afterward. Even with a careful and thorough breast exam it is possible for a clinician (or for you) to miss a lump that is present. Results are even more likely to be inaccurate if the exam is quick or perfunctory. **A thorough exam requires several minutes and good concentration, whether the examiner is you or your clinician.**

For mammography, coming to a persuasive conclusion about overall benefit and risk has been a more complex and controversial task. Potential, or even theoretical, risks of x-ray exposure and substantial costs must be weighed against benefits. **Experts today, however, make recommendations for mammography that are more forceful and more unanimous than was the case even in 1980 because:**

- Research studies are now completed that report significant health benefit from routine mammography. Women who receive screening are less likely to die of breast cancer.
- Mammography has been steadily improved. Advances in x-ray technology have made films more accurate and results clearer, and at the same time have reduced the dose of x-ray exposure.

Many clinicians and professional health organizations endorse the current American Cancer Society recommendations regarding mammography. Some experts, however, feel that the research documentation available does not support quite such an aggressive x-ray regimen. And it is entirely possible that screening recommendations may change as results of further studies are reported.

Only a small minority of U.S. women are actually undergoing the screening exams and x-rays that are recommended, so **it is quite likely that your own screening will need to be intensified even if you decide on a very conservative regimen** (2). **Decide** is the key word. Mammography should be assessed like any other health issue and it is your decision. Mammography benefits and risks are discussed in detail in a later section of this chapter. **No matter what mammography schedule you decide is right for you, be sure that you also follow through with the breast self-exam and clinician exam part of your screening plan.**

Breast Cancer Risk Factors.   Paying attention to danger signs, and conscientiousness about self-exams, clinician exams, and a personal mammogram schedule are important for all women because **most breast cancers occur in women with no specific risk factors.** These are absolutely essential steps for any woman who does have one or more risk factors. The most important risk factors are:

- Previous breast cancer
- Close family history of breast cancer (especially mother and/or sister)

The following additional risk factors are based on statistical association; their precise importance is not yet clear.

- High dietary fat intake
- Drinking alcohol
- Hyperplasia or atypical hyperplasia (two fairly uncommon forms of fibrocystic breast disease)
- Previous radiation treatment or chemotherapy (some types)
- Previous carcinogen exposure or impaired immune response (after organ transplant, for example)
- DES (diethylstilbestrol) treatment during pregnancy (DES mothers)
- Menstrual periods before age 12 or after age 55
- Menstrual cycles for more than 40 years
- Obesity
- Previous uterine cancer
- First pregnancy after age 30, or no pregnancies
  (You'll notice injury isn't on this list, and neither is caffeine or wearing—or not wearing—a bra.)

It is not yet clear whether use of birth control Pills affects your breast cancer risk. Most large studies have shown no increased breast cancer risk for women who have used Pills, but some researchers have found a somewhat higher risk for Pill users, especially those who have taken Pills for 8 to 12 years or more. This controversy is discussed in detail in Chapter 13. Conscientious attention to monthly breast self-exam and to periodic clinician exams and mammography screening are clearly essential for current and former Pill users, as they are for all women.

You will need to take responsibility yourself for being certain you do have the exams and screening you need. Don't wait for your clinician to remind you, or expect that someone else will make the arrangements. Do it yourself!

Examining Your Breasts

Any clinician will tell you that women find their own breast lumps most of the time. It is rare for a clinician to find a lump that a woman has not first discovered herself. You are the best person to examine your breasts because you know your own breast tissue much better than your clinician does if you examine yourself regularly. And you are the only person you know who will certainly be around once a month when it is time for your breast examination.

Almost all clinicians recommend that women do a breast self-examination (BSE) once each cycle, and for most women that means about once every four weeks.

The best time to do your exam is right after your menstrual period when your estrogen levels are low. A high level of estrogen sometimes causes breast swelling and tenderness that can make it difficult for you to do a careful, accurate exam. If your period begins on Monday, for example, mark your calendar to do your exam the following Monday. If your periods are very irregular or if you do not have periods for some reason (hysterectomy or menopause, for example), pick a date for your exam each month. Use your birthday, the first day of the month, or any day that is easy to remember.

OVERCOMING NATURAL RESISTANCE

Few women enjoy examining their own breasts. After all, you might find something, and that is a completely understandable worry.

I've examined my breasts each and every month for at least 10 years, and I still have to *make* myself do it every time! I always do it *in the morning of a weekday*, so I know I can call my doctor *immediately* if I find anything. I don't think I could do it at night.

—WOMAN, 33

It would be less frightening to find a lump that wasn't there a month ago than to find a lump that wasn't there a year ago. And there is some research evidence to show that faithful self-exams do help. In one study, women who did self-exams at least once a month had substantially lower risks for breast cancer death: 75% were alive after five years compared to 57% of women treated for breast cancer who did not report frequent self-exams (3). Other studies have documented similar self-exam benefits although some studies have not been able to find a benefit. Investigators believe that regular breast self-exams clearly helped women find breast cancer at an earlier, more treatable stage.

Breast cancer is most common in women over 35 but can occur in young women as well. If you begin examining your breasts as a teenager, you will be an absolute expert on your own breast tissue by the time you reach the age when breast cancer is a significant risk. Many clinicians advise young women to begin BSE as soon as they begin having menstrual periods, and for sure by age 20.

Breast lumps are fairly common, and at least eight out of ten lumps are not cancer. See your clinician at once if you find a lump. You may avoid anxious, worrying nights. There is absolutely nothing to be gained by waiting to see if your lump goes away. You need an exam, and you need your clinician's advice immediately. Read Chapter 37 to learn how your clinician will evaluate and treat you should you find a lump.

STEPS IN BREAST SELF-EXAM

A thorough breast exam has three stages: (1) observing your breasts in a mirror; (2) examining your breasts while you are lying down; and (3) examining your breasts while you are sitting or standing.

Observing Your Breasts in a Mirror.   Stand in front of a mirror that has good lighting and let your arms hang relaxed at your sides. Is there any change in the direction your nipples are pointing? Does either nipple seem unusually drawn up into the breast? Do you see any skin areas that are dimpled or reddened? Is there an area of skin with enlarged, coarse pores, skin that looks somewhat like an orange peel? Do you have a persistent rash or skin eruptions in the nipple area? Report any of these changes to your clinician promptly.

Put both hands on your hips and push down. Do your chest muscles contract about the same amount? (They should.) Does any skin area dimple when you press down? (It shouldn't.) **Put your hands in front of your chest at about heart level and press your palms together. Then raise your arms straight above your head.** Check each time for muscle contraction and dimpling.

Squeeze each nipple gently. Is there any discharge at all? It is not uncommon to have some nipple secretions after delivery, miscarriage, or abortion, or if you take birth control Pills. Women whose sexual patterns include a great deal of breast stimulation may develop a nipple discharge. Not all nipple discharges indicate illness, but you should **discuss any nipple discharge with your clinician.**

Breast Exam—Lying Down.   When you lie flat on your back, your breast tissue spreads out over your rib cage and it is easier to feel deep tissue layers with your fingers.

Lie down with a pillow under one shoulder and put your arm on that side behind your head. You will first examine the breast on the same side as your raised arm. (Putting your arm behind your head stretches chest muscles so that you will have a firmer surface to press downward on.) **Feel every part of your breast by pressing your fingertips on a spot and then moving your whole hand in a small circle so that the breast tissue slides back and forth under the skin** (see Illustrations 5-2 and 5-3). You can move your hand around in any pattern you like as long as you examine all parts of your breast. Try thinking of your breast with an imaginary grid or checkerboard marked on it. Begin at the top and check each square in a row till you reach the bottom. Then move to the next imaginary row and check downward again. Repeat the process horizontally, checking each square across. Go all the way to the middle of your chest, all the way up to your collarbone, and all the way under your arm. Be sure to check directly under your nipple.

You may notice that glands are a little more prominent in the outer half of your breast than the inner half (see Illustration 5-4). This is normal. **Examine your armpit carefully for enlarged lymph nodes.** An enlarged node would feel like a rounded, firm bump. If you find an enlarged node in your armpit, talk to your clinician promptly.

If your breasts are large, it may be hard to feel all the way down to your chest wall, especially when you are checking the lower half of your breasts. Use your other hand to shift your breast around so that you can check each part.

Repeat the entire procedure for your other breast. Your behind-the-head arm becomes your examining arm, and vice versa.

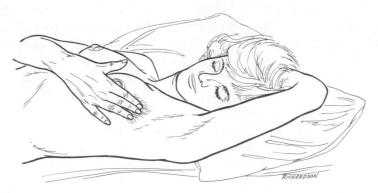

ILLUSTRATION 5-2   Use your fingertips to feel each area of the breast.

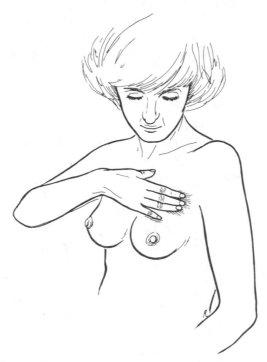

ILLUSTRATION 5-3   Repeat your exam in a standing or sitting position. Also, remember to check for nipple discharge.

Breast Exam—Sitting or Standing.   It is important to repeat exactly the same examination steps while you are sitting or standing, because a sitting or standing position creates a different distribution of breast tissue. During a shower is an excellent time for self-exam. Abnormalities may be more obvious when your skin and hands are

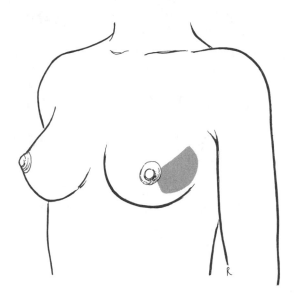

ILLUSTRATION 5-4   Normal glands are likely to be most prominent in the outer half of your breast.

wet and your fingers can glide easily over your breast tissue. Some lumps are easier to find while you are lying down, and other lumps are more apparent when you are sitting or standing.

WHAT YOU CAN LEARN FROM YOUR BREAST EXAM

You can examine your breasts to **watch for danger signs** and to **detect any change** since your exam four weeks ago. Certainly you will feel more confident about your ability to spot a change when you've done 40 exams than when you've done 3.

The first time I examined myself I didn't know *what* I was doing! I felt about 20 places I thought were lumps! I thought everything was supposed to feel smooth, and I sure didn't feel smooth.

So I went to my doctor; she checked me, and said my breasts were normal.

After about ten months I got the hang of it, finally. I learned where I'm smooth and where I'm kind of grainy. Now I think I would spot something different without much trouble.

—WOMAN, 19

If you feel uncertain about your first few exams, forge ahead. You *will* get good at it. If you're worried, you can ask your clinician to examine your breasts first to verify that you really are normal. You may be able to find a class on self-exam, or there may be an education center in your area specifically for breast self-exam. Also, a chance to practice using a breast model may help you hone your skills and give you the confidence you need.

Lumps can be round and smooth, or quite irregular. They can be movable or fixed. There may not be a true lump at all, but rather a place that feels thicker or stringier than usual. **Never assume that thickening in the breast is just muscle development because you're getting new exercise; there are no muscles in the breast. Report any change to your clinician.**

For some women, breast self-exam is easy, but for others it can be quite a challenge. If you have fibrocystic breast characteristics, you may find the dense, nodular consistency of your breast confusing. So will your clinician. One advantage you have, though, is the opportunity to do your exams every month. With practice you will be able to identify changes more accurately than anyone else. So for you, self-exams are especially important. Be sure to read about changes in diet and treatment that may reduce your fibrocystic problems. These are discussed in detail in Chapter 37. Reducing your dietary fat and avoiding foods and beverages that contain caffeine, tea, and chocolate may help, and your breasts may become less difficult to examine.

Mammography

Mammography, x-ray of the breast, may be recommended as a routine test or as part of the evaluation of a lump or breast problem. **Mammography is the only test currently available that can detect many cancers of the breast before a lump is big enough to feel.** Mammography may detect cancer as much as two years before a lump would be evident, and some experts believe that breast cancer deaths for women aged 50 to 64 can be reduced by one third through mammography screening (4).

For your exam, each breast will be compressed firmly against the x-ray plate, and two different views will probably be needed. **The procedure is mildly uncomfortable because of pressing the breast flat against the plate, but takes only a few minutes.** You may be asked to wait until the film has been developed and checked for clarity, and a repeat film may be taken if the initial views are not satisfactory. Usually this occurs because of a technical problem, so there is no reason for alarm.

The radiologist (physician x-ray specialist) will review your films to identify abnormalities or any questionable areas that may require follow-up. A lump or mass is likely to be evident on your mammogram (although some lumps are not), and **the radiologist may be able to detect a lump so small or deep in the breast that it cannot be felt.** A lump the size of a BB, for example, might be missed by you or your clinician, but probably would be quite clear on a mammogram. The radiologist will also look for other x-ray signs of trouble such as tiny calcium deposits called calcifications. Some types of calcifications are associated with cancer, and may be evident even before a lump can be seen on a mammogram.

Like any medical test, mammography is not infallible, and does sometimes miss evidence of disease and provide a false-negative report. Some experts believe that in a program with good x-ray equipment and experienced radiologists, the false-negative rate should not exceed 10% (5). The x-ray report cannot provide a final diagnosis. A mass that is obvious by examination may be invisible on x-ray. Conversely, a scary and suspicious area on the x-ray may prove to be entirely benign when biopsy results are obtained. False-positive and false-negative results are one of mammography's serious disadvantages (see "Mammography: Weighing Benefits and Risks" later in this chapter). On the whole, though, x-ray findings correlate fairly well with biopsy findings.

Your films and the radiologist's report will be sent to your clinician or surgeon for review. She/he will contact you to discuss the results and decide what further steps, if any, are needed.

ABNORMAL MAMMOGRAMS: WHAT NEXT?

If your mammogram is suspicious for cancer, then the need for biopsy may be quite clear. Depending on your mammogram results, your radiologist may recommend an ultrasound examination, which can make the important distinction between fluid-filled and solid lumps. A fluid-filled cyst is almost always benign and may require no further treatment. Occasionally a cyst will require a simple needle puncture and draining of fluid. If your cyst is too small or too deep to be felt by your clinician, the radiologist may be asked to drain the cyst using ultrasound. These procedures are described in Chapter 37.

My mammogram wasn't normal, but it "probably wasn't anything to worry about" either, they said. I could have a biopsy or wait, they said, "whatever I'd feel best about." It took me several conversations with the radiologist and my own internist to feel like I even understood what my mammogram results might mean. It came down to deciding what would give me the most peace of mind. I had a biopsy. Everything was normal. I paid $600 for that peace of mind, and I'd probably do it again.

—WOMAN, 40

The dilemma in decision making occurs when a mammogram is just slightly suspicious, or a questionable area is identified. Mammography is a very sensitive technique, but interpretation is not always clear-cut, and of course, your own personal risk factors and feelings should be considered as well. This is sometimes an agonizingly hard decision for a woman. If a tiny area is somewhat suspicious, then what should be done? Another mammogram after three to six months might be one option. By comparing the two sets of films, the radiologist should be able to detect even minimal change. For a woman with very high breast cancer risk (previous cancer in the other breast, for example) immediate biopsy might be indicated. These are the tough decisions, and seeking a second opinion may be a reasonable precaution if you have trouble making a decision.

Mammography is most accurate for a woman who has medium-sized, soft breasts. Dense breast tissue, most likely to be found during the reproductive years, is dense on x-ray film too, and subtle abnormalities may not be evident. **The mammography designation for this density problem is dysplasia**; it is often the term radiologists use to describe the mammogram of a woman who has thick, rubbery breast tissue typical of fibrocystic breast disease. Fibrocystic breast problems do not mean that mammography is useless, just somewhat less sensitive. Fibrocystic breast problems are discussed in Chapter 37, and in the previous section on breast self-exam.

MAMMOGRAPHY: WEIGHING BENEFITS AND RISKS

Research to assess mammography benefits has compared death rates from breast cancer for women who receive routine screening to rates for women who do not. Also, studies have determined the number of **unsuspected** cancers found by mammography, that is, cancers treated early because of x-ray detection in women who did not have a lump large enough to feel and had no other danger signs of cancer. Another benefit, more difficult to assess in statistics, is the fact that **treatment required for early cancer is less aggressive than treatment for more advanced disease.** Surgery may be less extensive, surgical complications less likely, and treatment with radiation or drugs may be avoided. This benefit is significant in reducing both financial and human costs.

Mammography risks are more difficult to assess in research than benefits. Possible harm from x-ray exposure probably comes to mind first. Research on risks of radiation at high doses does exist, but **experts can only guess (estimate) the possible effects of the very low radiation doses involved in mammography.** Possible radiation risks, however, are almost certainly not the most important mammography risks to consider. Consequences of false-negative and false-positive mammography results and complications of biopsy and of breast surgery that occur because of mammography are more significant.

Research on Mammography Benefits.   One of the early studies of mammography, conducted by the Health Insurance Plan of Greater New York (HIP) two decades ago, found that **breast cancer deaths were reduced by 25% to 30% for women over 50 years of age who participated in an annual screening program** for 10 to 15 years. Results of this study led to the recommendation that screening should be done annually for all women after age 50. Breast cancer death rates for women under age 50 in this study were the same in the screening group and the control group, but about 20% of cancers detected by mammography among women under age 50 were otherwise unsuspected (6).

The HIP study was a carefully designed and reputable study, and its conclusions were based on accepted statistical methods. Critics, however, point out that about one third of the cancers in the screening group were detected not by screening but by the same methods used in the control group. These were the interval cancers, found because a woman noticed one or more of the danger signs or her clinician found the cancer at an exam. So in fairness, the HIP study should be considered a study of mammography screening plus excellent access to routine care compared to excellent care access alone. Mammogram screening alone would not have shown the relative benefit the study found.

Recent studies in Europe have also reported that routine mammography can reduce cancer death rates. Researchers in the Netherlands (7) concluded that annual mammograms reduced cancer deaths by more than 50% for women 35 years and over, and a 31% decline in deaths was reported by Swedish researchers for women undergoing single-view mammograms every two to three years (8). Once-a-year screening reduced the risk of death from breast cancer by 70% for women in a Utrecht study (9).

Despite these encouraging research conclusions, it is important to remember that details of research design and built-in biases can profoundly affect results. It is possible, for example, that women who were willing participants in screening also differed in other, unidentified ways from women who were not screened, and that mammography itself should not be credited with the entire benefit observed.

Instead of comparing cancer death rates the national Breast Cancer Detection Demonstration Project (BCDDP) evaluated cancer extent at the time of diagnosis to assess mammography benefit. Typical rates of lymph node spread for women not participating in screening programs are 50% or more at the time cancer is detected. A lower rate of lymph node spread for participants in a screening program correlates with earlier detection, and provides indirect evidence that screening is beneficial. The BCDDP reported in 1982 that more than 35% of cancers in women less than 50 years of age and 42% of cancers after age 50 were detected by mammography alone, and that less than 20% of women with breast cancer had evidence of spread to nearby lymph nodes at the time of their surgery (6).

On the whole, studies of cancer death rates support the concept that mammography screening is of benefit, and so does the BCDDP study of breast cancer extent. Research data available, however, probably do not allow a precise estimate of how much benefit can be expected nor an exact schedule for optimal mammography screening. It is also clear that mammography alone is not sufficient. Remember that at least one third of all breast cancers are detected in between scheduled screenings, so women and their clinicians must be alert for danger signs. It may be that part of the apparent benefit in screening programs is the fact that participants have good access to knowledgeable clinicians when problems arise in between scheduled screenings.

Radiation Risks.   So far there is no actual research evidence that mammography causes cancer. Radiation and x-ray exposure in general, though, are known to be significant risks for many types of cancer. Studying these risks is difficult because the time between exposure and subsequent appearance of cancer may be 10 years or more. Also, the rate for spontaneous breast cancer is so high that the contribution of a small number of cases caused by x-ray would be almost impossible to confirm.

Experts use statistics on the effects of higher-dose radiation exposure to estimate what the maximal risk might be for mammography and other diagnostic x-ray studies. Radiation dose is measured in rads. Increases in breast cancer risk have been shown for women exposed to 100 rads or more; women in these studies were exposed either through x-ray treatment in the past for tuberculosis or other infection, or through accidental industrial radiation. Radiation at this high dose is more hazardous for women less than 35 years old at the time of exposure, and risk persists throughout life (10). Risk is also cumulative, so a woman who has already been exposed to excessive radiation because of an accident or very extensive medical x-rays may need to minimize further exposure if at all possible.

Modern mammography techniques require approximately one tenth of 1 rad for each breast. Older mammography methods and xeromammography involved somewhat higher exposure, approaching 1 rad for screening.

By plotting risk curves backward toward zero or low-dose exposure, and studying radiation effect curves in animals, researchers estimate that perhaps 1 extra case of breast cancer each year might be expected among every 3 million women exposed to 0.1 rad by mammography at age 40 (10). This risk is similar to the death risk of traveling 10 miles in a car or smoking one eighth of one cigarette.

Cumulative risk, for screening beginning at age 40 and following the American Cancer Society recommendations, might be responsible for as many as 1 to 8 cancers out of the 900 that would be expected for every 10,000 women. Screening meanwhile might allow early detection, and possibly save the lives of 30%—270 of the 900 cancer victims. You have every right to ask your radiologist exactly how many rads of exposure will be required, and even how modern the x-ray equipment itself is, and when it was last inspected and calibrated.

False-Positive and False-Negative Mammogram Results.   False-negative mammogram results occur when cancer is present but is not detected on the x-ray. The mass may have been too small to identify, or an abnormality present on the film may have been incorrectly categorized. There is no way to determine what percentage of mammography results are falsely negative. False-negative results, however, do occur, and are dangerous, particularly if further evaluation and treatment are delayed because of the reassurance of a normal mammogram report. For this reason, biopsy should not be deferred or postponed when a woman has one or more of the breast cancer danger signs even if mammography is normal.

False-positive mammogram results also entail health risks. A mammogram report that is suspicious for cancer means that biopsy will be done. If the biopsy is benign, this is an example of false-positive mammogram results. **False-positive results and higher breast biopsy rates are an inescapable consequence of mammography screening.** When many abnormalities are evident only on mammography, it is obvious that more biopsies will be performed to evaluate them. The rate of false-positive results with mammography, however, is higher than it should be for an ideal screening test. Interpreting mammography films is a tricky and subtle task. Most experts feel that at least 90% of biopsies should be benign; if the percentage is lower, then too few biopsies are being done and some cancers may be missed.

For a woman, biopsy is a significant event. Medical risks of the procedure are low, but worry, discomfort, and time away from normal activities are all involved. Medical costs, too, are significant.

In the worst possible case a false-positive mammography result could be followed by a false-positive or overinterpreted biopsy diagnosis and result in breast surgery that might not have been necessary. It makes sense to be especially cautious about a decision that involves further surgery such as partial mastectomy or mastectomy if the tumor is very small or is classified as in situ or borderline cancer. **Taking time for a second review of your biopsy slides or a second opinion about treatment would be entirely reasonable.**

Deciding About Mammography. **Your decision about a mammography schedule deserves careful thought, and it is your decision to make.** Many health experts and many clinicians, including the authors of this book, believe that the American Cancer Society recommendations are reasonable. It is entirely possible, however, that recommendations may change as new research is reported. It may be that less frequent screening would provide similar benefit, or that some women would benefit from more frequent screening.

Weighing benefits against possible risks is difficult because precise measurement of benefits and of risks is a thorny research task. It may not even be possible. Research design can almost always be criticized and possible biases are inevitable. Whether or not the benefits of mammography screening are as high as initial researchers have concluded remains to be seen. Fortunately, however, serious health risks appear to be few. Nevertheless, it is important to be aware of possible risks, and consider them as you decide on your own schedule.

Whatever schedule you choose, it makes sense to be sure that your mammograms are done with the most modern, high quality equipment available and that they are evaluated by a radiologist with extensive experience in interpreting them. It is appropriate to ask about both of these issues before your x-rays are taken.

Also, it is important to remember that false results are possible. **Mammography is not magic.** A cancer could be missed in your x-ray or could develop in between scheduled exams. If you have a lump or danger sign, you need prompt and thorough evaluation no matter what your last mammogram found. Being sure you have a good medical resource available so you can arrange prompt care when you need it may be just as important as your x-rays in minimizing your personal breast cancer risks.

ALTERNATIVE SCREENING METHODS

An ideal cancer screening test would be simple, sensitive, inexpensive, and free of possible adverse effects. Obviously mammography falls short of these criteria. Considerable research has been directed to developing alternative tests based on heat, or light, and ultrasound.

Thermography, a technique for measuring heat radiated from breast tissue, has been tested quite extensively. Breast abnormalities may be apparent in a heat recording, but the technique has not been successful as a screening test (11). Thermography cannot reliably detect small abnormalities, and gives an unacceptably high rate of false-positive results: an abnormal test report when there is actually no significant disease present. This technique was originally included in the U.S. breast screening study (BCDDP) described previously, but was abandoned in 1977. Improvements in heat sensing techniques may be possible, however, and research is continuing.

Breast **transillumination,** a technique for identifying abnormal patterns of light transmission, and **ultrasound,** the use of sonar wave reflections to detect areas of differing density, are also possibilities for the future. Ultrasound is already useful in determining whether a palpable lump is a fluid-filled cyst or a solid mass. **Magnetic resonance imaging** (called MRI) is another new technique that may be useful in the future. Expensive equipment is required for MRI, but radiation exposure is not involved.

FUTURE ISSUES IN BREAST CANCER

Faithful screening cannot prevent cancer, or cure it. Real success in combating its menace will require better understanding of the disease, and probably changes in our lifestyles as well. Strong evidence links breast cancer risk to affluence and dietary habits, and it is never too soon (or too late) to make healthful changes part of your own breast cancer strategy. Reducing dietary fat and alcohol, and being more conscientious about fresh vegetables that provide a full range of vitamins, may be particularly significant in breast cancer risk, as well as many other aspects of health.

REFERENCES

1. American Cancer Society: Mammography guidelines 1983: Background statement and update of cancer-related checkup guidelines for breast cancer detection in asymptomatic women age 40 to 49. *Ca—A Cancer Journal for Clinicians* 33:255, 1983.

2. Howard J: Using mammography for cancer control: An unrealized potential. *Ca—A Cancer Journal for Clinicians* 37:33–48, 1987.
3. Foster RS, Costanza MC: Breast self-examination practices and breast cancer survival. *Cancer* 53:999–1005, 1984.
4. National Health Service: Screening for breast cancer: A report to the health ministers of England, Wales, Scotland and Northern Ireland. *Lancet* 1:575–576, 1987.
5. Newsome JF, McLelland R: A word of caution concerning mammography. *Journal of the American Medical Association* 255:528, 1986.
6. Baker LH: Breast cancer detection demonstration project: Five-year summary report. *Ca—A Cancer Journal for Clinicians* 32:194–225, 1982.
7. Verbeek ALM, Holland R, Sturmans F, et al: Reduction of breast cancer mortality through mass screening with modern mammography. *Lancet* 1:1222–1224, 1984.
8. Tabar L, Gad A, Holmberg LH, et al: Reduction in mortality from breast cancer after mass screening with mammography. *Lancet* 1:829–832, 1985.
9. Collette HJA, Rombach JJ, Day NE, et al: Evaluation of screening for breast cancer in a non-randomised study (the DOM project) by means of a case-control study. *Lancet* 1:1224–1226, 1984.
10. Feig SA: Radiation risk from mammography: Is it clinically significant? *American Journal of Radiology* 143:469–475, 1984.
11. Moskowitz M: Thermography as a risk indicator of breast cancer: Results of a study and a review of the recent literature. *Journal of Reproductive Medicine* 30:451–459, 1985.

CHAPTER 6

Charting Menstrual Cycles

The cyclic ups and downs in a fertile woman's hormone levels produce subtle but detectable body signs. Body temperature rises and falls, vaginal discharge changes in quality and quantity, abdominal twinges come and go, all in a cyclic pattern. Almost all women notice some sort of predictable ebbing and flowing month after month.

*Many women can relate outward signs to internal hormone events with astonishing precision. Your ability to notice and use cyclic signs can be enhanced by learning **charting skills**. These skills enable you to **detect** many cyclic changes, to **record** changes accurately, and to **interpret** cyclic records correctly. Menstrual cycle charting skills can be used:*

- *To predict a woman's fertile days so she and her partner can avoid intercourse or use birth control on those days to avoid unwanted pregnancy*
- *To predict a woman's fertile days so she and her partner can have intercourse at the appropriate times to maximize the chances of planned conception*
- *To aid in the diagnosis and treatment of a couple's impaired fertility*
- *To aid in the diagnosis and treatment of the premenstrual syndrome*
- *To document cyclic patterns over time so that a woman can predict when her menstrual periods are expected and note changes in her body's patterns promptly*

*Charting menstrual cycles is **work**. In many cases, records are most meaningful when signs are charted **each and every day, month after month**. Women who are*

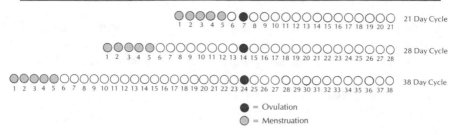

ILLUSTRATION 6-1   When cycle length varies in a fertile, ovulating woman, it is the phase *before* ovulation that changes. The number of cycle days *after* ovulation remains the same—usually about 14 days.

willing to be diligent about charting acquire a degree of body wisdom that can genuinely enhance reproductive health and autonomy. Beyond that, they often come to respect and appreciate their body rhythms in a new way as they learn to listen—to attend—with heightened skill.

Women are fertile, as a general rule, for a week or so during each cycle, and that week usually falls about halfway between two menstrual periods. Although an egg lives only about 24 hours after it leaves the ovarian follicle, sperm can survive two, three, or even more days in the woman's reproductive tract. To allow several days for sperm survival on each side of ovulation, we arbitrarily say women are fertile for about a week. You can indeed have intercourse on Saturday, ovulate on Sunday, and conceive on Monday.

For all of history before the 1930s, it was commonly believed that women were fertile during and immediately after menstruation. (Not such a dumb conclusion, because bleeding is associated with estrus and mating in other mammals.) Finally, in the 1930s, scientists on opposite sides of the world, Ogino in Japan and Knaus in Austria, demonstrated the crucial facts about the timing of human ovulation: **ovulation occurs quite consistently 14 days (plus or minus 2 days) before your next menstrual period begins,** whether your cycles are 21 days long, 28 days long, or 35 days long (see Illustration 6-1). (Read that sentence again, because that simple fact is the keystone of human reproductive physiology.) Their information was used to devise calendar-based formulas for calculating and predicting fertile days for women—the early ''rhythm'' charts.

Another piece of the puzzle fell into place in the 1940s when Ferin in Belgium first recommended that women using calendar rhythm double-check the reliability of their calculations by taking their temperature each day. **Body temperature is related to hormonal fertility cycles and is normally higher after ovulation than during the first half of the cycle.**

The quantity and quality of a woman's normal cervical mucus and vaginal discharge also undergo cyclic changes. Mucus secreted from glands that line the cervical canal changes in response to estrogen. Increasing secretions may be noticeable a few days before ovulation, and on ovulation day, women usually have a wet-feeling, clear, slippery discharge; at other times discharge is either absent or is thick, cloudy, and scant.

Other Signs of Ovulation. Some women have dark red or brownish spotting shortly before, during, or after ovulation as the uterine lining responds to a sudden drop in estrogen.

I always know when I'm ovulating. I'm kind of tender on one side, and it hurts for about half a day. When Jack and I were first married, we had intercourse one night and the next morning I had my ovulation pain. I told him right then I was pregnant, and I was right!

—WOMAN, 30

About one fifth of women can actually feel ovulation, or at least its aftereffects. They notice a distinct pain, low in the abdomen on one side or the other, that lasts for a few minutes or even up to 24 hours. It can be on one side one month and then switch, or appear on the same side for several months in a row. The technical word for it is mittelschmerz, German for midcycle pain, and it is great for identifying, but not predicting, ovulation. Pain can occur just before, during, or after ovulation.

Some women are able to examine a vaginal discharge sample carefully and determine whether ovulation signs are present. Try stretching a discharge sample, either between your thumb and index finger or between two hands as you would a rubber band. Near the time of ovulation you may be able to stretch cervical mucus 3 inches or more before it breaks. Clinicians call this stretching phenomenon spinnbarkeit. It probably enables sperm to swim through the cervix more easily.

Other women note cyclic changes in the position and feel of the cervix when it is examined with a finger in the vagina. The cervix may feel low and close to the vaginal opening for much of the cycle, then seem high and harder to reach during fertile days. The cervical os or opening may feel somewhat more dilated during fertile days, and the whole cervix may seem softer to the touch than usual. Not all women find it useful to check for cervical changes as part of their routine charting efforts.

If you have a microscope around the house (a child's model is fine), try spreading discharge thinly on a glass slide. Let it dry, then look at it under low or medium magnification. If you can spot ferning patterns you have another clear signal that ovulatory cervical mucus is present. A ferning pattern as seen under the microscope is shown in Illustration 6-2.

Charting Aids. Sensitive at-home urine tests are available (no prescription needed) to detect the surge in LH hormone just before ovulation. When the surge is detected, it

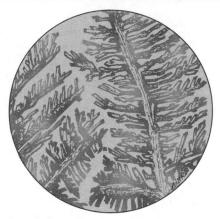

ILLUSTRATION 6-2   Cervical mucus dries in a ferning pattern at the time of ovulation.

is an indication that ovulation will occur within 24 hours. Using the LH kits is somewhat time-consuming, and fairly expensive, but results are accurate if you follow the directions carefully.

Tests based on the changing properties of cervical mucus or even changes in other body secretions are being developed. Ovulatory discharge is thinner—less viscous—than discharge at other times in the cycle and its chemical composition is altered. It may be that in the future you will be able to buy simple instruments that test a discharge sample for its viscosity or chemical properties so that you can know immediately whether or not you are fertile. If these charting aids are as accurate as some developers claim, detecting ovulation will become easier in the future. Because such products have appeared and quickly vanished in the past, talk to your clinician before you make a substantial financial investment.

Basic Charting Instructions

Making sense of your cyclic changes is likely to seem tough in the beginning, but should get easier by the third, fourth, or fifth cycle. Just as women who first begin breast self-examination often feel they don't have a clue about what they're doing, you may feel lost in the early cycles. Be patient with yourself. You will almost certainly get better.

CORNERSTONES OF CHARTING

Charting is wonderfully flexible, and you can usually modify someone else's formal instructions to meet your own needs. Only a few rules are hard and fast, and they are cited in this section. (Even these aren't carved in marble.)

You Probably Need an Instructor. This chapter doesn't tell you all you will need to know about charting skills, and probably a 300-page book wouldn't either. There are too many times you need to take your own charts to an expert and ask, "What on earth does this mean?" Start with your clinician, health department, or local Planned Parenthood as you search for a qualified counselor. Most certified counselors have been trained in using charting skills for contraception, so they may be called natural family planning or fertility awareness counselors. They are likely to know about charting for other purposes as well.

Recording Lots of Signs Usually Reveals a Clearer Picture. Some women chart only periods and body temperature. Others record a dozen or more events every cycle, including intercourse, daily weight, cervical mucus, position and texture of cervix, and as many personal cyclic signs as they are aware of, from headache to sex drive changes to appetite changes. Record what seems to meet your needs.

Charting Is a Daily Undertaking. At least in the first few cycles you will need to make a commitment to record events each and every day. A temperature recording every three or four days simply doesn't tell you enough. Experienced charters are sometimes able to cut back on chart entries later on (starting record keeping on cycle day 5 or so, for example), but others continue careful daily charting for years.

Usually Patterns Emerge, but Sometimes Not. You won't know in the beginning whether daily charting is going to tell you what you want to know, so you will have to be patient. **Remember that no chart can tell you exactly when ovulation occurs**. You can almost certainly learn to be a skilled recorder of **objective** signs such as temperature and weight fluctuations. Learning to be good with the **subjective** signs—quality and quantity of mucus, mood shifts, energy level—is harder. If after six or so months you still feel lost, and interpretation eludes you, back off your charting. Patterns simply aren't there for some women. Certainly reliable patterns won't be there for very young women who don't yet menstruate, women on Pills, breastfeeding women, and women who are nearing or past menopause.

CALENDAR CHARTING

The theory of calendar charting is that a record of your past cycles can be used to predict your future cycles. This skill is most helpful for women who use charting to plan or to avoid pregnancy, because it helps predict fertile days.

Calculate your fertile days each cycle, as soon as your menstrual period starts. Consult your past calendar or charts and find the shortest and longest cycles you have had in the most recent six to eight months. (Your first day of menstrual bleeding or even light spotting is the first day of a cycle. The last day before a period is the last day of a cycle.) Use the fertile days chart in Illustration 6-3 to predict your first and last

HOW TO CALCULATE FERTILE DAYS

If your shortest cycle has been:	Your first fertile day is:	If your longest cycle has been:	Your last fertile day is:
21	3rd Day	21	10th Day
22	4th	22	11th
23	5th	23	12th
24	6th	24	13th
25	7th	25	14th
26	8th	26	15th
27	9th	27	16th
28	10th	28	17th
29	11th	29	18th
30	12th	30	19th
31	13th	31	20th
32	14th	32	21st
33	15th	33	22nd
34	16th	34	23rd
35	17th	35	24th

Day 1 = First day of menstrual bleeding

ILLUSTRATION 6-3

fertile days for the present cycle. Begin counting from the day your present period started, and mark your chart with your predicted fertile days. A sample calculation is shown in Illustration 6-4:

• On July 21 this woman's period started, so she sat down to calculate and predict her fertile period for her present cycle
• She looked back at her previous charts to find the shortest and longest cycles in the most recent eight cycles (bottom left corner of chart)
• Her May 27 to June 20 cycle was shortest: 25 days
• Her June 21 to July 20 cycle was longest: 30 days
• Next she consulted her fertile days chart, the same as Illustration 6-3. She learned that her first fertile day is day 7; her last fertile day is day 19.
• Then, beginning with July 21, the first day of her present cycle, she counted forward to day 7 and marked her first fertile day, July 27
• She counted on to day 19 and marked her last fertile day, August 8
• All the days from July 27 through August 8 will be fertile days

The calendar method gives you your earliest clue for the beginning of fertile days, so keep your records carefully. Temperature and/or mucus changes may give you a clearer, and earlier, idea of the **end** of your fertile days, so you may be able to declare your fertile days over earlier than your calendar prediction recommends. Accumulate six to eight months of good records before you begin relying on your calculations to predict fertile days, and continue faithfully to record your days of bleeding as long as you use the fertile days chart.

TEMPERATURE CHARTING

Your goal with temperature charting is to identify the low-then-high biphasic pattern in your basal body temperature (bbt) that signals an ovulatory cycle. (Basal body

Cycle Day	Date	Daily Weight	Blood (X)	No Discharge (X)	Discharge (X)	Describe discharge when present	Intercourse (X)	Headache	Other Events / Comments
1	7/21	120	X					O	
2	7/22	120	X					O	
3	7/23	120	X					O	
4	7/24	121	X					I	
5	7/25	120		X			X	O	
6	7/26	120		X				O	
7	7/27	121		X			X	O	
8	7/28	120		X				O	
9	7/29	121			X	Thick		O	
10	7/30	120			X	Thick	X	O	
11	7/31	120			X	Clear		O	
12	8/1	120			X	Clear		O	
13	8/2	121			X	Clear, lots		O	
14	8/3	120			X	Clear		O	
15	8/4	120			X	clear		O	
16	8/5	120		X				O	
17	8/6	121		X				O	
18	8/7	121		X				O	
19	8/8	123		X			XX	O	
20	8/9	123		X				O	
21	8/10	125		X				2	Took Advil
22	8/11	125		X				2	Took Advil
23	8/12	124		X				2	
24	8/13	124		X				1	
25	8/14	122		X				2	
26	8/15	122		X		Thick	X	O	
27	8/16	121		X		Thick		O	
28	8/17	120	X					O	
29	8/18								
30	8/19								
31	8/20								
32	8/21								
33	8/22								
34	8/23								
35	8/24								

(Column heading notes: CYCLE DAY — First day of menstrual bleeding is cycle day 1. BASAL BODY TEMPERATURE — Measure in morning first thing before you get out of bed. Circle daily temperature. Connect the daily circles. DAILY WEIGHT — Measure in the morning undressed, before eating. OTHER EVENTS — Use these blocks for frequent entries such as medications, common symptoms. X = present. Additional Comments. The label "Fertile" appears along the left margin spanning cycle days 9–16.)

Calendar Calculations

Shortest cycle in last 8: _____ days. First fertile day in this cycle is cycle day _____.
Longest cycle in last 8: _____ days. Last fertile day in this cycle is cycle day _____.
Cycle length for this cycle _____ days. (Complete at end of cycle.)

Name _____
Month _____
Year _____

© Reproductive Health Resources, 1986

ILLUSTRATION 6-4   A textbook example of a completed chart for a normal menstrual cycle. Most women's patterns are not nearly this clear and easy to interpret. In this case, basal body temperature (bbt) is classically biphasic and mucus patterns are consistent with bbt. The woman has premenstrual headaches and weight gain.

temperature is the lowest temperature reached by a healthy person during waking hours.) A drop in temperature **sometimes** precedes ovulation by about 12 to 24 hours, and a **sustained rise almost always follows for several days**. Body temperature rises under the influence of progesterone, which is produced by the ovary's corpus luteum only **after** ovulation. (See the description in Chapter 2 of the cycle's basic hormonal events, if you'd like to know more about progesterone, the corpus luteum, and other cyclic factors.) Your upward **temperature shift does not give you any advance warning** of approaching ovulation, but it **does give clear after-the-fact evidence** of when ovulation has occurred and fertile days are over.

Take your temperature each morning before you get out of bed after at least three hours' sleep. You can take oral, vaginal, or rectal temperatures, but be consistent and always use the same site. If possible use a special bbt thermometer rather than a standard fever thermometer. A bbt thermometer registers a maximum of 100 degrees so each degree is larger and easier to read. Take a reading after five full minutes and record your temperature on your chart (see Illustration 6-4). Use a line to connect each consecutive day's reading with the last. You can purchase a bbt thermometer in a drugstore without a prescription. Charts are available in family planning clinics, and through agencies such as the one listed in this chapter's "Resources" section, and are often sold along with bbt thermometers in drugstores. Be careful to store your bbt thermometer away from heat.

Not all women have easily identifiable biphasic—low then high—bbt patterns. One study found that 6 out of 30 women had no identifiable bbt pattern in a cycle when hormone tests clearly documented ovulation (1), and even women who can usually identify the biphasic pattern may be thwarted by a cold, an early morning nightmare, flu, jet lag, or a 6 A.M. diaper change. Days go by, and you wait for The Pattern to materialize. Don't guess. If there's no pattern, don't draw any conclusions.

Assume fertile days are over when your bbt is elevated 0.4 to 0.8 degrees Fahrenheit over your readings for the six or so days preceding the rise, and your reading stays elevated for at least three days, and probably several days longer. If you can't identify a sustained rise, you may not have ovulated in that cycle. Generally a true postovulatory bbt rise will persist 10 days or even longer.

CERVICAL MUCUS CHARTING

In order to chart cervical mucus and vaginal discharge effectively, you must become familiar with your own discharge patterns so that you can spot the changes that herald ovulation. Changes in the mucus produced by your cervix are easiest to detect by noting variations in the discharge that appears just at the entrance to your vagina. After menstruation and before ovulation, normal vaginal discharge either is absent, or is white, cloudy, or yellowish in color, scant, thick, and sticky. A few days before ovulation, the volume of discharge increases and it becomes creamy rather than sticky. Close to or at ovulation, discharge becomes clear, abundant, elastic, and quite wet and slippery, much like raw egg white. Ovulation probably occurs about 24 hours after the last day of abundant, slippery discharge. If you are using charting to avoid pregnancy, however, you need to assume that ovulation could occur anytime in the two days before and two days after your wet mucus peak. You can assume that your fertile period is over four days after your last abundant, slippery discharge day.

Keep a record of the quality and quantity of your vaginal discharge each day as you pass through your cyclic phases. Check at the entrance to your vagina with a finger or with bathroom tissue. Note whether any discharge is present, and note its color, consistency, and amount. Note also whether you have a sensation of wetness around the entrance to your vagina. If you notice different types of discharge characteristics on the same day, record the more fertile sign. Those who interpret mucus signs very strictly say that if you note any mucus at all, assume that is a fertile day for you.

Ovulation can occur during your menstrual period, especially if you have long menstrual periods and short cycles. Menstrual blood would mask the discharge changes you look for to predict ovulation. You may have a few relatively discharge-free days following your period, when you notice little or no discharge around your vulva. Women with very short cycles may not have any discharge-free days; preovulatory discharge changes may begin during or immediately after menstruation.

Days between the fourth day after your last discharge day and the beginning of your next menstrual period are likely to be relatively free of discharge. Any discharge would probably be cloudy, thick, sticky, and scant again, a fairly reliable sign that your fertile days are over.

Mucus changes seem to appear in a recognizable pattern even among women whose cycles are otherwise irregular. Charting mucus changes is not without problems, however. Checking for changes in discharge may be unpleasant for some women. Douching makes it practically impossible to notice discharge changes, and sometimes it is difficult to tell semen from a slippery discharge. Abnormal discharges that result from infections can mask normal changes, and medications such as creams and suppositories can throw you off track as well. Lubrication—natural or store-bought—can also mask the nature of the discharge.

Charting Skills for Birth Control

Couples who use charting skills for birth control use the calendar, bbt, mucus changes, and/or other signs to identify fertile days, then either avoid intercourse or use a method of birth control such as a diaphragm, condom, or sponge on days when pregnancy is possible. When charting is used for birth control it may be called fertility awareness, rhythm, natural family planning, or any number of other names.

EFFECTIVENESS

Charting is only moderately effective for preventing pregnancy when couples have unprotected intercourse both before and after ovulation; it can be extremely effective when unprotected intercourse is limited to postovulatory days only. In nine separate studies, failure rates of 3% to 30% have been documented for users of calendar, mucus, and bbt methods, alone or in various combinations. A failure rate of less than 1% was found in a West German bbt study when couples had unprotected intercourse only after bbt patterns showed that ovulation had passed. According to a 1982 summary report of the International Fertility Research Program, "Overall results have neither been good enough to convince those who doubt the usefulness of the method, nor poor enough to dim the enthusiasm of those who promote it." Experts at the World Health Organization suspect that sexual risk taking during fertile days accounts for more accidental pregnancy than does inability to interpret chart records accurately (2).

INSTRUCTIONS

Use every possible sign you can to find your fertile days. At a minimum you'll want to use your calendar, bbt, and mucus changes.

Use the fertile days chart (Illustration 6-3) to set your first fertile day each cycle. Remember that calendar calculations usually give you earlier fertile days warning than other methods. If you have had any cycles in the last six to eight months that were shorter than 25 days, you may want to be extra careful and assume all your preovulatory days are fertile.

Meanwhile, keep an eye on your discharge changes and check your bbt. Use these two calculations together (last discharge day just before, and elevated temperature just after) to bracket ovulation. Wait four full days to make sure that your temperature remains elevated and that you have identified your last discharge day accurately. If you think your bbt and discharge signals are definite and clear, it is safe to ignore your chart-calculated "last fertile day" and assume that your fertile days are over beginning three full days after ovulation as documented by bbt, or four days after as documented by last discharge day. If you don't have clear bbt and discharge signs, however, assume that you are fertile until after your last calendar and chart-calculated fertile day, and continue to check for increasing or wet discharge. If they occur, you must assume you are having a delayed ovulation, and are fertile.

If illness, travel, or life's general chaos obscures your patterns, don't guess. Abstain from intercourse or use another method of birth control. Remember that most accidental pregnancies occur in the first half of the cycle, when couples have unprotected intercourse two, three, or four days before ovulation. Your charting will be much more effective if you limit unprotected intercourse to after-ovulation days only. And if your recorded signs do not all agree, don't guess. Your temperature and mucus should make sense with the calendar, and with each other. If they don't, it is not reasonable to assume that you are safe. The grand combination of signs you are monitoring is shown in Illustration 6-5.

PROBLEMS AND RISKS

Sexual spontaneity can be pretty significantly restricted, and frustration is no doubt a common problem. Some 31% of couples in one British study found abstinence "frequently difficult" (3). Some people dislike a feast-or-famine sex life (others like it

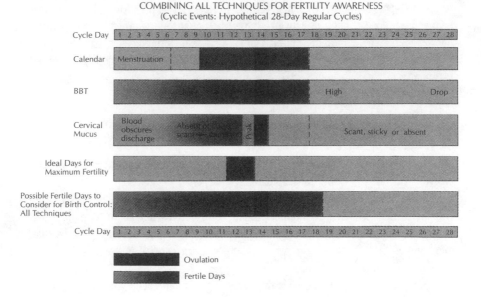

ILLUSTRATION 6-5   Use all three techniques—calendar, basal body temperature, and discharge changes—for the best results. (Reproductive Health Resources, Inc. Used with permission.)

fine). It helps to remember that abstaining from intercourse does not necessarily mean abstaining from sex. Oral sex, mutual masturbation, and other forms of sexual pleasuring need not be avoided on fertile days. Even intercourse needn't be avoided on fertile days if you use condoms, foam, a sponge, or a diaphragm at these times.

Charting is not a birth control method that you can use halfway; **it does you no good to "sort of" keep a bbt or mucus chart.**

If pregnancy does occur, the risk may be somewhat greater than average that an old egg will be fertilized because the couple has either avoided intercourse or used another method of birth control until they believed that fertile days were over. It has been well documented in animal studies that the fetal abnormality rate is higher than average when pregnancies result from old eggs (3). Research involving humans, however, is too limited to determine whether the same might apply to accidental pregnancy conceived late in the cycle.

A U.S. researcher reviewed all the published evidence on this issue in 1984, and reported that this problem "is not likely to be a major hazard" with charting for birth control, and that more data analysis is needed to finally determine an answer. His review found that the risk of miscarriage, stillbirth, and birth defects may be two to four times greater with conception outside the expected fertile days, but that "the evidence is by no means conclusive" (4).

Old eggs may be the biggest concern. Other factors may be old sperm, the pregnant woman's age, and any history of miscarriages and abnormalities. Some couples faced with an accidental postovulatory pregnancy might choose abortion, but for many couples who use charting, abortion is not a comfortable option.

In the teen years and premenopausal years especially, cycles can be very irregular. Women who have markedly irregular cycles sometimes find it hard to use charting for birth control. Cycles that fluctuate widely may mean you have only a very few "safe" days a month, and there goes romance.

CONTRAINDICATIONS

A contraindication is a medical condition that renders inadvisable or unsafe a course of treatment that might otherwise be recommended. There are no true contraindications to charting for birth control. There are some problems and risks, which are discussed in the preceding section.

ADVANTAGES

Charting is completely safe and very inexpensive; you need buy only a thermometer and charts for recording your temperature. It is acceptable to the Catholic Church and some other religious groups that oppose other contraceptive methods. It gives you an opportunity to tune in on and understand your cyclic patterns, and it may open up new areas of sexual pleasuring for you and your partner.

Charting Skills for Pregnancy Planning

I used to scoff at sex-by-timetable babies, but both our kids were conceived in the very first month we tried. And we went right by the charts.

—WOMAN, 29

Several months of detailed cycle charts will help enormously when you are ready to time intercourse to maximize chances for conception, and good bbt records will give you a good early clue to when pregnancy is underway.

Charts that show a clear low/high biphasic bbt pattern and mucus changes consistent with the temperature patterns also give you very good evidence that you **are** ovulating and **when** you are ovulating, so you can make reasonable predictions about

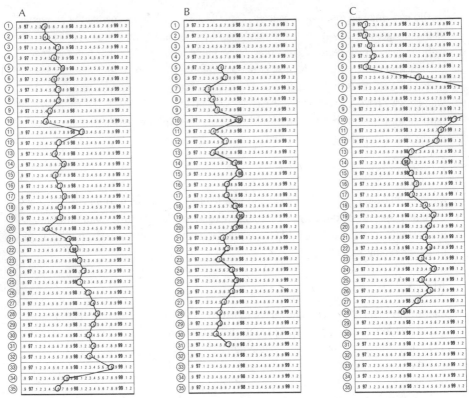

ILLUSTRATION 6-6 A: A long, ovulatory cycle. One early and one late spike on days 11 and 33, each caused by sleeping late on weekends. The charter will disregard both temperatures.
B: A cycle with no ovulation. Temperature stays low with no biphasic pattern.
C: A normal ovulatory cycle with a biphasic pattern. Time of ovulation obscured by fever and flu. The charter would need good mucus signs to help pinpoint ovulation time.

when to have intercourse. **Try to have intercourse every day beginning about five days before you expect ovulation and continue until your bbt shows a postovulatory rise.** (For some couples who have problems because of low sperm count, intercourse every other day may be recommended.) One clear sign to tell you when to begin frequent intercourse is the appearance of clear, slippery, abundant fertile mucus, so **if fertile mucus appears earlier than five days before ovulation, forge ahead.** Conception is more likely to occur with intercourse just **before** rather than just after ovulation (5), so focus your efforts on the early side of ovulation. Make sure you have intercourse at least three times during your predicted fertile period. (See Chapter 10 for more advice about optimal conditions for conception. Look especially at the section "How to Increase Your Chances of Pregnancy.")

Keep faithful daily bbt records when you are trying to conceive. A postovulatory temperature rise that is sustained for 18 or more days is an excellent tip-off to early pregnancy.

Charting Skills
for Impaired Fertility

It didn't take Bob and me long to figure out the problem. Three months after I started recording my bbt and periods we realized I wasn't ovulating.

—WOMAN, 32

When couples seek help with getting pregnant, fertility specialists usually try to start with tests that yield a lot of information, and that at the same time are inexpensive and harmless. A series of cycle charts costs nearly nothing, can do no harm, and sometimes yields much of the answer to a fertility problem.

About 20% of the time, fertility impairment is related to infrequent or absent ovulation. Women who do not ovulate usually have irregular periods and even skip periods occasionally, but sometimes anovulatory cycles look a lot like ovulatory ones on a calendar.

Bbt charts give a much clearer indication of ovulation. Most women who ovulate will show a bbt pattern that is consistently low before ovulation and high afterward. Women who don't ovulate tend to have a steady but meandering bbt pattern throughout the cycle. Ovulatory and nonovulatory temperature patterns are demonstrated side by side in Illustration 6-6.

If you have been trying to conceive without success, start immediately to record your bbt and mucus every day. You will have a head start on your diagnosis, and may even uncover a solution for yourself. Fertility impairment is discussed at length in Chapter 10.

Charting Skills
for Premenstrual Syndrome

I was sure I had headaches just before my period each month, but when I actually recorded my periods and my headaches on a chart, there was no particular cyclic headache pattern at all. So much for my PMS theory. Turned out to be an allergy to dust that flared up when I did heavy housecleaning.

—WOMAN, 33

Although there is no hard and fast definition of premenstrual syndrome (PMS), most researchers agree that headache, breast tenderness, depression, or any other problem must be cyclic, and that there must be at least a brief symptom-free interval in each cycle if the problem is to be diagnosed as PMS. Your first task, therefore, is to begin careful charting of any symptoms you believe may have a cyclic pattern. You will need to relate your symptoms to your menstrual periods as a bare minimum, and ideally you will want to relate them to bbt and mucus changes as well so that you can connect symptoms to ovulation patterns.

Illustration 6-4 shows a premenstrual weight gain and headache pattern. If such a pattern were to recur for several cycles, PMS is a very reasonable diagnosis. There are at least 25 commonly reported physical and emotional manifestations of PMS, and many more that are less common. Some women find PMS pretty manageable, while others are utterly incapacitated. You are the best judge of whether your symptom seems to be cyclic, even if it seems unlikely. Careful charting for three to six cycles will give you the answer; it just may be that your occasional inability to keep up with your keys is indeed a cyclic malady!

When you have charted evidence that your symptoms are cyclic, you are ready to search for an appropriate therapeutic solution. These PMS issues are discussed in detail in Chapter 30.

SUGGESTED READING

Aguilar, Nona: *The New No-Pill No-Risk Birth Control.* New York: Rawson Associates, 1986. Current, thorough, and detailed charting instructions, particularly geared to contraception.
Kass-Annese, Barbara, and Danzer, Hal C.: *The Fertility Awareness Workbook.* Redondo Beach, Calif.: Patterns Ltd., 1984.
Nofziger, Margaret: *The Fertility Question.* Summertown, Tenn.: The Book Publishing Co., 1982. Good instructions for charting bbt, mucus changes, and other signs, particularly in the service of understanding impaired fertility.

RESOURCES

Order blank 8 1/2 x 11-inch menstrual cycle charts like the ones used in the illustrations in this chapter from Printed Matter Inc., P.O. Box 15246, Atlanta, Ga. 30333. One year's worth (13 cycles) for $4.00, which includes shipping costs, or a tear-off pad of 50 charts for $6.00, which includes the shipping.

REFERENCES

1. Moghissi KS: Accuracy of basal body temperature for ovulation detection. *Fertility and Sterility* 27:1415–1421, 1976.
2. Hatcher RA, Guest FJ, Stewart FH, et al: *Contraceptive Technology, 1986–1987.* New York: Irvington Publishers, 1986. Refers to all direct citations in preceding paragraph.
3. Ross MA, Piotrow PT: Birth control without contraceptives. *Population Reports,* Ser I, No 1, June 1974. Washington, D.C.: George Washington University Medical Center.
4. Gray RH: Aged gametes, adverse pregnancy outcomes and natural family planning: An epidemiologic review. *Contraception* 30:297–309, 1984.
5. Dixon GW, Schlesselman JJ, Ory H, et al: Ethinyl estradiol and conjugated estrogens as postcoital contraceptives. *Journal of the American Medical Association* 244:1336–1339, 1980.

7

Recommendations for Routine Health Care

Do you need an annual checkup? What routine tests are worth your money? The purpose of this chapter is to summarize current recommendations for routine health care. These include your own personal health promotion tasks as well as specific medical examinations and lab tests that are recommended for normal, healthy women.

*The value of any routine exam or test should be determined by calculating the number of **unsuspected problems** discovered by testing, and comparing the risk and cost of testing to the years of life and medical costs saved by early identification and treatment. Determining whether or not a specific test is of value is not a simple matter; it requires sophisticated statistical information about the actual experiences and outcomes for large numbers of people who are tested. Also, value depends on factors such as your age and the overall incidence of the disease in question. It is not surprising, therefore, that proving overall benefit is a very difficult research task, and very few exams and tests actually have well-documented benefit/risk assessments. Routine screening recommendations also change over time as new information is gathered, disease prevalence shifts, or new screening methods that are more accurate or have lower risks and costs are developed.*

As you read about the leading causes of death for women your age it will be obvious that what you do yourself to safeguard your health is by far the most important part of routine care. Being faithful about routine checkups is of value, but your lifestyle decisions are even more crucial.

Also, remember that these recommendations are meant for the normal, healthy times in your life. If you are at higher risk than normal for a specific problem, then you may need more frequent exams or additional tests. An abnormal Pap test six months ago may mean you are at high risk for several years until the problem is put to rest. Some problems mean that you are at high risk throughout your life: women with a strong family history of heart disease, bone strength loss (osteoporosis), or breast cancer, for example, need more careful surveillance. So do women with a close family history of colon or rectal cancer as well as DES mothers and offspring (women treated with diethylstilbestrol during pregnancy and their exposed sons and daughters; see Chapter 42).

If you are having symptoms, then your care is no longer determined by routine recommendations. Symptoms are your clinician's most important clues in diagnosing significant medical problems, so don't delay your evaluation. Recommendations for routine care are based on the assumption that you will recognize the times when you are not normal and routine. If symptoms occur, it is up to you to seek care promptly and to follow through with whatever evaluation is needed for your problem.

Leading Causes of Death

Looking at the ten leading causes of death for women in your age group may help in setting your health priorities, for these same problems are also leading causes of illness or disability. It makes sense to focus prevention efforts on health problems that are statistically most common, and on problems for which prevention is possible. Most of the top ten meet these criteria.

Table 7-1 shows the leading causes of death for four age groups. Except for coronary heart disease and chronic lung disease, which are important for older women, and murder, pregnancy, and birth defects, which primarily affect younger women, the most important causes of death are similar throughout a woman's life. What changes is their rank order, and the overall likelihood of death.

Also, it is interesting to realize that health risks such as pregnancy or birth control Pill complications are not at the top of the risk lists. These issues receive considerable emphasis in newspapers and magazines, and certainly can impact well-being or cause illness, but their contribution to a woman's risk of death is relatively small. The risk that a healthy young woman who does not smoke might die from birth control Pill complications is much, much less than her risk of dying from problems on the top 10 list.

FIRST PRIORITY ISSUES

Before you turn to the section on specific health measures for your age group, take time to assess the issues that are important for women (and men) of all ages. These are lifestyle choices or health habits that you control yourself.

TABLE 7-1

LEADING CAUSES OF DEATH

(Deaths among 100,000 Women in one year)

FOR WOMEN 15 TO 24		FOR WOMEN 25 TO 44	
Auto accidents	17	Cancer	29
Other accidents	4	Heart disease	11
Murder	6	Auto accidents	10
Cancer	5	Suicide	8
Suicide	4	Other accidents	6
Heart disease	2	Murder	6
Birth defects	1	Stroke	5
Stroke	1	Liver disease (alcohol)	4
Flu/pneumonia	1	Flu/pneumonia	2
Pregnancy/birth	0.5	Diabetes	2
TOTAL[a]	52	TOTAL[a]	102

FOR WOMEN 45 TO 64		FOR WOMEN 65 AND OVER	
Cancer	269	Heart disease	1,945
Heart disease	171	Cancer	782
Stroke	37	Stroke	520
Liver disease (alcohol)	20	Flu/pneumonia	129
Lung disease	18	Arteriosclerosis	98
Diabetes	17	Diabetes	98
Other accidents	10	Lung disease	96
Suicide	9	Other accidents	56
Auto accidents	9	Kidney disease	46
Flu/pneumonia	8	Overwhelming infection	30
TOTAL[a]	654	TOTAL[a]	4,330

[a]For each age group, other uncommon causes of death account for the difference between the top ten causes listed and the total. All other cause categories, however, have fewer deaths than the categories that are listed.

SOURCE: "Deaths and Death Rates for 10 Leading Causes of Death in Specified Age Groups, by Color and Sex: United States, 1982." National Center for Health Statistics, Department of Health and Human Services, Public Health Service.

Safe Driving and Seatbelts.   The importance of auto accidents in death and serious illness is obvious in Table 7-1. Wearing seatbelts and choosing a taxi if you drink alcohol are probably more important safeguards for your health than *all* your well-patient visits to the doctor.

Don't smoke, buckle up, lose weight, don't drink and drive, eat healthy, get exercise. . . . Even kids in grade school know all that! The problem isn't knowing what to do, it's doing what you know! Old bad habits die hard.

—WOMAN, 41

Smoking. Cigarettes have a terrible impact: smoking places you at risk for both cancer and heart disease, and can cause chronic lung disease such as emphysema. Your smoking also endangers the health of your family because of its toxic effects on a fetus during pregnancy and risks caused by secondhand smoke for those who live with you. Even hormone patterns are affected by smoking: women who smoke have lower than average estrogen hormone levels and earlier menopause. They also have more problems with skin wrinkles. But if you are able to stop smoking, your risks will drop quite rapidly. If you are choosing one health task to begin with, this should be it. Make stopping a priority—more than once if necessary. And ask for help. Your clinician can refer you to reputable programs designed to help you stop.

Getting Your Life Straightened Out. Social situations can be dangerous to your health. Murder most often occurs as the result of conflict between family members or people who know each other well, so make it a priority to get help before conflict reaches dangerous intensity. Marital or family counseling may be an option. If physical abuse is a problem in your family, a program or shelter for battered women in your community may be a resource for refuge or for counseling and support as you work to get past this problem. Also, be sure your home does not contain a gun. For every criminal killed with a handgun, 100 noncriminals are killed through murder or suicide.

Minimizing STD Risks. Sex can be dangerous to your health. If you are not celibate or half of a strictly monogamous, permanent relationship, then learning about STD (sexually transmitted disease) risks is essential. The list of STDs is long and includes life-threatening illnesses such as cervical cancer, hepatitis, and AIDS (acquired immunodeficiency syndrome). Being selective and cautious is key, and using condoms could save your life. Condoms drastically reduce your risk for acquiring an STD if you are exposed; using condoms as a routine practice whenever you have intercourse is an entirely reasonable idea.

Depression. Your psychological health profoundly influences your physical health. Problems with depression, especially, deserve a high priority, just as any other significant medical symptom does. Talk to your clinician, and get help. Therapy and sometimes medication are quite likely to be successful. Severe depression is serious; suicide is a very real medical problem for women of all ages. If you are seriously depressed, you won't necessarily cry all the time, and the cause of depression may not be clear. Typical symptoms include sleep pattern disturbances, eating pattern disturbances, fatigue, feeling sad and hopeless, inability to concentrate, and having frequent thoughts of suicide.

Gandhi said that there is more to life than increasing its speed, but many of us find it hard to slow down. Stress-related problems are so prevalent that a whole industry of stress reduction has come into being since the mid 1970s. Researchers now understand which life events are most likely to cause anxiety, physical symptoms of stress, and depression. Leading that list, in roughly descending order, are:

- Death of a spouse
- Divorce
- Marital separation
- Jail term
- Death of a close family member
- Personal illness or injury
- Marriage
- Being fired at work
- Reconciliation with mate
- Retirement
- Change in health of a family member
- Pregnancy
- Sexual difficulty
- Gain of new family member
- Business readjustment
- Change in financial status

When these or other events trigger depression or other signs of stress that are hard for you to manage on your own, your physical health is likely to suffer. Your clinician, therapist, or a stress reduction specialist can help you construct your own personal approach to banishing stress and enhancing peace of mind.

Drinking.   Cirrhosis of the liver caused by excessive alcohol consumption is in the top ten causes of death for women aged 25 to 64. Alcohol also contributes directly to deaths caused by auto and other accidents and to problems with high blood pressure and stroke, as well as cancer risk. Alcohol problems can be overcome. Alcoholics Anonymous groups are a source of support in almost every community, and your clinician can help you find other reputable programs in your area to help you.

Many people who have problems with alcohol also have problems with cigarettes, tranquilizers, and drugs such as cocaine or marijuana. You may feel you are caught in a web, or that you can enjoy yourself only when you alter your consciousness chemically. Think about this pattern and talk it over with a counselor or clinician. The health price is high, and is likely to increase over time. These are hard problems to tackle, but many, many people have tried and succeeded.

Diet and Exercise.   Researchers believe that improvements in diet quality and commitment to exercise have contributed to this country's dramatic decline in heart disease deaths since the mid 1970s. Diet is also a significant factor in many types of cancer and in arteriosclerosis. Blood pressure is influenced by diet and exercise, and high blood pressure contributes to your risks for stroke and heart disease. Being overweight is one serious blood pressure risk factor. Excess salt (sodium), inadequate calcium, and excessive alcohol may also play a role in blood pressure problems.

Most of us weren't taught sound nutrition principles as children, so we must unlearn old patterns as adults and **join the national trend toward a diet lower in fat, moderate in protein, and high in fiber and complex carbohydrates such as whole grains and vegetables.** Finishing all the food on your plate does not help starving children anywhere, even if the food has cost $15 at a restaurant. Avoid foods high in saturated fats or cholesterol; reduce your consumption of red meat and liver; instead, eat fish or vegetarian meals. Minimize your consumption of processed meats such as bologna and hot dogs, fried foods, and charcoal-broiled foods. Remember that one egg yolk contains about 275 mg of cholesterol, enough to take up your whole day's allotment. Variety and plenty of fresh (not processed) foods help insure adequate vitamins and minerals. Reducing cancer risk may be another important benefit of healthy nutrition. Effects of diet and vitamins on cancer are described in Chapter 41.

Exercise is beneficial in three ways. First, **it will make you feel more energetic and optimistic, and you will sleep better.** Second, exercise is crucial in allowing your body to maintain an ideal weight. Your body needs at least 20 to 30 minutes of vigorous exercise every other day to keep your appetite/weight thermostat functioning properly. And third, exercise **helps your heart** build and maintain its own circulatory channels and reserve strength.

Preventing Accidents.   It is normal to have moments of carelessness or less than ideal coordination, but a little foresight can help you avoid accidents. Be aware, for example, of times when your reactions may be slowed by fatigue, medications, or alcohol. Risky activities should be postponed for better moments.

Home safety inspection is especially important for older women. Correct slippery floors, anchor throw rugs that slide, install adequate handrails for stairs, and add grab bars for the tub or shower to help prevent serious injuries due to falls. Also, medical problems or medications that cause dizziness, faintness, or impaired alertness or vision should be discussed with your clinician and corrected or changed if at all possible.

Routine Health Exams, Tests, and Immunizations

If you are an average woman, with no current symptoms and no ongoing, significant disorder (such as diabetes), then it is very unlikely that even the most lengthy and detailed physical examination will detect any unsuspected, serious disease. The same is true for extensive laboratory and x-ray studies. Probably you do not have a serious disorder, and if you do, it is as yet at an undetectable stage. This is the reason that the "executive exam" concept has been discredited: the statistical likelihood that information gained will be helpful to health is too low. Your health is better served by using the money to buy several new low-fat cookbooks, repair the back porch guardrail, join a local swimming club, or take a wonderful stress-reducing vacation.

Even if the financial cost of exams and tests is not an issue for you, your plan for routine care still deserves careful consideration because health risks may be involved as well. Screening procedures can potentially cause harm if the procedure itself has a risk (such as x-ray) or the procedure falsely identifies you as abnormal, when you are actually normal, and further evaluation involves more—and perhaps riskier—tests or procedures. If you and your clinician are surprised by an abnormal result, there is a very good chance that the result is actually not correct for you. Errors can occur, and most screening procedures single out at least some normal people along with the abnormal ones the test is designed to detect. Careful assessment of the precision of the test, and repeat testing to be sure the result is accurate, are entirely appropriate. These steps are absolutely essential before undergoing surgery or any evaluation procedure that involves significant risk.

There are, however, simple screening measures that are of definite health value, and many women are missing their possible benefit. So cynicism about the concept of a complete executive checkup should not necessarily influence your assessment of the value of routine "well-person" care. The value of routine care depends on what is done, and on what you do with the information gained.

Research proof of health benefit, in general, is clearest for simple and low-risk tests like blood pressure measurement. The value of health counseling is harder to measure in statistics, but has the potential for the most important personal health benefits because prevention is its goal.

The physical exam portion of a routine, well-person checkup is quite brief. Probably most important is the time spent to review your own lifestyle factors that impact health. A routine visit is also a good time to discuss any symptoms or changes you may have noticed in the last year, and any events that need to be added to your personal and family health history. The purpose of this review is to identify any new risk factors you have that may require further evaluation or a change in your ongoing surveillance plan. By seeing your clinician on a regular basis you can also stay up-to-date with any new medical research findings that might be applicable specifically to you and any new general recommendations such as diet guidelines that may be clarified in the future.

Another by-product of routine care is the opportunity to get to know your clinician. If urgent care is needed, it will be easier for you to arrange promptly, and you will have the confidence that your clinician knows you as well.

When you are well, try thinking of your clinician as a personal health counselor or coach. Ideally, a routine visit can be a positive, upbeat experience. Your clinician's job is to help you analyze your own overall health priorities and to help you find ways to make whatever lifestyle changes may be needed. Major change is a difficult job—and even fine-tuning can be tough; support from your clinician as well as suggestions for resources or referrals may make a difference.

PERIODIC EXAMS AND TESTS

The following recommendations for specific exams and tests have been drawn from multiple sources (see "Sources" list at the end of this chapter). These guidelines are intended for the healthy times in your life, when you have no medical symptoms, and for average "normal" women. If you have one or more of the risk factors shown in Illustration 7-1, you may need additional exams or tests related to that specific problem, or you may need more frequent surveillance.

In some cases, medical opinions are quite unanimous about appropriate ages and frequency for testing; in other cases, recommendations differ. So do not be surprised, or dismayed, if your clinician's recommendations are not identical to those described here.

Routine Annual Exams.

AGE 20 TO 40: Every one to three years
AGE 40 AND OVER: Every year

An exam every year makes sense for most women. The American Cancer Society recommendations for routine cancer detection require an exam each year for women (and also men) 40 and over, and most women 20 to 40 will need to see their clinician once a year anyway for Pap testing. Your routine checkup should include:

• Health history review
• Risk factor identification
• Lifestyle assessment and counseling
• Measurement of blood pressure, weight, and height
• Breast exam
• Pelvic exam
• Skin exam, check for thyroid gland abnormalities or enlarged lymph nodes, check for cancer in the mouth
• Rectal exam (women 40 and over)

Breast Cancer
- Previous breast cancer
- Close family history of breast cancer (mother, sister)
- Age over 40
- Some types of Fibrocystic Breast Disease (hyperplasia, atypical hyperplasia)
- Previous radiation treatment or chemotherapy
- Exposure to carcinogens, impaired immune response
- DES exposure in pregnancy (DES mothers)
- High dietary fat intake
- Menstrual cycles for more than 40 years
- Impaired fertility, no pregnancy, first pregnancy after age 30
- Uterine cancer
- Alcohol consumption

Colo-rectal Cancer
- History of benign or malignant colo-rectal tumors (including adenomatous polyps)
- Ulcerative colitis
- Diet high in fat, low in fiber, low in calcium
- Family history of colo-rectal cancer or hereditary polyps
- History of genital cancer

Cervical Cancer (risk factors for Vulvar and Vaginal Cancer are similar)
- Previous CIN (cervical intraepithelial neoplasia, also called dysplasia)
- Genital wart virus infection (some strains)
- Previous vulvar or vaginal cancer
- Exposure to a male whose previous partner had cervical cancer or CIN
- Exposure to a male partner who has (or had) penile cancer
- Exposure to more than 1 male partner (increases with increasing number of lifetime partners)
- Smoking cigarettes
- DES exposure during fetal life (DES daughter)
- Birth control Pills used 4 years or more
- Previous herpes, gonorrhea, other sexually transmitted infections
- First intercourse before age 18 to 20
- First pregnancy before age 18 to 20

Lung Cancer
- Smoking
- Asbestos exposure

Heart Disease and Stroke:
- Smoking
- Age over 35, risk increases substantially after menopause
- Diabetes
- High blood pressure
- High cholesterol
- Family history of heart disease or diabetes
- Obesity
- Inadequate physical activity

Ovarian Cancer
- Age over 40
- Family history of ovarian cancer (especially mother, sister)
- Previous cancer of the colon or rectum, or hereditary intestinal polyps
- Ovulation for more than 40 years
- Impaired fertility, no pregnancies, first pregnancy after age 30
- Menopause after age 55
- Talcum powder exposure (vaginal area)
- Previous breast cancer or benign breast disease
- Hypothyroidism
- Obesity
- High blood pressure
- Endometriosis
- Asbestos exposure
- Excessive coffee consumption
- Mumps or rubella in childhood/adolescence
- Close family history of uterine cancer (mother, sister)
- Caucasian, especially Jewish ethnicity

Uterine Cancer
- Obesity
- Age over 40
- Uterine hyperplasia (adenomatous)
- History of abnormal uterine bleeding
- Postmenopausal treatment with estrogen alone
- Impaired fertility, few or no pregnancies
- History of infrequent or absent ovulation
- Polycystic ovary disease
- Uterine polyps
- Previous radiation treatment
- Diabetes
- Breast, ovary, or bowel cancer
- Menopause after age 52
- High blood pressure
- Family history of uterine cancer
- Hypothyroidism
- Previous use of sequential birth control Pills

ILLUSTRATION 7-1

Your routine exam is an important chance for you and your clinician to identify any specific risk factors you may have for cancer, heart disease, or other problems, and to help you assess the healthiness of your lifestyle. For this, your past and current health history and your social history are more important than your physical exam. Don't be surprised if your clinician does not look into your ears and eyes, or check your reflexes. Ear exam is a standard part of a pediatric checkup because ear infections are common during childhood, but for adults this is not the case. Similarly, examination of the eyes is essential when problems occur, or when high blood pressure or diabetes is present; otherwise, it does not contribute significant medical information about a healthy adult. Steps in your routine physical exam, just like recommendations for screening tests, are (or should be) chosen because of their *value in detecting unsuspected problems.*

Pap Tests.

AGE UNDER 20: Every year after beginning sexual intercourse
AGE 20 AND OVER: Every year
Every 3 years, low-risk only

The medical community is not in complete agreement about how often women should have Pap smears. The American Cancer Society, the American College of Obstetricians and Gynecologists, and the National Institute of Child Health and Human Development each have slightly different recommendations for Pap smear intervals.

The current **American Cancer Society (ACS)** recommendation is that a woman have her first Pap smear soon after she begins having intercourse or when she reaches age 20, whichever comes first. She should have the test repeated a year later. If both tests are normal, she can then begin to have Pap smears at three-year intervals. ACS notes that women who begin intercourse at an early age (before 20), who are exposed to multiple sex partners, or who have other risk factors such as prenatal DES (diethylstilbestrol) exposure (DES daughters, see Chapter 42) need Pap smears annually. Women who are "relatively inactive sexually" may prefer the longer interval.

The **American College of Obstetricians and Gynecologists (ACOG)** continues to recommend annual Pap smears for most women because, among other reasons, the test is inexpensive and incorrect results can occur. Pap test results can be normal even in the presence of precancerous cervical disease or cancer as often as 15% to 40% of the time, and early cervical disease is much easier to treat and cure than advanced disease. Annual screening is especially recommended for high-risk women. The ACOG policy states that "extending the screening interval in the low-risk group should be an informed choice arrived at by the patient and her physician." ACOG defines women at low risk for cervical cancer as those who do not begin intercourse before age 18 to 20, are not exposed to multiple sexual partners, and are not DES daughters.

The National Institute of Child Health and Human Development (NICHD) agrees with ACS that Pap smears should begin as soon as a woman is sexually active, should be repeated in one year, and can then be extended to three-year intervals if both tests are normal. Their panel was not able to reach agreement on screening intervals for high-risk women, which NICHD defines as women who begin intercourse before age 18, who have multiple sexual partners, or who are of lower socioeconomic status. DES daughters may need Pap smears before they are sexually active, if intercourse is delayed beyond the teen years. If a woman has two normal tests after age 60, "further screening appears to be unproductive," says NICHD.

For most women these recommendations all mean that Pap smears should be done annually because most women are at high risk using these definitions. Although the term "multiple partners" is not specifically defined, a woman's risk for developing cervical cancer increases significantly with exposure any time during life to any more than one male partner who is himself strictly monogamous. Also, sexual exposure that occurred years in the past for yourself or your partner can confer a continuing risk.

Accurate assessment of sexual exposure is a thorny task. Forthright reporting of current and past sexual relationships is difficult for many women, and it is doubly difficult for a clinician to assess secondhand the possible exposure risk the woman's partner may contribute. Many clinicians feel the wisest course is to recommend annual Pap smears for all women.

Inaccurate Pap smear results is another potential pitfall with longer Pap smear intervals. Ideal conditions for obtaining a smear and Pap smear accuracy problems are discussed in Chapters 4 and 35.

STD Testing.

ALL AGES: Every year if at risk

Testing for sexually transmitted diseases (STDs) including chlamydia, gonorrhea, and syphilis is reasonable for all sexually active women at least once during early adult years; repeat testing is appropriate annually, or more often for any woman exposed to more than one male sexual partner, or whenever symptoms occur. Testing for AIDS (acquired immunodeficiency syndrome) is also appropriate if you are a member of a high-risk group or you have a male sexual partner who is at risk. Risk categories are discussed in Chapter 28. You will probably have to ask for STD testing yourself. Many clinicians do not ask about STD risk because they fear offending the patient.

Anemia Testing.

AGE 15 TO 50: Every five years if at risk

Women who have had anemia (low red blood cell count) in the past, have prolonged or very heavy periods, or have inadequate dietary iron are at risk for anemia. Routine anemia tests such as hemoglobin or hematocrit (blood count) are recommended every five years for women at risk so anemia can be detected and treated.

Blood Lipid Assessment.

AGE 20 TO 50: Every four to five years if at risk
AGE 50 AND OVER: Every four to five years

An initial blood test for hereditary lipid (blood fat) excess is recommended during childhood. Women at risk for cardiovascular disease and/or excessive blood lipid levels because of personal or family history of early heart attack, high blood pressure, stroke, or diabetes should be tested every five years beginning at about age 20. Routine testing every four to five years is recommended for all women beginning at age 50. You should fast (no food) for 14 hours prior to your blood test. The sample will be analyzed for cholesterol and/or triglyceride level, and other simple tests such as fasting blood sugar may be performed at the same time. If your tests results are abnormal and you are considering medication to treat the problem be sure your test is repeated. Laboratory variablility can be a problem, especially in determining cholesterol levels.

Mammography.

AGE 35 TO 40: One initial exam
AGE 40 TO 50: Every one to two years
AGE 50 AND OVER: Every year

Following these American Cancer Society recommendations for routine mammography screening can reduce your risk of dying from breast cancer. Mammography is discussed in detail in Chapter 5.

Bone Density Assessment.

AFTER MENOPAUSE: Every one to two years if at risk

The risk of osteoporosis, bone strength loss that results in fragile bones and dowager's hump, is greatest for nonblack women during the postmenopausal years. After menopause, whether it occurs normally at about age 51 or at an earlier time because of surgery, a woman's natural hormone production is diminished or lost and loss of bone density may be accelerated. Women who do not take hormone replacement medication after menopause are at risk for osteoporosis. Additional risk may be conferred by other factors as well (see Chapter 34).

Bone density assessment using photon absorptiometry is a reasonable screening measure for women who do not use hormone replacement medication after meno-pause. If the initial test result shows low bone density, or repeated evaluations show rapid bone loss, then the advantages and disadvantages of hormone treatment can be reassessed, as well as other measures to counteract loss of bone strength.

Stool Blood Tests.

AGE 50 AND OVER: Every year

Chemical tests to detect traces of blood in your stool are recommended annually beginning at age 50. Occult (inapparent) bleeding can be an early warning sign for colon cancer. Your clinician may check for occult blood after your routine rectal exam, and home kits for self-testing are also available without prescription at your pharmacy.

Sigmoidoscopy.

AGE 50 AND 51, then every three to five years

Sigmoidoscopy allows your clinician or a specialist in gastroenterology to see the lining of your rectum and lower colon through an illuminated, flexible tube. The American Cancer Society recommends sigmoidoscopy beginning at age 50 to detect early colon and rectal cancer and to identify men and women with intestinal polyps who are at high risk for cancer. After two normal exams, one year apart, sigmoidoscopy should subsequently be repeated every three to five years. People at high risk because of ulcerative colitis, intestinal polyps, or a family history of colon cancer may need screening even earlier in life.

Glaucoma Testing.

AGE 40 AND OVER: Every four to five years

Glaucoma causes increased pressure inside the eye and can lead to blindness. Testing is a painless and simple office procedure, but you may need to see an ophthalmologist or optometrist for the test.

Hearing Assessment.

AGE 40 AND OVER: Every one to five years

Hearing loss is common and may be unnoticed especially if it involves primarily one ear. Simple office assessment is an appropriate part of a routine annual exam for women age 40 and over, and audiogram testing should be done every five years or more frequently if office assessment or symptoms suggest hearing loss. An audiogram determines your hearing sensitivity at different sound wave frequencies (pitches). It is a simple and painless procedure, but you will probably need to see a hearing specialist for the test.

Dental Examinations.

AGE 20 AND OVER: Every one to two years

Faithful visits to the dentist are important for health as well as for your teeth. Tooth and gum disease can impact health, and part of your routine dental exam is a careful check for early signs of oral cancer.

OTHER PERSONAL PREVENTIVE HEALTH TASKS

In addition to routine screening tests, there are several preventive health steps that apply to all women, and screening tests that should be considered at least once during your adult years.

Breast Self-exam.   Every woman needs to learn breast self-examination, and should check her own breasts once a month beginning at about age 20 and continuing for the rest of her life. Breast self-exam is described in detail in Chapter 5.

Self-surveillance for Cancer Danger Signs.   Regular self-exams to check the appearance of your moles or warts and to look for lumps in your neck or elsewhere are a wise precaution. The following danger signs, listed by the American Cancer Society, mean that you need prompt evaluation by your clinician.

• Abnormal bleeding or discharge, especially after menopause
• A lump that persists more than a few weeks
• A sore that does not heal within two weeks (on your body or in your mouth)
• A change in bowel or bladder patterns
• Persistent hoarseness or cough
• Indigestion or difficulty swallowing
• Change in a wart or mole

Any wart in the vaginal area demands attention. Genital wart virus is a sexually transmitted infection, so your warts are contagious, and you may be at risk for cervical cancer.

Personal Record keeping.   Keep a written health record for yourself. It can help you remember important personal and family history factors as well as the dates of any significant illnesses or surgery you have had. Ask your clinician for a copy of the hospital surgery report and the pathologist's report if you have surgery or a biopsy, and keep them in your file. Keep a record of your exam dates, blood pressure, weight and height, and any significant exam results, as well as routine lab test results such as blood count, cholesterol, or triglycerides.

Calcium Balance.   Maintaining adequate calcium intake throughout life is an essential step in preventing osteoporosis, bones too fragile to withstand normal stresses. Insufficient calcium intake may also play a role in problems with high blood pressure. Prior to menopause, an overall daily intake of 1,000 mg is sufficient for adult women, except during pregnancy and breastfeeding, when 1,500 mg is needed. A total of 1,200 mg is an appropriate goal for teenage women. After menopause, daily calcium intake should be 1,500 mg (women taking postmenopausal hormone replacement need 1,000 mg). Take calcium supplements if your consumption of dairy products is low or borderline. Supplements at this dose are safe unless you have serious kidney disease or rare parathyroid gland problems (see Chapter 34). If you rely on three glasses of milk daily for calcium, be sure it is nonfat (skim) milk; otherwise you will exceed your cholesterol and fat allowance for the day!

TB Testing.   A skin test for tuberculosis is appropriate for most women at least once during the early adult years; testing should be repeated if symptoms occur or TB exposure is above average.

Electrocardiogram (ECG).   An ECG provides your clinician with a permanent record of the electrical patterns your heart produces with each heartbeat. It is not recommended as a routine annual test procedure because your ECG is not likely to predict future abnormalities. A baseline ECG, recorded once between the ages of 40 and 45, however, may be helpful as part of your medical record. If you have heart problems later in life, a new ECG can be compared with your baseline to identify subtle changes.

IMMUNIZATIONS

Rubella.   Every woman should be immunized against rubella (German measles) or tested to document her immunity **before her first pregnancy** is conceived. Immunity is permanent thereafter.

Tetanus–Diphtheria.   Immunization against tetanus and diphtheria is usually begun in childhood with DPT vaccine that also protects against pertussis (whooping cough). Continuing immunity against tetanus and diphtheria requires booster shots every 10 years throughout life.

Measles and Mumps.   Adults born before 1956 are considered immune to measles, since it was an almost universal childhood infection before vaccine became available. The same is true for mumps, although mumps vaccine may be given to adults, especially men, who are considered susceptible.

All adults born in 1957 or later should receive measles vaccine unless they have a definite record of previous vaccination with live-measles vaccine or lab tests show definite immunity. Those vaccinated between 1963 and 1967, when inactivated-measles-virus vaccine was used, should be revaccinated with live-measles-virus vaccine. Vaccine combining measles, mumps, and rubella (MMR) is used if the person is likely to be susceptible to more than one of the three diseases; one vaccination provides lifetime protection.

Influenza (Flu).   Annual immunization against influenza is recommended for younger adults who have a serious illness or chronic disease such as heart, lung, or kidney disease, diabetes, or persistent anemia; it is recommended annually for all adults age 65 and over.

Pneumococcus.   Immunization against the most common form of pneumonia (caused by the **pneumococcus** bacterium) is recommended for younger adults who have serious illness or chronic disease, and for healthy adults age 65 or over. A one-time injection of vaccine is recommended for immunity.

Hepatitis.   Immunization to provide long-term immunity against hepatitis B is recommended for people at high risk of exposure to the disease, including some health care workers, clients, and staff at institutions for the mentally retarded, people planning foreign travel to areas where hepatitis B is prevalent, and sexual partners of those who have hepatitis B. Risk groups and immunization procedures are described in detail in Chapter 28.

Other Vaccines.   Immunization against **polio** is recommended during childhood. Adults who have not been previously immunized should receive vaccine only if exposure to polio is anticipated because of international travel or close contact with polio patients.

Immunization against **meningitis** may be recommended along with antibiotic treatment for those in close contact with a meningitis patient, and for those traveling to areas where the disease is prevalent.

Vaccination against **smallpox** is no longer recommended. The world was declared free of smallpox in 1980 by the World Health Organization and proof of immunity is no longer required for international travel.

Proof of immunization against **yellow fever** and **cholera** may be required for travel to certain countries. Advance planning is necessary: more than one vaccine dose may be needed. You may also want to consider protection against **hepatitis, cholera, rabies,** and **plague** prior to travel if your plans are exotic or if you are at risk of exposure because of work or hobbies. Vaccination against **tuberculosis** is recommended for some health care workers and **anthrax** vaccine is recommended for those who work with imported animal hides, hair, or bristles.

For detailed information on vaccine recommendations, travel requirements, and where to go for vaccinations, you can contact your state, county, or city health department.

ASSESSING YOUR RISK FACTORS

Risk factors for leading killers are shown in Illustration 7-1. For women, just as for men, heart disease is number one. The second-ranked cause of death is cancer, and lung cancer fatalities top the list for women as well as for men. Almost all lung cancer (about 90%) is caused by smoking. Next is breast cancer (Chapter 41 covers breast and reproductive tract cancers in detail). Colon and rectal cancer causes 15% of cancer deaths in women, and uterine cancer and ovarian cancer each cause 5%. Ovarian cancer is less common than uterine cancer, but treatment is less effective. Cancer of the cervix causes less than 1% of women's cancer deaths. Cervical cancer precursors are fairly common, but treatment is highly effective so true cancer is quite rare.

This book covers only breast and reproductive tract disease in detail. See "Suggested Reading" at the end of this chapter for good sources on nongynecologic illnesses.

As you review these lists of risk factors, remember that they are based on statistical association, not necessarily cause and effect. **It's entirely possible for someone with none of the known risk factors to develop heart disease or a cancer. Conversely, having all the risk factors does not mean that the problem is inevitable.** Until the actual causes of a problem are known, science can only use statistics to identify people who may benefit from more frequent or more extensive screening tests.

RESOURCES

This brief list is intended as a starting point. Dozens of organizations, hundreds of books, and probably thousands of pamphlets address the issues in this chapter. Extensive resources are likely to be found in your own community through the public library, local health department, and local chapters of national organizations.

American Cancer Society
The national organization and local affiliates provide educational materials as well as patient services and rehabilitation resources. Find your local chapter in the telephone book or write to the national headquarters: American Cancer Society, 90 Park Avenue, New York, N.Y. 10016.

American Heart Association
The American Heart Association Cookbook (ed 3, New York: Ballantine Books, 1980) includes clear and very helpful chapters on principles of nutrition, and how-to advice for a healthy diet, as well as practical recipes and menu plans. It also lists local Heart Association chapters.

American Institute for Cancer Research
This national research and education organization publishes a newsletter and public information pamphlets including a summary of dietary guidelines recommended by the Committee on Diet, Nutrition, and Cancer of the National Academy of Sciences. For a list of publications, write to American Institute for Cancer Research, Washington, D.C. 20069.

SUGGESTED READING

Brody, Jane: *Jane Brody's Nutrition Book.* New York: W.W. Norton & Co., 1981; and,
Brody, Jane: *Jane Brody's The New York Times Guide to Personal Health.* New York: Times Books, 1982. Two comprehensive and exceedingly clear references. Topics include nutrition and exercise, with well-documented, specific recommendations, and a wide range of common health issues. Resources and suggested reading are included for each topic, and can help you assess problems such as alcohol, depression, or drugs, and find appropriate help.
Cooper, Patricia J (ed): *Better Homes and Gardens' Women's Health and Medical Guide.* Des Moines: Meredith Corporation, 1981.
Ornish, Dean: *Stress, Diet and Your Health.* New York: Holt, Rinehart and Winston, 1983. A comprehensive personal program for preventing and/or treating heart disease. Stress reduction techniques and nutrition recommendations are described in detail.
Tapley, Donald F; Weiss, Robert J; and Morris, Thomas Q., et al (eds): *The Columbia University College of Physicians and Surgeons Complete Home Medical Guide, Consumers Union Edition.* Mt. Vernon, N.Y.: Consumers Union, 1985. An excellent home health encyclopedia.

SOURCES

The American College of Obstetricians and Gynecologists: Periodic cancer screening for women. *ACOG Statement of Policy as Issued by the Executive Board of ACOG,* June, 1980.
American Cancer Society: ACS report on the cancer-related health checkup. *Ca—A Cancer Journal for Clinicians* 30:194–237, 1980.
Brendler SJ, Tolle SW: Fecal occult blood screening and evaluation for a positive test. *Western Journal of Medicine* 146:103–105, 1987.
Bunting GF: Guidelines for the periodic health examination. *Postgraduate Medicine* 79:49–56, 1986.

Canadian Task Force on the Periodic Health Examination: The periodic health examination. *Canadian Medical Association Journal* 121:1193–1254, 1979.

Centers for Disease Control: Adult immunization: Recommendations of the Immunization Practices Advisory Committee. *Morbidity and Mortality Weekly Report, Supplement* Vol 33, No 1S, 1984.

Collen MF, Garfield SR, Richart RH, et al: Cost analyses of alternative health examination modes. *Archives of Internal Medicine* 137:73–79, 1977.

Frame PS, Carlson SJ: A critical review of periodic health screening using specific screening criteria. Part 1: Selected diseases of respiratory, cardiovascular, and central nervous systems. Part 2: Selected endocrine, metabolic, and gastrointestinal diseases. Part 3: Selected diseases of the genitourinary system. Part 4: Selected miscellaneous diseases. *Journal of Family Practice* 2:29–36, 123–129, 189–194, 283–288, 1975.

Grobbee DE, Hofman A: Effect of calcium supplementation on diastolic blood pressure in young people with mild hypertension. *Lancet* 703–706, 1986.

Hamburg DA: Disease prevention: The challenge of the future. *American Journal of Public Health* 69:1026–1033, 1979.

Olsen DM, Kane RL, Proctor PH: A controlled trial of multiphasic screening. *New England Journal of Medicine* 294:925–930, 1976.

Ory HW: Mortality associated with fertility control. *Family Planning Perspectives* 15:57–63, 1983.

Robin ED: *Matters of Life and Death: Risks vs. Benefits of Medical Care.* New York: W.H. Freeman & Co., 1984.

Roemer MI: The value of medical care for health promotion. *American Journal of Public Health* 74:243–248, 1984.

8

❖

Recognizing the Early Signs of Pregnancy

Early diagnosis gives us the chance to have a filling instead of a tooth extraction, or hypertension pills instead of kidney failure. With pregnancy the benefits of early diagnosis are incalculable. When pregnancy is welcome news, good prenatal care can begin immediately, and you can protect the embryo during early pregnancy when it is most vulnerable to countless physical and chemical agents. When pregnancy is not welcome news, you can have an early, safe abortion procedure.

And yet many pregnancies progress utterly unacknowledged until they are a third over, or even more. We are all risk takers, and we exempt ourselves from the law of averages. If 100 average couples have intercourse without birth control for a year, about 80 to 90 will become pregnant. Pregnancies can occur with intercourse during days you thought were "safe," with or without birth control, even when risk taking worked last month and the month before. It is embarrassing to get caught with risky behavior showing, and it is very easy to wait. "Maybe my period will start tomorrow."

Some women wait because they fear being told that they are not pregnant. When a period is late after months of trying to conceive, it is natural to hold tight to hope and excitement. "I'll go in next week."

Waiting doesn't make pregnancy happen, and it doesn't make pregnancy go away. It just gives risks a toehold. Early diagnosis of pregnancy benefits every woman, and each sexually active woman needs to know the early signs of pregnancy and how to get medical confirmation of pregnancy.

An exam and pregnancy test in the early weeks of pregnancy may also save your life. Ectopic pregnancy, which means the embryo has implanted outside the uterine cavity, can lead to severe internal hemorrhage and even death if it is not detected early. Rates for ectopic pregnancy are climbing steadily in the United States, and it now ranks as a leading cause of death during pregnancy. Other pregnancy problems, too, may be prevented or treated more successfully if pregnancy is diagnosed early. You need to learn about possible pregnancy problems and their danger signs discussed in the last section of this chapter.

Almost all pregnancy tests are accurate when your period is about two weeks late. When you wait longer than that to see your clinician, you are stalling, and the stakes are simply too high for that. "Am I pregnant?" Surely this is one of the most important, life-changing questions a woman ever asks. Promise yourself to ask it promptly.

Early Signs of Pregnancy

The more attuned you are to your body and to your cycle, the earlier you are likely to notice pregnancy changes. **Symptoms that often occur during the first 6 to 12 weeks are:**

• Missed period(s)
• Breast and nipple tenderness; breast swelling
• Fatigue
• Queasiness or nausea; sensitivity to smells; vomiting and/or gagging
• Urinary frequency; waking up at night to urinate
• Slightly elevated body temperature; 99 to 100 degrees Fahrenheit by mouth
• Mood swings; possibly increased sex drive
• "Glowing countenance"; happiness gets a boost from extra-active facial oil glands
• Unusual food cravings; clinicians call this "pica" (the Latin word for magpie, a bird that eats anything). Unusual cravings for ice, clay, or cornstarch may be a warning that your body is deficient in iron or other important nutrients. Talk to your clinician about your cravings so that she/he can check you for anemia.

Most women begin to have pregnancy symptoms two to three weeks after conception: the week after a period should have started. **You may develop all the above symptoms, or one, or none of them.** You may feel exactly as you did during a previous pregnancy, or the pattern may be entirely different. These changes are caused by the hormones that your reproductive system is churning out. Within a few days after conception, the tiny placenta begins to produce human chorionic gonadotropin (HCG), the pregnancy hormone. In addition, the ovary that released your newly fertilized egg continues to produce large amounts of progesterone.

An overdue period is usually the first clear-cut sign of pregnancy, but not always. Some women have "false" periods and bleed even though they are pregnant. Sometimes a period arrives but is not quite normal—perhaps light, or late. It is not unheard of for a woman to have two or even three periods in early pregnancy. These periods usually occur at about the time you would expect a normal period.

There are many reasons for missed periods other than pregnancy. Women on strict weight-loss diets occasionally miss periods, as do women who failed to ovulate in the previous cycle. Travel, a significant life change like moving or starting school, emotional upset, or illness can temporarily interrupt your cycle. It is fairly common for a woman using birth control Pills to miss a period. Continue your regular Pill schedule for the next cycle if you are sure you haven't missed any Pills (see Chapter 13). If you may have missed a Pill or two or have other pregnancy symptoms, however, stop your Pills, use another method of birth control, and have a pregnancy test and exam promptly.

In sum, pregnant women don't always miss periods, and missed periods don't always signal pregnancy. The presence or absence of the other pregnancy signs is important, and a pregnancy test and an exam are necessary for a definite diagnosis— yes or no—regarding pregnancy.

By week 12, some of the early signs of pregnancy may subside; others may persist. Additional pregnancy signs after the 12th week of pregnancy are:

• Breasts increase in size; bras don't fit
• Nipples darken
• Chloasma; spotty darkening appears on the forehead, on the cheekbones under the eyes, and on the upper lip
• Lower abdomen protrudes; waistbands are tight; pants are too tight to fasten comfortably at the waist
• Weight gain increases
• Vaginal discharge increases; greater susceptibility to yeast infections (see Chapter 23 for treatment)
• Fetal movement begins about weeks 18 to 20; first noticeable as an intermittent flutter, then graduates to serious kicking

Some of these signs reflect the physical impact of an enlarging uterus and others reflect the continuing high hormone production.

EVERY WOMAN KNOWS

The old saw has it that "every woman knows" when she is pregnant. Some women do, but some women don't. Some simply don't spot the signs, or ignore them, or are misled. For example:

Some women ignore early signs of pregnancy because they believe that they can't become pregnant. Perhaps you didn't become pregnant in the past when you had intercourse without birth control, or perhaps you were misled by something your clinician said.

I had chlamydia two years ago, and the doctor I went to said my tubes were infected. He went on and on about how I wasn't going to be able to have children later on if I wasn't careful. I just figured he meant I was sterile, but I had to have an abortion last summer.

—WOMAN, 20

When our son was born, we were told we couldn't have any more children because of my tilted uterus. We accepted the fact, I got my degree, and taught for a year. Then I found out I was pregnant. Our lifestyle that had been so free changed drastically with the birth of our daughter.

—WOMAN, 38

Some women assume that a tipped uterus means impaired fertility, but it does not. Clinicians' warnings can be taken more literally than they are intended and lead a woman to assume that intercourse without birth control will be safe. **No clinician can determine with certainty that you are fertile, and similarly, it is almost impossible for a clinician to be certain that you are not fertile unless you have had a hysterectomy.**

Women who stop birth control Pills may misinterpret a missed period and other signs of pregnancy as the body's readjustment to being off Pills. The error can be compounded when Pill users wrongly assume that Pill protection extends for some vague period of time after they stop Pills. **Most women resume normal hormone cycle patterns within a few days after taking their last Pill,** and ovulation usually occurs within two or three weeks. (See Chapter 13 for advice on planning pregnancy after Pills.)

Some women fail to recognize pregnancy because they had intercourse only on "safe" days. **It is impossible to be absolutely accurate in calculating your safe days** even if you live in a research lab. Ovulation can occur earlier or later than expected if your cycle is disrupted for some reason. You may not have any hint of the change until pregnancy occurs.

My niece was so sure she was "safe" that she told everybody she had an abdominal tumor! She believed that until the baby started kicking!

—WOMAN, 50

Pregnancy Testing

Sensitive tests can detect pregnancy hormone in your urine or blood as early as 8 days after conception, in other words, 6 days **before** your next period would be due. Tests that can confirm pregnancy at the time your period is due are widely available, and standard urine slide tests can confirm pregnancy 28 days after conception, when your period is two weeks overdue.

So by the time your period is about two weeks late or when you have other early signs of pregnancy, it is definitely time for pregnancy confirmation.

Confirming pregnancy is a two-step procedure that includes both a pregnancy test and a pelvic exam to verify the pregnancy test result and to estimate how far along in pregnancy you are. Neither step alone gives a conclusive answer. Uterine enlargement can be caused by conditions other than pregnancy, and pregnancy test results can be incorrect. Only when the results of your test and your exam confirm each other is your clinician able to give you a definite yes or no diagnosis. During the first 12 weeks of pregnancy an experienced clinician should be able to determine the length of your pregnancy accurately. She/he will judge from the size of your uterus and the dates of your recent menstrual periods.

Accurate, specific determination of pregnancy dates is important, whether you plan to continue your pregnancy or are thinking about abortion. **If your clinician is not able to give you a definite diagnosis in the number of weeks, after a pelvic exam, then she/he will probably recommend an ultrasound evaluation.** Using sonar (sound waves), soft tissue structures inside your abdomen, including your uterus, should be visible. About six weeks after your last normal period, a pregnancy sac should be clearly visible inside the uterus. Sonar measurements of the sac, or later of fetal size, should provide an accurate estimate of pregnancy dates.

DATING FROM LMP

One bit of inside information you need in any discussion of pregnancy has to do with the all-important LMP. **"LMP" means last menstrual period, the date your last normal menstrual period started.** More than likely it will be one of the first things your clinician will ask about. It is medical tradition to date the beginning of pregnancy from the LMP because the LMP is the most recent provable and recordable event in your reproductive life.

EXAMPLE: Your period began January 1. It was normal. You had intercourse once in January, on the 14th. Your period, due around the first of February, was late. You had a positive pregnancy test on Valentine's Day.

Your clinician will tell you on Valentine's Day that you have a pregnancy of six weeks' size. In medical language, your pregnancy "began" January 1.

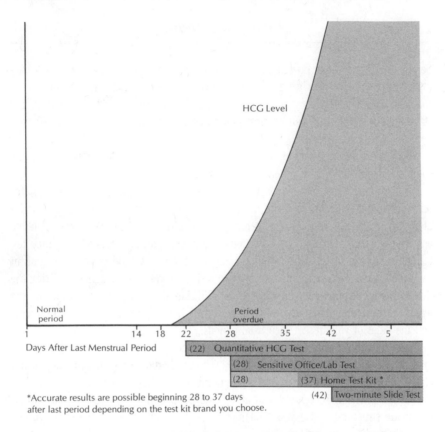

HCG Level

Normal
period

Period
overdue

1   14   18   22   28   35   42   5

Days After Last Menstrual Period   (22)   Quantitative HCG Test

(28)   Sensitive Office/Lab Test

(28)   (37) Home Test Kit *

*Accurate results are possible beginning 28 to 37 days   (42) Two-minute Slide Test
after last period depending on the test kit brand you choose.

ILLUSTRATION 8-1   Blood pregnancy tests are accurate as early as eight days
after conception—before your next period is even due.

You know and your clinician knows that your pregnancy actually began with
intercourse on January 14, but everything and everybody in the medical world
consistently uses the LMP system of dating, so you may as well get used to it. (In your
heart of hearts you can secretly subtract two weeks for the true age of your developing
embryo.)

PREGNANCY TESTING METHODS

Human chorionic gonadotropin (HCG), the pregnancy hormone, is easily detectable in
your blood serum and urine throughout the first five months of pregnancy. All
pregnancy tests use chemical procedures to detect the presence of HCG. Rabbit tests
have not been used in years. Illustration 8-1 shows how HCG levels rise during the first
few weeks of pregnancy, and when the common pregnancy tests will be accurate
(counting from your last menstrual period).

Two-Minute Slide Test. A simple urine slide test can accurately detect pregnancy 42 days after your last normal period started: in other words, when your period is about two weeks late if you normally menstruate once a month. A two-minute urine slide test is the least expensive pregnancy test option; it is designed to show a positive result when your pregnancy hormone level reaches 1,500 to 2,000 units (milli-International-units per milliliter, to be precise). Incorrect results, however, are possible if your urine contains protein or other contaminants (see the section on incorrect results later in this chapter). Simple urine slide tests are very commonly used, and likely to be available at your clinician's office, family planning clinic, or local health department.

Sensitive Office Urine and Blood Tests. Several types of highly sensitive tests are available through medical offices or laboratories. Tests suitable for office use can accurately determine whether or not you are pregnant at about the time your period is due, or two weeks after conception. Sensitive office urine tests are slightly more expensive than the ordinary urine slide test, but are accurate for a pregnancy hormone level as low as 50 units. They take advantage of monoclonal antibodies, a miracle of high-tech manufacturing, to detect minute amounts of HCG very accurately.

In addition to earlier sensitivity, these tests have a second important advantage in accuracy. The monoclonal antibodies are much less likely to react with chemicals other than HCG, so **false-positive results are rare.** The two-minute slide test may show a positive result for a woman who is actually not pregnant, but instead has abnormal protein in her urine, or traces of certain medications. The sensitive monoclonal tests are not nearly as likely to be fooled.

Quantitative HCG Tests. Sophisticated laboratory procedures called radioimmuno-assay (RIA) can be used to determine the exact amount of HCG present in a blood sample. RIA results should be available within one or two days. RIA is substantially more expensive than simpler pregnancy tests, but may be very helpful if your clinician suspects an ectopic pregnancy or impending miscarriage. Steps in evaluating these problems are described later in this chapter.

Home Pregnancy Test Kits. You can buy a do-it-yourself pregnancy test from the drugstore without a prescription. Kits can detect pregnancy somewhat earlier than a two-minute slide test. Some can be used as early as the day your period would be due; others are not accurate until your period is nine days overdue (see Table 8-1). Home tests are fairly expensive but quite simple to use. **Following directions carefully, however, is absolutely essential for accurate results.** In one study, researchers found that 20% of the women using home kits had falsely negative results. In other words, the test result was negative even though they actually were pregnant (1). An even larger percentage of women, 35%, had falsely negative results with tests performed before their menstrual period was at least nine days late.

TABLE 8-1
HOME PREGNANCY TEST KITS

NAME	EARLIEST ACCURATE RESULTS[a]	TIME FOR TEST
Advance Colorstick	Period 3 days overdue	30 minutes
Fact	Period 3 days overdue	45 minutes
Daisy 2	Period 3 days overdue	45 minutes
Acu-Test	Period 9 days overdue	2 hours
Answer	Period 9 days overdue	1 hour
Answer 2	Period 3 days overdue	1 hour
BeSure	Period 9 days overdue	2 hours
First Response	Same day period is due	20 minutes
EPT—New and Improved	Period 3 days overdue	2 hours
EPT Plus	Period 9 days overdue	1–2 hours
Predictor	Period 9 days overdue	1 hour
Q Test	Same day period is due	16 minutes

[a]The "overdue" day recommended for earliest accurate results *assumes* that your last cycle would have been exactly 28 days long. If your true cycle length is more than 28 days, your test results *may not be accurate* this early.

SOURCE: Adapted from Batzer FR: Guidelines for choosing a pregnancy test. *Contemporary OB/Gyn* 26 (special issue:Technology 1986):37-52, 1985.

TABLE 8-2
PREGNANCY TEST OPTIONS

COST	TYPE OF TEST	SPECIMEN NEEDED	TIME	EARLIEST ACCURATE RESULTS (DAYS AFTER LMP)
$ 5–15	Two-minute slide test	urine	2 minutes	42 days
$10–15	Home pregnancy test kit	urine	3–120 minutes	28–37 days
$10–20	Sensitive office/lab test	urine or blood	2–30 minutes	28 days
$15–20	Quantitative lab test	blood	30–120 minutes[a]	22 days

[a]The lab is likely to process only one batch daily, so results may not be available for 24 hours or more.

SOURCE: Adapted from Batzer FR: Guidelines for choosing a pregnancy test. *Contemporary OB/Gyn* 26 (special issue: Technology 1986):37-52, 1985.

If your test result is negative you should plan to have another test about a week later if your period still has not started. You can use another home test kit, or better still, see your clinician for a pregnancy test and exam.

Also remember that all types of urine pregnancy tests are most reliable if you use your first morning urine. Since early morning urine is the most concentrated, the concentration of HCG will be highest, and will be easier to detect than in urine samples taken later in the day.

Home pregnancy tests are very popular and have some big advantages. Delay in confirming pregnancy may be minimized, and you have the convenience and privacy of testing in your own home. On the other hand, you won't have any way to avoid some of the uncommon factors that can cause pregnancy test errors, and there is no such thing as a do-it-yourself pelvic exam to verify your urine test results. You will still need to see your clinician for an exam either way. **If your home test is positive, you need early verification of your pregnancy dates. If it is negative, you will want to find out what has delayed your period.**

ARRANGING A PREGNANCY TEST

Pregnancy test options are summarized in Table 8-2. You can use a home test kit or you can see your regular clinician, go to a family planning clinic, or go to an abortion clinic for a pregnancy test. **Be sure to record the date of your pregnancy test and the specific brand or type used,** and whether your results are positive or negative. This information may be very helpful later if there is any question about your pregnancy dates. If your test is done at a clinician's office or lab, you will need to ask what type of test has been done. Was the test designed for accuracy at 42 days (1,500 to 2,000 pregnancy hormone units) or was it a more sensitive test (50 units) that should be accurate 28 days after your last period?

Pregnancy testing is available without an appointment at some clinics. It is best to call first for instructions, because you may be advised to bring in a specimen of your first morning urine for your test. Put your specimen (half a cup is plenty) in a clean glass jar, cover it, and store it in the refrigerator to prevent growth of bacteria until you leave for the clinic or doctor's office.

Take your menstrual calendar with you. You will be asked about your recent periods, recent sexual activity, and birth control methods. Think through the last two or three months and mark down all the dates you can reconstruct, especially the first day of your last two normal periods.

Have a pelvic exam, if at all possible, when you have your pregnancy test. The exam can confirm that your dates are accurate and help insure that your test result (either positive or negative) is correct. False test results are possible, especially with the two-minute slide test. An exam is especially important if you are having symptoms such as pain, spotting, or bleeding. These could be danger signs of possible pregnancy problems described in the next section.

TABLE 8-3

INCORRECT RESULTS WITH A URINE SLIDE TEST

TEST RESULT IS NEGATIVE BUT THE WOMAN ACTUALLY IS PREGNANT

Test performed too early or too late in pregnancy
Test performed incorrectly
Urine too dilute
Specimen stored too long before testing
Hormone level is low because of ectopic pregnancy or miscarriage

TEST RESULT IS POSITIVE BUT THE WOMAN IS NOT PREGNANT

Blood or protein in the urine (kidney or bladder infection, for example)
Test performed on the day of ovulation (high LH level)
The woman has started menopause (high LH level)
Test performed incorrectly
Test performed too soon after previous pregnancy
Urine contains traces of drugs such as heroin or methadone, or
     medications such as some antidepressants or tranquilizers

SOURCE: Adapted from Saltzman L, Policar MS: *The Complete Guide to Pregnancy Testing and Counseling.* San Francisco: Planned Parenthood Alameda/San Francisco, 1985.

If your test results and exam don't jibe, or the presence or absence of pregnancy symptoms doesn't fit with your test result, then further evaluation is essential.

INCONCLUSIVE OR INCORRECT PREGNANCY TEST RESULTS

Chemical pregnancy tests are not infallible and pelvic examination may be inconclusive, especially very early in pregnancy when the HCG level is too low to be detected and your uterus has not yet become noticeably enlarged. If your urine test is negative and your pelvic exam is inconclusive, then you can either have a more sensitive urine or blood pregnancy test or simply wait another week and repeat the urine test and pelvic exam. If your clinician suspects that results of your urine slide test may be incorrect (see Table 8-3), then a more sensitive (and accurate) urine or blood test should be arranged.

Special Warning. In the past, clinicians sometimes used progestin pills as a test for pregnancy. Progestin pills taken for five consecutive days or a progesterone shot will trigger bleeding if you are not pregnant. If you are pregnant, no bleeding will occur.

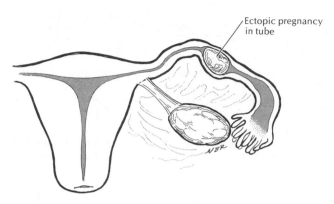

ILLUSTRATION 8-2   This ectopic pregnancy implanted in a fallopian tube.
Pregnancy test results with a two-minute urine slide test may be positive or
negative, but a sensitive office or lab test can detect the pregnancy.

This is no longer an acceptable way to diagnose pregnancy. Instead, a pregnancy test
should be used.

It is best to avoid taking hormones during pregnancy, even though research
evidence on the effects of hormone exposure is contradictory. Early studies concluded
that progestin may cause fetal abnormalities in as many as 1 in 1,000 pregnancies
exposed; more recent studies have not confirmed this finding (see Chapter 13).
Nevertheless, there is no reason to take any risk.

If progestin treatment is recommended to bring on your period, and you think there
is any chance you might already be pregnant, have a sensitive pregnancy test first.
Then you can begin your progestin treatment without worry.

Signs of Trouble in
Early Pregnancy

ECTOPIC PREGNANCY

Ectopic pregnancy is a significant hazard for women in the early months of pregnancy,
and early diagnosis may save your life. **An ectopic pregnancy is one that implants and
begins to grow outside the uterine cavity.** Ectopic implantation occurs in about 1% of
pregnancies. Most occur inside one of the fallopian tubes, as shown in Illustration 8-2.
As tubal pregnancy advances, it stretches the tube and can cause tearing or tubal
rupture. Symptoms of ectopic pregnancy usually begin at about the seventh or eighth
week. Tubal rupture can cause sudden, massive internal bleeding, and is a serious
complication. **Ectopic pregnancy hemorrhage is a leading cause of pregnancy-related
death.**

8:3   EARLY PREGNANCY DANGER SIGNS

Possible Ectopic Pregnancy

Sudden intense pain, or persistent pain, or cramping in the lower
   abdomen, usually localized to one side or the other
Irregular bleeding or spotting with abdominal pain when your
   period is late or after an abnormally light period
Fainting or dizziness that persists more than a few seconds. These
   may be signs of internal bleeding. You will not necessarily have
   any bleeding from your vagina if you have internal bleeding.

Possible Miscarriage

Your last period was late, and bleeding is now heavy, possibly with
   clots or clumps of tissue; cramping is more severe than usual
Your period is prolonged and heavy—5 to 7 days of "heaviest" days
You have abdominal pain and fever

Contact your clinician immediately or go to a hospital emergency
room if you develop any of these signs.

A woman who has an ectopic pregnancy often has a positive pregnancy test, **but not always**. Your clinician may find that your uterus is smaller than it should be according to your menstrual dates, and sometimes it is even possible to feel an enlarged tube. Ectopic pregnancy may also cause intermittent bleeding or spotting during early pregnancy. Many times, however, early ectopic pregnancy occurs with no symptoms, or with symptoms that are very subtle.

Think about ectopic pregnancy any time you suspect you could be pregnant and develop any of the danger signs in Illustration 8-3. Call your clinician or go to an emergency room at once if you develop any of these signs. You could have a real medical emergency on your hands, and will very likely need emergency abdominal surgery. **Be sure your clinician or the emergency room staff is aware that you think you could be pregnant.**

Causes of Ectopic Pregnancy.   In 1970, the rate for ectopic pregnancy was less than 1 in 200 pregnancies; in 1983 the rate was a little more than 1 in 100 (2). Rates are highest for pregnant women age 35 to 44, when about 1 pregnancy in 50 is ectopic. Researchers suspect that increases in ectopic pregnancy are related to **increases in rates for pelvic infection and for sexually transmitted infections.** Other risk factors play a role as well. You and your clinician should be especially alert for possible ectopic pregnancy if you have any of the following risk factors:

• Previous pelvic infection (PID)
• Previous abdominal or pelvic surgery

• Previous repair surgery to correct damaged fallopian tubes
• Previous tubal ligation
• Previous tubal ligation repair surgery
• Pregnancy conceived with an IUD (intrauterine device) in place
• Pregnancy conceived while taking progestin-only Minipills
• Pregnancy conceived despite morning-after hormone treatment
• DES daughter (exposed to diethylstilbestrol during fetal life)
• Previous ectopic pregnancy

Steps in Evaluating Possible Ectopic Pregnancy.   You and your clinician are likely to suspect possible ectopic pregnancy on the basis of your medical history risk factors and symptoms you may be having. **An overdue menstrual period and pain are the two most common symptoms.** Pain may be subtle at first, but is likely to be quite severe if tearing of the fallopian tube causes internal bleeding. Pain may be one-sided or it may be diffuse; shoulder pain can also occur if internal bleeding causes irritation of the abdominal lining at the top of the abdomen. **Abnormal vaginal bleeding or spotting occurs in about 50% to 80% of cases,** and 5% to 10% of women notice abnormal-looking tissue in their vaginal bleeding. Pregnancy symptoms such as breast tenderness and nausea are also present in 10% to 25% of cases (3).

Tenderness in the area of the tube and ovary is likely to be obvious during pelvic exam, but a mass large enough to feel is evident in only half of ectopic pregnancy cases. **Severe bleeding leads to faintness, weakness, and a drop in blood count.** Diagnosis before this stage, however, is highly desirable. In some cases ectopic pregnancy is first suspected when an abortion procedure is performed and no pregnancy tissue is found inside the uterus.

If symptoms are severe or significant internal bleeding is suspected, then immediate hospitalization will be necessary. Otherwise, the tests you need can be arranged outside the hospital. Evaluation will probably begin with a quantitative pregnancy test and an ultrasound assessment. HCG levels are likely to be lower than expected, but definitely positive for the presence of pregnancy. With ultrasound (see Chapter 4 for a description of ultrasound) your clinician will be looking for a normal pregnancy sac safely inside your uterus. The likelihood of simultaneous ectopic and normal pregnancy is very low. In some cases a pregnancy sac inside the tube can be clearly identified. There may be indirect evidence of an ectopic pregnancy such as a mass in the area of a fallopian tube or a blood pool at the bottom of your abdominal cavity (your clinician calls it the cul-de-sac). **Ultrasound is not 100% accurate in diagnosing ectopic pregnancy,** however, so further evaluation may be necessary.

If results of your initial tests are suspicious or your symptoms are persistent, then laparoscopy is likely to be the next step. With laparoscopy (see Chapter 48), your surgeon can inspect your uterus, tubes, and ovaries through a lighted tube inserted just below your navel. Laparoscopy is classified as major surgery and requires general anesthesia, but worth it because ectopic pregnancy should be evident with laparoscopy, and laparoscopy is the most accurate diagnostic procedure available. If ectopic pregnancy is found, your surgeon will remove the laparoscopy instruments and proceed with abdominal surgery (laparotomy, also described in Chapter 48) to remove the pregnancy and repair the tubal damage.

Surgery Options for Ectopic Pregnancy. Immediate surgery is necessary, even life-saving, when ectopic rupture is already causing significant internal hemorrhage. There may not even be time for initial evaluation steps or laparoscopy as described above.

When symptoms are not severe and there is no evidence of blood loss, **a calmer and slower approach may be possible.** In some cases ectopic pregnancy may even stop growing and degenerate on its own with no intervention required. In that case the elevated pregnancy hormone levels will gradually return to zero over the following week or two. Researchers suspect that spontaneous degeneration of an ectopic pregnancy followed by disappearance of pregnancy hormone and physical symptoms occurs quite commonly during the very early weeks of pregnancy.

If your initial pregnancy hormone level is below 250 milli-International-Units per milliliter, you have no symptoms of tubal rupture, and laparoscopy shows a pregnancy in your tube that is less than 2 cm in size with no bleeding or distention of the tube, your surgeon may be willing to **postpone** further surgery for a few days to see whether the pregnancy will degenerate on its own. You will need to have close observation in the hospital while you wait, with daily pregnancy hormone level tests to watch for any further rise in pregnancy hormone production. Using this approach, one researcher found that only 3 out of 14 patients required further surgery, and the average hospital stay for observation in the other 11 cases was 4 days (4). Alternatively, it may be possible for your surgeon to remove the pregnancy during laparoscopy by aspirating it through the laparoscopy instruments (5).

In most cases, though, you will need surgery to remove the pregnancy. If your ectopic pregnancy is more advanced, waiting in hope that the pregnancy will abort would be risky because rupture and severe internal bleeding are more likely to occur with each passing week and catastrophic bleeding can occur very suddenly. **Your life may be in jeopardy in just a few hours.**

When ectopic pregnancy is diagnosed early, **conservative surgery to remove only the pregnancy and spare the tube may be possible.** By making a surgical slit in the tube (salpingostomy) the surgeon may be able to tease the pregnancy free and leave the tube in place to heal. It may even be possible for your surgeon to repair previous fallopian tube damage from infection at the time of the surgery.

If your ectopic pregnancy is large, or the involved tube is severely damaged, it may not be technically feasible to preserve it. In that case, your surgeon will remove the tube along with the pregnancy (salpingectomy).

Every effort should be made to preserve your ovary on that side, even if its fallopian tube must be removed. Without its own tube the ovary does not contribute much to your future likelihood of success with conceiving a pregnancy on your own, and its presence may even decrease your natural fertility since ovulation cycles from that side are less likely to result in conception. But your chances for success using in vitro fertilization may be higher with two ovaries, and future problems might necessitate surgery to remove your other ovary. Whatever damage led to your ectopic pregnancy means your risk for future problems, possibly involving your other tube and ovary, is higher than average.

Prognosis.　　Future pregnancy success after an ectopic pregnancy is very likely. You are at risk for having another ectopic, but if you have at least one tube and ovary remaining, a normal uterine pregnancy and normal birth are good possibilities. Rates for subsequent pregnancy success depend on the severity of previous damage (that may have been responsible for your ectopic) and on the type of ectopic surgery that was necessary in your case.

As many as 80% to 85% of women can expect future pregnancy success if their initial ectopic pregnancy was detected early, before rupture, and treated with salpingostomy so that they didn't lose the tube. Pregnancy rates are lower, 45% to 75%, for women who lost a tube or tube and ovary, and even lower for women who have extensive evidence of previous damage (3).

Ectopic Pregnancy in Other Locations.　　Almost all ectopic pregnancies are located in one of the fallopian tubes. In rare cases, however, a pregnancy might implant at the junction between the tube and uterus (called the cornu), on the cervix, on an ovary, or in the abdominal cavity. Surgery to remove the pregnancy is necessary in these rare cases also.

MISCARRIAGE (SPONTANEOUS ABORTION)

At least 15% of all pregnancies end in miscarriage (spontaneous abortion), and the vast majority occur before the 12th week of pregnancy. Something goes wrong, and your body has the good sense to call everything off before the going gets worse. **You need prompt medical care for a miscarriage.** Call your clinician or go to an emergency room if you develop any of the danger signs shown in Illustration 8-3.

Even if your miscarriage is complete, you need to see your clinician to have your blood Rh type determined. If you are Rh-negative, you will need treatment, within 72 hours if possible, with Rh immune globulin to prevent Rh problems in future pregnancies (see Chapter 18). Common brand names for this drug are RhoGAM, Gamulin Rh, and HypRho-D. Your clinician will also want to be sure that all the fetal and placental tissue has been expelled from your uterus, because infection is much more likely if tissue remains in your uterus.

ABNORMAL PREGNANCY

Your clinician may use terms like "blighted ovum" or "missed abortion" to describe a pregnancy that really isn't a pregnancy. If an embryo starts to grow and then development stops, there may be evidence of pregnancy hormone, thickened uterine lining tissue, and even placenta tissue, but no fetus. This problem may be first suspected when an ultrasound evaluation fails to show the fetus at a time in pregnancy when it should be visible. Abnormally low HCG levels or an HCG level that does not increase as rapidly as it should may be a clue. Bleeding, spotting, or early signs of miscarriage may also occur.

Once you and your clinician are certain the pregnancy is not progressing normally, a vacuum aspiration procedure similar to the technique used for early abortion (see Chapter 18) may be recommended because the presence of dying tissue inside your uterus increases your risk for developing an infection.

Molar pregnancy is another rare type of abnormal pregnancy. With molar pregnancy, growth of placental tissue is excessive, and a normal fetus is almost never present. Grape-like clumps of placenta tissue form, and may even be expelled spontaneously through the vagina. The size of your uterus may increase more rapidly than it should for your pregnancy dates as placenta tissue grows. The excessive placental tissue also produces very high levels of HCG, so a quantitative pregnancy test can help your clinician confirm the diagnosis. Ultrasound will show that your uterus is filled with homogeneous clumps of tissue, with no evidence of a fetus or pregnancy sac.

Vacuum aspiration will be recommended to remove the molar pregnancy, and in most cases no further treatment will be needed. Persisting molar tissue or spread of molar tissue to other organs can occur, and in rare cases a malignant form of this disease, called choriocarcinoma, subsequently develops. This cancer is almost certain to be curable.

Conscientious follow-up after molar pregnancy is obviously essential. You will need to have quantitative pregnancy tests repeated frequently until your HCG level returns to zero, and then periodically thereafter. In about 20% to 30% of cases, HCG fails to return to zero or rises again after an initial drop. In this situation further evaluation and treatment to eradicate the molar tissue is necessary (6).

PREGNANCY WITH AN IUD IN PLACE

If you have an IUD in place and are pregnant, you face a significant risk of both miscarriage and uterine infection (although your pregnancy may continue in a completely normal way, unaffected by the IUD). Infection risk is particularly serious, however, because illness can have a very rapid onset and develop literally overnight into a life-threatening, massive infection. It is infection risk that leads many clinicians to advise that you seriously consider abortion if you become pregnant with an IUD in place. Whatever decision you make, be sure to see your clinician as soon as you suspect pregnancy. If you plan to continue your pregnancy, the IUD should be removed if at all possible. Be sure to read about IUD pregnancy in Chapter 14.

See your clinician at once if you have an IUD and develop possible signs of infection such as abdominal pain, fever, or abnormal bleeding or discharge. And if you suspect that you could be pregnant as well, run, don't walk. You may need to be admitted to a hospital for antibiotic therapy.

Importance of Early Diagnosis

If you plan to continue your pregnancy, early diagnosis gives you an opportunity to avoid the multitude of physical and chemical agents that can harm a developing embryo so you can have an optimal pregnancy (see Chapter 9).

If you are pregnant and don't want to be, legal abortion is both safe and widely available in early pregnancy. If you are not clear in your mind whether abortion is the right choice for you, your local Planned Parenthood agency can probably refer you to pregnancy counselors who can help you evaluate the pros and cons. Remember that abortion is safer and cheaper early in pregnancy; so try to make your decision as quickly as you can. (See Chapters 16 and 18 for a complete discussion of pregnancy decision making and locating reputable abortion services.)

If you are not pregnant and would like to be, talk with your clinician or with the staff at your family planning clinic. They can give you advice and refer you to specialists who treat fertility problems, if necessary. Many of the problems that cause infertility can be resolved, and sometimes counseling alone does the job. (See Chapter 10 for a discussion of common fertility problems.)

If you are not pregnant and you breathe a sigh of relief, reevaluate your birth control status, especially if you have been relying on luck or on one of the less reliable methods of birth control. This may be an ideal time to make some new contraceptive resolutions. Ask yourself whether you might be better off with another method, possibly a more effective one. Chapters 11 through 14 provide a complete description of the most popular methods of birth control. Ask your clinician or ask at your family planning clinic for advice. If you and your partner don't have a method you trust and feel comfortable with, it could be pregnancy testing time again in a couple of months, and no one enjoys the sweaty palms and sleepless nights of a pregnancy scare.

REFERENCES

1. Doshi ML: Accuracy of consumer performed in-home tests for early pregnancy detection. *American Journal of Public Health* 76:512–514, 1986.

2. Atrash HK, Hughes JM, Hogue CJR: Ectopic pregnancy in the United States 1970–1983. *CDC Surveillance Summaries,* August 1986, Vol 35, No 2SS, 1986.

3. Weckstein LN: Current perspective on ectopic pregnancy. *Obstetrical and Gynecological Survey* 40:259–272, 1985.

4. Carp HJA, Oelsner G, Serr DM: Fertility after nonsurgical treatment of ectopic pregnancy. *Journal of Reproductive Medicine* 31:119–122, 1986.

5. Pouly JL, Mahnes H, Mage G, et al: Conservative laparoscopic treatment of 321 ectopic pregnancies. *Fertility and Sterility* 46:1093–1097, 1986.

6. Lurain JR, Brewer JI, Torok EE, et al: Natural history of hydatidiform mole after primary evacuation. *American Journal of Obstetrics and Gynecology* 145:591–595, 1983.

9

❖

Planning for An Optimal Pregnancy

About 6 million pregnancies begin in the United States each year. Some are planned, but more are accidents. These pregnancies variously end in births, miscarriages, or abortions, as shown in Illustration 9-1. This chapter concerns itself with the 3.6 million of those pregnancies that result in births each year, and how human behavior influences their outcome.

*About 95% of the time, full-term pregnancy ends with a healthy, normal baby and a healthy mother. Overall, about 5% of babies are born with one or more congenital abnormalities. Most abnormalities are minor, but 2% of babies have more serious problems. Most pregnancy complications and most newborn abnormalities occur **despite the best efforts** of parents and health care providers. Others, though, can be prevented. Following the recommendations in this chapter can help you maximize your chance for a successful pregnancy and a healthy baby.*

Pregnancy Precautions

Ideally, your planning and precautions should start well before you conceive. Several months, or even longer, may be needed to assess special problems or make needed changes in your lifestyle. You will want to be sure, for example, that you are immune to rubella well in advance of pregnancy. If you are not, it's best to arrange for rubella vaccine at least three months before you begin trying to conceive. Similarly, if you

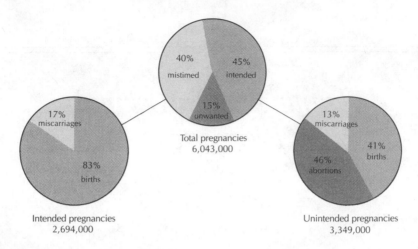

ILLUSTRATION 9-1 Almost half of all pregnancies are planned (or at least intended).

have a serious medical condition like diabetes, advance planning to be sure your blood sugar is in good control before you conceive may reduce the risk that your fetus will be adversely affected.

As soon as you start trying to conceive you will want to be especially conscientious about these **precautions recommended for all women during pregnancy**:

- **Avoid exposure to potentially toxic agents** including:
  Alcohol, smoking, caffeine
  X-ray of the abdominal area
  Illicit drugs
- **Do not take any medications**—prescription or over-the-counter—until you have discussed possible pregnancy risks with your clinician
- **Make a healthy diet a top priority.** A restricted diet or weight loss can be dangerous for your fetus.
- **Take a prenatal multivitamin daily.** Begin at least a month before you plan to conceive, if possible. Do not take megadose vitamins (or mega-anything-else).
- **Review your work and leisure activities.** Be sure your daily exercise and physical exertion are moderate, but not excessive.
- **Avoid anything that might cause your body temperature to be elevated** such as saunas, hot tubs, steam rooms, or exposure to viral illness that could be avoided
- **Review medical and family histories** for you and your baby's father to assess whether prenatal testing might be advisable, and to identify any pregnancy risk factors that may require special surveillance during pregnancy
- **Have a pregnancy test and see your clinician as early as possible** in pregnancy. Assessment of pregnancy dates is most accurate if you have an exam within two weeks after your first missed menstrual period. If you plan to have prenatal genetic testing, accurate date assessment is especially important.

9:2   EARLY PREGNANCY DANGER SIGNS

Possible Ectopic Pregnancy

Sudden intense pain, or persistent pain, or cramping in the lower
    abdomen, usually localized to one side or the other
Irregular bleeding or spotting with abdominal pain when your
    period is late or after an abnormally light period
Fainting or dizziness that persists more than a few seconds. These
    may be signs of internal bleeding. You will not necessarily have
    any bleeding from your vagina if you have internal bleeding.

Possible Miscarriage

Your last period was late, and bleeding is now heavy, possibly with
    clots or clumps of tissue; cramping is more severe than usual
Your period is prolonged and heavy—5 to 7 days of "heaviest" days
You have abdominal pain and fever

Contact your clinician immediately or go to a hospital emergency
room if you develop any of these signs.

• **Do not eat raw meat or drink raw goat milk,** and **avoid contact with cat fecal
matter.** Someone else will have to be in charge of the kitty litter, and it should be
disposed of daily.
• **Try to minimize your risk of STD exposure.** Using condoms during pregnancy is
entirely reasonable if you have any doubts about possible exposure to any sexually
transmitted infection: STDs can cause serious and even lethal fetal and newborn
complications.
• **Watch for danger signs of possible pregnancy complications** (see Illustration
9-2). Spontaneous abortion (miscarriage) and ectopic (tubal) pregnancy are likely to
cause symptoms within the first month or two of pregnancy; steps for evaluation and
treatment are described in Chapter 8.

Reasons for each of these recommendations are discussed in detail in the following
sections, along with advance-planning steps you may want to consider. Although there
are thousands of research studies concerning pregnancy risk factors and outcome,
many gaps still remain. It is entirely possible that you may have good questions for
which there are no satisfactory answers, and in some areas such as nutrition and
vitamins, the information available is less specific and less definite than it ideally
should be. We know more about the effects of some rare industrial chemicals than we
do about common vegetables. Also, the complexity involved in pregnancy assessment
means that **no book chapter can be a substitute for your own personal evaluation
with a careful clinician.** Consultation with your clinician well in advance is especially

TABLE 9-1
FETAL DEVELOPMENT TIME LINE

Day 1[a]	The first day of your last normal menstrual period
Day 11–13	Intercourse on these days is most likely to lead to conception
Day 14	A mature egg is released from your ovary
Day 14–15	One sperm enters the egg to form a fertilized egg
Day 14–17	The fertilized egg divides into 2, 4, 8, 16 . . . cells, and becomes a tiny embryo during its 3-day journey through the fallopian tube to the uterus
Day 17–18	Embryo implants on the wall of the uterus
Day 20–24	A sensitive blood pregnancy test can detect pregnancy hormone (HCG) produced by the tiny placenta
Day 28	Your expected menstrual period fails to occur, or is abnormally light, so you suspect you may be pregnant; a sensitive urine pregnancy test can detect HCG to confirm your pregnancy
Day 28–70	Critical exposure time for toxic agents. Major organ systems form and develop during this interval
Day 70–280	Body structures complete their development and the fetus grows in overall size
Day 280 (40 weeks)	Birth

[a]Hypothetical 28-day cycle

important if you have significant medical problems or have had previous pregnancy complications.

The information in this chapter is limited to prepregnancy planning and precautions for early pregnancy. An important goal for your first prenatal care visit is to identify any risk factors or problems in your particular case and plan for the precautions and care you will need during the remainder of your pregnancy. So be sure that you understand your clinician's recommendations clearly. Also, extensive information is available on many aspects of pregnancy. The "Suggested Reading" list at the end of this chapter may help you find answers to the dozens of questions you will surely have about pregnancy, delivery, and breastfeeding.

EXPOSURE TO TOXIC AGENTS

Lord knows, I never was the body-is-a-temple type! I smoke, *love* to drink, crave junk food. I was scared I wouldn't be able to clean up my act when the time came. It's amazing, though. It really wasn't too hard to behave when I was pregnant. For almost a *year* I was Ms. Clean!

—WOMAN, 24

Toxic agents can affect pregnancy success in several entirely distinct ways. If the toxin interferes with sperm production or maturation of a woman's eggs, then impaired fertility may make conception unlikely or impossible. If exposure damages chromosomes inside the sperm or egg, the fetus may receive abnormal genes that result in miscarriage or birth defects. Exposure during pregnancy may affect the fetus directly, causing abnormal development; the effects that occur depend on the specific toxic agent, the dose of exposure, and the precise time in pregnancy that exposure occurs. **Effects are generally most severe for toxic exposure during the first four months of pregnancy,** when major organ systems are forming. Later in pregnancy, more minor defects may be triggered or overall growth impaired (see Table 9-1).

Alcohol.   Alcohol in your bloodstream traverses the placenta in full strength so your fetus is directly exposed whenever you drink. Fetal alcohol syndrome is a cluster of birth defects including mental retardation, heart defects, and abnormal structure of the face that affects about 50% of babies born to alcoholic mothers. Research studies confirmed this link for women who drank 3 ounces of alcohol or more daily (six cocktails or six glasses of wine or six beers) throughout pregnancy. Similar problems, however, were found for 10% of babies born to women drinking 1 or 2 ounces daily, and drinking in amounts as low as 2 ounces per week has been linked to higher than average rates for miscarriage (1). There is no research evidence to show that an occasional glass of wine is harmful, but there is no evidence to prove it is safe, either. There are also no data to determine what effect, if any, a single episode of heavy drinking early in pregnancy might have.

- **Eliminate alcohol as soon as you begin trying to conceive.** At a minimum, limit alcohol to an occasional, small amount, especially during the last two weeks of each cycle, when you might already be pregnant, and absolutely avoid drinking binges.
- **If you need help in overcoming alcohol dependence,** tackle this problem before you decide on pregnancy

Caffeine. In animal studies, caffeine has been linked to birth defects. So far, human research has not associated caffeine consumption with birth defects, but women who consumed more than 150 mg of caffeine daily (equivalent to 36 ounces of cola or 1 1/2 cups of coffee) in one study had miscarriage rates that were double the expected rate (2). Caffeine, and other chemically similar xanthines, are found in coffee, nonherbal tea, cola, cocoa, chocolate, and in many medications, including pain relievers such as Excedrin, Anacin, and Fiorinal, as well as cold remedies, and appetite suppressants.

• **Eliminate caffeine and other xanthines as soon as you begin trying to conceive.** At a minimum, limit caffeine to 100 mg (one mild cup of coffee) daily.

Smoking. Smoking cigarettes during pregnancy is associated with increased risks for miscarriage, pregnancy complications such as premature separation of the placenta from the uterine wall, and fetal death during pregnancy. Babies born to mothers who smoke during pregnancy have lower than normal birth weight and size, and are more likely to die during the first few days after birth. Smoking exposes the fetus to nicotine and other toxic chemicals in smoke, and also decreases the oxygen-carrying capacity of red blood cells because carbon monoxide from smoke attaches to the blood cells, displacing oxygen.

The adverse effects of smoking are greater for women who smoke 15 to 20 cigarettes or more daily, compared to those who smoke less. Also, risks may be somewhat mitigated for a smoker who is able to stop or drastically reduce smoking during pregnancy, even if several months have already passed. The effort is especially worthwhile since an infant living in a household where a parent smokes has higher than normal risks for illnesses during the first years of life.

• **Stop smoking as far in advance of pregnancy as possible** (years or decades are best). Eliminate smoking from your home. At a minimum, reduce smoking to your absolute minimum, below five cigarettes daily. Make the effort even if you are already pregnant.

Illicit drugs. Research on the pregnancy effect of illicit drugs is very limited because accurate data about illegal behavior are hard to ascertain. **Marijuana** can cause fertility problems for men, but no specific congenital defects have been linked to its use. Researchers suspect that marijuana smoke, like cigarette smoke, may impair fetal growth and lead to low birth weight. A recent, small study of women who used **cocaine** during pregnancy found higher than average rates for miscarriage, and several instances of premature placenta separation that occurred immediately after cocaine injection (3). Babies also showed evidence of neurologic abnormalities within the first three days after birth. No specific fetal problems have been documented for **amphetamine (speed)** exposure during pregnancy, but its secondary effects on appetite and diet would be unhealthy for pregnancy. **Narcotic (heroin)** use is definitely associated with high risks for premature birth and growth retardation, and a baby born to an addicted mother is likely to be born addicted as well.

• **Stop using illicit drugs** as far in advance of pregnancy as possible. At a minimum, eliminate drugs from your life as soon as you begin trying to conceive.
• **If you need help in overcoming drug dependence,** tackle this problem before you decide on pregnancy.

X-ray Exposure.   Exposure to high levels of radiation that might occur with a serious accidental industrial exposure or with radiation treatment for cancer would be likely to cause fetal death or serious congenital abnormalities (birth defects). Moderate x-ray exposure (1 to 10 rads) that might occur with extensive diagnostic x-rays of the abdomen or pelvis may also be associated with a slight increase in risks for congenital defects, especially if exposure occurs before the 16th week of pregnancy. Exposure to this level of radiation during fetal life may also confer approximately doubled risks for later development of childhood leukemia. With proper shielding using a lead apron to cover the abdomen and pelvis, x-rays of the chest or extremities, mammography, and dental x-rays should not pose any added risk during pregnancy.

Medical procedures that involve the use of radioactive drugs, thyroid scan, or lung scan, for example, should be avoided during pregnancy if at all possible. These substances can enter the fetal bloodstream and subject developing fetal tissue to toxic radioactivity exposure.

• **Avoid x-ray exposure of the abdomen and pelvis** whenever possible. If serious illness or injury necessitates x-rays, the total dose should be kept as low as possible, and shielding should be used if feasible.
• **Avoid any medical test or procedure that involves the use of a radioactive drug.**

Hazardous Chemicals.   Adverse reproductive effects of hazardous chemicals, primarily through occupational exposure, is an extremely important issue in prepregnancy planning. At least 50 commonly used industrial chemicals are known to impair reproduction in animals, and millions of workers in the U.S. are exposed to substances known or suspected to cause adverse reproductive outcomes. Table 9-2 lists common chemicals and substances that may have toxic effects on reproduction.

Unfortunately, research to clarify risks for human exposure is quite limited. Studies so far have documented excessive rates for spontaneous abortion (miscarriage) among laboratory and chemical workers, and among workers exposed to lead, ethylene oxide, and anesthetic gases (4), as well as among nurses exposed to drugs used for cancer treatment (5).

Assessing your own risks may not be a simple task. If you suspect that there may be an exposure hazard at your workplace, you, your employer, or your labor union can request assistance in evaluating the problem. Contact your state health department or

TABLE 9-2
COMMON CHEMICALS AND SUBSTANCES THAT MAY CAUSE ADVERSE REPRODUCTIVE OUTCOMES

Dibromochloropropane (DBCP)	Formaldehyde	Organohalide pesticides
Cadmium Lead	Waste anesthetic gases	Styrene
Chloroprene	Carbyl	Vinyl chloride
Ethylene glycol	Toluenediamine Dinitrotoluene	Methylmercury
Ethylene oxide Ethylene dibromide	Glycol ethers	Carbon disulfide

the National Institute for Occupational Safety and Health, Hazard Evaluation and Technical Assistance Branch, 4676 Columbia Parkway, Cincinnati, Ohio 45226.

Exposure to hazardous chemicals can also occur at home. Solvents used for some hobbies and agricultural chemicals used for home gardening require the same precautions against exposure that would be needed for their use in an industrial setting.

Experts are reassuring about one-time, limited exposure that might occur for a pregnant woman who walks past a neighbor's yard where pesticide has recently been used. Avoiding exposure completely is desirable, but a brief accidental encounter should not be a cause for alarm.

• **Avoid exposure to potentially hazardous chemicals altogether** if at all possible before and during your reproductive years (both women and men). If your occupation involves possible exposure, follow safety precautions scrupulously.
• **Be sure that potential hazards at your workplace are evaluated** thoroughly and that safety procedures, as well as equipment and protective clothing, are up to recommended standards and are used

Radiofrequency/Microwave Radiation. Researchers suspect that exposure to radiofrequency/microwave radiation may have adverse reproductive effects, possibly as a result of local heat effects. Temperature elevation of only a few degrees can impair sperm production, and may also adversely affect a developing fetus. Equipment that may emit high levels of radiofrequency/microwave radiation (RF) includes RF induction heaters used to treat and test metals, RF welding equipment, and RF heat sealers used in the plastics, rubber, and tire industries, and in wood products, shoes, and furniture. RF exposure also may be high near broadcast antennas for AM, FM, or TV stations, radar equipment at airports or military installations, and mobile communication equipment used in personal automobiles, buses, ambulances, and police and military vehicles. Medical equipment used for diathermy may expose the patient and medical staff to significant RF.

Radiation emission standards for home (and industrial) microwave ovens are set and monitored by the Food and Drug Administration. Risks for RF exposure or possible heat injury are negligible as long as the oven's safety features are intact, including its lining and case and an automatic off switch activated when the door is opened.

Radiation from Television and VDT's.   Possible radiation hazard from television screens or video display terminals (VDT's) has received considerable national attention. Experts consulting for the Food and Drug Administration reviewed available data on measured radiation emissions and concluded that the amount of harmful ionizing radiation released during normal operation is negligible, and even under the worst possible conditions fetal exposure from this source would be lower than exposure from the natural background radiation we all experience walking around outdoors (6). Clusters of spontaneous pregnancy loss that have been reported, FDA experts concluded, were due to random statistical chance or to causes other than the mothers' work with VDT's.

MEDICATIONS DURING PREGNANCY

Any medication—prescription, over-the-counter, or homemade, herbal, or "natural"—might potentially affect pregnancy. Serious congenital abnormalities as the result of the use of some drugs during pregnancy have been clearly documented in humans, but for many drugs human research hasn't been done, and potential risks are not known. For a few drugs, safety in pregnancy is well enough established that your clinician may feel comfortable about approving their use.

Your clinician is almost certain to recommend that you **avoid all medications unless treatment is medically necessary.** Drugs designed to relieve symptoms of a cold or flu, for example, are not really essential. A stuffy nose is unpleasant, but using decongestants that cause blood vessel constriction may not be desirable during pregnancy. Even aspirin should be avoided, especially during the last few months of pregnancy. Aspirin can cause delayed blood clotting and result in excessive blood loss at the time of delivery, and may also interfere with normal labor patterns.

Be sure that any clinician who cares for you is aware that you are pregnant and that possible pregnancy risks are specifically considered in deciding on your treatment. Some very common medications, including tetracycline and the acne medication Accutane (isotretinoin) must be avoided in pregnancy. Drugs in the penicillin family can be prescribed safely during pregnancy, and sulfa drugs are a reasonable choice early in pregnancy. Sulfa drugs, however, should not be used during

TABLE 9-3
COMMON MEDICATIONS THAT CAN CAUSE BIRTH DEFECTS[a]

Androgens (male hormones)

Some antibiotics:
tetracycline
streptomycin
aminoglycosides (gentamicin and
kanamycin)
erythromycin estolate (Ilosone)
nalidixic acid (NegGram)
nitrofurantoin (Furadantin)

Some anticoagulant drugs:
dicumarol
warfarin (Coumadin)

Some antiepilepsy drugs:
diphenylhydantoin (Dilantin)

Benzodiazepines (Valium, Librium)

Some cancer chemotherapy drugs:
methotrexate
aminopterin

Chlorpropamide

Corticosteroids (including
steroid cream or ointment)

Diethylstilbestrol (DES)

Isotretinoin (Accutane)

Lindane (Kwell)

Lithium

Meprobamate (Miltown)

Podophyllin

Thalidomide

Some thyroid drugs:
propylthiouracil
iodide
methimazole (Tapazole)

Tolbutamide

Trimethadione (Tridione) and
paramethadione (Paradione)

Valproic acid (Depakene)

[a]Specific toxic effects depend on the drug, dose, and timing of exposure. These drugs should be avoided during pregnancy unless treatment is absolutely necessary and no satisfactory alternative can be found.

SOURCES: American College of Obstetricians and Gynecologists: Teratology. *ACOG Technical Bulletin*, No 84, 1985.
Safety of antimicrobial drugs in pregnancy. *Medical Letter on Drugs and Therapeutics* 27:93–95, 1985.
Hales D, Creasy RK: *New Hope for Problem Pregnancies*. New York: Berkley Books, 1984.
Rayburn WF, Zuspan FP, Fitzgerald JT: *Every Woman's Pharmacy*. Garden City: Doubleday Books, 1984.

the last weeks of pregnancy because they can cause newborn jaundice. Table 9-3 lists common medications that are known to cause birth defects.

In some cases, your ongoing treatment for serious medical problems can be altered to reduce pregnancy risks. In other cases, continued treatment will be needed despite known hazards that your medication may pose. If you have a serious medical condition that requires medication, consult with your clinician before you begin trying to conceive to plan the best management strategy in your case.

NUTRITION

A well-balanced diet, with at least three meals each day, is essential for optimal fetal development. Protein is particularly important, and a consistently positive calorie balance so that you are taking in more calories than you actually need. Your fetus relies on nutrients and vitamins in your bloodstream, so skipping breakfast and/or lunch means at least a temporary deficit in the raw materials she/he needs for development.

Your weight should increase gradually and continuously throughout pregnancy, and a good pregnancy outcome with a healthy baby is correlated statistically with a total gain of at least 25 pounds. Weight gain of at least 30 pounds is recommended for a woman who is below normal weight at the beginning of her pregnancy. **Weight loss because of intentional (or unintentional) dieting is dangerous for your fetus.**

Low birth weight babies are at high risk for mental retardation and developmental abnormalities, and low birth weight is strongly associated with pregnancies in which the woman doesn't gain enough weight. **Weight gain below 20 to 25 pounds is proof that nutrition has not been adequate during pregnancy.**

At full term, the weight of your baby and the placenta accounts for 9 to 11 pounds, your uterus weighs about 2 pounds, and increases in your blood volume and body fluid accounts for about 9 pounds. This weight (20 to 22 pounds) will be quickly shed in the first few weeks after delivery. Increased breast size adds about 4 pounds to your weight and will persist during breastfeeding. Calorie demands of milk production are high, so the additional 5 to 10 pounds you may retain after pregnancy will be needed to get started with breastfeeding. **Women who do breastfeed are likely to find it easier to get back to their normal prepregnancy weight**, however, and lose the extra 5 to 10 pounds in the first few weeks.

The quality of nutrition is important as well as the quantity. A balanced diet with ample protein and complex carbohydrates such as grains and vegetables is optimal. Empty calories, from food high in refined sugar or fat, are undesirable because it is preferable to "spend" the calories on foods that have better nutritional value. Adequate calcium intake through dairy products or calcium supplements is also essential during pregnancy and breastfeeding (specific recommendations are discussed in the following section). The storied craving for pickles may not be so strange after all, because pregnant women do have an increased need for salt. Do your best not to overindulge an unusual food craving, and keep balance in your diet. Pica—an abnormal craving for and consumption of one particular substance—is sometimes a problem for pregnant women, and nutrition suffers. For help in planning menus and recipes see "Suggested Reading" at the end of this chapter.

Food Additives.   Pregnancy is a good time to be especially careful about reading labels on food packages. Although research is maddeningly scarce about the effects of food additives on people (pregnant or not), caution does make sense. Of course you

TABLE 9-4
FOOD ADDITIVES TO AVOID
DURING PREGNANCY

AVOID	
Artificial colors	Brominated vegetable oil (BVO)
Blue No. 1	
Blue No. 2	Caffeine
Citrus Red No. 2	Quinine
Green No. 3	
Red No. 2	Saccharin
Red No. 3	Sodium nitrate
Red No. 40	
Yellow No. 5	Sodium nitrite

USE CAUTION	
Artificial color Yellow No. 6	Mono- and diglycerides
Artificial flavorings	Monosodium glutamate (MSG)
Butylated hydroxyanisole (BHA)	Phosphoric acid and phosphates
Carrageenan	Sodium bisulfite
Heptyl paraben	Sulfur dioxide

SOURCE: Brody J: *Jane Brody's Nutrition Book.* New York: W.W. Norton & Co., 1981, p. 487. Jane Brody credits part of her list to "Chemical Cuisine," a poster prepared by the Center for Science in the Public Interest. She notes that for some items on the "Avoid" list, "there is no known clear-cut risk, but the chemicals have been poorly tested and serve no essential role." Testing for some items on the "Use Caution" list "has been inadequate or has raised suspicions of a possible hazard and safer substitutes are available."

can very nearly eliminate any worry about additives if you eat only fresh food, but additives are ubiquitous in prepared food. Table 9-4 offers reasonable guidance for additives to avoid, particularly during pregnancy.

VITAMINS AND MINERALS

Most women in the U.S. probably have adequate vitamin intake without need for supplements. Amazing as it may seem, research data are not available to show what role, if any, minor vitamin and mineral deficiencies may play in human pregnancy. Pregnancy does, however, stress your nutritional reserves, so routine (**not** megadose) multivitamin supplements are a simple and inexpensive insurance policy. Also, small studies in Great Britain have found a reduced risk for spina bifida and other neural tube birth defects when pregnant women took routine multivitamins and iron three times daily for at least 28 days before conceiving and during the first two months of pregnancy (7). The vitamin used provided a daily total of vitamin A, 4,000 International Units; vitamin D, 400 International Units; thiamine, 1.5 mg; ascorbic acid (vitamin C), 40 mg; folic acid, 0.36 mg; ferrous sulfate equivalent to 75.6 mg of iron; and calcium phosphate, 480 mg.

Some U.S. nutrition experts take a more conservative position, and recommend that supplementation during pregnancy is of proven value only for folic acid (0.3 to 1 mg daily) and iron (30 to 60 mg daily). Nonprescription vitamin products contain no more than 0.8 mg of folic acid (800 micrograms), so prescription prenatal vitamins will be necessary if you want a single product containing 1 mg. Alternatively you could take a nonprescription prenatal multivitamin plus an additional nonprescription folic acid tablet. You can find what you need with low-cost, nonprescription vitamin and mineral supplements.

Adequate **calcium** intake is essential during pregnancy, and a total daily intake of 1,500 mg is necessary to maintain positive calcium balance. Otherwise, calcium bone stores may be in jeopardy. Maintaining calcium intake will require strong emphasis on dairy products, and/or faithfulness about calcium supplements. An 8-ounce glass of milk contains about 300 mg of calcium, so at least three or four glasses daily will be needed. **Magnesium** deficiency in animals is linked to fetal malformations and pregnancy loss. Deficiency in humans is probably not common, but some researchers suspect that it may play a significant role in pregnancy complications and may possibly pose a risk for birth defects. Some also recommend assessment of **zinc** intake, and supplements if necessary to insure a total of 10 mg to 20 mg daily.

Some experts recommend **fluoride** supplements during pregnancy (1 mg daily), especially for women who live in areas where water is not fluoridated. Exposure to adequate fluoride during fetal development may be of benefit in increasing the resistance of your child's tooth enamel to cavities later in life.

Megadose Vitamins.   Excessive vitamin intake can cause severe fetal problems. High doses of vitamin A (100,000 International Units or more daily) and of vitamin D (500,000 International Units or more daily) can cause birth defects, and excessive vitamin C can cause problems during early infant life. During pregnancy it is wise to avoid megadose (meaning more than ten times the recommended daily allowance, or RDA) treatment of any kind, and to forgo any other dietary or supplement practices that involve unusually excessive intake of any one product or substance. Diversity and moderation are sensible safety precautions in an area where so much is unknown.

• Talk to your clinician about starting multivitamins several months before pregnancy
• During pregnancy a recommended daily vitamin/mineral intake, through food or supplements, includes iron (30 to 60 mg), folic acid (0.8 to 1 mg), calcium (1,500 mg), and magnesium (450 mg)
• Do not take megadose vitamins

EXERCISE

Vigorous physical exercise helps maintain good muscle strength and optimal heart and lung capacity. Exercise is safest, most beneficial, and least likely to cause muscle strain and pain when your exercise program is regular and frequent, every other day at least. Ideally your exercise should be strenuous enough to raise your pulse to 120 beats per minute, but no higher than 140. Sustain this level for no more than 10 or 15 minutes at a time; then reduce exertion or rest for 5 to 10 minutes before resuming. Be sure you are not out of breath at any time: if you can talk comfortably, your exertion level is not excessive. A short burst of intense exercise is not desirable, especially during pregnancy.

Prolonged, intense exercise can be harmful during pregnancy as well. Prolonged, strenuous exercise raises your body temperature, and any activity that results in an elevated temperature should be avoided, especially during the first few months of pregnancy, because internal body temperature of 102 degrees Fahrenheit or more can cause birth defects. Body core temperature during pregnancy is already about one half degree Fahrenheit higher than normal, and strenuous exercise sustained for as little as 30 minutes may be enough to cause an undesirable rise in body temperature. Also, any oxygen deficit is undesirable since adequate blood flow and oxygen are essential for fetal well-being, so you don't want to get out of breath.

Specific guidelines for pregnancy exercise and a pregnancy home workout program are available from the American College of Obstetricians and Gynecologists (see ''Resources'' at the end of this chapter).

Your clinician may recommend restricted physical activity if you have had pregnancy complications in the past or develop medical problems during your present pregnancy. Also, you will be advised to **completely avoid potentially dangerous activities such as skiing, mountain climbing, horseback riding, and scuba diving.** Changes in your body balance and joints that occur during pregnancy increase your risk for injury with these activities, and surgery or medical treatment required for management of serious injuries can be hazardous for pregnancy.

WORK, PHYSICAL EXERTION, AND STRESS

During normal pregnancy most women are able to continue to work productively until labor begins, and are able to resume work safely within a few weeks after delivery (8). Limiting paid employment will not be recommended unless tasks involved in the woman's job are more hazardous than activities of normal daily life, or special pregnancy risk factors are present. **Restricted work activities or even rest at home may be recommended for a woman who develops medical complications** such as high blood pressure or signs of premature labor during pregnancy, a woman who has had previous miscarriages or premature deliveries, or a woman who has a serious medical problem such as heart or kidney disease (9).

TABLE 9-5
GUIDELINES FOR STRENUOUS WORK
DURING PREGNANCY

ACTIVITY	TIME IN PREGNANCY THIS WORK SHOULD BE DISCONTINUED (IN WEEKS OF PREGNANCY COUNTING FROM FIRST DAY OF LAST MENSTRUAL PERIOD)
Prolonged standing	
More than 4 hours daily	24
Intermittent standing	
More than 30 minutes per hour	32
Stooping/bending below knee level	
More than 10 times per hour	20
2 to 10 times per hour	28
Climbing ladders and poles	
4 or more times daily	20
Less than 4 times daily	28
Climbing stairs	
4 or more times daily	28
Repetitive lifting	
More than 10 pounds	20
5 to 10 pounds	24
Intermittent lifting	
More than 10 pounds	30

Full-term pregnancy is 40 weeks. Similar activities at a less strenuous level may be continued through 40 weeks.

SOURCE: Council on Scientific Affairs: Effects of pregnancy on work performance. *Journal of the American Medical Association* 251:1995–1997, 1984.

Very little research information is available to determine what effects, if any, various kinds of jobs may have on pregnancy, so recommendations are quite vague, and further research is certainly needed. General guidelines for women whose work involves strenuous physical exertion are shown in Table 9-5. Researchers suspect that persistent strenuous physical exertion late in pregnancy may be a risk factor for premature delivery and low infant birth weight. Similarly, **working more than 40 hours weekly may be a factor in adverse pregnancy** outcomes for the pregnant woman and/or her offspring (10).

There is a wide range in the degree to which the normal physical effects of pregnancy impact different women, and experience in the workplace may vary as well.

TABLE 9-6　INFECTIONS THAT MAY HAVE ADVERSE PREGNANCY EFFECTS

TYPE OF INFECTION	STEPS FOR PREVENTION	TYPE OF INFECTION	STEPS FOR PREVENTION
May Cause Birth Defects		**May Cause Infant Illness**	
Rubella (German measles)	Vaccination	Polio	Vaccination
Measles	Vaccination	Tetanus	Vaccination
Chicken pox	Avoid exposure	Hepatitis B	Avoid exposure, including STD[a]
Mumps (?)	Vaccination	Cytomegalovirus	Avoid STD[a] exposure; practice good hygiene after contact with infants and children
Influenza (?)	Avoid exposure	Streptococcus group B	Avoid STD[a] exposure
Toxoplasmosis	Avoid exposure to cat fecal matter, raw meat, and raw goat milk	Herpes type 2	Avoid STD[a] exposure; monitor herpes cultures during pregnancy
Cytomegalovirus (CMV)	Avoid STD[a] exposure; practice good hygiene after contact with infants and children	Chlamydia	Avoid STD[a] exposure; test or treat before or early in pregnancy
Syphilis	Avoid STD[a] exposure; test and treat before or early in pregnancy	Gonorrhea	Avoid STD[a] exposure; test or treat before or early in pregnancy
		Mycoplasma	Avoid STD[a] exposure
		Ureaplasma	Avoid STD[a] exposure

(?)Indicates that definite risk is not confirmed
[a]Sexually transmitted disease

SOURCES: American College of Obstetricians and Gynecologists: Immunization during pregnancy. *ACOG Technical Bulletin No 64*, 1982.
Sweet RL: Chlamydia, group B streptococcus, and herpes in pregnancy. *Birth* 12:17–23, 1985.
Elliot DL, Tolle SW, Goldberg L, et al: Pet-associated illness. *New England Journal of Medicine* 313:985–995, 1985.

For some, early pregnancy is a pleasant, symptom-free experience; for others, pregnancy nausea and fatigue can be quite overwhelming. Fatigue and fluid retention may be severe enough in late pregnancy to interfere with even simple activities, or they may be entirely absent. Ultimately, work recommendations must be made on the basis of individual assessments.

Stressful life events, too, may impact pregnancy. A study of 224 women in England documented an increased risk for premature labor among those who experienced serious illness, illness of a family member, death of spouse or friend, separation or divorce, physical abuse, or loss of income while they were pregnant (11).

INFECTION

Some types of infection a woman may acquire during pregnancy can spread to her fetus and cause miscarriage or severe birth defects. Risks for these problems are highest if infection occurs during the first three months of pregnancy; infection later in fetal life may pose little threat. Other types of infection can be passed from the mother to the baby during pregnancy or at birth and cause illness during the first few days of life, or even later in infancy or childhood.

Rubella.   Many virus infections pose potential hazards during pregnancy (see Table 9-6), but rubella, commonly called German measles, is the most significant because it causes severe defects in as many as 50% of exposed fetuses if infection occurs during the first three months of pregnancy. Rubella risk can be entirely prevented by vaccination prior to pregnancy.

Any woman who has not previously been vaccinated against rubella should be tested for immunity and/or vaccinated at least three months before planning to conceive. A history of an illness believed to have been rubella is not reliable evidence of immunity; the symptoms of rubella cannot be accurately distinguished from symptoms of many other viral illnesses.

A blood test to check rubella immunity status is routinely done for all women as part of the initial pregnancy evaluation. A woman who is not immune and develops symptoms of viral illness during early pregnancy can be retested to detect rubella exposure. Rubella vaccination during pregnancy is not recommended, although there is no evidence that the vaccine has adverse effects on the fetus. Fetuses exposed accidentally to vaccine have not shown increased risks for birth defects.

• Check your rubella immunity status at least three months before trying to conceive. If you have not previously been vaccinated, or there is any doubt, arrange for vaccination.
• Be sure that you are up-to-date on all the recommended routine immunizations. Vaccination against polio, rubella, measles, and whooping cough is normally completed in childhood. Tetanus immunization (combined with diphtheria) must be repeated every ten years.

Toxoplasmosis. Some 30% to 80% of domestic cats show evidence of past infection with this microscopic parasite, and so do 30% of adult humans, so it is very common. Humans acquire the parasite by ingesting (accidentally) parasite cysts from cat fecal matter, raw meat, or raw goat milk. During pregnancy someone else must be in charge of daily kitty litter box changes, and you must avoid raw goat milk and cook meat to a temperature of at least 149 degrees Fahrenheit. Also, remember to wash your hands thoroughly after handling raw meat, after gardening (which might expose you to cat feces), and after accidental contact with cat feces if it does occur.

An adult who acquires this parasite may have no apparent symptoms, or only a mild illness with swollen lymph glands, fever, headache, and malaise. An initial attack that occurs during the first six months of pregnancy will cause some problems after birth for a majority of exposed fetuses, and birth defects in about 15%.

Cytomegalovirus (CMV). CMV infection is extremely common among children as well as adults, and it can be spread through contact with saliva, blood, feces, and other body secretions of an infected person as well as through sexual intimacy. The exposure risk is especially high for people who work with children in health care facilities or day care centers, where contact with diapers or respiratory secretions is likely. Thorough hand washing after contact, and attention to good hygiene, are especially important for women who work in such facilities during pregnancy. There are, as yet, no accepted guidelines for screening tests, treatment, or CMV vaccination.

Other Viral Infections. A woman who develops symptoms of possible viral infection during pregnancy, or is exposed to hepatitis, should report these problems immediately to her clinician. Evaluation may be needed to document rubella exposure or infection with toxoplasmosis or cytomegalovirus. In the case of hepatitis, postexposure treatment with immune globulin may be needed.

Sexually Transmitted Agents. Syphilis, gonorrhea, chlamydia, and herpes infections all adversely affect pregnancy and are readily transmitted between adults through sexual intimacy. Sexual transmission is also an important means of spread for hepatitis, cytomegalovirus (CMV), streptococcus group B, mycoplasma, and ureaplasma, and a possible route for the spread of AIDS (acquired immunodeficiency syndrome). All of these have potentially hazardous pregnancy consequences. Syphilis and CMV can infect the fetus during pregnancy and cause severe congenital defects; the remaining virus and bacterial diseases listed above can be transmitted directly from the mother to her fetus during pregnancy or delivery and lead to serious illness during the baby's newborn period or later in life. Some also cause serious problems for the woman during pregnancy or increase her risk for severe infection after delivery.

The importance of avoiding sexually transmitted diseases (STDs) before and during pregnancy is obvious: the stakes are high. Exposure to multiple sexual partners, now or in the past, for you *or* for your partner, is the most important determinant of STD risk.

During pregnancy, do all you can to minimize or eliminate STD exposure risk; using condoms just to be sure is an entirely reasonable idea.

- **Arrange testing to detect unsuspected infection** before you begin trying to conceive. Be scrupulous in completing any treatment needed for both you and your partner.
- **Be sure your clinician is aware of past STD problems, especially any history of herpes** for you or your partner

If you or your partner have active, recurrent **genital herpes**, or even if either of you have had herpes attacks in the past, testing during the last part of your pregnancy will be needed to detect any herpes recurrence. If you have active herpes sores, or your culture tests are positive at the end of pregnancy, cesarean section delivery will be necessary to avoid exposing your baby to the virus during a vaginal delivery. Be sure that your clinician is aware of this problem, and that culture tests are done at the appropriate times.

The risk of herpes infection for an infant whose mother has **recurrent** herpes is quite low even if exposure to herpes sores does occur at the time of birth. Researchers in one study concluded that no more than 8% of such infants would become infected (12). These babies are probably protected by the pregnant woman's anti-herpes antibody. **The risk is much higher, however, if the pregnant woman acquires herpes for the first time during her pregnancy.** About 50% of infants exposed during birth to the herpes sores of a primary (initial) attack develop serious neonatal herpes infection. So preventing herpes during pregnancy is especially important for a woman who has never had genital herpes. **Scrupulous precautions are essential if an uninfected woman has a partner who does have herpes attacks.**

AIDS is quite rare among women but has terrible consequences for an exposed pregnancy. A woman who has the disease or is a silent virus carrier is likely to transmit it to her fetus, leading to fatal illness during infancy. Needle sharing among drug users is the most common cause of AIDS among U.S. women. Sexual intercourse with a man who has the disease or is in a high-risk group, however, also exposes women to AIDS risk. Risk factors are described in detail in Chapter 28. **Testing to detect antibody evidence of exposure to AIDS is essential for any woman who has one or more risk factors.** Testing should be done before trying to conceive. Pregnancy is not wise for a woman who has evidence of AIDS exposure.

HEREDITARY DISORDERS/GENETIC SCREENING

Some birth defects are caused by abnormal chromosomes that can be transmitted from one generation to the next. For some hereditary problems, the presence of just one abnormal chromosome in a pair will transmit disease even though the other chromosome in the pair is normal. In other cases, an offspring has no outward signs

TABLE 9-7
BIRTH DEFECTS CAUSED
BY ABNORMAL CHROMOSOMES

Polydactyly (extra fingers or toes)

Huntington's chorea

Cystic fibrosis

Sickle cell anemia

Thalassemia (hereditary anemia)

Tay-Sachs disease

Hemophilia

Duchenne's muscular dystrophy

Down's syndrome

Klinefelter's syndrome

Turner's syndrome

Inborn errors of metabolism
(about 100 rare enzyme disorders including
galactosemia and phenylketonuria)

of disease unless both chromosomes in the pair—one from each parent—are abnormal. The offspring can nevertheless transmit an abnormal chromosome to the next generation. An individual who has an inapparent abnormal chromosome is called a carrier.

Some hereditary disorders are the result of one chromosome abnormality, and some involve simultaneous abnormalities in several chromosomes. Some also occur when the process of chromosome replication is disrupted and the sperm cell or egg cell contains an extra chromosome or part of a chromosome is missing. Down's syndrome (mongolism) occurs when an embryo has three copies of chromosome 21 instead of two (trisomy 21). Severe chromosome errors are likely to cause miscarriage. Examples of congenital disorders caused by abnormal chromosomes are shown in Table 9-7.

Some genetic disorders are strongly linked to specific ethnic groups. Sickle cell anemia, thalassemia (also called Mediterranean anemia), and Tay-Sachs disease are examples. Fortunately, individuals who are carriers for these disorders can be identified by simple blood tests before pregnancy. If both partners are carriers, each of their offspring will have a 25% chance of having the disease, and a 50% chance of being a carrier. Testing can be done early in pregnancy to determine whether or not the fetus is affected.

- If you and your partner are Jewish, arrange for Tay-Sachs testing well in advance of pregnancy
- If you and your partner are black, Asian, or of Mediterranean origin, arrange for blood tests, called hemoglobin electrophoresis, for both of you to determine whether you are carriers for sickle cell anemia or thalassemia

Chromosome abnormality risks may also be linked to the age of each parent. Small chromosome changes or mutations that occur in the sperm of older men cannot be detected by tests now available, but major chromosome number errors such as Down's syndrome can be detected. The risk of Down's syndrome increases as the woman's age increases.

Inheritance patterns for hereditary disorders can be quite complex. Specialists in genetic counseling can review family histories for both you and your partner to assess the statistical likelihood that your offspring will be affected, and to determine whether prenatal diagnostic testing may be advisable. In some cases, blood tests for you or your partner may be recommended to determine whether you are carrying an abnormal chromosome.

Genetic counseling is available through taxpayer-supported genetic centers. Your clinician can obtain a free directory of genetic centers from the National Foundation—March of Dimes, Box 2000, White Plains, New York 10602.

Arrange for genetic counseling well in advance of pregnancy if:

- You are 35 or older
- You already have had a child with a birth defect
- You or your partner has a birth defect or genetic disorder or a family history of birth defects or genetic disorders
- You have had three or more miscarriages, or your partner has fathered several pregnancies ending in miscarriage

Counseling is reasonable even if you are not certain whether a birth defect in your own history or your family history was caused by a hereditary problem. The counselor can help you learn the answer. Remember also that some defects may have multiple causes: cleft lip and abnormalities in the development of the spinal cord and brain are examples. The cause(s) of spinal cord and brain defects is not known, but hereditary factors may play a role. Prenatal testing (see the next section) can help detect these problems.

PRENATAL DIAGNOSIS

It is possible to detect major chromosome abnormalities such as Down's syndrome and certain other genetic disorders through diagnostic tests in early pregnancy. Genetic counseling beforehand is essential to determine which specific tests may be appropriate.

Hundreds of different genetic problems can be detected prenatally, and that number will undoubtedly increase. Hundreds of other fetal problems cannot be detected. **Even if you were to have every imaginable prenatal test and all your test results were normal, you are by no means guaranteed a healthy infant.** Testing isn't—and probably never will be—that good.

Amniocentesis.   By analyzing a sample of fluid drawn from the amniotic sac surrounding the fetus—a procedure called amniocentesis—it is possible to evaluate fetal chromosomes and to test for chemical abnormalities that identify some genetic disorders. Amniotic fluid contains living cells that have sloughed off the fetus, and these cells can be cultured in a laboratory to encourage their multiplication for study. Samples for study are obtained by inserting a thin needle through the skin on the woman's abdomen directly into the amniotic sac. No incision is required. **Major defects in chromosome structure or number such as Down's syndrome can be detected.** Amniocentesis is usually performed at about 16 weeks of pregnancy, and analysis requires an additional 3 to 4 weeks. New techniques to allow earlier amniocentesis are now being evaluated at some research centers. Ultrasound is used in conjunction with amniocentesis to find the location of the fetus inside the uterus and identify an accessible area where fluid can be obtained.

Amniocentesis risks for both fetus and mother are quite low. Amniocentesis can trigger Rh factor incompatibility problems, so treatment with an injection of RhoGAM may be recommended if the woman is Rh negative. Overall, miscarriage or stillbirth risks are probably increased about 0.5% to 1% for women who undergo amniocentesis compared to women who do not (13).

Chorionic Villus Sampling.   This procedure is a newer alternative to amniocentesis available at some genetic centers. Cells in the developing placenta have the same chromosomes as the fetus, and a small sample from the placenta surface (chorionic villi) can be removed without jeopardy to placenta function or fetal development. To obtain a tiny sample of chorionic villi, a narrow flexible tube is inserted through the cervical canal and guided to the placenta by ultrasound (see below for more on ultrasound). A placenta sample is aspirated by vacuum, and chromosome analysis is carried out in the lab.

Chorionic villus sampling is usually performed between the 9th and 12th weeks of pregnancy, and chromosome analysis results with this technique may be completed within a few days. Analysis of the cell sample goes much more quickly than with amniocentesis because a larger sample of fetal cells is immediately available for analysis than with amniocentesis, although there may still be a delay of three weeks in some cases to allow the cell sample time to multiply in culture. A six- to eight-week time savings over amniocentesis is a major advantage for most couples who consider genetic screening.

At first, the test seemed about like having a Pap smear, but the clamp on my cervix caused uterine contractions, and we had to wait 20 or 30 minutes for another try before a good sample was obtained. My cervix was pretty sore that night, but I felt fine after that. I did have some spotting for two weeks, but they assured me that it was from my cervix, and not from my uterus.

The worst part was having a full bladder for the ultrasound. Also, I worried about the increased risk of infection and miscarriage, since the test had to be repeated in my case because of my cramping. The best part of the chorionic villus biopsy was being able to have it done at least six weeks earlier than amniocentesis—and the joy I felt when they told me our baby is a normal girl.

—WOMAN, 41

Chorionic villus sampling risks and complications are not well documented in the mid 80s, but may be higher than amniocentesis risks. As with amniocentesis, researchers suspect that slightly increased rates for spontaneous miscarriage will be the most significant risk for the procedure.

Alpha-Fetoprotein Monitoring.   Alpha-fetoprotein is a protein produced by the fetus during pregnancy. In normal pregnancy, the protein is present in high concentrations in the fetal bloodstream and in smaller amounts in the amniotic fluid. Low levels are also present in the pregnant woman's blood.

Abnormally high levels of alpha-fetoprotein in amniotic fluid occur when the fetus has a significant **neural tube defect,** or one of several other less common congenital abnormalities. A neural tube defect means that a malfunction in early fetal development causes birth defects that affect the spinal cord and/or brain. Spina bifida is one type of neural tube defect. A high amniotic fluid level can be detected by amniocentesis testing, and abnormally high levels of the protein also may be detected in the pregnant woman's blood. **Abnormally low alpha-fetoprotein levels may indicate that the fetus has Down's syndrome.**

A test performed at 16 weeks of pregnancy on the pregnant woman's blood can identify almost all cases of serious neural tube defects, and many unsuspected cases of Down's syndrome. Unfortunately the test is not very specific, so **many women with abnormal initial test results actually have pregnancies that are entirely normal.** When the test is used as a routine screening measure for all pregnancies, approximately 50 women out of 1,000 have an abnormally high alpha-fetoprotein result at 16 weeks. True fetal abnormalities, however, will be found in only about 2 of the pregnancies (14). For this reason, repeat testing, ultrasound evaluation, and, in some cases, amniocentesis will be necessary to determine for sure whether an abnormality is present.

Ultrasound.   It is possible with sonar equipment to construct an electronic picture of internal soft-tissue structures, simply by moving instruments over the skin. During pregnancy, ultrasound can provide a good view of your uterus, the amniotic sac, and the moving fetus within. As early as five to six weeks into pregnancy a fluid-filled space inside your uterus should be clearly visible with a small dense streak inside it. Within a few more days it should be possible to see a tiny pulsating heartbeat, and by seven or eight weeks of pregnancy the fetal outline should be distinct enough to measure. By nine to ten weeks, measurement of fetal size provides an accurate assessment of fetal age, so an accurate prediction about a delivery date can be made.

Ultrasound is clear enough and precise enough that **some birth defects can be identified quite accurately by the time the pregnancy reaches 20 weeks or so.** Neural tube defects, for example, or severe heart or kidney defects, can be confirmed in many cases. Ultrasound also can be used to monitor fetal growth and development during pregnancy. This is helpful if dates are uncertain or pregnancy problems that interfere with growth are suspected.

Ultrasound may be recommended to help evaluate situations such as threatened miscarriage, possible ectopic (tubal) pregnancy, or suspected twin pregnancy. It is also used with amniocentesis or chorionic villus sampling to pinpoint the location of the fetus and placenta before sampling begins, and as one step in evaluating abnormal alpha-fetoprotein results.

So far, no adverse effects have been documented in infants or women from ultrasound during pregnancy. Studies of animals, however, have shown adverse effects with ultrasound energy at very high levels, and further research will be necessary to determine whether the lower levels used for medical testing may have subtle or long-term effects that are not yet known (15). Most specialists do not view ultrasound as a hazard, and the procedure is very commonly used, and very helpful in pregnancy.

MEDICAL PROBLEMS AND PREVIOUS PREGNANCY COMPLICATIONS

Serious medical problems such as heart disease, kidney disease, or blood clotting disorders may mean that pregnancy risks are high for both the woman and the developing child. Pregnancy may affect the severity of the disease, or the disease and its treatment may affect pregnancy. Pregnancy in a diabetic woman, for example, is likely to alter insulin requirements, and can cause several kinds of fetal abnormalities including excessively high birth weight. Twelve-pound babies are not uncommon for diabetic women. Medications used for treatment of epilepsy, asthma, rheumatoid arthritis, and excessive thyroid production may cause fetal problems.

Careful assessment and planning prior to pregnancy is essential, and consultation with a specialist in high-risk pregnancy (a perinatologist) prior to conception is a reasonable precaution.

Good control of diabetes early in pregnancy is especially important. When diabetes is out of control, rates for birth defects may be two to four times higher than for nondiabetic pregnancy, and the damage is greatest during the first few weeks of fetal life (16). **Normal blood sugar levels before conception and during the early weeks can reduce the birth defect risk to normal levels.**

Prepregnancy screening for diabetes is also a reasonable precaution for women who have one or more of the following diabetes risk factors: strong family history of diabetes (parent or sibling), previous diabetes during pregnancy, high blood pressure, overweight (20% or more above ideal weight), age 35 or older, sugar in urine with routine fasting urine testing, previous unexplained stillbirth, an infant with congenital malformations, or an infant who weighed nine pounds or more at birth.

- **If you have diabetes, work with a perinatologist and with your clinician to make sure that your diabetes is in good control before you conceive and during the first two months of pregnancy**
- **If you have one or more diabetes risk factors, arrange for diabetes testing before pregnancy**

Advance planning is also reasonable when serious complications have occurred in a previous pregnancy. Testing may be needed prior to pregnancy, and plans for intensive surveillance during pregnancy may be recommended for a woman who has had problems such as multiple miscarriages, previous late miscarriage or stillbirth, a low birth weight or premature baby, or blood pressure problems during pregnancy. DES daughters also may need special pregnancy surveillance.

- **Arrange for consultation with a perinatologist before conceiving if you have a serious medical problem or have had previous serious pregnancy complications**

Surgery requiring general anesthesia is also a potential hazard during pregnancy. If at all possible, surgery should be avoided, especially during the first three months.

If you anticipate that you may need elective surgery because of dental problems or recurring gallbladder attacks, for example, try to resolve these problems before trying to conceive.

Other Pregnancy Planning Issues

SEX PRESELECTION

Effective and reliable ways to assure the birth of a girl or the birth of a boy have been sought since time immemorial. Medically, a reliable sex preselection technique would be of potential value in helping couples who carry an abnormal sex chromosome that causes one of the rare sex-linked birth defects. Hemophilia is one example.

Several do-it-yourself formulas for influencing the statistics that otherwise provide boys and girls in about equal numbers have been developed. One of the best known, by Rorvik and Shettles, involves careful timing of intercourse in relation to estimated ovulation, use of mildly acid or alkaline douches, and rules for depth of penile penetration and orgasm for the woman. These rules are intended to exploit the slight differences between a sperm that carries an X chromosome, which will result in a female fetus if it is the one to reach a woman's egg first, and a sperm that carries a Y chromosome, which will result in a male fetus. The Y chromosome is somewhat smaller than the X, so Y sperm are slightly lighter and swim slightly faster. Sperm that carry an X chromosome, on the other hand, are slightly hardier.

Research on the effectiveness of do-it-yourself methods is limited (practically nonexistent). The success rates reported by their proponents are based on anecdotal reports, mainly letters from successful couples. Since at least 50% would be successful anyway, evaluating the meaning of such statistics is impossible. The techniques are not likely to be harmful, but experts are not enthusiastic about their effectiveness. Some of the formulas, in fact, contradict evidence from studies of couples who conceive with artificial insemination. Slight shifts in the 50/50 ratio do occur with different days of insemination in relation to ovulation, but not necessarily in the direction that would be predicted by the do-it-yourself methods. And for practical purposes, a shift of 1% or 2% is not helpful enough. Also, following do-it-yourself rules means restricting intercourse severely around the time of ovulation. For couples with limited fertility especially, this is undesirable.

Technologic methods for sex preselection, already available in some centers, also are based on the slight differences between X and Y sperm. These involve artificial insemination using a sperm from the father that has been treated in the laboratory to select a sperm sample that is predominantly X or predominantly Y. The Ericsson method uses a laboratory column like an obstacle course so that faster-swimming Y sperm, likely to reach the end sooner than X sperm, are found in high concentration in a sample from the end. Other laboratory techniques are being developed as well, and some may be able to favor conception of a girl. For further information, contact a specialist in fertility in your area, or the American Fertility Society; they should be able to help you locate the fertility center nearest you that offers this service.

PREGNANCY AND AGE

There are no clear-cut age limits for ideal childbearing. Risks for maternal and infant complications are lowest when both parents are between the ages of about 20 to 35; risks are probably somewhat higher both early and late in the reproductive years. Age also affects fertility—the couple's chances for success in becoming pregnant—and risks for genetic abnormalities.

TABLE 9-8
MOTHER'S AGE AND RATES FOR
CHROMOSOME ABNORMALITIES
(Number of abnormal infants per 10,000 births)

AGE	DOWN'S SYNDROME	TOTAL CHROMOSOME ABNORMALITIES
15	10	22
20	6	19
30	11	26
35	32	56
40	111	158
45	405	537

SOURCE: Adapted from: Hook EB: Rates of chromosome abnormalities at different maternal ages. *Obstetrics and Gynecology* 58:282–284, 1981.

As you read the following sections the reasons why couples and clinicians are concerned about late or early childbearing will be clear. Data available, however, cannot answer the crucial questions you are probably asking. Research evidence cannot tell you, for example, precisely how long you can delay trying to conceive without jeopardizing your chances for successful pregnancy.

Unless you have medical problems, or risk factors for impaired fertility, no special surveillance is necessary before about age 35. If childbearing is a high priority for you, planning that includes pregnancy sometime before 35 is a reasonable precaution. By age 40, genetic risks (for both women and men) and declining fertility are very significant issues. **Couples who delay trying to conceive until age 35 to 40 are not as likely to achieve their childbearing goals,** and may be pressed to complete childbearing before age 40 if they are planning two or more ideally spaced children. Successful pregnancy is certainly a possibility; most experts, however, would not encourage waiting until 40.

Birth Defects. Fear of genetic defects such as Down's syndrome (mongolism) is likely to be at the top of the list for couples considering late pregnancy. It is a reasonable concern. Rates for major abnormalities that can be detected through chromosome analysis increase quite sharply when the woman is 40 years old or older, and there is a moderate increase beginning at about age 35 (see Table 9-8). The extra chromosome in Down's syndrome comes from the man's sperm in some cases, and there may be a **slight** increase in Down's risk for elderly fathers (17). Prenatal diagnostic testing, however, is not recommended specifically in relation to the father's age. Statistical evidence of a clear association is lacking, and the magnitude of the risk increase, if any, is probably small.

• **Arrange for amniocentesis or chorionic villus sampling (see the section entitled "Prenatal Diagnosis") if you are 35 years old or older when you conceive.** A pregnancy test and exam will be needed as early in pregnancy as possible so these procedures can be scheduled at the correct week of pregnancy.

For a woman between the ages of 35 and 44 who would abort her pregnancy should a severe birth defect be detected, prenatal diagnosis can reduce the risk of bearing a child with a severe birth defect to the same risk level younger women face.

Men over age 40 have significantly increased risks for genetic mutations that cause disorders such as achondroplasia (dwarfism), Marfan's syndrome (a condition that affects the heart and causes very long arms, legs, fingers, and toes), and neurofibromatosis (Elephant Man's disease). Overall rates for these rare diseases increase throughout the father's reproductive years, and at age 40 the risk that a fetus will be affected by one of them is about 3 to 5 in 1,000 (18). This risk is equivalent to the Down's syndrome risk a woman faces at age 35. Unfortunately, chromosome analysis cannot detect genetic mutation disorders such as these.

• **Plan to complete your childbearing before you and your partner reach 40 years of age**

Pregnancy Complications.   Traditional teaching is that serious pregnancy complications such as high blood pressure and hemorrhage after birth are related to the pregnant woman's age as are serious fetal problems such as premature birth and infant death. **These precepts are based on overall national data, and on scholarly analysis of statistics that are now quite old.** The frequently cited maternal death rates in Table 9-9, for example, are based on statistics from the 1970s. Similarly, the classic research analysis of age and adverse fetal outcome was published in 1974, and was based on data encompassing several decades (19), and more recent reviews as well must rely on data from the past (20).

There is no doubt that these meticulous analyses were correct. What is in doubt now is how relevant their conclusions may be for women today who delay childbearing intentionally or complete a pregnancy very early in the reproductive years. **Reproductive health risks are strongly influenced by factors such as poverty, inadequate nutrition, and lack of good medical care,** and many of the very young and older women in the classic statistical studies faced severe health disadvantages. Many, for example, were women undergoing a fifth, sixth, or even tenth pregnancy, despite terrible poverty. So in retrospect, many researchers believe that factors **other than age** were probably responsible for some, or perhaps even most, of the increased risk observed.

Another pitfall in applying old data to the present is the steep decline in risks over time. Illustration 9-3 shows that maternal death rates in the U.S. have dropped from

TABLE 9-9
MATERNAL DEATH RATES IN THE UNITED STATES
BY AGE OF THE WOMAN

AGE	RATE PER 100,000 LIVE BIRTHS (U.S., 1972–1974)
15–19	11.1
20–24	10.0
25–29	12.5
30–34	24.9
35–39	44.0
40–44	71.4

Death rates now are significantly lower than the rates found in this study: overall, about 8 deaths occur for every 100,000 live births. Rates in this table do, however, show that risks may be affected by the mother's age.

SOURCE: Tietze C: New estimates of mortality associated with fertility control. *Family Planning Perspectives* 9:74–76, 1977.

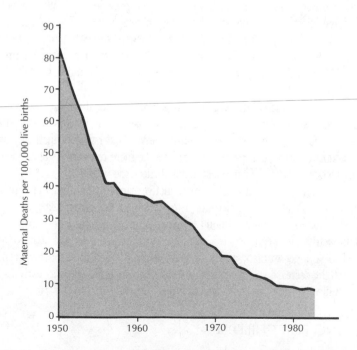

ILLUSTRATION 9-3   The risk of death a woman faces during pregnancy has been reduced dramatically, even in the last 30 years.

83 to less than 10 deaths for every 100,000 live births just since 1950. **Your overall risk of death from pregnancy now is less than one eighth the risk your mother probably faced.** So even if the risk for older women is double or triple the average risk, it is still very low. Risk curves for infant mortality show similar declines.

There is little new research to suggest what the true risks of delayed, or very early, childbearing may be. One 1985 study in Los Angeles, however, found that **overall risks for adverse pregnancy outcome for women 35 and older were not significantly higher** than risks for women 20 to 25 years old (21). Women 35 and older in this study did not have an increased incidence for stillbirth or early infant death, or for premature births or infants requiring intensive care. This study also did not find any increase in rates for prolonged labor among older women, although other studies have reported this effect. Older women were more likely than younger ones to have surgical delivery: 41% of first-time older mothers, compared to 23% of young first-time mothers, underwent cesarean section. Older mothers also had higher rates for diabetes and high blood pressure in pregnancy, and for breech position at the time of delivery.

In another study of women 40 years old or older at the time of delivery, **diabetes and high blood pressure problems were also found,** and were linked to fetal risks including higher rates for stillbirth. Women in this study who were not overweight (150 pounds or less at the time of delivery), however, had no higher pregnancy or fetal risks than a comparison group of normal women aged 20 to 30 (22).

Recent analysis of national statistics from Sweden provides a slightly less optimistic picture of age effects. Fetal and early infant death rates were low in all age groups of women (about 10 per 1,000 births total) but risks were somewhat higher for women less than 20 years of age and for women 35 to 39 years of age. Risks for premature delivery and low birth weight were also higher for women 35 and older (23).

Fertility.   Difficulty achieving pregnancy is actually one of the most important issues in delayed childbearing. Gynecologic problems that may impair fertility—endometriosis or fibroid tumors, for example—are more common among older women than they are early in the reproductive years, and sperm problems may be more common in older men. Intercourse frequency, a crucial factor, also tends to decrease with age.

Aging changes may directly affect reproductive capacity in ways that are not yet understood. The likelihood of conception is quite low for a woman nearing menopause even if she does have regular monthly cycles and ovulation is occurring. Overall success in achieving pregnancy is definitely lower for women who are 40 or older compared to younger women, and a gradual decline in fertility probably begins even earlier. A slight decrease in conception rates has been demonstrated as early as age 35 in some studies. Fertility problems are described in detail in Chapter 10.

PLANNING FOR CHILD SPACING

Medically, a very short interval between successive pregnancies is undesirable. Risks for prematurity, low birth weight, and death during fetal life or early infancy are higher than average for a baby conceived within the first six months after the birth of a sibling. In some studies, an increased risk persisting as long as 18 to 36 months has been shown (24).

Research data regarding birth interval, however, are similar to data for age risks. No one knows whether these conclusions, based on national and international overall rates, are applicable for healthy women with fully adequate nutrition and access to good medical care. Also, the magnitude of the risk increase with a short pregnancy interval is probably quite small compared to other risk factors. In one 1974 study, for example, the overall rate for low birth weight among white women was 5.4%; the rate for white women with less than six months between prior delivery and conception was 6.4% (25).

A more important consideration in child spacing is the psychic and social impact that the birth of a sibling will have on children you already have and on your family life. Experts in child development, as well as experienced mothers, will tell you that children born close together are a real strain on family resources, especially during the first few years. Spacing of at least two years or so is probably preferable.

STOPPING BIRTH CONTROL

If you have been using a diaphragm, sponges, foam, or condoms, no advance planning will be needed when you decide to conceive. Just stop! You can stop any time during a cycle that you want to. Also, there is no need to be concerned if you use your spermicidal barrier method and later find out you had already conceived. One scary study implicating spermicide exposure in birth defects was published in 1981 (26). Intensive research efforts since that time, and careful review of all research data available, provide good reassurance. No other researchers have found an adverse effect and experts believe that the 1981 study results are invalid because of flaws in research design (27).

If you have an IUD in place for birth control, you will need to see your clinician to have it removed. This is an office procedure that is usually less painful and quicker than IUD insertion. There is no evidence that conception immediately after IUD removal would be harmful to you or a fetus. If you are able to plan ahead, though, it is reasonable to have your IUD removed a month or two before you plan to conceive. Your uterine lining should be entirely back to normal within that time, and you can use condoms or another barrier method temporarily for the time you are waiting.

If you have been using birth control Pills and stop them, it is quite likely that you will ovulate within about two to four weeks after taking your last Pill. If you stop Pills at the end of a pack you will have a Pill period, and your next normal period (on your own) should begin four to six weeks after your Pill period. Although there is some conflicting research reported, most experts feel that conceiving in your first cycle presents no special hazards for fetal abnormalities. Conceiving immediately, however, may be a problem in determining accurate dates for your pregnancy. This, in turn, could result in premature delivery if pregnancy complications occur that necessitate cesarean section. Your clinician may have no way to be certain exactly when conception occurred.

Ideally, you should plan to stop taking Pills two to three months before you begin trying to conceive. This will allow time for your own natural cycles to return, your uterine lining will reflect your own hormone patterns, and your clinician will be better able to determine accurate dates for your pregnancy. You can use condoms or another barrier method during your two- to three-month wait.

Although former Pill users and women who have never used Pills do eventually have conception rates that are quite comparable, a small percentage of Pill users experience a longer delay in conceiving than they would like after they stop Pills. Because becoming pregnant in the first year or two after stopping Pills is difficult for a few women, it is reasonable to allow yourself plenty of time to conceive, especially if you are already over 30 years old or have any other reason to suspect extra trouble with conception. Simply stop Pills 6 to 12 months before you'd like to conceive.

I wanted to allow *plenty* of time to get pregnant since I was pushing 32, so I stopped Pills in February, even though ideally I wanted to get pregnant in October. Well, I got pregnant in June. Better early than late. Or never.

—WOMAN, 32

Another Pill concern is inadvertent fetal exposure to Pill hormones early in pregnancy. Exposure can and does happen when a Pill user doesn't realize right away that she's pregnant and continues her Pills. Most experts believe that the risk of birth defects is quite low from this type of hormone exposure, perhaps increasing the normal birth defects risks by no more than 1 per 1,000 births (28). Remember that the average birth defect risk is already about 30 per 1,000 births. Of course, you will want to avoid fetal exposure to all hormones if at all possible. That means you should avoid taking progesterone hormone, which clinicians sometimes prescribe to bring on a late period. This is not an appropriate intervention if you are trying to become pregnant.

CONCEIVING

If you are healthy, and have no reason to suspect fertility problems, all you need to do is stop birth control and keep track of your menstrual period dates. Be sure to write them down. It may be a lot harder to remember them accurately than you might imagine. If you wish, you can chart your basal body temperatures to pinpoint your most fertile days each month (see Chapter 6). Your chart will also help you identify pregnancy. If your temperatures rise with ovulation and stay up for more than 15 to 18 days, chances are good you are pregnant. Pregnancy testing is a must, and an exam early in pregnancy is also. Schedule your appointment within one or two weeks after you miss your first period, and earlier if you are having any problems.

If you do not conceive in the very first month or two, there is no reason for worry. The chance of pregnancy in any one cycle is no more than about 25% even when all factors are totally normal. Overall, about 80% of couples can expect to conceive within the first 12 months of trying.

Waiting and trying does not make sense, however, if you have any of the following reasons to suspect impaired fertility:

• You are over 30
• You aren't menstruating regularly. Irregular menstrual cycles may mean that you are not ovulating regularly, so trying to conceive without treatment is unlikely to be successful.
• You have had three or more miscarriages or your partner has fathered three or more pregnancies that ended in miscarriage
• You or your partner has had infections that can decrease fertility, such as pelvic infection for you and prostate infection for your partner
• You or your partner suspects for some reason that there may be a fertility problem. For example, pregnancy did not occur in a previous marriage despite efforts to conceive.
• You or your partner was exposed to DES (diethylstilbestrol) or you have a problem such as endometriosis or uterine fibroids that can interfere with fertility
• You have used an IUD in the past, or have had appendicitis or previous abdominal surgery; all of these carry a risk of damage or scarring involving the tubes or uterus

If any of these factors apply in your case, read Chapter 10 and see your clinician early or even before you decide to try to conceive. Tests and the help you may need can be started right away, and you may avoid months of delay and disappointment.

As soon as you begin trying to conceive you need to remember the danger signs of possible problems in early pregnancy (see Illustration 9-2). Miscarriage is very common, especially during the first few weeks of pregnancy. If you suspect pregnancy and have any signs of miscarriage, see your clinician promptly. At a minimum, you will need a blood test to determine your Rh type. If you are Rh negative, treatment with an Rh immune globulin such as RhoGAM can insure against problems in future pregnancies. Also, rates for ectopic (tubal) pregnancy are high and climbing. Prompt evaluation for bleeding and/or pain in early pregnancy could save your life.

SUGGESTED READING

Bing, Elisabeth, and Colman, Libby: *Having a Baby After 30.* New York: Bantam Books, 1980. Issues and special concerns of delayed childbearing. Discusses medical considerations as well as feelings and emotional aspects.
Brody, Jane E.: *Jane Brody's Nutrition Book.* New York: W.W. Norton & Co., 1981.

Cronin, Isaac, and Brewer, Gail Sforza: *Eating for Two: The Complete Pregnancy Nutrition Book.* New York: Bantam Books, 1983. Good resource for nutrition during pregnancy, including cooking hints and recipes.

Ewy, Donna, and Ewy, Rodger: *Guide to a Healthy Pregnancy.* New York: E.P. Dutton, 1981. Covers prenatal care, choices in care givers and facilities, fetal development, and changes in pregnancy. Includes sections on nutrition, prenatal exercises, and a glossary and bibliography.

Freeman, Roger K., and Pescar, Susan C.: *Safe Delivery: Protecting Your Baby During High Risk Pregnancy.* New York: Facts on File, 1982. Thorough, readable discussion of issues related to high-risk pregnancies: what constitutes "high risk," prenatal care and advice, tests and procedures used to identify and deal with problems, and psychological effects of high-risk pregnancies.

Gots, Ronald E., and Gots, Barbara A.: *Caring for Your Unborn Child.* New York: Bantam Books, 1977. Covers fetal development, nutrition, use of drugs and medications (in pregnancy and for labor), infections, and environmental hazards.

Hales, Dianne, and Creasy, Robert K.: *New Hope for Problem Pregnancies.* New York: Berkley Books, 1984. Up-to-date information on management of high-risk pregnancy, including prepregnancy planning and what to expect during and after pregnancy.

Kitzinger, Sheila: *The Complete Book of Pregnancy and Childbirth.* New York: Alfred A. Knopf, 1980. Covers conception, pregnancy changes and care, options for care providers, labor and options for birth, nutrition and exercise, relaxation techniques, hospital procedures.

Klaus, Marshall H., and Kennell, John H.: *Bonding: The Beginnings of Parent–Infant Attachment.* New York: Mosby, 1980. Research and insight into the process of attachment between parents and newborns, including information on special situations.

La Leche League International: *The Womanly Art of Breastfeeding* (ed 3). New York: Times Mirror, A Plume Book, 1981. Thorough and practical advice on breastfeeding, including techniques, getting started, nutrition, dealing with problems, and special circumstances.

Llewellyn-Jones, Derek: *Breastfeeding—How to Succeed.* London: Faber & Faber, 1983. Excellent resource for nursing mothers. Discusses physiology and techniques, and provides answers to commonly asked questions.

Price, Anne, and Bamford, Nancy: *The Breastfeeding Guide for the Working Woman.* New York: Simon & Schuster, 1983. Discusses successful breastfeeding from the working mother's viewpoint, including helpful suggestions and problem solving.

Price, Jane: *You're Not Too Old to Have a Baby.* New York: Penguin Books, 1977. Important considerations in late parenthood—careers and life changes, family relationships, the "reproductive time clock," medical considerations, and options for prenatal care and birth.

Rayburn, William F.; Zuspan, Frederick P.; and Fitzgerald, Jeanne T.: *Every Woman's Pharmacy.* Garden City: Doubleday & Co., 1984. Concise but comprehensive information on medications and effects during pregnancy and breastfeeding.

Scher, Jonathan, and Dix, Carol: *Everything You Need to Know About Pregnancy in the 1980's.* Garden City: Doubleday & Co., 1985. Answers to common questions about pregnancy, beginning before conception and continuing week by week through pregnancy and delivery.

Shapiro, Howard: *The Pregnancy Book for Today's Woman.* Mount Vernon, N.Y.: Consumers Union in arrangement with Harper & Row, 1983. Discusses pregnancy and childbirth in a question and answer format, with good sections on nutrition, use of drugs and medications during pregnancy, and exercise, sports, and fitness in pregnancy.

Simkin, Diana: *The Complete Pregnancy Exercise Program: The Step-by-Step Illustrated Guide to a Healthy, Fit Body During Pregnancy and After.* New York: Mosby, 1980. When, why, and how to exercise. Routines for prenatal and postnatal exercises. Common pregnancy problems and concerns.

RESOURCES

The American College of Obstetricians and Gynecologists, in collaboration with Dr. Art Ulene, has produced two home-exercise programs designed for pregnant and postnatal women. The *Pregnancy Exercise Program* and the *Postnatal Exercise Program,* available on video cassettes, record albums, and audio cassettes, can be purchased in selected pharmacies and through your clinician, or by mail order. For more information you can write to ACOG Pregnancy Exercise Programs, c/o Feeling Fine Programs, 3575 Cahuenga Blvd. West, Suite 440, Los Angeles, California 90068.

REFERENCES

1. Kalter H, Warkany J: Congenital malformations. *New England Journal of Medicine* 308:491–497, 1983.
2. Srisuphas W, Bracken MB: Caffeine consumption during pregnancy and association with late spontaneous abortion. *American Journal of Obstetrics and Gynecology* 154:14–20, 1986.
3. Chasnoff IJ, Burns WJ, Schnoll SH, et al: Cocaine use in pregnancy. *New England Journal of Medicine* 313:666–669, 1985.
4. Centers for Disease Control: Leading work-related diseases and injuries—United States, disorders of reproduction. *Morbidity and Mortality Weekly Report* Vol 34, No 35, September 6, 1985.
5. Selevan SG, Lindbohm M-L, Hornung RW, et al: A study of occupational exposure to antineoplastic drugs and fetal loss in nurses. *New England Journal of Medicine* 313:1173–1177, 1985.
6. Food and Drug Administration: Video display terminals and pregnancy. *FDA Drug Bulletin* 14:8, 1984.
7. Seller MJ: Periconceptional vitamin supplementation to prevent recurrence of neural tube defects. *Lancet* 1:1392–1393, 1985.
8. The American College of Obstetricians and Gynecologists, Committee on Obstetrics, Maternal and Fetal Medicine, and the Ad Hoc Task Force on Pregnancy and Work: Pregnancy, work, and disability. *ACOG Technical Bulletin,* No 58, May, 1980.

9. Council on Scientific Affairs: Effects of pregnancy on work performance. *Journal of the American Medical Association* 251:1995–1997, 1984.

10. Chamberlain, G: Effect of work during pregnancy. *Obstetrics and Gynecology* 65:747–750, 1985.

11. Newton RW, Hunt LP: Psychosocial stress in pregnancy and its relation to low birth weight. *British Medical Journal* 288:1191–1194, 1984.

12. Prober CG, Sullender WM, Yasukawa LL, et al: Low risk of herpes simplex virus infections in neonates exposed to the virus at the time of vaginal delivery to mothers with recurrent genital herpes simplex virus infections. *New England Journal of Medicine* 316:240–244, 1987.

13. O'Brien WF: Midtrimester genetic amniocentesis. A review of the fetal risks. *Journal of Reproductive Medicine* 29:59–63, 1984.

14. Prenatal detection of neural tube defects. *ACOG Technical Bulletin* No 99, December 1986.

15. National Institute of Child Health and Human Development: Panel issues recommendations on ultrasound use during pregnancy. *NICHD Research Highlights and Topics of Interest* May, 1984.

16. Gabbe SG, Niebyl JR, Simpson JL (eds): *Obstetrics: Normal and Problem Pregnancies.* New York: Churchill Livingstone, 1986.

17. Hook EB: Rates of chromosome abnormalities at different maternal ages. *Obstetrics and Gynecology* 58:282–284, 1981.

18. Friedman JM: Genetic disease in the offspring of older fathers. *Obstetrics and Gynecology* 57:745–749, 1981.

19. Nortman D: Parental age as a factor in pregnancy outcome and child development. *Reports on Population/Family Planning* Number 16, August, 1974, New York: The Population Council.

20. Hansen JP: Older maternal age and pregnancy outcome: A review of the literature. *Obstetrical and Gynecological Survey* 41:726–742, 1986.

21. Kirz DS, Dorchester W, Freeman RK: Advanced maternal age: The mature gravida. *American Journal of Obstetrics and Gynecology* 152:7–12, 1985.

22. Spellacy WN, Miller SJ, Winegar A: Pregnancy after 40 years of age. *Obstetrics and Gynecology* 68:452–454, 1986.

23. Forman MR, Meirik O, Berendes HW: Delayed childbearing in Sweden. *Journal of the American Medical Association* 252:3135–3139, 1984.

24. Winikoff B: The effects of birth spacing on child and maternal health. *Studies in Family Planning* 14:231–245, 1983.

25. Eisner V, Brazie JV, Pratt MW, et al: The risk of low birth weight. *American Journal of Public Health* 69:887–893, 1979.

26. Jick H, Walker AM, Rothman KJ, et al: Vaginal spermicides and congenital disorders. *Journal of the American Medical Association* 245:1329–1332, 1981.

27. Bracken MB: Spermicidal contraceptives and poor reproductive outcomes: The epidemiologic evidence against an association. *American Journal of Obstetrics and Gynecology* 151:552–556, 1985.

28. Ory HW, Forrest JD, Lincoln R: *Making Choices: Evaluating the Health Risks and Benefits of Birth Control.* New York: Alan Guttmacher Institute, 1983.

Overcoming Impaired Fertility

Pregnancy is the quite miraculous result of innumerable complex physiologic events occurring over 20 years or more.

An egg destined to contribute half the genetic blueprint for a new life begins its journey many years before. A woman is born with all the eggs she will ever have, about 1 to 2 million of them. Her eggs remain immature and dormant in her ovaries until puberty brings the hormonal patterns responsible for final egg maturation. Then, for about 30 years, just one or two of her eggs undergo final maturation each month. After its release (ovulation), the egg is capable of undergoing fertilization for approximately 12 hours. Ovulation also must be perfectly timed to coincide with optimal development of the uterine lining to nurture and provide safe haven for a tiny embryo, about the size of a pinpoint, that arrives in the uterus three to six days or so after ovulation if fertilization does occur.

Sperm, each one carrying half the chromosomes a new human being needs, have a longer and more arduous journey, and are provided in much larger numbers—many millions daily. Beginning at puberty new sperm cells are continuously produced, and fertility for men may be possible for 70 years or even longer. Sperm cells originate in the testicles, and require approximately ten weeks to reach maturity. Essential nutrients are provided by the secretions of the prostate gland and seminal vesicles. This fluid, seminal plasma, contributes most of the volume to semen.

Ejaculation is the beginning of a long journey for sperm. Perhaps 100 million sperm are deposited in the vagina with each ejaculation; fewer than 200 are likely to succeed in traversing the cervix, uterus, and the length of the fallopian tube, a journey of about 8 inches. Most sperm never reach the cervix; of those that do enter the cervix, probably fewer than half reach the uterine cavity. During their journey, sperm undergo final steps in maturation with changes in the chemical composition and structure of the chromosome-containing sperm head. These essential steps prepare the sperm to fuse with the surface of the egg cell. Once ejaculated, sperm probably retain their capacity to fertilize an egg for 24 to 72 hours, and sometimes longer.

The day before ovulation, the woman's pituitary gland releases a sudden pulsating surge of luteinizing hormone (LH), which triggers the final preparation for egg release. Then, 24 to 36 hours later, the mature follicle on the surface of her ovary spontaneously bursts, releasing a tiny plume of fluid and a single egg somewhere near the open end of her fallopian tube. The frond-like fimbriae at the end of her tube are ready to capture the egg, and rhythmic movements of the ciliated cells that line the tube create a continuous current in the tubal fluid that helps the egg begin its journey toward the uterus.

***If sperm are available in the fallopian tube, fertilization is possible.** One or several sperm may, quite by accident, swim up against the surface of the egg, and one will be the first to penetrate the outer egg membrane. Immediate release of chemicals just under the surface of the egg blocks penetration by any additional sperm. **The newly formed embryo begins development in the fallopian tube during the first three to six days of its existence.** By the time it arrives at the uterus it will have undergone many cell divisions, but no real overall growth. Just barely visible to the naked eye, it will be ready to implant in the uterine lining and begin growth after two or three more days. And within seven days or so after fertilization the developing placenta produces enough pregnancy hormone (HCG, human chorionic gonadotropin) to be detected by sensitive blood tests.*

It is hard to know just how many people have impaired fertility. Based on the number of people who seek help for this problem, **most experts estimate that 10% to 15% of couples have impaired fertility.** Whether or not fertility problems are increasing is not clear, but more and more couples are seeking medical treatment for fertility. And some potential causes of impaired fertility are definitely on the increase (1). As you read about the causes of impaired fertility, you will recognize at least one familiar problem: rising rates for sexually transmitted disease. Intentional delay of childbearing until later in the reproductive years can also contribute to impaired fertility, and some researchers are also concerned about the possibility that environmental toxins may play a role in the fertility problems that couples experience.

In the area of infertility, great progress has been made in diagnosis and in treatment, and prevention is receiving increasing medical emphasis. Patients and clinicians are weighing possible effects on fertility carefully as choices are made about birth control and management of common gynecologic and urologic problems. Even more important, men and women are becoming more aware of, and concerned about, the fertility consequences of decisions they make in daily life.

Fertility involves two people, and fertility evaluation should include both partners from the very beginning. Usually it is possible to identify one primary reason for impaired fertility. In about 40% of couples, infertility is caused by a male factor, and in about 40% the cause is a female factor (2). In the others, a combination of factors is involved, or it is impossible to identify the specific problem.

There is good reason for hope even if you do have a fertility problem. Research in the last decade has brought major improvements in techniques for fertility evaluation and treatment. Even couples who have believed pregnancy impossible may have new options to consider.

As soon as you start trying to conceive you need to be aware of the special precautions that make sense in early pregnancy. You might begin by reading Chapter 9, "Planning for an Optimal Pregnancy."

And one more warning. Just as no test or medical expert can give you certain assurance that future pregnancy will be possible, **there is no way to be absolutely certain that you are infertile.** Pregnancy is unlikely if you have severe tubal damage or a very low sperm count, but even under these circumstances pregnancies do occasionally occur. So if you do not want to be pregnant, you will need to think carefully about birth control, even if you have impaired fertility.

In the meantime, you may want to consider the following precautions to help protect your future fertility.

MINIMIZING YOUR RISKS FOR FUTURE FERTILITY PROBLEMS

There are many practical steps you can take to protect your future fertility options. Most apply to both men and women.

• **Avoid risking exposure to sexually transmitted diseases**

• **If you are less than 25, use condoms faithfully,** because you are in a high-risk age group for sexual infections. If you are a young teenager, the best way to protect your future fertility is to avoid intercourse entirely.

• **Use condoms for the first three to six months of any new relationship,** and whenever either of you has more than one partner

• **Limit your number of sexual partners.** That includes your own partners and your partner's other partners as well.

• **Do not have intercourse with a partner who has possible symptoms** of sexually transmitted infection

• **Skip intercourse or use condoms if you have the slightest doubt** about infection risk, even if you are also taking birth control Pills

• **If infection does occur, be sure that both (or all) partners** are treated with a full course of antibiotics

- **Be sure your medical care is thorough** if you have problems with infection (men and women) or with abnormal Pap tests (women)
- **(For women) Avoid using an IUD** (intrauterine device); birth control Pills, a diaphragm, or condoms are better choices if future fertility is at all important to you
- **(For women) Be sure you are immune to rubella**
- **(For women) Attend promptly to any gynecologic problems** that develop, especially symptoms such as pain, cramps, abnormal bleeding, vaginal discharge, or warts
- **(For men) Attend promptly to any urologic problems** that occur, especially symptoms such as penile discharge, urinary burning, bleeding, pain, or warts
- **Make a reproductive life plan**, and reevaluate it periodically; if possible, allow for childbearing earlier rather than later in your reproductive years
- **Think of sterilization surgery (tubal ligation or vasectomy) as an absolutely permanent and irreversible decision**
- **Discuss beforehand the possible impact on your fertility** of any surgery or medical treatment you are considering. If surgery is necessary for an ectopic pregnancy or ovarian cyst, for example, every effort should be made to preserve both ovaries and both fallopian tubes.
- **(For men) Be sure you have had mumps immunization**, preferably in childhood
- **Avoid risking genital trauma**. Use appropriate protective gear and good judgment in sports and other potentially dangerous activities. Testicular injuries for men are particularly common.
- **Avoid illicit drugs** (including marijuana), excessive alcohol consumption, and exposure to environmental and industrial toxins

WHEN TO SEEK MEDICAL HELP

Experts define infertility as "the inability to conceive after trying for one year," and they usually counsel patience for couples who have been trying for only a few months.

In some situations, it doesn't make sense to wait. Seek help for fertility problems earlier if you would like to conceive and:

- **You are over 30.** Fertility declines with age, and childbearing is somewhat safer for you and your baby before you reach your mid-thirties.
- **You aren't menstruating regularly.** Irregular menstrual cycles may mean that you are not ovulating regularly, so trying to conceive before treatment is unlikely to be successful.
- **You have had three or more miscarriages** or your partner has fathered three or more pregnancies that ended in miscarriage
- **You or your partner have had infections** that can decrease fertility, such as pelvic infection for you and mumps or prostate infection for your partner
- **You or your partner suspect for some reason that there may be a fertility problem.** For example, pregnancy did not occur in a previous marriage despite efforts to conceive.
- **You or your partner was exposed to DES** (diethylstilbestrol) or you have a problem such as endometriosis or uterine fibroids that can interfere with fertility

• **You have used an IUD in the past,** or have had appendicitis or previous abdominal surgery; all of these carry a risk of damage or scarring for your tubes or uterus

Causes of Impaired Fertility

Medical factors are likely to be the cause of your fertility problem, but human factors are important too. You are likely to receive well-meaning advice from family and friends. It helps to have a clear idea of what is true and what is not.

MYTHOLOGICAL CAUSES OF IMPAIRED FERTILITY

Psychological stress can be severe enough in rare cases to cause hormone abnormalities that stop ovulation, depress sperm production, or significantly alter intercourse frequency. Otherwise, though, **there is no evidence that psychological problems are a cause of fertility impairment.** Studies have also shown that **pregnancy rates are not higher after adoption, nor after D&C** (uterine scraping)(2). Thyroid or clomiphene fertility pill treatment "just in case" is also useless. A certain number of couples who are being evaluated, or have had evaluation with no specific problem found, will spontaneously conceive on their own. These are the couples who conceive after adoption or "just in case" treatment, and they would have conceived anyway. And there is no reason to believe that quitting your job or resting will improve fertility, unless infrequent intercourse is a factor in your problem and you **begin to have intercourse more often because of the changes you make in your life.** Of all the common advice, taking a vacation (at the right time) may make the most sense. Many couples find that they have more time, energy, and inclination for intercourse when they are on vacation.

Possible causes of impaired fertility described in this section are listed in Table 10-1. Some are very common, others quite rare. We begin with intercourse timing because this often receives less emphasis than it deserves. It is a very common problem. Male problems, also very common, are followed by female problems as they can affect each part of the woman's reproductive system. Evaluation and treatment options are described in the later sections of this chapter.

TIMING AND FREQUENCY OF INTERCOURSE

In most cases, intercourse is necessary for pregnancy. Exceptions are pregnancy conceived through artificial insemination, in vitro fertilization (IVF), and gamete intrafallopian transfer (GIFT). **If you are having intercourse once or twice a week it is entirely possible that you are missing your fertile days all or many months.** This is

TABLE 10-1
POSSIBLE CAUSES OF IMPAIRED FERTILITY

TIMING AND FREQUENCY OF INTERCOURSE

AGE OF PARTNERS

IMPAIRED SPERM PRODUCTION OR SPERM FUNCTION

Chromosome or genetic
  abnormality
Testicular tumor
Trauma, vasectomy
Retrograde ejaculation
Toxic chemicals and drugs
High altitude or temperature
Varicocele
Infection
Thyroid deficiency
Excessive prolactin or adrenal
  hormone

OVULATION OR HORMONE DISTURBANCES

Irregular or absent ovulation
Unruptured follicle syndrome
Excess prolactin
Luteal phase defect
Inadequate cervical mucus
Toxic chemicals and drugs

VAGINAL, CERVICAL, AND UTERINE PROBLEMS

Congenital abnormalities in
  structure
Fibroids
Cone biopsy, cryosurgery
Infection
Antibodies
Acidity

FALLOPIAN TUBE DAMAGE

Infection
Previous surgery

ENDOMETRIOSIS

ANTISPERM ANTIBODY PROBLEMS

DES-EXPOSED OFFSPRING

REPEATED MISCARRIAGE
Uterine abnormalities
Hormone problems
Chromosome abnormalities
Infection
Antisperm antibody problems
Incompetent cervix
Toxic chemicals and drugs

---

quite a common problem, and its impact on fertility is self-evident (see Table 10-2).

For most women, ovulation occurs in mid to late morning (3). **The ideal time for intercourse is the day or evening before ovulation occurs.** This timing will assure that sperm are present in the fallopian tubes when the egg is released, ready to fertilize it a few hours later when it is perfectly matured. The difficulty in timing intercourse is that pinpointing the exact day of ovulation is not easy, so you will probably need to be sure you have intercourse at least three times during your fertile week each cycle. Illustration 10-1 shows that **conception rates are highest with intercourse one, two, or three days before the day of ovulation.**

Having intercourse too frequently is a very rare cause of impaired fertility. After each ejaculation sperm count is temporarily lowered, but for a man with normal sperm

TABLE 10-2
FERTILITY AND INTERCOURSE FREQUENCY

INTERCOURSE TIMING (COUPLES OF ALL AGES)	% OF COUPLES WHO CONCEIVE WITHIN 6 MONTHS
Less than once weekly	17
Once weekly	32
Twice weekly	46
Three times weekly	51

SOURCE: Keller DW, Strickler RC, Warren JC: *Clinical Infertility*. Norwalk: Appleton-Century-Crofts, 1984. Keller's data are drawn from MacLeod and Gold's work on male fertility, which is cited in Keller's text.

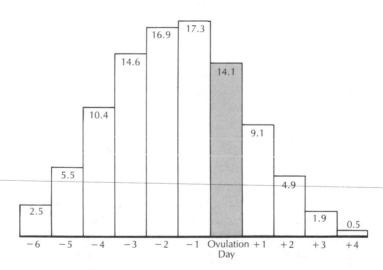

Each bar represents the percentage of couples who would conceive after intercourse once on a given day near ovulation. That is, 14 out of 100 couples who had intercourse once on ovulation day would be expected to conceive.

ILLUSTRATION 10-1   The best intercourse time for fertility is the day *before* ovulation. Next best are two and three days *before*.

production, the slight decrease is insignificant. If chronic low sperm count is a problem, then it is reasonable to allow at least 36 to 48 hours between ejaculations during the fertile days each month; otherwise, **intercourse every day is preferable**.

Intercourse frequency is something to think about and something to keep track of on a chart if you suspect this may be a factor for you. You may be surprised to find

TABLE 10-3
FERTILITY AND AGE OF MALE PARTNER

MAN'S AGE[a]	% OF COUPLES WHO CONCEIVE WITHIN 6 MONTHS
Less than 25	75
25–29	48
30–34	38
35–39	25
40 and older	23

[a]"Husband" is the term researchers used in this study.

SOURCE: Keller DW, Strickler RC, Warren JC: *Clinical Infertility*. Norwalk: Appleton-Century-Crofts, 1984. Keller's data are drawn from MacLeod and Gold's work on male fertility, which is cited in Keller's text.

that you and your partner have quite different recollections about frequency, and that neither of you is accurate. Changes in your life and priorities may be needed to give you the strength and opportunity to have a real chance for pregnancy.

FERTILITY AND AGE

Age has a definite, but not clearly understood, relationship to fertility for both men and women. For men, there is no specific, clear-cut biological endpoint to reproductive function. For some, fertility may persist through the 60s or even 70s. **Gradual decline in the statistical likelihood of conception, however, can be documented for men starting in the mid 20s.** Table 10-3 shows the decreasing likelihood of conception within six months for men 25 years of age and older. This decline may be partially explained by the gradual accumulation of fertility problems within the male population as elapsing time increases the proportion of men affected by sperm production disorders. It also reflects the important impact of the partner's age and of intercourse frequency on fertility. Intercourse frequency generally decreases as the age of the partners increases.

For women, menopause—usually at about age 51—is a clear and definite end for the reproductive phase in life. Although pregnancy can occur in the immediate premenopausal years, **fertility is substantially reduced in the preceding decade so that the probability of pregnancy after age 45 is very low.**

As menopause approaches, a woman is likely to have less frequent ovulation. Absence of ovulation, however, does not entirely explain the reduction in fertility. Pregnancy is unlikely even when ovulation can be documented. Changes may occur in

TABLE 10-4
FERTIILTY AND AGE OF FEMALE PARTNER

AGE	% WHO CONCEIVED[a] WITHIN 12 INSEMINATION CYCLES
18–25	94
26–30	84
31–35	69
36–40	57
41–44	56

[a]Some of these women experienced subsequent miscarriage, a problem that increases with age. Statistics on full-term pregnancy success would therefore show a slightly greater difference between younger and older women.

SOURCE: Virro MR, Shewchuk AB: Pregnancy outcome in 242 conceptions after artificial insemination with donor semen and effects of maternal age on the prognosis for successful pregnancy. *American Journal of Obstetrics and Gynecology* 148:518–523, 1984.

the uterus with aging that interfere with implantation, or age may affect the process of egg maturation in a way that is not yet apparent to researchers.

In the real world, **pregnancy success for older women is usually influenced by the age of her partner and intercourse frequency as well as the effects her own age may have.** There is some statistical information, however, on the isolated effect of her age. A widely publicized French study of pregnancy rates following artificial insemination documented a gradual reduction in the likelihood of conceiving within 12 insemination cycles. Fertility declined somewhat for women over 30 and substantially for women over 35. The same age pattern was confirmed in a subsequent Canadian study. Pregnancy rates were higher in the Canadian study, probably because women with ovulation problems were treated to induce ovulation and fresh, rather than frozen, donor semen was used. The Canadian findings are summarized in Table 10-4.

Reviewing historical population data and national fertility surveys in the United States in 1965, 1976, and 1982, demographers concluded that **the likelihood of success in achieving pregnancy for women decreases gradually and steadily from the mid-twenties until the late thirties or early forties, and then decreases sharply.** This review found no evidence that intentional delay in childbearing or contemporary STD epidemics had significantly altered overall fertility patterns, and provides some reassurance to those who are considering postponed childbearing. The average time required to conceive is greater for older women, but eventual success is likely. At age 20 to 24, the risk that a woman will be unable to bear a child is about 5%; at age 30 to 35 the risk is no more than 16% (4).

"How old is too old?" is a question I hear every single day. I'm not really sure what to say—I try to be quite reassuring. There is no definite age cutoff for successful pregnancy: 36 is not really different than 34, scientifically speaking. But I do worry because if a 34-year-old woman does have trouble becoming pregnant there isn't a whole lot of time to intervene and try to help. I wish that our educational and social systems would provide a good time for childbearing a little earlier in a woman's life.

—GYNECOLOGIST

IMPAIRED SPERM PRODUCTION OR SPERM FUNCTION

Semen evaluation is likely to be the first test your clinician will order when you begin evaluation. The single most common cause of infertility is production of too few sperm, or too few normal sperm.

Complete Absence of Sperm. The term for this problem is **azoospermia**. It is quite rare (except after vasectomy), and rare disorders may account for it. A man with azoospermia is likely to be aware of the problem already if the cause is a chromosome or genetic abnormality, a congenital abnormality such as undescended testicles, or cystic fibrosis. Mumps infection that occurs after puberty permanently affects sperm production in about 25% of its victims. Severe testicle injury, tumor, or scarring from a previous episode of sexually transmitted disease can also stop sperm production entirely.

Some men who have diabetes or have had surgery involving the prostate gland or urethra (see Illustration 10-2) have impaired fertility because ejaculation fluid containing the sperm escapes backward into the bladder. This is called *retrograde ejaculation* and occurs when the sphincter, the circular band of muscle that normally closes the base of the bladder just before and during ejaculation, fails to function properly. Medications for high blood pressure can also cause this problem. It is possible that a man with retrograde ejaculation might not be aware of the problem. In some cases, part of the semen is released normally through the penis, while the remainder escapes to the bladder. Ejaculation problems may also cause infertility for a man who has congenital hypospadias (a birth defect in which the urethral opening is located at the base of the penis), or severe sexual dysfunction that precludes intercourse or ejaculation inside the vagina. Some men find that the sex-on-demand requirements of fertility treatment cause temporary impotence.

Sperm Production That Is Consistently Low. Often this very common problem is accompanied by abnormalities in sperm shape and function as well. In

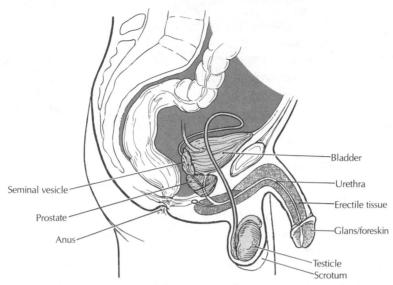

ILLUSTRATION 10-2   Normal reproductive function depends on the brain as well as the reproductive organs. In addition, hormones from the thyroid and adrenal glands are also essential for normal reproductive function.

some cases a specific cause can be identified—and possible causes are numerous. In 25% to 50% of cases, however, the reason for the problem is not evident despite careful evaluation (5).

The number and quality of new sperm being formed on any particular day can be influenced by current events in a man's life. It is not surprising, therefore, that fairly **wide fluctuations in both sperm count and quality occur over time**. Today's ejaculated sperm reflect conditions of approximately ten weeks ago when those sperm were first being formed.

Alcohol and drugs probably rank high among the causes of semen problems. Illicit drugs, especially marijuana, some medications (including certain antibiotics, cimetidine for treating ulcer disease, and sulphasalazine for colitis), alcohol, and nicotine can all cause a temporary reduction in semen quality (6,7)—temporary, that is, if the exposure is temporary. Consistently low sperm quality can result if any or all of these substances are part of daily life.

Information on the precise effect of marijuana in humans is quite limited. Research has suggested that chronic use may cause a decrease of 30% to 40% in testosterone production, and may also have a direct effect on the sperm-producing cells in the testicles. In one small study, **men who used marijuana daily for one month experienced a 35% decline in sperm production**, with reduction in motility and the percentage of normal sperm shapes as well (5). Sperm abnormalities in animal studies of marijuana effects show alterations in the protein structure of the sperm head. This could occur with no change in the part of the sperm that carries the chromosomes. There is no conclusive research, however, to give assurance about possible chromosome damage, so it is possible that marijuana exposure could cause an increase in birth defects or spontaneous miscarriage.

Occupational and environmental exposure to chemicals and other toxins is probably an important cause of semen problems (8), but is not yet fully understood. Some researchers believe that these agents are at least partly responsible for increasing problems with male infertility among couples seeking treatment. Deleterious effects have been documented for lead exposure, as well as for hydrocarbons such as DBCP in the petroleum industry (9,10), and glycolethers commonly used in industrial and household solvents (11). Pesticides and herbicides may also be toxic to sperm production. Dioxin, Kepone, and the herbicide 2,4,5-T are of particular concern. Men using these agents at work may be aware of their exposure; as chemicals sprayed on crops move into the water supply or food chain, though, thousands may be unwittingly exposed. Read Chapter 9 for more details on toxic exposure and its relation to fertility and pregnancy outcome.

The physical environment is also important to testicle function. High altitude and high temperature adversely affect semen quality. **Temporary illness, such as flu, that involves fever can cause severe but temporary depression in sperm production.** Use of a hot tub or sauna conceivably could cause this problem, as could consistent wearing of tight underwear or a scrotal support, although research is limited in this area.

Until recently, **varicocele**, varicose veins in the testicle, was believed to be a common cause of poor semen quality (see Illustration 10-3). Researchers suspected that the presence of dilated scrotal veins might raise the temperature in the testicles, and thus cause poor sperm production. Approximately 10% to 15% of men have varicocele, and it is found in as many as 25% of men with fertility problems (2).

The actual importance of varicocele as a cause of infertility, though, is now being questioned by many fertility specialists. One recent study showed no significant difference in pregnancy rates between men who did have varicocele and those who did not, and found that surgery repair did not alter the pregnancy rate (2); significant improvement in pregnancy rates, however, was documented in another large study for men who had low counts initially and were treated with varicocele repair (12). If varicocele is found in evaluation of abnormal semen production, surgery to correct it will probably be recommended. If semen is normal, however, surgery to correct varicocele is not mandatory. Routine semen evaluation and exams to insure that the situation is stable may be all that is necessary.

If varicocele is discovered in childhood or adolescence, then surgical repair is probably wise. **Varicocele may impair normal growth of the testicle involved,** and may interfere with hormone function and fertility later on (5).

Serious medical illness can cause depressed sperm production. Some examples include long-term illness such as colitis or rheumatoid arthritis, as well as short-term illness or injury that is severe. Some experts believe that severe psychological stress can also affect semen quality (5).

Overall health and nutritional status no doubt play a role in fertility for men. Severe

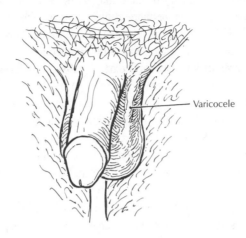

ILLUSTRATION 10-3   Varicocele can be corrected in most cases with simple surgery, and repair is *sometimes* followed by improvement in semen quality.

nutritional deprivation as well as true vitamin deficiency cause measurable impairment of sperm production in animals. **There is no evidence, however, that extra vitamins or nutritional supplements can improve semen for men who have a normal diet.**

Reproductive Tract Infection.   Infection damage severe enough to cause blockage in sperm pathways (vas deferens or epididymis) is a clear cause of infertility. Obstruction is not common, but the damage is likely to be permanent. Similarly, infection that destroys part or all of the testicle or the prostate gland can permanently impair semen production.

It is also possible that a less severe infection, or unrecognized infection that is persistent, could also cause sperm problems. Men with abnormal sperm function are more likely to have infection-fighting white blood cells present in semen than are men with normal fertility (13). These cells may reflect infection in the urethra, seminal vesicles, prostate, or epididymis. **The presence of bacteria or infection-fighting cells in the semen could affect sperm** directly, and infection might also interfere with the ability of the prostate gland to produce the normal secretions it contributes to semen. Prostate secretions are essential for normal sperm survival and motility, and may also play a role in preventing formation of antibodies against sperm.

In some cases a specific bacterial cause such as gonorrhea or chlamydia or mycoplasma infection can be identified. (See Chapters 25 and 29 for more information about these problems.) In other cases bacterial cultures are not successful—either no active bacteria are present, or the ones responsible for the problem cannot be grown with culture techniques available. When white blood cells are found, treatment with antibiotics is a reasonable idea even if the man has no obvious symptoms of infection.

Prolonged treatment of a month or more may be necessary to eradicate mycoplasma, and bacterial resistance to one or more antibiotics is possible. Follow-up cultures are therefore crucial. Also, since these are sexually transmitted diseases, both (or all) partners need to be treated at the same time. Recurrence of infection is common, so periodic cultures make sense as a part of subsequent fertility treatment.

Hormone Abnormalities.   Alterations in hormones are not a common cause of semen problems. Levels of testosterone, the primary male hormone, are almost sure to be entirely normal, as are sex drive and sexual functioning. Semen is also likely to appear completely normal to the naked eye. Most of the fluid in semen originates from the prostate gland and seminal vesicles, and the sperm-containing fluid from the testicle is only a small part of the total volume.

Hormone testing may not be recommended unless there have been other signs of hormone problems such as failure to undergo puberty or chronic impotence, or if complete evaluation has shown no other cause for impaired semen. In rare cases, unsuspected thyroid abnormalities or elevated production of prolactin by the pituitary gland is found.

OVULATION OR HORMONE DISTURBANCE IN WOMEN

Infrequent or Absent Ovulation.   Problems with ovulation are found in about 20% of couples with fertility impairment. Fortunately, success in treating this problem is good. Any woman who is not having menstrual periods (amenorrhea) or has infrequent or irregular menstrual patterns should suspect this problem. She will need systematic evaluation, whether or not she wishes to be pregnant, to be sure that she does not have a serious medical problem such as a pituitary gland tumor. Steps in evaluation and treatment of amenorrhea and of irregular menstrual patterns are described in detail in Chapters 32 and 33. For most women a serious problem or clear-cut hormone defect is not found.

Subtle hormone abnormalities can disturb ovulation. Many women have temporary disturbances in their cyclic patterns because of stress, dieting, or athletic training, and for some, cyclic disruptions may be a fairly consistent part of life for a long period of time. Thyroid problems, usually low thyroid production, can also interfere with ovulation, as can some medications, such as the tranquilizers Stelazine and Thorazine.

If ovulation occurs only 2 or 3 times each year rather than 12 or 13 times, it is obvious that fertility will suffer. Treatment to induce ovulation is essential for women who do not ovulate at all, and is also used to insure that ovulation occurs at reasonable intervals and at a predictable time.

Ovulation is essential for pregnancy. During the preovulatory maturation phase, the egg destined for release undergoes its final steps in maturation, neighboring cells form a fluid-filled cyst to surround it, and biochemical changes in the egg's surface prepare it to fuse with a sperm. If hormone preparations for ovulation fail to occur, eggs will remain dormant, or perhaps begin to mature but then stop maturing before the necessary changes are completed.

An immature egg is not capable of fertilization or subsequent normal embryo development. Even if egg maturation occurs, however, hormone abnormalities can also interfere with essential steps in the release of the egg, fertilization, and successful implantation in the uterine lining. **Unruptured follicle syndrome** is an example of such a problem. This term is used when ovulation patterns documented by a woman's temperature records and blood hormone levels appear normal, yet the egg follicle fails to release its egg. The problem might be suspected when ultrasound studies (sonar used to create a picture of the woman's ovaries) show persistence of the follicle cyst and no fluid release. One small study found ultrasound evidence of unruptured follicle syndrome in 9% of cases of unexplained infertility (14). Hormone treatment similar to that used for ovulation induction has been recommended for this extremely uncommon problem (15).

Excess Prolactin. Prolactin is the pituitary hormone responsible for breast milk production. When prolactin production by the pituitary gland is very high, ovulation is likely to be blocked altogether. A test for prolactin level is one of the first steps in fertility evaluation. Slight elevations in prolactin levels may occur without causing ovulation failure, but still interfere with fertility (16). Prolactin testing multiple times during the menstrual cycle may be necessary in order to find the small and temporary prolactin elevations involved. If no other cause for impaired fertility is found, multiple prolactin tests for this problem should be considered. Medication to lower prolactin levels is likely to be effective.

Luteal Phase Defect. Insufficient progesterone production by the ovary's corpus luteum after ovulation—in the cycle's luteal phase—is a fairly rare cause of infertility and/or repeated miscarriage. Normal progesterone patterns are essential in preparing the uterine lining for implantation and early embryo growth. **Inadequate luteal phase is diagnosed in less than 5% of women with impaired fertility** (2). In some cases the length of the postovulatory phase is shortened, and in some cases the normal 13- to 14-day length is maintained but the level of progesterone is lower than normal. This problem may be suspected if the time between ovulation and the following menstrual period is 11 days or less, or when endometrial biopsy shows that actual maturation of the uterine lining is 2 days or more behind the expected pattern for that cycle. Progesterone hormone levels that are low during the time of expected peak production may also suggest impaired corpus luteum performance.

This problem is often corrected by the same techniques used for ovulation induction. Alternatively, treatment with progesterone hormone injections or suppositories may be recommended.

Inadequate Cervical Mucus.   Copious, slippery cervical mucus is essential for sperm to be able to traverse the inch-long cervical canal. Cervical mucus problems can be caused by infection, antibodies, hormone abnormalities, or an insufficient amount of cervical gland tissue. Mucus production by the tiny glands that line the cervical canal is a direct response to estrogen stimulation. Peak estrogen levels occur just before ovulation, and are responsible for the profuse mucus secretion that facilitates sperm migration into and through the cervical canal. Mucus production at other times in the cycle, when estrogen levels are lower, is greatly reduced, and the canal secretions are likely to be thick and relatively impermeable to sperm. Even if impaired cervical mucus production is caused by some other problem, hormone treatment to improve it may be suggested. Ovulation induction treatment may also help correct mucus problems, or in some cases, cause mucus problems.

Toxic Chemicals and Drugs.   For men, exposure to drugs and toxic chemicals can directly affect ongoing sperm production, and hence can be a significant factor in fertility. For women, exposure to drugs and chemicals significantly impacts a fetus during pregnancy, but toxic exposure is less clearly understood as a factor in impaired fertility. A woman's eggs are already formed and dormant, so unless the toxic substance affects hormone patterns and ovulation, it may be less likely to reduce her likelihood of conception. Read Chapter 9 for more information on toxic exposure and its relation to fertility and pregnancy outcome.

VAGINAL, CERVICAL, AND UTERINE PROBLEMS

Structural abnormalities, such as a double uterus, partially divided uterus, or a vaginal septum (a thin membrane dividing the vagina in half), could interfere with contact between the sperm and egg or with implantation of the embryo. These problems are quite rare, and can often be surgically corrected.

Normal variations in size and position of the uterus are extremely unlikely to be a cause of infertility. A uterus that angles backward in the pelvis—called a retroflexed or tipped uterus—or one that is small, is almost certain to be entirely normal, and should function fine for purposes of conception and pregnancy. Terms like "juvenile uterus" or "infantile uterus" are not meaningful diagnostic categories: normal uteri come in a range of sizes, including quite small.

Structural abnormalities caused by trauma, infection, or gynecologic disorders are more common than congenital ones, and are found in approximately 15% of couples who have fertility problems. The normal female reproductive system is shown in Illustration 10-4. Fibroid tumors (leiomyoma) in the uterine wall, for example, can interfere with implantation and result in apparent infertility or repeated early miscarriage. The abnormal bleeding sometimes caused by fibroids and uterine polyps

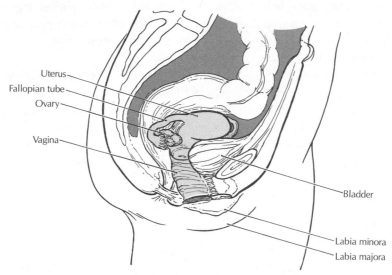

Uterus
Fallopian tube
Ovary

Vagina

Bladder

Labia minora
Labia majora

ILLUSTRATION 10-4   Normal reproductive function depends on the reproductive organs, plus normal thyroid and adrenal hormone production and precise cyclic regulation by the pituitary gland and hypothalamic centers in the brain.

probably also interferes with fertility. **Scar tissue**—called adhesions or synechiae—inside the uterine cavity or in the cervical canal can also impair fertility.

Damage to the cervical canal or to the mucus glands that line it can severely reduce normal mucus production and thus affect fertility. **Surgical treatment involving the cervix such as cone biopsy** for precancerous cell changes or cancer can cause severe narrowing or stenosis of the canal and loss of mucus function, as can damage during childbirth. Laser cautery or freezing (cryosurgery) for cervical disorders can also cause this problem.

Active infection involving the cervix can affect mucus production at the time and may cause permanent damage to the glands. Cervical mucus is also a site for immunologic and chemical problems. **Antibodies** against sperm are present in the cervical mucus of some women, and can severely hamper sperm survival and motility. The **acidity of cervical mucus** is also important to sperm survival. Vaginal secretions are normally too acid for sperm to survive; abundant, less acid, cervical mucus is essential as a safe haven. In rare cases, a woman's cervical mucus is too acid for sperm survival.

Cervical Incompetence.   A birth defect or trauma to the cervix during previous surgery or full-term delivery may result in premature dilation of the cervical canal and miscarriage. The normal cervix is buttressed by strong muscular and fibrous tissue that remains firmly closed until the forceful contractions of labor are underway. An incompetent cervix dilates with minimal force, painlessly, without obvious uterine contractions. Typically, an incompetent cervix causes fairly late miscarriage, often in the second or even third trimester. Once cervical dilation occurs, rupture of the amniotic membranes follows and labor is triggered.

If cervical incompetence is suspected because of previous late miscarriage or your gynecologic history, then careful monitoring will be recommended in early pregnancy. **Ultrasound can be used to detect early warning signs of cervical changes.** Miscarriage can often be prevented by placement of a strong suture around the cervix to hold it closed until the end of a pregnancy. This procedure is called cerclage and is usually delayed until ultrasound shows normal fetal development at about 12 weeks of pregnancy.

FALLOPIAN TUBE DAMAGE

For approximately 20% of couples with fertility problems, damage to the fallopian tubes is a primary or contributing factor. The tubes provide the pathway between the ovary and the uterus. Sperm must travel through a tube to meet the egg just inside the open end of the tube, and the newly forming embryo makes the return trip down the tube to reach the uterine cavity. In addition to a pathway, **the fallopian tubes provide an environment essential for sperm function and for early embryo development.** The tubes are lined with cells that secrete mucus and fluid, and with ciliated cells whose microscopic projections (cilia) wave to create a constant current in the tubular fluid.

Damage to the fallopian tubes that blocks the ends of the tubes or completely obstructs them is a clear cause of infertility. **Severe pelvic inflammatory disease, adhesions, endometriosis, and surgery to remove an ectopic (tubal) pregnancy are quite common causes of blocked tubes.** (See Chapter 25 for more on pelvic inflammatory disease.)

Damage to the inner structure or function of the tube lining cells can also result in infertility, even if the pathway is not completely blocked. This is the reason that surgery to repair damaged tubes is not uniformly successful. It may be possible to create an open pathway, but there are no current techniques to restore normal tube lining cells once they are lost. Illustration 10-5 shows normal and damaged fallopian tube linings.

ENDOMETRIOSIS

Endometriosis means growth of endometrial tissue outside the uterine cavity. Endometrial cells respond to normal hormone patterns with monthly growth and then shedding or bleeding, no matter where they are located. In endometriosis, one or more patches or implants of endometrial tissue are found on the fallopian tubes, ovaries, outer surface of the uterus, bladder, bowel, or peritoneal lining. Depending on the size and location of the implants, the monthly bleeding that occurs may cause no symptoms at all or may cause pain, abnormal bleeding, scar tissue, and infertility.

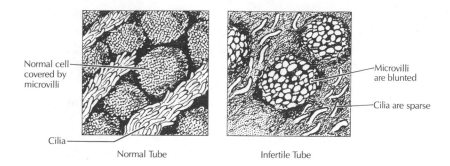

Normal cell covered by microvilli

Microvilli are blunted

Cilia are sparse

Cilia

Normal Tube   Infertile Tube

ILLUSTRATION 10-5 Mucus-producing cells, responsible for creating a constant gentle current inside the fallopian tube, can be permanently destroyed by infection. Without them, normal tube function is lost and the woman may be unable to conceive even though the tube pathway is open.

When endometriosis is severe, large blood-filled cysts and extensive scar tissue may completely block the area around one or both ovaries and/or fallopian tubes. Mechanical obstruction by endometriosis is a clear cause of infertility. Many experts believe, however, that **fertility may be impaired by endometriosis even if it is not extensive** and the pathways are open (2). Blood, white blood cells, and scavenger macrophages associated with endometriosis patches could affect sperm or an egg directly, or biochemically active substances such as prostaglandin hormones released by endometriosis tissue could affect the function of the tubes or developing follicle in the ovary. Treatment for endometriosis may involve surgery and/or hormones to suppress growth of the implants and is described later in this chapter. Further information on the causes, symptoms, and management of endometriosis is presented in Chapter 36.

IMMUNOLOGIC PROBLEMS

Antibodies are a normal part of the body's defense system. The immune system identifies foreign invaders such as bacteria, and forms antibodies coded to the specific culprit. Antibodies coat the invader and mark it for attack by white blood cells and other infection fighters.

Fertility problems are caused by antibodies against sperm in less than 5% of couples. **Both men and women can produce antisperm antibodies,** and in either case the antibodies can severely impair sperm function. Antibodies coating sperm cells interfere with their motility and forward progress; they also may block the sperm's ability to fuse with and fertilize the egg. Women with antisperm antibodies are also more likely to have early miscarriages.

Successful pregnancy is a fairly complex undertaking for the woman's immunologic system. Her body must recognize both sperm and embryo as immunologically foreign ("not me") but *okay,* and arrange for suppression of her normal body defenses that would attack any other "not me" invader. There is some evidence that men and women who are very similar immunologically (have high histocompatibility) may have problems with failure of this suppression system. Possibly the woman's body is less able to make the initial "not me" identification of sperm and/or embryo, and so fails to suppress later defenses.

In normal circumstances sperm do not actually enter the woman's body tissues at all, but trauma during intercourse or other factors may alert her immunologic defenses and trigger antibody production. In some cases the woman produces antibodies to all sperm; in other cases the reaction is limited to sperm from one specific partner. Antibodies may be present in the woman's bloodstream and/or in her cervical mucus.

Some men develop antibodies against their own sperm, particularly after vasectomy. Infection and trauma may also be causal factors when this problem occurs.

Treatment of antibody-related fertility problems may involve placement of washed semen inside the woman's uterus to bypass cervical mucus antibodies or donor insemination. Treatment to reduce antibody production such as with cortisone or intentional immunization with sperm has also been tried on an experimental basis.

DES (DIETHYLSTILBESTROL) EXPOSURE

Between 1940 and 1971 DES was used during pregnancy in the (incorrect) belief that this hormone could prevent miscarriage. Depending on when in pregnancy the DES treatment was begun, DES daughters and sons may have structural abnormalities in the reproductive organs that affect fertility. DES daughters also have an increased risk for vaginal cancer and for cervical cancer, which potentially impair fertility. For DES sons, an increased incidence of testicular abnormalities, reduced sperm count and percentage of normal sperm shapes, and impaired motility have been documented (17).

Not all DES offspring experience problems, and not all fertility problems they have are caused by DES. Further information on the special problems DES offspring face, and recommendations for medical surveillance, are presented in Chapter 42.

REPEATED MISCARRIAGE

Repeated loss of pregnancy because of miscarriage is a special category of impaired fertility. For the couple, this problem is often more stressful than other fertility problems because the elation of early pregnancy is followed by loss and grieving. For the clinician, the fact that conception occurred is very reassuring; chances for subsequent successful pregnancy even after several miscarriages are high. Your clinician will probably use the term spontaneous abortion to describe miscarriage.

Spontaneous miscarriage is extremely common. If very early miscarriages are counted, then the "normal" rate for miscarriage is probably close to 50% (2). Most

TABLE 10-5
RISK OF SPONTANEOUS PREGNANCY LOSS

NUMBER OF PREVIOUS MISCARRIAGES	RISK OF LOSS IN THE NEXT PREGNANCY (% MISCARRIAGES)
0	12
1	24
2	26
3	32
4	26

SOURCE: Keller DW, Strickler RC, Warren JC: *Clinical Infertility*. Norwalk: Appleton-Century-Crofts, 1984. Keller's data are drawn from Warburton and Fraser's work on miscarriage risk, which is cited in Keller's text.

women are not aware of pregnancy until two or three weeks after conception when pregnancy symptoms begin and the expected menstrual period is delayed, so the very common early losses are never even recognized. Most of them simply seem like periods that are a little late or a little heavy. The typical "normal" rate cited for miscarriage is about 15%, the rate for loss between 4 and 20 weeks of pregnancy. Because spontaneous loss is so common, most clinicians would reassure a couple following one or two miscarriages. The statistical probability is that no significant medical problem is involved. Data for pregnancy outcome following previous miscarriage support this conclusion (see Table 10-5).

Evaluation for possible medical causes of miscarriage is usually recommended for a couple when three or more miscarriages have occurred. Some of the problems already discussed in this section can cause repeated miscarriage, such as structural abnormalities of the uterus, cervix, or vagina; structural damage from infection, fibroid tumors, or endometriosis; abnormal thyroid or progesterone hormone levels; toxic exposure; and antibody problems. Other possible causes are considered in the following paragraphs.

Chromosome and Genetic Abnormalities.   Researchers believe that chromosome and gene abnormalities are a very common cause of miscarriage. In many cases, the abnormal chromosomes originate from just the single egg or the sperm that fused to begin the pregnancy. Perhaps one or more chromosomes accidentally were omitted or duplicated as that specific egg or sperm was formed. In this case, all the other eggs or sperm that each partner produces may be entirely normal.

Alternatively, the woman or the man may be a carrier for one or more chromosome problems. Each body cell contains 23 pairs of chromosomes. An abnormality in one chromosome is quite likely to be masked if the other member of that pair is normal. So a woman or a man could "carry" an abnormal chromosome with absolutely no evidence of any problem. When germ cells are formed, however, each one—whether egg or sperm—receives just one chromosome from each pair. Half of the eggs or sperm, therefore, would be normal, the other half abnormal.

Detectable chromosome abnormalities are found in about 10% of couples who have two or more miscarriages when chromosome analysis (karyotyping) is performed on a blood specimen from each partner. Even if chromosome abnormalities are found, subsequent normal pregnancy may be possible. If pregnancy does occur, however, prenatal genetic testing should be considered to look for detectable genetic or chromosomal abnormalities in the fetus. If the male is found to have chromosome abnormalities, donor insemination is a possible choice, as would egg donation if the female is affected.

Mycoplasma Infection.   Infection with mycoplasma organisms may be a silent cause of infertility or of early miscarriage. Mycoplasma organisms can be sexually transmitted and can be present in a woman's cervix or uterus without causing symptoms the woman would be likely to notice. If cultures of the man's urethra or woman's cervix confirm the presence of mycoplasma, then treatment with antibiotics such as doxycycline and/or erythromycin is indicated. Studies of pregnancy outcome after treatment for mycoplasma have shown excellent improvement (18).

How to Increase Your Chances of Pregnancy

If you don't fit any of the categories described at the beginning of this chapter in the section "When to Seek Medical Help," you might first try some of the following suggestions on your own. Many fertility experts agree with Masters and Johnson that leading causes of fertility problems are not having intercourse often enough, and/or not having intercourse at the right time in your menstrual cycle.

• Keep a careful record of your menstrual cycles. Use your menstrual records, basal body temperature, cervical mucus (see Chapter 6), and LH monitoring kit to pinpoint your ovulation time as accurately as possible. Watch especially for the low/high biphasic pattern in your basal body temperature to be certain that you are ovulating.
• Avoid douching, and do not use lubricants on or before your fertile days. Lubricants can kill sperm. Don't even douche with plain water before or after intercourse. And, of course, don't use contraceptive products. Spermicidal cream or jelly used for lubrication also greatly reduces the chance of pregnancy.
• Have intercourse once every 24 to 36 hours during your fertile days. At a minimum, begin with intercourse three days before the earliest day that your ovulation might occur. You will need to use calendar calculations to know when to begin. Continue having intercourse once every 24 to 36 hours until the rise in your basal temperature and mucus signs show that ovulation has occurred.

- Use the "missionary" position, lying on your back with your partner above, for intercourse on fertile days if your uterus angles toward the front of your body (anteverted), as it does in 70% of women. If your uterus is angled toward your back (retroverted) lying on your stomach may be a better position for conception; you can check with your clinician or a fertility specialist.
- After intercourse lie still for at least 20 minutes, or an hour if possible. Your goal is to insure that the pool of semen in your vagina stays in contact with the opening of your cervix for a reasonable period of time.

  What is a reasonable period of time? There is no scientific research to answer the question. Sperm may enter the cervical canal and even reach the uterus and tubes within minutes. However, the sperm pool in the vagina initially coagulates and then liquefies after 20 minutes or so. It seems reasonable to allow time for sperm to reach the cervix whenever this is feasible. If your schedule permits only a few minutes of lying still, so be it. Intercourse is more important than the lying still part.
- Put a pillow under your hips during and after intercourse to help semen stay in the back part of your vagina
- When your partner is about to ejaculate, he should stop thrusting and penetrate as deeply as he can so that semen is deposited deep in your vagina. Most of the sperm are in the first few ejaculated drops. Immediately after ejaculation, your partner should withdraw his penis slowly and carefully.

Male ejaculation is essential for fertility. Conception can occur without female orgasm, but no one knows what role female orgasm may play in enhancing the likelihood of pregnancy.

How Your Clinician Can Help

It wasn't easy, saying it out loud for the first time. "We can't get pregnant." At the doctor's office I grabbed Ray's hand and his was as clammy as mine!

—WOMAN, 33

Your own clinician may be able to evaluate your fertility problem, or you and your partner may be referred to a fertility specialist. Your evaluation will begin with a complete medical, sexual, and social history for you and for your partner. Be prepared to answer many detailed and personal questions; your clinician will need to know, for example, your intercourse frequency and the positions and sexual techniques you use. Thorough physical exams for you and perhaps your partner, and a pelvic exam for you are likely to be next. Your clinician may refer your partner to an internist or urologist for his exam. After that, you and your clinician can plan for the tests that will be needed to determine the cause or causes of impaired fertility in your particular case.

Throughout your evaluation, your clinician will be looking for problems that might impair these essential components of fertility:

- **Adequate sperm** production and semen delivery (impaired for 40% of couples who seek fertility evaluation)
- **Regularly occurring ovulation** (impaired for 20%)
- **A functional pathway** through the cervix, uterus, and fallopian tubes and a uterine environment able to sustain embryo implantation and growth (impaired for 30%)
- **Intercourse frequency** and timing that allows an opportunity for conception (impaired for many couples, percentage unknown)
- **Cervical mucus** that is adequate in amount and composition (impaired for less than 5%)
- **Adequate progesterone** production during the luteal phase, the 14 days after ovulation, of each cycle (impaired for less than 5%)
- **Reproductive tracts for both partners that are free of infection** or immunologic problems, and are supported by normal overall nutritional and health status (impaired in less than 5%)

Multiple fertility problems are often identified, so the percentages above total more than 100%. For about 5% to 10% of couples studied, no specific cause of infertility can be found; as yet unknown causes of fertility impairment may be involved, or they may not really have impaired fertility.

STEPS IN FERTILITY EVALUATION

The first ten steps in fertility evaluation can be completed within four to six weeks.

Your evaluation, of course, is entirely elective. No medical emergency exists, so you and your partner should be the ones to decide when and how aggressively you want to work on this issue. **There is no medical reason, however, to prolong the evaluation process beyond a few weeks.**

If a clear problem such as absent ovulation is found in the early steps of evaluation, your clinician may recommend treatment for that problem for three to six months before proceeding with further testing. If pregnancy occurs, the problem is solved. If pregnancy does not occur, though, you will need to return to the evaluation process.

If you do not have an obvious problem for preliminary treatment, and want answers with the least delay and minimum number of visits to your clinician, you will need to understand and follow through on the proper scheduling for your visits and tests. **Results of the tests are meaningful only if they are done at the correct time in the menstrual cycle.** Time intervals for testing are shown in Table 10-6 for a typical couple starting the fertility evaluation process.

TABLE 10-6
TIMING FOR TEN INITIAL FERTILITY
EVALUATION PROCEDURES

Any time	• Initial visit for **history and physical exam; infection tests** done at this time
Menstrual bleeding	• Begin recording temperatures on **bbt chart** • Have **semen analysis**; remember to avoid ejaculation for 2 days prior to semen test • Call to schedule hysterosalpingography and postcoital test
After bleeding stops but before ovulation	• Have **hysterosalpingography** during this interval • Remember to avoid intercourse or ejaculation for 2 days prior to postcoital test; normally these would be excellent intercourse days since the likelihood of conception is quite high
Ovulation day or the day before	• These are ideal days for **postcoital test**; if you cannot predict when ovulation will occur, make a guess (on the early side) and have your test anyway. It can be repeated every other day until ovulation signs are clear.
5 to 10 days after ovulation	• Blood test for **progesterone** should be done during this interval; *prolactin*, TSH, and T_4 are tested at the same time
11 to 13 days after ovulation	• **Endometrial biopsy** should be done during this interval

After the initial evaluation is completed you may need additional tests to pinpoint the cause of a problem discovered, or to assess the extent of the problem and the best approach for treatment. Often, though, treatment can be started in the meantime.

Fertility Testing Procedures

SEMEN ANALYSIS

They sent me down the hall to the bathroom with a jar. Not even the Dallas Cheerleaders would have made that any easier!

—MAN, 29

Semen analysis is a standard step in every fertility evaluation, even if the man involved has fathered previous pregnancies. It should be repeated periodically throughout evaluation and treatment to make sure that no new problems have arisen.

Your partner will collect an entire ejaculate in a clean, dry container and take it to the laboratory within 30 to 60 minutes. Ideally, the specimen should be collected by masturbation without any lubrication, at or near the laboratory, after 48 hours of no ejaculation. The specimen must be kept at body temperature, protected from temperature extremes, until the laboratory exam is done. If masturbation is not successful, a special sheath can be used during intercourse to collect the specimen. Regular contraceptive condoms are not satisfactory because they may have a deleterious effect on sperm. Using withdrawal during intercourse is also unsatisfactory: the first few drops of semen released are often lost, and they may contain the highest concentration of sperm.

In routine semen evaluation, the semen volume and thickness will be measured, and a sample will be examined under a microscope to determine the sperm count, the percent of sperm that are moving (motility), and the percent of sperm that are normal in shape (morphology). A normal semen specimen will total about 1/2 teaspoon (2 cc) or more. At least 60% of the sperm should be actively moving, and at least 60% should be normal in shape. Normal ranges for sperm count are more controversial. Overall sperm counts for normal men can be as high as 100 to 200 million per cc. Men who have consistent counts of at least 20 million sperm, however, may have normal fertility (2). Counts below 10 to 20 million are likely to be associated with abnormal motility and shape, and reduced fertility.

If the initial semen evaluation is poor or borderline, it should be repeated. Poor results that persist more than ten weeks indicate that the problem is not a temporary reaction to flu or life events. Because there is considerable variation in sperm measurements from one week to the next, some researchers suggest making a final determination based on three separate semen samples each two weeks apart for a reliable profile (19).

Routine semen evaluation should also check for white blood cells in semen and for abnormal motility patterns or sperm clumping that might indicate sperm antibody problems or infection. Semen normally coagulates into a thick lump soon after ejaculation, and then liquefies 15 to 20 minutes later. Failure to liquefy properly, with persistent thick or coagulated semen, should also be obvious at the time semen analysis is attempted.

New, more sophisticated techniques for semen analysis can be used to obtain greater precision in sperm evaluation. Using a video camera attached to a microscope, the number of sperm and percent that are motile can be counted accurately rather than estimated. Also, speed and direction of motility can be measured, and abnormal patterns of motility more easily identified. Sperm shape can also be plotted precisely (20). Certain sperm shape abnormalities such as long tapered heads and amorphous shapes may suggest that varicocele or the temporary stress of an illness with fever is causing the problem (21). Specialized tests such as the hamster egg penetrance assay may also help identify subtle sperm abnormalities.

BASAL BODY TEMPERATURE (BBT) CHARTS

Your clinician will ask you to record your bbt each day and will review your bbt charts with you to look for a clear low/high biphasic pattern that indicates ovulation. **You can begin charting your bbt even before you see your clinician to save time.** A clear low-then-high biphasic cycle pattern will demonstrate that you are ovulating and will help pinpoint the time of ovulation. (See Chapter 6 for complete charting instructions.) Illustration 10-6 shows a typical bbt chart for one cycle. Don't be surprised if your charts are a little hard to interpret. **Many women do not have an identifiable drop before ovulation, and the rise pattern may be gradual.** Some women with normal ovulation have no clear rise at all. If your bbt charts are not clear-cut, your clinician may recommend additional tests to find out for sure whether you are ovulating. Your clinician will ask you to record when you have intercourse so that you can determine whether you are timing intercourse correctly. Accurate bbt charts, even if they are confusing, are very important for any fertility evaluation and will also be needed later, during treatment.

POSTCOITAL TEST (HUHNER'S TEST)

A postcoital test evaluates a woman's cervical mucus by sampling a mucus specimen soon after intercourse at the time of ovulation to look for healthy, motile sperm in healthy cervical mucus. Although tricky to plan, it's a simple, quick procedure that provides essential information about both male and female fertility factors. Postcoital testing is a routine part of initial fertility evaluation.

For accurate results, **proper timing for this test is key.** If the test results are good, then there is no need to worry about it further. If the test results are borderline or poor, though, the problem may simply be improper timing. **Postcoital test results are quite likely to be poor for normal couples if the test is done too early or too late** in the woman's menstrual cycle.

The ideal time for cervical mucus evaluation is one, two, or three days before ovulation, and about two to eight hours after intercourse. Intercourse and ejaculation should be avoided for 24 to 48 hours prior to that time. Mucus collection is painless. Your clinician will use a narrow pipette (medical eyedropper) or thin plastic tubing to collect a few drops of mucus from your cervical canal and will examine your mucus under a microscope. She/he should be able to see adequate numbers of sperm in the mucus, and at least half the sperm should be moving actively.

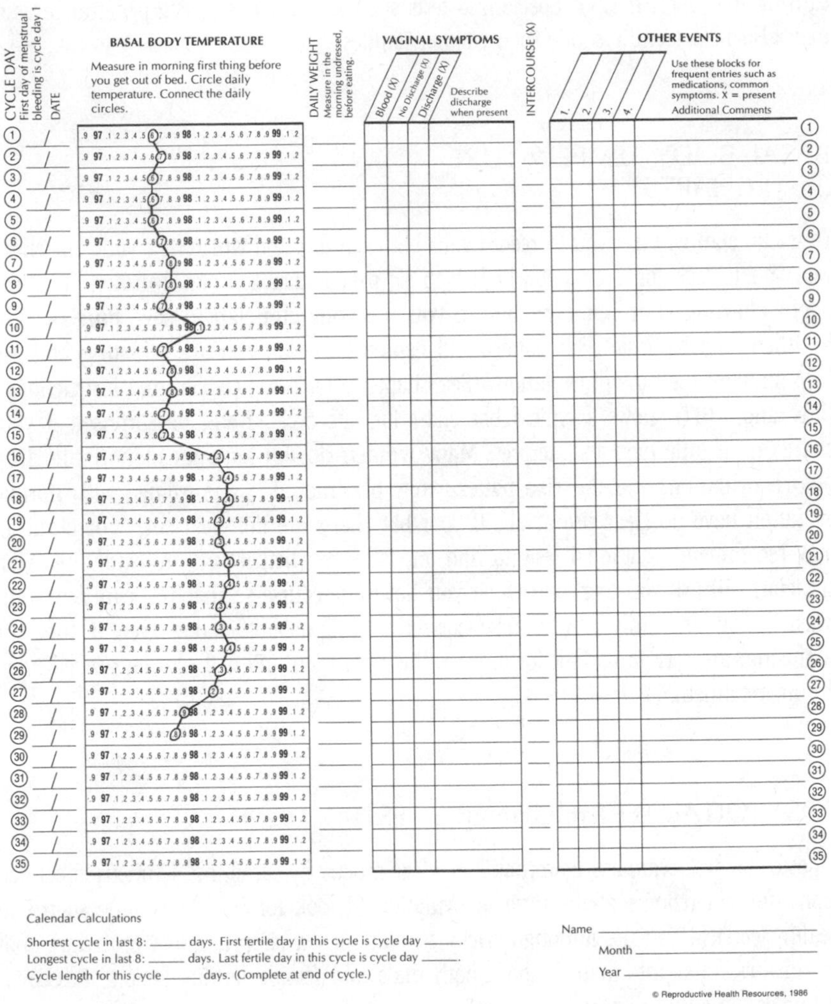

| CYCLE DAY First day of menstrual bleeding is cycle day 1 | DATE | BASAL BODY TEMPERATURE Measure in morning first thing before you get out of bed. Circle daily temperature. Connect the daily circles. | DAILY WEIGHT Measure in the morning undressed, before eating. | VAGINAL SYMPTOMS Blood (X) / No Discharge (√) / Discharge (X) / Describe discharge when present | INTERCOURSE (X) | OTHER EVENTS 1. 2. 3. 4. Use these blocks for frequent entries such as medications, common symptoms. X = present Additional Comments |

Calendar Calculations

Shortest cycle in last 8: _____ days. First fertile day in this cycle is cycle day _____.
Longest cycle in last 8: _____ days. Last fertile day in this cycle is cycle day _____.
Cycle length for this cycle _____ days. (Complete at end of cycle.)

Name _____
Month _____
Year _____

© Reproductive Health Resources, 1986

ILLUSTRATION 10-6   This woman has a fairly clear biphasic pattern, with a sustained rise beginning on her cycle day 16. She ovulated on day 15. Her temperature was a little high on day 10 because she did not wake up until 9:30 A.M., so this temperature is ignored.

Your clinician will also examine the consistency of your mucus, which should be abundant, thin, and slippery during your fertile days. Mucus should be clear and free of abnormal cells. Your clinician may measure the mucus's ability to stretch in a long thin strand, called **spinnbarkeit**, up to 3 inches or more in length. Good ovulatory mucus forms a crystalline ferning pattern as it dries on a microscope slide. If your mucus is scant, thick, and sticky, you may need more tests to be sure that you are ovulating and to find out when in your cycle ovulation is occurring. If your mucus is consistently poor, then you may need specific treatment for this problem.

If your cervical mucus contains no sperm, your clinician will examine a sample of vaginal secretions to see if sperm are present at all. Sperm in the vagina are not likely to be motile because the acidity of vaginal secretions is unfavorable for sperm survival. **If no sperm at all are present, though, then you and your partner may need help with intercourse technique, or your partner may need testing for retrograde ejaculation.**

When properly timed postcoital testing shows only a few sperm, or sperm that are not moving, then further evaluation will be needed. Just how many motile sperm should be present is quite controversial. **More than 20 active sperm in each microscope high-power view area is a clearly excellent test result. Some experts feel that even one or two active sperm should be considered a normal result** (2), while others would consider a count of five or less as abnormally low (21). Poor postcoital test results may occur because of low sperm count or motility, poor cervical mucus quality, or sperm antibody problems.

ENDOMETRIAL BIOPSY

A small shred of uterine lining (endometrium) can be examined by a pathologist to confirm that you are ovulating and to assess whether your cyclic uterine lining development pattern is normal. Your clinician will **schedule endometrial biopsy for the last few days of your cycle just before you expect your period.** Endometrial biopsy is usually part of an initial fertility evaluation, and is especially important if your bbt charts are not clear-cut or if the remainder of your fertility evaluation has been normal.

Endometrial biopsy is an office procedure. Most women find it slightly or moderately uncomfortable. To perform the biopsy your clinician will need to stabilize your cervix with a small clamp called a tenaculum and insert a slender tubular biopsy instrument though your cervical canal into your uterus. The sharp edge on the inner end of the biopsy instrument scrapes away a thin sliver of uterine lining tissue as it is gently withdrawn. Local anesthesia can reduce discomfort from the cervix, but crampy pain during and for a few minutes after biopsy is quite common. (See Chapter 4 for more information about this procedure.)

Since endometrial biopsy is done at the very end of a normal cycle just before your expected period, it is possible that conception has already occurred and the uterus contains a tiny growing embryo. The risk of disrupting a pregnancy is very low (2), and the correct timing in a menstrual cycle is essential for meaningful interpretation by the pathologist. Complications such as infection or uterine perforation are possible with endometrial biopsy, but are very rare. **Abdominal or lower back pain, fever, and excessive bleeding after this procedure are the danger signs of infection, and should be reported immediately to your clinician.** Temporary light bleeding, however, is not unusual.

TESTING FOR INFECTION

Tests to check for gonorrhea, chlamydia, and mycoplasma infections are often recommended early in fertility evaluation for both men and women. Testing is essential if white blood cells are found in semen or in cervical mucus, or if symptoms of infection such as abnormal discharge or pain are present. Specimens for these tests are obtained from the woman's cervix, and the man's urethral opening, with a sterile cotton swab. Massage of the prostate gland is sometimes helpful in obtaining a small drop of prostatic fluid for culture; rectal cultures may also be recommended. Specimens are submitted to a laboratory for processing, and results are not available for several days.

MEASUREMENT OF HORMONE LEVELS

A blood test to measure your progesterone level, taken five to ten days after you think ovulation has occurred, helps your clinician confirm that ovulation did occur. A progesterone result of 5 ng/ml (nanograms per milliliter) or more substantiates ovulation. Your clinician may also want to verify that your progesterone **peak** is at least 10 ng/ml. Lower peak levels suggest that inadequate corpus luteum function may be a problem.

Prolactin, and the thyroid hormone T_4, and TSH (thyroid-stimulating hormone) are usually measured in the initial fertility evaluation as well. If you are having irregular menstrual periods, or ovulation failure is suspected, your clinician may need additional hormone test results to be certain that you don't have a serious underlying medical or hormone disorder.

HYSTEROSALPINGOGRAPHY

Hysterosalpingography is a procedure used to determine whether your fallopian tubes are blocked or scarred. **This test will be scheduled one or two days after the end of a menstrual period,** after you have stopped bleeding, but before ovulation. Either your physician or a radiologist (physician x-ray specialist) will perform the procedure in the x-ray department of a hospital or in a radiology facility. The radiologist will position you on a table, insert a small tube into your cervical canal, and inject x-ray dye through the tube into your uterus. The radiologist will watch the dye on the x-ray screen as it fills your uterus and moves out into your fallopian tubes. Abnormalities in the shape of your uterus or tubes will be apparent, and tubal obstruction will be evident as well. After several hours the dye should spread throughout the pelvis. **You may be asked to return for an additional x-ray several hours later or the next day** to check for scar tissue in your abdomen. A pocket of dye near the end of a tube may indicate obstruction or scar tissue near the ovaries.

Both oil-base and water-base x-ray dyes are commonly used for hysterosalpingography. Some fertility specialists recommend the use of Ethiodol, an oil-base dye, because women who have oil dye hysterosalpingography have slightly higher fertility during the next six months (2). Water-base dye, on the other hand, does not seem to increase fertility. Medical risks of hysterosalpingography with either type of dye are low. If modern x-ray techniques such as image intensification fluoroscopy are used and the minimum number of still films taken, the overall x-ray exposure should be reasonably low. Accidental dye injection into the bloodstream could potentially cause serious problems, but is extremely rare. Fluoroscopy allows the radiologist to see exactly where the dye is going. Dye that passes through a normal, open, fallopian tube and into the peritoneal cavity must be gradually absorbed by the body. Theoretically, the slower absorption of oil-base dye might affect the risk of scar tissue formation around spilled dye. Scar tissue formation from such a cause is rare (2).

A more serious issue with hysterosalpingography is infection risk. Manipulation of any kind involving the cervix and uterus increases the risk that infection may spread upward from the surface of the cervix and cervical canal into the uterus and fallopian tubes. If symptoms or physical exam suggests infection, then treatment to eradicate the infection should be initiated and hysterosalpingography delayed for at least two to three months. Hysterosalpingography should be skipped altogether and laparoscopy performed instead if there is a definite history of previous pelvic inflammatory disease (PID). You will want to avoid any risk of triggering a recurrence of your PID. And if there is any question of previous infection, your clinician will want to use water-base rather than oil-base dye, and prophylactic antibiotic treatment will be considered.

Expect some discomfort during hysterosalpingography. In most cases, however, local anesthesia is not needed. Your clinician may use a clamp on your cervix to hold it steady during the procedure, and the clamp may cause some cramps. Dye pressure in your uterus and tubes may cause pain as well.

Hysterosalpingographic assessment of tube obstruction is about 75% accurate (22). If the results aren't clear or if obstruction does seem to be causing your fertility problem, your clinician will probably recommend laparoscopy.

LAPAROSCOPY

Laparoscopy is a surgical procedure that permits your clinician to look through a lighted tube at your ovaries, tubes, uterus, peritoneal lining, adjacent bowel, and bladder. The laparoscope is inserted into the abdomen through a 1-inch incision just below your navel (see Chapter 48). General anesthesia is usually required, but recovery is rapid and overnight hospitalization is rarely necessary. Your fertility specialist will be able to see whether the outside of your fallopian tubes is scarred. She/he can inject dye during laparoscopy and watch the dye traverse your tubes and empty from their ends. Other abnormalities such as fibroid tumors in your uterine wall (leiomyoma) or endometriosis should also be apparent. Laparoscopy allows your surgeon to identify them and document their severity. If you do have tubal damage, your surgeon can assess whether surgical correction is likely to be successful.

Laparoscopy is recommended as part of the initial fertility evaluation instead of hysterosalpingography for a woman who has had previous pelvic inflammatory disease. Laparoscopy is also recommended if hysterosalpingography results suggest tubal damage, or when no cause for impaired fertility has been found.

Laparoscopy is categorized as major surgery because the laparoscopy instruments enter the woman's abdominal cavity. Risks with laparoscopy, however, are low. Internal bleeding, as well as damage to the bowel, bladder, or reproductive organs, is possible with this procedure, as are anesthesia complications. Risk statistics for laparoscopy are presented in Chapter 48.

HYSTEROSCOPY

Hysteroscopy is a procedure that permits your surgeon to examine the interior of the uterine cavity through a narrow lighted optical tube. The tube is inserted through the cervical canal up inside the uterus while you are positioned as for a pelvic examination. In most cases, general anesthesia will be recommended for this procedure, and it will be performed in a hospital operating room or outpatient surgical facility. Overnight hospitalization is not usually necessary. Your clinician may refer you to a specially trained gynecologist in your community or nearby for this procedure.

Hysteroscopy can be used to identify sources of abnormal uterine bleeding such as polyps, or for evaluation and/or removal of scar tissue or adhesions that are suspected as a cause of impaired fertility. Hysteroscopy is discussed in detail in Chapter 46.

ANTIBODY TESTING

If abnormal sperm motility patterns or poor postcoital test results suggest antibody problems, or if no other cause of fertility impairment is found, then testing for the presence of antisperm antibodies will be recommended. Antibody evaluation requires blood samples from both partners as well as samples of semen and of cervical mucus. Laboratory studies can identify and determine levels (called titers) for antisperm antibodies present in any of these specimens. Results for agglutinating, or clumping, antibodies and for immobilizing antibodies will be reported separately. Subsequent treatment options depend on the antibody level and the type of antibody present, as well as on the specific source of the antibodies.

MUCUS PENETRANCE TESTS

Microscopic study of the ability of sperm in a small semen sample to enter and swim through a drop of mucus on a microscope slide can be used to assess sperm function and/or the quality of a woman's midcycle fertile mucus. If sperm are being evaluated, then the test will be done with both the patient's semen and semen from a donor known to be fertile. Alternatively, cervical mucus from a woman known to be fertile can be used for comparison when the goal is to evaluate the woman's mucus.

HAMSTER EGG PENETRANCE ASSAY

For normal fertility sperm must be capable of **binding** to the protective layer around the egg and then **fusing** with the surface of the egg. Microscopic evaluation can identify abnormalities in sperm shape and motility, but cannot identify defects in binding and fusing ability. Your clinician may use terms such as **capacitation** or **acrosome reaction**, the chemical and structural changes essential for binding, fusing, and fertilization that sperm normally undergo after ejaculation. One technique to evaluate capacitation and acrosome function, hamster egg penetrance, is used by many fertility centers. Fresh hamster eggs, prepared by removing the surrounding "zona" layer, are exposed to human sperm. The percent of eggs penetrated by sperm being tested is compared to the percent penetrated by sperm from a donor known to be fertile. Penetrance scores of 10% or lower are predictive of continued fertility impairment. The test, however, is not foolproof. Low penetrance results are sometimes found for men with normal fertility.

DETECTING OVULATION

Bbt charts provide indirect evidence of ovulation. The sustained rise in temperature is caused by progesterone, and progesterone is produced only after ovulation occurs. Bbt charts are often difficult to interpret, however, and may not pinpoint the time of ovulation very precisely. Similarly, **blood tests for progesterone level can confirm that ovulation has occurred,** but do not show exactly when it was. Daily ultrasound measurements of ovarian follicles, and daily blood tests for luteinizing hormone (LH) level can be used to determine exactly when ovulation is occurring. Both of these, however, are cumbersome and expensive.

Urine LH tests are a good alternative. Approximately 24 to 30 hours before ovulation, a tremendous increase in LH secretion by the pituitary gland occurs. The level of LH present in the bloodstream rises immediately, and the level present in urine rises a few hours later. By testing one or more urine samples daily during the few days before ovulation is anticipated, **the precise timing of the LH rise** can usually be detected. Urine assay tests are now widely available through medical laboratories, and home test kits are available in drugstores for sale without prescription. Home kits are fairly expensive, but simple to use; each urine sample is tested by dipping a test strip into the urine and recording the change in color on the strip.

IF ALL YOUR TESTS ARE NORMAL

If fertility evaluation fails to identify the reason or reasons for your apparent infertility, try not to be discouraged. Be sure that your evaluation was thorough, and that each step was done correctly. Then breathe a sigh of relief and be patient. A recent study of "infertile" couples who had normal results for bbt charting, hysterosalpingography, postcoital test, and semen analysis found that 76% **became pregnant within two years and 87% within five years with no treatment at all.** For them, the time required to achieve pregnancy was longer than for "normal" couples, but the eventual success rate was excellent (23). Most infertility specialists would recommend laparoscopy as well as the basic tests used in this study, however. With laparoscopy included as part of a complete evaluation, less than 5% of couples are likely to face the frustrating diagnosis of "unexplained" infertility.

Treatment for Fertility Problems

When impaired fertility is the result of a male problem, there are four basic treatment options:

• Surgery or medical treatment to improve semen quality or semen delivery
• Artificial insemination
• In vitro fertilization and embryo transfer (IVF-ET)
• Gamete intrafallopian transfer (GIFT)

Artificial insemination using donor semen, AID, is the sole treatment possibility if sperm production is entirely absent. Many couples with other male problems also choose AID because success with achieving pregnancy is high, and does not involve lengthy medical intervention or waiting.

   When impaired fertility is the result of a female problem, there are six basic treatment options:

• Hormone treatment to induce ovulation and/or correct other hormone abnormalities
• Surgery to repair cervix, uterus, or fallopian tube structural problems or damage
• Surgery or medical treatment to control endometriosis
• Treatment to correct or circumvent cervical mucus problems
• In vitro fertilization and embryo transfer (IVF-ET)
• Gamete intrafallopian transfer (GIFT)

In addition to these treatment options, **alternative avenues to parenthood also deserve consideration.** For many couples adoption may be a more reasonable choice than a lengthy struggle with fertility treatment. These decisions involve intensely personal, and quite complex, ethical and practical issues. Don't be surprised if you and your partner find the decision-making process difficult. Alternative parenthood options and child-free living are discussed at the end of this chapter, along with suggestions for coping with the stress of fertility evaluation and treatment.

The goal of fertility treatment is to maximize all the components necessary for pregnancy. Even if there seems to be one primary problem in your case, it is reasonable to do whatever you can to improve any other problems as well.

Be sure to keep intercourse timing in mind throughout your treatment. Pregnancy is not likely, even for couples with normal fertility, if intercourse is infrequent. If you do not have intercourse during your most fertile days, one to three days before ovulation, in just about every cycle, then your chance of success is greatly reduced no matter how excellenttherest of your treatment is.

Also be sure that any infection problems you may have are promptly treated. Infection diagnosed in the initial part of your evaluation will presumably be treated. Infection can recur, however, either because of reinfection or because initial treatment fails to eradicate the organisms completely. Be sure to report any suspicious symptoms promptly to your clinician, and ask for testing and/or retreatment if you suspect for any reason that you may have a new problem.

The following sections describe possible medical and surgical treatments for male problems and female problems, artificial insemination, and in vitro fertilization.

IMPROVING SEMEN QUALITY AND SPERM PATHWAYS

Medical or surgical treatment may be of help for male problems caused by:

• Toxic effects of drugs, smoking, scrotal heat
• Tumor in the testicle or prostate gland
• Traumatic or surgical injury to the sperm pathways (including previous vasectomy)
• Varicocele
• Insufficient thyroid hormone
• Elevated prolactin levels
• Excessive adrenal gland activity
• Insufficient pituitary release of reproduction-stimulating hormone

Treatment for any of these problems will require patience. Even if treatment is entirely successful, the evidence of success will be delayed. New, **improved sperm cannot appear in the semen until about two to three months after treatment** has succeeded. This creates a problem for you and your clinician because you will not be able to tell right away whether your problem has been solved. It also means that pregnancy success is likely to be delayed 9 to 12 months or more—allowing time for your treatment, then three months for new sperm production, then a reasonable opportunity for conception to occur.

As an initial part of your treatment, your clinician will advise you to limit exposure to potentially sperm-toxic drugs and heat. Even if other obvious problems are present, this is a very good time to quit smoking, limit alcohol, and skip marijuana, hot tubs, and saunas. Also avoid prolonged use of a scrotal support or tight clothing, and consider using a cooling fiber pad for driving if your life involves more than a little time behind the wheel. If you are taking medications for a serious medical problem, consultation between your fertility clinician and your other clinician(s) may make it possible to change your drugs or dosage to minimize fertility side effects.

Surgical Repair of the Vas Deferens or Varicocele.   If surgery is necessary, your evaluation and treatment will probably be managed by a urologist. Ideally, microsurgical techniques should be used for repair of sperm pathways or for vasovasostomy (reconnection of the vas deferens after previous vasectomy). Success rates for creating an open pathway and proving the reappearance of sperm in semen after vasovasostomy are high—80% or better, but are probably somewhat lower if repair is attempted for infection damage. Success in achieving pregnancy, however, is not as good. Overall pregnancy rates of 50% to 65% are typical after vasovasostomy, although somewhat better success rates may be realistic if the previous vasectomy did not remove excessive vas tissue, and the interval between vasectomy and repair is not long.

Men who have undergone vasectomy, or have injury or infection causing vas blockage, often develop antisperm antibodies. Antibody production is likely to persist after repair surgery, and impairs fertility even if sperm production is resumed (24).

Vasovasostomy is likely to involve hospitalization and general anesthesia for surgery, although some surgeons do utilize local anesthesia and/or outpatient surgery facilities. The surgery itself may require several hours and postoperative rest is needed to facilitate the best possible healing. Activities will be restricted, and a suspensory support to immobilize the scrotum will be required for two weeks or so following surgery.

Surgery to repair varicocele is somewhat simpler. Through a small incision at the crease of the leg, the vein leading downward to the involved testicle is located and tied. One or both testicles may be involved. This surgery can be performed with either general or local anesthesia in a hospital or outpatient surgery facility.

Hormone Treatment for Men.   For hormone problems, a urologist with special interest in fertility or an endocrinologist (hormone specialist) would be appropriate referral choices. Treatment with thyroid hormone pills is successful in restoring semen quality for the very rare man who has definite thyroid deficiency. Adrenal hormone abnormalities will also require further evaluation, but are amenable to treatment.

Evaluation of excessive prolactin production by the pituitary gland will probably necessitate x-rays and possibly a CAT scan (computer assisted x-rays, called computerized axial tomography) of the skull to be certain that a pituitary gland tumor is not the culprit. Treatment with bromocriptine (Parlodel) is likely to be effective. Further information about this drug, including possible side effects, is presented later in this chapter. It is also used to achieve ovulation for women who have elevated prolactin levels.

Insufficient pituitary release of gonadotropins, the stimulating hormones that trigger and sustain normal testicular function in men, is a rare problem, but can be treated successfully in many cases. Frequent injections of stimulating hormones over a period of several years, however, may be necessary.

Empirical Treatment.   If no specific cause has been found for subfertile semen, and elimination of heat and toxic exposure has not been followed by improvement, then some clinicians would consider empirical treatment with stimulating hormones such as clomiphene, human menopausal gonadotropin (HMG), or human chorionic gonadotropin (HCG). If no improvement occurs, then treatment with testosterone would be tried (21).

The word "empirical" here means that no clear research evidence shows whether these treatments are more effective than a placebo. And since no specific problem has been identified, there is also no physical or chemical rationale for how the treatment might exert its effect. Other fertility experts oppose empirical treatment (2), and feel that the successes observed after empirical treatment would have occurred anyway. It also may be unfair to encourage couples to persist in lengthy treatment programs with no definite reason to expect success. Alternatives such as artificial insemination or adoption may be more reasonable.

TREATMENT TO INDUCE OVULATION

Medical treatment for women who do not ovulate at all, or ovulate infrequently, is usually quite straightforward, and very likely to be successful. The same treatment is also commonly used to correct inadequate luteal phase problems and cervical mucus problems. Once your clinician is sure that you don't have a pituitary gland tumor or an underlying serious medical disorder, and that your prolactin level is normal, then your treatment will probably begin with clomiphene.

I remember those weeks as a time of utter concentration on my ovaries, and ovaries are *very* strange objects for obsession! There's lots to pay attention to, though, to take those pills the right way.

—WOMAN, 36

Clomiphene Citrate (Clomid or Serophene) Treatment.   Clomiphene citrate is similar in structure to a synthetic estrogen, but has only very weak estrogen effects. It acts directly on the hormone regulatory process in the brain to cause increased pituitary hormone release, which in turn triggers ovulation.

Clomiphene treatment involves taking clomiphene tablets daily for five days beginning on day 2, 3, 4, or 5 of a menstrual cycle.

If you are not having menstrual periods, then oral progestin tablets such as Provera will be used to induce bleeding before your first treatment cycle. A typical treatment plan might begin with 10 mg of Provera daily for five days. Bleeding should start within a few days after your Provera is finished—no more than 14 days at the most. The first day of bleeding is counted as cycle day 1, and clomiphene is usually started on cycle day 5. If your initial Provera treatment fails to induce bleeding, then further evaluation will be necessary to determine the cause of your failure to bleed. Read Chapter 33 for more information about this problem.

Once your clomiphene treatment is successful in inducing ovulation, your own cycles will trigger menstrual flow each month, so you will not need further Provera treatment. Your initial dose of clomiphene is likely to be 50 mg daily; if your basal body temperature and/or serum progesterone level show that ovulation has not occurred, then the dose is increased to 100 mg, then 150 mg, and finally 200 mg daily. Provera treatment may be needed in between clomiphene courses as your dose is increased. You may fail to have menstrual bleeding until the clomiphene you are taking is sufficient to trigger ovulation. Lower doses of Clomid may also be an option, especially if your response to a standard 50-mg dose is excessive.

Your clinician will probably schedule you for an examination each month just before you begin the five-day clomiphene treatment to check for excessive stimulation of the ovaries and to be sure that you have not already conceived. **If your ovaries are tender or enlarged, then further treatment must be delayed** until they return to normal. This problem, called hyperstimulation, occurs in less than 1% of women undergoing ovulation induction with clomiphene. Table 10-7 summarizes side effects and possible complications of drugs used to induce ovulation. Side effects are not common and rarely are so severe that treatment must be stopped. **Vision problems—spots or flashes or blurred vision—are uncommon, but stop clomiphene and call your clinician if these symptoms occur.**

Clomiphene should not be used if a woman is allergic to the drug, or if menopause or premature menopause is the cause of her absent ovulation. This ovarian failure can be easily detected by a blood test for the pituitary hormone FSH. If the follicle-stimulating hormone level is 40 ng/ml or more, then ovarian failure is the problem. Also, you should not take clomiphene if you are already pregnant. There is no evidence that clomiphene taken during pregnancy causes fetal abnormalities in humans, but laboratory studies show that high doses given to animals during early pregnancy may cause fetal problems.

Chromosome abnormalities have also been found in human eggs obtained for study after clomiphene treatment. Whether or not similar chromosome abnormalities would also be found without clomiphene treatment, however, is not known. Researchers suspect that chromosome abnormalities are common in normal cycles as well, and are responsible for early pregnancy losses (miscarriages) that are also very common during the first few days and weeks of pregnancy (25).

Pregnancies conceived when ovulation is induced by clomiphene do not show an increased risk of congenital defects. **The frequency of twin pregnancy (5% to 10% of clomiphene pregnancies) is slightly higher than normal,** but multiple pregnancy (triplets, quadruplets, quintuplets) is rare (2).

Intercourse timing will be key while you are taking clomiphene. Ovulation should occur between five and ten days after your last clomiphene tablet. Your bbt chart will help you pinpoint the day. As you begin, assume that ovulation could be as early as five days after your last clomiphene dose. If you began clomiphene on cycle day 5, your ovulation day could be as early as day 14 or as late as day 23; most commonly it is day 17 or 18. **Begin having intercourse every 24 to 36 hours on day 11 and continue until you see a temperature shift** that shows you have ovulated. Illustration 10-7, a typical clomiphene cycle, indicates optimal timing for intercourse.

Clomiphene can restore normal fertility by inducing ovulation, but does not make women superfertile, so **treatment must be continued for a reasonable time to allow an opportunity for conception to occur.** Throughout treatment you will need to monitor your response to clomiphene to be sure that you are continuing to have ovulatory cycles consistently every month. Bbt charts, with serum progesterone tests one week after ovulation if charts are not clear, are the simplest ways to monitor for ovulation.

Overall, treatment of women who are appropriate candidates for clomiphene results in ovulation for 80% and pregnancy for 40%. For couples who have no other fertility problems besides failure to ovulate and who persist in their treatment, pregnancy rates are higher—up to 80% or more. As many as 55% to 75% may conceive in the first three successful treatment months. Treatment should be continued for at least six to nine months, and all other factors corrected. If no pregnancy has occurred at that time, then **further evaluation such as laparoscopy is reasonable** to identify unsuspected endometriosis or tubal damage, as is ultrasound after ovulation to identify the rare occurrence of the unruptured follicle syndrome.

From the patient's point of view, clomiphene treatment is fairly straightforward. Drug costs are likely to be $25 to $100 per month for the 5 to 20 clomiphene tablets required, and one office visit will be needed each month to check for excessive ovarian stimulation.

Human Menopausal Gonadotropin (Pergonal) Treatment. If clomiphene is not successful, then injections of Pergonal, a more potent hormone stimulator, may be a possibility. Pergonal should only be administered by an experienced specialist. You will need close medical supervision and frequent examinations while you are taking Pergonal. **The dose of Pergonal must be adjusted very precisely, on an individual basis,** to minimize the chance of multiple pregnancy and to avoid overstimulation of your ovaries, which could cause severe ovary swelling.

TABLE 10-7
POSSIBLE SIDE EFFECTS AND COMPLICATIONS OF DRUGS USED TO INDUCE OVULATION

CLOMIPHENE CITRATE (BRAND NAMES: CLOMID, SEROPHENE)

Significant side effects: Stop taking clomiphene if these symptoms occur:

Visual symptoms—blurring, spots, or flashes, or diminished vision
Excessive ovarian stimulation, swelling and severe pain

Other side effects:

Hot flushes	Weight gain
Abdominal discomfort	Dizziness
Abnormal vaginal bleeding	Frequent urination
Breast tenderness	Itching
Nausea or vomiting	Hair loss
Nervousness, insomnia	Abnormal liver function test results
Depression, fatigue	Twin pregnancy (10%)
Headache	Multiple pregnancy (1%)
	Inadequate luteal phase

All of clomiphene's side effects are believed to be reversible as soon as the medication is discontinued.

Contraindications: Do not take clomiphene if:

you suspect you are already pregnant
you have liver disease, or history of liver disease
you have abnormal vaginal bleeding, and its cause has not been determined

HUMAN MENOPAUSAL GONADOTROPIN (BRAND NAME: PERGONAL)

Significant side effects: Pergonal treatment must be stopped if these symptoms occur:

Severe ovary swelling
Fluid or bleeding inside the abdomen
Fluid in the lungs
Artery blood clots (stroke)
Inadequate luteal phase

Other side effects:

Twin pregnancy (20%)
Multiple pregnancy (5%)

Contraindications: Do not take Pergonal if:

you suspect you are already pregnant
you have abnormal vaginal bleeding, and its cause has not been determined
you have enlarged ovaries or ovarian cysts
you have a pituitary gland tumor
you have premature menopause
absent ovulation *is not your only fertility problem*

BROMOCRIPTINE MESYLATE (BRAND NAME: PARLODEL)

Side effects:

Nausea, vomiting	Nasal congestion
Headache	Constipation
Dizziness, lightheadedness	Diarrhea
Fatigue	Low blood pressure
Abdominal cramps	

Contraindications: Do not take Parlodel if:

you are allergic to Parlodel
you are allergic or sensitive to ergot drugs such as Hydergine

Warning: Bromocriptine can affect blood pressure, and possible vascular disease complications have been reported including stroke and heart attack. Whether these problems were caused by bromocriptine is not known. If you have high blood pressure or a history of serious heart or vascular disease, possible benefits and risks should be weighed carefully before treatment.

HUMAN CHORIONIC GONADOTROPIN (BRAND NAME: PROFASI)

Side effects:

Headache	Fluid retention: this may aggravate
Irritability	existing heart or kidney disease,
Restlessness	epilepsy, migraine, or asthma
Depression	Breast enlargement
Fatigue	Pain at the injection site

Contraindications: Do not take Profasi if:

you are allergic to human chorionic gonadotropin

SOURCES: FDA-approved product labeling. *Physicians' Desk Reference* (ed 40). Oradell, N.J.: Medical Economics Co., 1986. Drugs that induce ovulation. *Medical Letter* 27:82–84, 1985. Scialli AR: The reproductive toxicity of ovulation induction. *Fertility and Sterility* 45:315–323, 1986. Iffy L, TenHove W, Frisoli G: Acute myocardial infarction in the puerperium in patients receiving bromocriptine. *American Journal of Obstetrics and Gynecology* 155:371–372, 1986.

CYCLE DAY (First day of menstrual bleeding is cycle day 1)	DATE	BASAL BODY TEMPERATURE (Measure in morning first thing before you get out of bed. Circle daily temperature. Connect the daily circles.)	DAILY WEIGHT (Measure in the morning undressed, before eating.)	Blood (X)	No Discharge (X)	Discharge (X)	Describe discharge when present	INTERCOURSE (X)	1	2	3	4	OTHER EVENTS (Use these blocks for frequent entries such as medications, common symptoms. X = present / Additional Comments)
1	/	9 97 1 2 3 4 5 6 7 8 9 98 1 2 3 4 5 6 7 8 9 99 1 2		X									
2	/	9 97 1 2 3 4 5 6 7 8 9 98 1 2 3 4 5 6 7 8 9 99 1 2		X									
3	/	9 97 1 2 3 4 5 6 7 8 9 98 1 2 3 4 5 6 7 8 9 99 1 2		X									
4	/	9 97 1 2 3 4 5 6 7 8 9 98 1 2 3 4 5 6 7 8 9 99 1 2		X									
5	/	9 97 1 2 3 4 5 6 7 8 9 98 1 2 3 4 5 6 7 8 9 99 1 2		X									Clomid 50
6	/	9 97 1 2 3 4 5 6 7 8 9 98 1 2 3 4 5 6 7 8 9 99 1 2		X									Clomid 50
7	/	9 97 1 2 3 4 5 6 7 8 9 98 1 2 3 4 5 6 7 8 9 99 1 2		X									Clomid 50
8	/	9 97 1 2 3 4 5 6 7 8 9 98 1 2 3 4 5 6 7 8 9 99 1 2											Clomid 50
9	/	9 97 1 2 3 4 5 6 7 8 9 98 1 2 3 4 5 6 7 8 9 99 1 2											Clomid 50
10	/	9 97 1 2 3 4 5 6 7 8 9 98 1 2 3 4 5 6 7 8 9 99 1 2											
11	/	9 97 1 2 3 4 5 6 7 8 9 98 1 2 3 4 5 6 7 8 9 99 1 2											
12	/	9 97 1 2 3 4 5 6 7 8 9 98 1 2 3 4 5 6 7 8 9 99 1 2						X					
13	/	9 97 1 2 3 4 5 6 7 8 9 98 1 2 3 4 5 6 7 8 9 99 1 2						XX					
14	/	9 97 1 2 3 4 5 6 7 8 9 98 1 2 3 4 5 6 7 8 9 99 1 2											
15	/	9 97 1 2 3 4 5 6 7 8 9 98 1 2 3 4 5 6 7 8 9 99 1 2						X					
16	/	9 97 1 2 3 4 5 6 7 8 9 98 1 2 3 4 5 6 7 8 9 99 1 2						X					
17	/	9 97 1 2 3 4 5 6 7 8 9 98 1 2 3 4 5 6 7 8 9 99 1 2						X					
18	/	9 97 1 2 3 4 5 6 7 8 9 98 1 2 3 4 5 6 7 8 9 99 1 2											
19	/	9 97 1 2 3 4 5 6 7 8 9 98 1 2 3 4 5 6 7 8 9 99 1 2						X					
20	/	9 97 1 2 3 4 5 6 7 8 9 98 1 2 3 4 5 6 7 8 9 99 1 2						X					
21	/	9 97 1 2 3 4 5 6 7 8 9 98 1 2 3 4 5 6 7 8 9 99 1 2											
22	/	9 97 1 2 3 4 5 6 7 8 9 98 1 2 3 4 5 6 7 8 9 99 1 2											
23	/	9 97 1 2 3 4 5 6 7 8 9 98 1 2 3 4 5 6 7 8 9 99 1 2											
24	/	9 97 1 2 3 4 5 6 7 8 9 98 1 2 3 4 5 6 7 8 9 99 1 2											
25	/	9 97 1 2 3 4 5 6 7 8 9 98 1 2 3 4 5 6 7 8 9 99 1 2											
26	/	9 97 1 2 3 4 5 6 7 8 9 98 1 2 3 4 5 6 7 8 9 99 1 2											
27	/	9 97 1 2 3 4 5 6 7 8 9 98 1 2 3 4 5 6 7 8 9 99 1 2											
28	/	9 97 1 2 3 4 5 6 7 8 9 98 1 2 3 4 5 6 7 8 9 99 1 2											
29	/	9 97 1 2 3 4 5 6 7 8 9 98 1 2 3 4 5 6 7 8 9 99 1 2											
30	/	9 97 1 2 3 4 5 6 7 8 9 98 1 2 3 4 5 6 7 8 9 99 1 2											
31	/	9 97 1 2 3 4 5 6 7 8 9 98 1 2 3 4 5 6 7 8 9 99 1 2		X									
32	/	9 97 1 2 3 4 5 6 7 8 9 98 1 2 3 4 5 6 7 8 9 99 1 2											
33	/	9 97 1 2 3 4 5 6 7 8 9 98 1 2 3 4 5 6 7 8 9 99 1 2											
34	/	9 97 1 2 3 4 5 6 7 8 9 98 1 2 3 4 5 6 7 8 9 99 1 2											
35	/	9 97 1 2 3 4 5 6 7 8 9 98 1 2 3 4 5 6 7 8 9 99 1 2											

Calendar Calculations

Shortest cycle in last 8: _____ days. First fertile day in this cycle is cycle day _____.
Longest cycle in last 8: _____ days. Last fertile day in this cycle is cycle day _____.
Cycle length for this cycle _____ days. (Complete at end of cycle.)

Name _____
Month _____
Year _____

ILLUSTRATION 10-7 This woman took clomiphene tablets daily for five days beginning on her cycle day 5. Since this was her first cycle on clomiphene, she began having frequent intercourse on day 12, in case ovulation occurred as early as day 15. Her temperature shift on day 18 shows that she actually ovulated on day 17.

Pergonal treatment should not be used if menopause or premature menopause or a large pituitary tumor is the cause of infertility. If a couple has other fertility problems in addition to ovulation failure, then Pergonal treatment may not be a reasonable undertaking. Side effects and possible complications of Pergonal treatment are listed in Table 10-7. **Hyperstimulation is more common when Pergonal is used than it is with clomiphene.** Your clinician will probably use ultrasound measurements of the developing follicles in your ovaries and frequent serum estrogen determinations to find the optimal dose for your Pergonal treatment, and to reduce the risk of hyperstimulation.

Ultrasound and estrogen levels can also help in assessing the maturity of your follicles and ovulation timing. In some cases an injection of human chorionic gonadotropin (HCG) is used to induce final egg maturation and ovulation. Ovulation will occur approximately 36 hours after HCG injection. **Plan for intercourse one to two days before ovulation.** Your clinician can help determine optimal timing for you.

Pergonal successfully induces ovulation for 90% of women treated, and 50% to 70% will become pregnant. Rates for multiple pregnancy are high, however, and cause significant pregnancy loss because of very premature birth. **Rates for twins as high as 20% and for triplets as high as 5% have been reported.** Improved treatment monitoring with ultrasound and measurement of estrogen levels may reduce this risk somewhat.

Pergonal treatment is an arduous and expensive undertaking. Multiple office visits, ultrasound exams, and blood tests will be required during each treatment cycle. The drug itself is expensive: treatment for one cycle may require 12 to 36 ampules of Pergonal at $30 or more each. The overall cost for one cycle may be $1,000 to $2,000 or more.

Combination treatment regimens, using clomiphene along with human chorionic gonadotropin and/or Pergonal, are being used more and more. Women who do not respond well to clomiphene alone may respond to a combination that employs HCG to trigger final maturation or low doses of Pergonal to boost the response just a little.

Gonadotropin-Releasing Hormone Pump.   For women who fail to ovulate with clomiphene treatment, the newly developed gonadotropin-releasing hormone (GnRH) pump may be an alternative to Pergonal treatment. Tiny surges of GnRH hormone are normally released by the hypothalamic hormone centers in the brain every few minutes throughout the day and night. These surges are necessary for normal production of the pituitary hormones that govern ovulation. The GnRH pump, about the size of a small portable radio, provides similar bursts of hormone every 90 minutes through a tiny plastic catheter placed just under the skin. During treatment, the woman carries the portable medication pump attached to her catheter with her throughout her normal activities. Initial reports on the use of GnRH pumps are encouraging: overall, ovulation was restored in 83% of treatment cycles and pregnancy occurred in 54% (26).

Bromocriptine (Parlodel).   When suppression of ovulation is caused by elevated prolactin levels, treatment with Parlodel is highly effective in restoring fertility. Parlodel directly inhibits secretion of prolactin by the pituitary. As the prolactin level returns to normal, the normal function of pituitary releasing hormones is restored and ovulatory cycles resume. Parlodel is quite likely to be effective in reducing prolactin levels even when a pituitary tumor is the cause of the problem, and the tumor is likely to shrink during treatment. If a tumor of 1 cm or more in diameter is present, however, pregnancy is not advisable. Pituitary tumor growth may be accelerated during pregnancy and might be dangerous to the woman. Her tumor should be treated with medication first, and pregnancy delayed until the problem is under control.

Parlodel treatment is likely to begin with one tablet (2.5 mg) daily, and then increase to two tablets daily after about a week. Side effects are common at the beginning of treatment, and even more gradual dose increases may be needed until tolerance is developed. Common side effects and possible complications are listed in Table 10-7. Some fertility experts recommend that Parlodel treatment be continued daily until pregnancy occurs; others recommend that treatment be stopped at ovulation each cycle and resumed when the next menstrual period begins. The latter approach is intended to avoid exposing an early pregnancy to the drug. No harmful fetal effects have been reported, however.

Prolactin release is likely to drop very quickly when the full Parlodel dose is reached. Ovulation resumes for at least 80% of patients, often within two months, and 75% of patients achieve pregnancy within six months. If ovulation has not resumed within two to three months, clomiphene treatment may be added while Parlodel is continued.

SURGICAL REPAIR OF THE UTERUS AND FALLOPIAN TUBES

The most common reason for a woman to consider fertility surgery is for repair of damage or obstruction caused by infection or endometriosis. Fibroid tumors in the uterine wall that interfere with implantation and congenital abnormalities in the shape of the uterus may also be reasons for surgery. Repair may also be considered for a woman who has previously undergone tubal sterilization surgery and wishes to have her fertility restored.

Surgical repair is sometimes carried out at the time of necessary surgery, to remove an ectopic pregnancy, for example. If the woman's medical condition permits, the additional anesthesia and surgery time required for repair of damage found incidentally during surgery may be reasonable. In most cases, however, repair surgery is elective. That is, the surgery will be planned in advance, and the decision to undergo surgery is entirely based on the patient's wishes.

Pelvic repair is major surgery. Hospitalization for several days and a recovery period of six weeks should be anticipated. A 4- to 5-inch abdominal incision will be required, and the surgery itself is likely to take several hours. Because surgery involves fairly lengthy anesthesia and surgical manipulations inside the abdominal cavity, complications are similar in kind and frequency to those experienced after hysterectomy or any other major abdominal procedure.

After pelvic repair surgery of any kind a woman faces a significantly higher risk of future ectopic pregnancy (see the section on ectopic pregnancy later in this chapter).

Clearly, your surgeon will not recommend pelvic repair surgery unless there is a reasonable chance that it will be successful in restoring fertility. You will almost

TABLE 10-8

TYPICAL REASONS FOR FERTILITY SURGERY

PROBLEM	% OF BLACK WOMEN	% OF WHITE WOMEN
Adhesions	44	22
Endometriosis	26	61
Reversal of previous tubal ligation	15	5
Uterine leiomyoma (fibroids)	12	3
Abnormal uterine shape	1	7
Other—includes repair or reconstruction of tubes	2	2

SOURCE: Buttram VC, Reiter RC: *Surgical Treatment of the Infertile Female*. Baltimore: Williams & Wilkins, 1985.

certainly need to undergo laparoscopy before a decision about repair surgery is made. With laparoscopy, your surgeon will be able to assess the extent and severity of damage, and give you some idea of how likely success would be with surgical repair. Also, evaluation of all other fertility factors should be completed prior to surgery. The presence of multiple factors may influence your decision about surgery. Surgery would not be recommended if you have any evidence of active infection.

Your surgeon's assessment of the extent of your damage and of the likelihood of success with repair are subjective. There are no fixed rules or quantitative tests that can be applied in making a decision for or against surgery. In general, success is most likely when the damage is not extensive, and there is a good portion of normal fallopian tube or tubes remaining. Success is least likely when damage is extensive, especially if the ends of the tubes near the ovary have been sealed shut and swollen by infection (hydrosalpinx) or by extensive endometriosis. Success rates with pregnancy following surgery have been as high as 77% when tubal damage is minimal and as low as 3% when damage is extensive (27).

The skill and experience of your surgeon also influence the likelihood that surgical repair will be successful. Be sure that the surgeon you select is someone who is trained in microsurgery techniques, and actually performs repair surgery on a regular basis. Microsurgery techniques involve the use of an operating microscope or magnification glasses, as well as very fine, small-scale surgical instruments and ultrathin suture material. Be sure your surgeon has the necessary equipment and skill available in the event that they are needed in your case.

Table 10-8 shows the reasons for fertility surgery among 968 patients at the Baylor School of Medicine. In each of these cases, surgery was presumably recommended on the basis of currently accepted subjective criteria for reasonable success, and the patient decided to go ahead with surgery. As you can see, endometriosis and removal of adhesions are both common reasons for fertility surgery. Surgery to repair or reconstruct the fallopian tubes is not common. Also, the reasons for surgery among black women differed significantly from those among white women.

Adhesions.   Often adhesions are the cause of obstruction, either alone or in combination with scarring from infection or endometriosis. **Adhesions are bands of scar tissue.** They can be very thin and filmy, like cobwebs, or quite thick and dense. Adhesion formation is part of the body's normal system of defense against infection or exposure to any irritating substance. The formation of adhesion tissue serves to wall off the offending intruder and to protect nearby structures from contact with it. The peritoneal lining that covers the inside of the abdomen and the abdominal surface of the bladder, uterus, and uterine ligaments is particularly prone to adhesion formation. Irritation from a previous attack of appendicitis or slight bleeding during previous surgery can trigger adhesion growth. So can pelvic infection and endometriosis.

Surgery to remove adhesions, **called lysis of adhesions or salpingolysis, is one of the more common kinds of fertility procedures.** If adhesions are removed that are holding the ovaries down against the pelvic walls and away from the tube openings, covering the surface of the ovaries or the tube openings, success in restoring fertility is quite likely. In some cases very thin adhesions can be removed during laparoscopy. For more extensive adhesions, however, standard pelvic surgery is required. Pregnancy rates reported after lysis of adhesions range from 30% to 50%; these rates also reflect the presence of additional underlying damage from infection or other disease that caused the adhesions to form.

Endometriosis.   Treatment of fertility problems caused by endometriosis may involve **surgery alone, hormone treatment alone, or a combination of both.** In choosing an optimal treatment plan, you and your clinician will consider how extensive the endometriosis is, as well as your age and your own preference for when pregnancy would ideally occur. If your endometriosis is minimal, you may not need any treatment at all.

Hormone treatment can be used prior to surgery to reduce the size of endometriosis patches and to reduce the local swelling and blood vessel buildup that occur in response to the patches. Surgery success after hormone treatment may be better than that of surgery used alone (28). On the other hand, hormone treatment will mean a delay of six months or so before surgery, and that delay may not be desirable, depending on the woman's age.

Hormone treatment is likely to involve suppression of menstrual cycles for six months or more with progestin or with danazol (Danocrine), a synthetic hormone that causes a marked reduction in estrogen levels. Danazol also has androgenic effects, and side effects are common. Most patients, however, are able to complete the full treatment course. **Both progestin and danazol are quite effective in stopping symptoms such as pain and abnormal bleeding** that are common among endometriosis sufferers. Another approach to hormone treatment, GnRH agonist, is also a possibility. This synthetic hormone is similar in structure to natural gonadotropin-releasing hormone (GnRH). It directly inhibits the release of pituitary hormones that are responsible for estrogen and progesterone production by the ovary. In effect, it induces temporary chemical menopause. Both of these approaches to hormone treatment are discussed more fully in Chapter 36. Hormone treatment alone may be quite successful if endometriosis is mild or moderate: pregnancy rates of 70% to 85% have been reported. A much lower rate, 35% to 40%, should be expected for severe endometriosis treated with hormone suppression alone, however (28). Also, later recurrence of endometriosis is quite likely.

The goal in conservative surgical treatment for endometriosis is to remove as much of the abnormal tissue as possible without risking damage to the organs involved, especially the bladder or bowel, and without creating bleeding or surgical trauma likely to cause adhesion formation afterward. In some cases, repair will involve removal of part or all of an ovary or tube if the endometriosis there is too advanced to repair. In conservative surgery, though, every effort will be made to leave both or at least one functioning ovary and tube in place, and the entire pelvis as free of endometriosis implants and damage as possible. This is time-consuming, meticulous surgery, and may require several hours in the operating room. Microsurgery techniques may also be involved.

After conservative surgery for endometriosis that is moderate to severe, pregnancy rates in the range of 40% to 60% are typically reported. Recurrence of endometriosis can occur after conservative surgery, and **approximately 25% of patients require another operation later for endometriosis problems** (21).

Tubal Reanastomosis and Tubal Repair.   Surgery to reverse previous tubal sterilization, **tubal reanastomosis, is reasonably successful when at least 5 cm of undamaged tube is available for the repair.** Assuming that the tubes are free of infection or damage other than previous sterilization surgery, and that the reanastomosis is carried out with microsurgery techniques in the middle portion of the tube, success in achieving pregnancy after repair may be as high as 60% to 75%. Somewhat lower success rates are reported for direct implantation of the tube into the uterine wall. If the remaining tube on either side of the previous surgery site totals 3 cm or less, repair will probably not be recommended, because success rates in this situation are low, and in vitro fertilization (see below) may be a more reasonable approach.

In some cases, surgical repair may be recommended to reconstruct tubes damaged by pelvic infection, abdominal infection such as appendicitis, or previous ectopic pregnancy. **Repair, called tuboplasty, in these situations is not as likely to be successful** in restoring fertility, however, as is reanastomosis. Even if the surgery does establish an open tubal pathway, **success with conception and pregnancy may be thwarted by irreversible damage to the delicate tubal lining.**

Before in vitro fertilization became available as an option, numerous surgical approaches to tube reconstruction were utilized, despite low success rates. Two-stage procedures, with placement of Teflon tubal splints at the initial surgery, and their removal at a second surgery several months later, were fairly common. Tuboplasty is less likely to be recommended today, however, unless the tubal damage to be corrected is not extensive and at least some normally functioning tube lining is likely to be present. **If the ends of the tubes near the ovaries are severely damaged, or sealed and swollen (hydrosalpinx), then surgery probably will not be recommended.** Tuboplasty surgery requires hospitalization, and involves a longer recovery time and greater surgical risk for the woman than does in vitro fertilization. It is also more expensive. To be a reasonable choice, tuboplasty should be considered only if the success estimate for surgery is at least as high as in vitro fertilization pregnancy rates.

Myomectomy.   Surgery to remove uterine leiomyomas (fibroids) is called myomectomy. In most cases, multiple tumors of varying sizes are involved. To remove the tumors, abdominal surgery with incisions into or through the wall of the uterus in one or more locations is necessary. Meticulous surgical technique is essential to reduce the chance of adhesion formation in the abdomen after surgery. Also, if the uterine incision is extensive, or multiple incisions are necessary, then **planned delivery by cesarean section may be necessary if pregnancy occurs.** Labor contractions may not be safe if the uterine wall is weakened by incisions.

Pregnancy success rates after myomectomy range from 40% to 60%. Problems with uterine fibroids can recur after surgery, however, and as many as 25% of patients will require additional surgery later because new tumors have formed (21). Fibroid tumors are discussed in detail in Chapter 40.

Repair of Abnormal Uterine Structure.   Minor congenital abnormalities in the structure of the uterus, cervix, or vagina are quite common and can often be repaired successfully if they are causing repeated miscarriage or interfering with fertility. Surgery to remove a septum in the uterus or to join the two horns of a bicornuate uterus is similar to myomectomy. Abdominal surgery, with an incision into the uterus followed by reconstruction, is required.

Ectopic Pregnancy.   Implantation of pregnancy in the fallopian tube, the most common site of ectopic pregnancy, is an important issue in fertility surgery because **the risk of ectopic pregnancy is higher than normal for any woman who has had fertility surgery.** Also, when ectopic pregnancy occurs, decisions must be made about the best surgical treatment, and those decisions influence subsequent fertility.

Ectopic pregnancy risk is high whenever there has been damage to one or both fallopian tubes. Infection, scarring, and surgery can all contribute to this risk. Following tubal reanastomosis, for example, 3% to 6% of patients may have ectopic pregnancies. Any woman who undergoes fertility surgery, therefore, should be aware of the ectopic pregnancy danger. Whenever she suspects she may be pregnant, she should arrange for a pregnancy test and exam as early in pregnancy as possible so that an ectopic pregnancy, if present, can be identified and treated before it becomes a surgical emergency.

If ectopic pregnancy is detected early, before its growth has ruptured the tube or caused internal bleeding, then conservative surgery to remove just the pregnancy may be possible. In some cases, the tube can be repaired successfully at that time; alternatively, a second surgery for repair may be considered after the pregnancy site has healed.

A woman who has a tube repaired after an ectopic pregnancy is at greater risk of having another ectopic pregnancy in that tube, and also in the other tube. **After one ectopic pregnancy, the likelihood of a subsequent ectopic is about 12% to 15% whether** the tube is repaired or removed (29). If future fertility is desired, it is reasonable to leave both tubes in place. If the tube cannot be saved, then at least the ovary should be left in place if at all possible. Having two ovaries present, even if one of them has no tube, is advisable because success with in vitro fertilization is better if two ovaries are available for egg retrieval. (Read more about ectopic pregnancy in Chapter 8.)

IMPROVING CERVICAL MUCUS

Cervical mucus problems caused by infection are likely to be identified and treated during the evaluation phase. Oral antibiotics for both (or all) partners will be successful in most cases. **Periodic reassessment to be sure that infection has been completely eliminated and does not recur will be needed** throughout fertility treatment.

If structural problems such as scarring or narrowing of the canal are the cause of impaired mucus, then dilation may be considered. A slender rod containing a water-absorbing chemical or made of dried and pressed seaweed (*Laminaria*) is inserted into the cervical canal, and the rod gradually expands as it absorbs moisture over the next few hours, gently dilating the cervical canal. Dilating rod insertion and removal are simple procedures that can be done in the office, with little or no discomfort. (See Chapter 18 for an illustration of dilation with laminaria.) Dilation is likely to be followed by treatment with estrogen to increase mucus production.

Cervical mucus gland activity is primarily governed by the level of estrogen present. Treatment with estrogen such as Premarin (0.6 to 2.5 mg daily) or ethinyl estradiol (approximately 50 mcg daily) for one week just before ovulation should produce a good mucus response. If treatment is successful in producing good mucus and a normal postcoital test, then it will probably be continued each cycle until conception occurs. If treatment is not successful, it may indicate that the cervical mucus glands have been irreversibly damaged, and **intrauterine insemination will be needed** (see the section on artificial insemination later in this chapter).

In rare cases, cervical mucus is too acid for sperm survival. If this is the case, douching with a dilute bicarbonate solution just prior to intercourse may be suggested.

The popular press has printed stories about the use of expectorant cough syrup as a treatment for thick, impenetrable cervical mucus, on the theory that if cough syrup makes respiratory system mucus runny, it will make cervical mucus runny as well. There is no evidence at all to support this home remedy.

CORRECTING LUTEAL PHASE PROBLEMS

Inadequate progesterone production by the ovary's corpus luteum after ovulation can be specifically treated with progesterone. Natural progesterone is rapidly destroyed by stomach acid, so treatment will require injections or vaginal or rectal suppositories. Treatment is started approximately three days after ovulation and continued daily until the next menstrual period, or if pregnancy occurs, until the sixth or seventh week of pregnancy. By that time the pregnancy is well established and its placenta is producing sufficient progesterone to support the continuing growth of the fetus.

CORRECTING ANTIBODY PROBLEMS

The role of antibody problems in fertility impairment is not yet fully understood. Antisperm antibodies present in cervical mucus, semen, or either partner's blood serum appear to reduce the likelihood of pregnancy, and increase the risk of miscarriage, but are not necessarily an absolute obstacle to pregnancy. **Antibody production fluctuates over time**. It is possible that when successful pregnancies do occur, they are the result of a temporary drop in antibody response.

The goal in treatment of antibody problems is to reduce antibody levels or bypass exposure to them. If antibodies are present only in cervical mucus, for example, then intrauterine insemination may be suggested.

If antibody production has been triggered by infection, treatment to eradicate the infection may reduce antibody levels as well. Cortisone treatment may be recommended for the partner producing antibodies in an attempt to reduce temporarily the overall antibody response.

Condom therapy was used in the past when the woman produced antisperm antibodies in the hope that her antibody levels would drop if condoms were used consistently for 6 to 12 months to prevent her from having any direct exposure to sperm. **This approach is no longer recommended**, because when exposure is resumed, the woman is likely to resume antibody production within a short time, and overall success with pregnancy was not improved with condom treatment.

There is little research data on pregnancy success with treatment for antibody problems. Better treatment options will require a better understanding of the role the immune system plays in reproduction.

ARTIFICIAL INSEMINATION

Artificial insemination procedures are named for the source of semen used. Acronyms to learn are:

• **AID**: Artificial Insemination using semen provided by (usually anonymous) Donor
• **AIH**: Artificial Insemination using semen provided by Husband

For artificial insemination, you will need to schedule an office visit one or two days before ovulation is anticipated. You will be positioned as for a pelvic examination, with a speculum in place. Your clinician will draw up the semen specimen into a plastic syringe, and gently expel it onto your cervix near the cervical opening. In some cases a plastic cup will be placed over your cervix to hold the semen against your cervix. Following insemination the speculum will be removed but you will need to lie still on the examining table for 20 minutes or so. After that you will be able to resume normal activities. If a cup is used, you can remove it that evening, wash it and return it to the office at your next visit so it can be sterilized for reuse.

Depending on how predictable your ovulation time is, **either one or two inseminations will be planned for each cycle.** You will need to keep good bbt records during your treatment. If timing is a difficult problem, then ultrasound measurements of your follicles or urine LH tests may help pinpoint ovulation. Artificial insemination can also be combined with treatment to induce ovulation, if that is necessary.

AIH (Artificial Insemination Using Your Husband's Semen).   If retrograde ejaculation, problems with intercourse technique, or severe sexual problems are the cause of impaired fertility, then AIH is a logical treatment option. In some cases your clinician may be able to teach you how to do AIH at home yourself.

AIH also provides your clinician an opportunity to enhance the semen specimen itself. Problems with excessive semen agglutination, or very high or very low semen volume, may be corrected in the laboratory by mixing semen with a specially prepared tissue culture medium and spinning it to obtain a sample of reasonable volume and consistency containing the active sperm. Alternatively, a technique called "swim up" can be used to obtain a specimen with actively motile (normal) sperm, leaving debris and abnormal sperm behind (30). These approaches may also be considered when antisperm antibodies are present in semen.

Unless specific problems are present with the male partner's ability to deposit semen in the female partner's vagina, however, there is no reason to believe that AIH is any more likely to result in pregnancy than is normal intercourse (31). AIH treatment as a last-ditch, "just in case" approach doesn't make sense.

AID (Artificial Insemination Using Donor Semen).   For couples who have male problems that cannot be treated, or have tried treatment without success, AID is the only other option for pregnancy. AID is also a very reasonable choice when:

• The male partner is Rh-positive, and the Rh-negative woman already has severe Rh sensitization

- The male partner is known to be a carrier of a serious genetic abnormality
- A single woman wishes to become pregnant
- A significant male problem is present, but the couple chooses not to undertake treatment

There are many reasons why a couple might choose AID in this last situation. Delay and expense are substantial considerations in treatment to improve or restore sperm production. If the woman is already in her late 30s, then waiting 12 months or more to find out whether her partner's treatment has been successful may reduce their overall chance for successful pregnancy because her fertility may decline while they are waiting.

On the other hand, donor insemination does involve personal, ethical, and practical considerations. Careful thought and a good joint decision by both partners are essential.

Donor insemination is also an option for a single woman who wishes to become pregnant, and many programs now provide this service (32).

Reputable programs provide donor insemination all across the country, and thousands of AID children are born each year. If you decide on AID, **look for a program that is thorough and cautious** in selection of donors. Your donor will be anonymous, but the **program should screen all donors with genetic and medical histories, physical exam, and, of course, tests to detect the presence of sexually transmitted infection.** Screening can reassure you that you are very unlikely to contract gonorrhea, chlamydia, syphilis, or AIDS (acquired immune deficiency syndrome) from donor semen. There are no completely foolproof screening tests for AIDS or any other sexually transmitted infections, so high-risk-group donors should be avoided. Donors whose ethnic background places them at risk should also be screened for Tay-Sachs disease, sickle cell anemia, and thalassemia. Men who are carriers of these or other known genetic problems should not be donors.

Concern about possible transmission of AIDS through donated semen has lead some experts to recommend that all donor semen be frozen and stored for at least three months. If the donor's blood shows no evidence of AIDS antibody three months after the sperm is collected, then the insemination recipient and her clinician can be quite confident that the semen sample is free of AIDS virus. This approach, however, means using frozen rather than fresh semen, and freezing may reduce insemination success rates. Also, AIDS risk with insemination is low, and other conscientious donor-screening measures probably can provide good protection (33).

Reported success rates for pregnancy following AID with fresh semen typically range from 75% to 85%, similar to rates for normal conception in average couples. If multiple fertility problems are involved, pregnancy rates are somewhat lower. **Approximately 50% of conceptions with AID occur within the first two to three months of treatment, and 90% within six months.** If AID has not been successful within three to six months, further fertility evaluation should be done to identify and correct additional problems. Unsuspected tubal damage or other female factors may be present.

Pregnancy outcome after AID is probably the same as that after normal conception. Reported rates for miscarriage, pregnancy complications, and birth defects among AID pregnancies are the same as those observed in the general population. So despite donor screening, AID cannot guarantee a normal baby, and probably does not reduce rates for birth defects except for couples who choose AID because of a known genetic abnormality carried by the male partner.

Intrauterine Insemination.   Intrauterine insemination means placement of sperm inside the uterine cavity. This procedure bypasses the cervical mucus, and gives sperm a 3- to 4-cm head start on their journey to the fallopian tube opening.

Semen contains numerous biochemicals such as proteins and prostaglandin as well as sperm, so it may be quite toxic to a woman if it is inserted directly into her uterus. For this reason, the sperm must be washed with tissue culture medium and separated from the other constituents present in semen to prepare an insemination specimen containing sperm but not seminal plasma. Sperm are suspended in tissue culture medium for placement. Either partner semen or donor semen can be used.

Intrauterine insemination may be used to bypass the function of cervical mucus when fertility is impaired because of inadequate mucus production. It may also be reasonable when antibodies are present in the woman's mucus or when the sperm count is low. Approximately 50% of sperm are lost during their journey through the cervix; if the entire sperm count from an ejaculate is placed inside the uterus, the effect is similar to a boost in the sperm count. Success rates reported with intrauterine insemination have ranged from 15% to 60% (34), and no doubt depend on the problem or problems being treated.

Frozen Semen.   Using precisely controlled, low-temperature freezing equipment, semen can be successfully frozen, maintained for long periods, and then thawed for use without losing its capacity to initiate normal pregnancy. Many programs take advantage of this technology in preparing AID specimens for later use if the desired donor is not available when needed, and some programs rely entirely on frozen AID specimens. **Freezing can also be used to prepare a partner's specimen for AIH if the** partner will be unavailable during the woman's fertile time (for example, traveling out of town).

Success rates for pregnancy with frozen semen are somewhat lower than for fresh semen, so additional treatment cycles to achieve pregnancy may be anticipated. Freezing is likely to decrease sperm motility, especially if semen quality is borderline or poor to start with, so pooling of multiple frozen semen specimens is not likely to be a successful approach in treatment of men with impaired sperm production.

Sperm Banking.   While many programs are able to provide freezing and temporary semen storage for use during fertility treatment, sperm banking is less widely available. Banking implies very long-term storage, with a commitment to maintaining the banked specimens at proper temperature, and access to the specimens by their owners months or years later. No accidental power failures, no bankruptcies.

Many couples ask about sperm banking as a way of hedging options when vasectomy is being considered. Although it is a logical question, sperm banking probably should not be viewed as a good alternative in this situation. If your future pregnancy desire is still enough of an issue to bring sperm banking to mind, then vasectomy should be delayed. There is no way to guess how many semen samples might be needed if other fertility problems in the future prevent successful conception in the first few cycles. Also, freezing may reduce motility in one or all samples, and bankruptcies can occur.

Sperm banking may be a reasonable option to consider, however, when surgery or medical treatment that may impair semen production is necessary, and the man wishes to have some hope of future fertility. Treatment with radiation or chemotherapy for cancer, and testicular tumor surgery, are examples of such situations.

IN VITRO FERTILIZATION AND EMBRYO TRANSFER (IVF-ET) AND GAMETE INTRAFALLOPIAN TRANSFER (GIFT)

In vitro fertilization and embryo transfer (IVF-ET) was developed as an option for couples with infertility caused by irreversible tubal damage. With IVF-ET, mature eggs obtained from the woman's ovary are mixed with sperm from her partner in the laboratory. The egg and sperm undergo fertilization and the first few hours of development in laboratory incubation. The tiny embryo (or embryos) is then inserted into the woman's uterus through her cervix for implantation and subsequent pregnancy development. **Pregnancy with IVF-ET involves the couple's own eggs and sperm** and, once established, is indistinguishable from pregnancy conceived in the traditional manner.

Irreparable tubal damage is the primary reason that couples undergo IVF-ET treatment. This approach, however, may also be a possibility for couples with:

• Very low sperm count
• Endometriosis
• Immunologic problems
• Unexplained infertility

An IVF-ET treatment cycle involves four main steps. The first step is **follicular development and ovulation monitoring.** In a normal cycle, one dominant egg follicle develops and at ovulation, only one mature egg is released. IVF-ET success rates are best when several mature eggs are available, so hormone treatment with clomiphene and Pergonal is used to stimulate simultaneous development of several follicles. Daily ultrasound and serum hormone measurements are used to find optimal hormone doses and to determine when the eggs are mature. When the egg follicles reach mature size, an injection of HCG (human chorionic gonadotropin) induces the final phases of egg maturation. **The second step in treatment, laparoscopic egg recovery,** is scheduled exactly 36 hours after HCG injection. The eggs must be retrieved just before ovulation would occur.

Laparoscopy allows the surgeon to locate the ovaries and identify each mature follicle. The follicles are easily visible on the ovarian surface; each mature follicle is a fluid-filled blister, approximately 2 cm in diameter, protruding slightly above the ovary surface. The egg aspiration needle, inserted through a tiny incision low in the abdomen, is used to vacuum out gently the contents of each follicle.

Laparoscopy requires general anesthesia and a hospital operating room or outpatient surgery facility (see Chapter 48 for a complete description of laparoscopy procedures and possible risks). Egg aspiration is likely to require 30 to 60 minutes of surgery time, but most women are ready to return home after two or three hours in the recovery room.

In some programs, egg aspiration guided by ultrasound is now being developed. A fine needle inserted through the woman's abdomen or vagina is visible inside the pelvis on the ultrasound monitor. Relying only on the ultrasound view, each mature egg follicle is punctured and its fluid withdrawn. With this technique, the need for general anesthesia and laparoscopy may be avoided. The relative success and safety of ultrasound aspiration, however, are not yet known.

Follicle fluid containing the egg or eggs is taken directly from the operating room to the laboratory to begin **the third step in IVF-ET: fertilization and embryo culture.** The follicle fluid is examined under the microscope to locate each egg. The egg is placed in a tissue culture medium in an incubator controlled for temperature, humidity, and gas atmosphere. After several hours of initial incubation, fresh sperm, prepared by washing and centrifugation, are added to the culture medium containing the egg. Fertilization and culture in the laboratory over the next 36 hours or so should result in one or more early embryos, each containing two to eight cells, about the size of the period at the end of this sentence.

The final step, embryo transfer, is scheduled approximately 48 hours after laparoscopy. The embryo or embryos are suspended in a drop of culture medium and drawn into a slender plastic catheter. With a speculum in place, the catheter is passed through the woman's cervical canal to the top of the uterine cavity, where the embryos are released. This procedure is not painful, and does not require anesthesia. After transfer, however, the woman will need to remain lying down for six to eight hours, and will then be allowed to return home to rest in bed for two days.

In order to undergo IVF-ET, the woman must have at least one ovary accessible for aspiration. If the surgeon cannot see the ovaries during laparoscopy because of dense adhesions or scarring, then egg retrieval may not be possible. The woman must also have a normal uterus. **The man must have at least some normal sperm.** Fertilization in the laboratory will require approximately 50,000 to 100,000 sperm.

The specific fertility problems being treated are important in predicting IVF-ET success. The number of eggs obtained and embryos replaced also influences success. **Overall rates for most programs range from 15% to 25% success in establishing early pregnancy** (35). Miscarriage after the first few weeks of pregnancy, however, may occur in as many as 30% of these pregnancies.

Age does not appear to be a significant factor in IVF-ET success (36), at least through age 40, and very little data exists on IVF-ET pregnancy rates for women over 40 because most programs exclude them. Serious medical problems that would make pregnancy or IVF-ET treatment more risky may also be a reason to decide against it.

It is too early to be certain about how IVF-ET may influence the risk of birth defects. The first IVF-ET baby was born in 1978, and since that time, several thousand babies have been delivered. So far, **the number and kinds of birth defects among IVF-ET babies have been the same as those that would be expected for children conceived in the usual way.**

What does IVF-ET entail from the couple's point of view? First, finding and registering for a program may require some research and travel. Reputable programs are now established in dozens of cities, however, and long waiting lists are no longer a major obstacle.

Your IVF-ET treatment cycle begins on the first day of a normal period. Hormone pills and/or injections will be needed daily beginning on day 2, 3, or 4. You may be able to arrange for these at home, however. Ultrasound and serum hormone measurements will be needed daily for about a week prior to egg recovery. For this phase, you will probably need to be seen daily at the program site itself. Your partner needs to be present at the time of laparoscopy because fresh semen will be used for fertilization. Embryo transfer will occur two days later, and after that you should be able to return home, although you may be advised to avoid strenuous activity for the following two weeks.

The major health risk of IVF-ET treatment is the laparoscopy itself. This, fortunately, is a low-risk surgical procedure, and complications are rare.

Financially, one IVF-ET treatment cycle requires your time for 10 to 12 days of frequent medical visits and possibly travel, and about $5,000 overall for the medications, hormone tests, ultrasound, and surgery involved. Some medical insurance plans do cover part or all of the medical costs, but many do not. Also, **achieving a successful pregnancy may require several treatment cycles.**

Future improvement in IVF-ET success and usefulness is expected as techniques to permit temporary embryo freezing are perfected, and new sperm treatment procedures are developed. Normal pregnancy after embryo freezing has already been achieved in Australia and in the U.S. With this approach, eggs retrieved and fertilized in one treatment cycle can be used for embryo replacement in several cyles, thus increasing the chance of successful pregnancy without the need for laparoscopy surgery each time.

IVF-ET also holds promise as a treatment for male problems. The number of sperm required for fertilization success in the laboratory is much lower than the number needed for conception with intercourse or insemination. Also, pretreatment with drugs or chemicals added directly to the sperm is possible.

An adaptation of IVF-ET technique, to allow surgical retrieval of eggs for laboratory mixing with the partner's sperm and immediate surgical replacement of the mixture in the end of the woman's tube, is also being explored. This approach, called gamete intrafallopian transfer, or GIFT, might be reasonable for a couple with male problems but no tubal damage, or for a couple with unexplained infertility (37). Fertilization and early embryo development would occur in the normal fallopian tube environment.

If you succeed with pregnancy through IVF-ET or GIFT, you will be able to return to your own physician for pregnancy care. Your program will probably recommend ultrasound and hormone tests early in pregnancy while the risk of miscarriage is highest, but no special care is required after that. If you are 35 or older, amniocentesis to check for normal fetal chromosomes will be recommended, just as it would for any other 35-year-old woman.

OTHER PARENTHOOD OPTIONS

The use of donated semen is a well-accepted and widely available treatment option. New fertility technology has made possible the use of donated eggs, or even a donated embryo. These treatment options have been the subject of intense controversy and debate. Although fundamentally similar to donated sperm, egg or embryo retrieval involves at least some risk for the woman donor, while semen donation is essentially risk-free for the donor. As yet, these approaches are not generally available, and their future role in infertility treatment will require considerable effort to resolve thorny legal and ethical controversies.

Somewhat more available are programs to provide a surrogate pregnancy mother. This approach involves the use of artificial insemination to impregnate a woman of normal fertility who is paid to carry the pregnancy to term and then relinquish the baby for adoption by the infertile couple. Couples considering this option have female infertility, or other medical concerns that make pregnancy inadvisable for the woman, but normal (or reasonable) male fertility. The husband's or partner's sperm are used for insemination.

Surrogate pregnancy, too, involves thorny legal, practical, and ethical issues. The surrogate mother faces significant medical risks that are an inescapable aspect of pregnancy, including at least some risk of death. And all parties involved must accept the possibility that the baby could have minor or serious abnormalities, and that someone will have to assume responsibility for parenthood nevertheless.

Adoption.   By far the most important alternative parenthood option is adoption. Many, many couples choose adoption rather than a prolonged or expensive struggle to overcome impaired fertility, and adoption can be a realistic possibility particularly for couples willing to adopt an older or hard-to-place child. Finding a normal newborn infant for adoption is not an easy task, and may necessitate some real effort and the help of an experienced adoption counselor or lawyer. Success, however, is quite likely within a reasonable period of time for couples willing to consider privately arranged adoption. State laws protect the rights of the relinquishing woman, the baby, and adopting parents, whether adoption is arranged independently or through a public agency. Private adoption does not necessarily carry any stigma of a black market situation. Remember that international adoption and adoption of slightly older children or children with medical problems are very reasonable possibilities to consider.

It makes sense to think about and discuss adoption as one logical option at the time initial fertility treatment decisions are being made. Depending on the fertility problems involved, and on your and your partner's personal feelings, adoption may be a better choice than treatment. The adoption alternative also deserves periodic reconsideration if treatment is not successful within a reasonable length of time.

Child-free Living.   It is never easy to alter personal goals, but some couples do manage it. The longing to be a parent gradually gets replaced with other life enrichments—career, friends, avocations—and there is fullness rather than emptiness. Bloom where you are planted.

Know when I realized I'd really settled in to child-free living? My friend Sara was describing their godawful muddy Saturday morning with *two* soccer games and a gymnastics meet all before 11 o'clock. At 11 o'clock Paul and I were still in bed reading the paper, listening to the rain, with one cat and one dog snuggled in with us. Not bad . . .

—WOMAN, 37

Coping with Fertility Evaluation and Treatment

When I think about it now, it was the hardest year in my life.

—MAN, 40

Remember Langston Hughes and "What happens to a dream deferred?"
It was a hellish time.

—WOMAN, 40

Fertility almost always has intense and very personal meaning for both men and women. As you and your partner begin to think about fertility, you may be surprised to find that it involves a distressing level of anxiety and often conflict. The two of you may agree about how much emphasis, time, money, and effort this problem deserves in your life, or you may not. And each of you is likely to have somewhat different reactions to and concerns about the specific tasks and decisions you may be facing. So even if you and your marriage were psychologically top-notch to start with, coping with fertility problems is quite likely to bring fairly severe stress.

Feelings of guilt and personal inadequacy are almost universal. Scientifically speaking, a fertility problem is not really different from, say, gallbladder disease or any other medical disorder, yet most people coping with gallbladder disease do not suffer in quite the same way with the self-blame or sense of not being a whole person that so often plagues fertility impairment couples. And sometimes medical procedures and terminology aggravate this problem. You may hear terms like "hostile" mucus or "infantile" uterus. They have no place in good fertility care. Such terms assault self-esteem, and do not express precise medical information. There is no evidence that your own attitudes—hostile or receptive—can really influence fertility problems.

Also particularly common are sexual problems. The necessity for sex on schedule, to match fertile days or medical appointments, is just about guaranteed to interfere with your sense of spontaneity, and can cause severe performance pressure. Consequently, sexual dysfunction is very common during fertility testing and treatment. It may be a quite normal reaction to the situation.

It is also hard to cope with the uncertainty of both evaluation and treatment. Planning is difficult when life consists of two-week intervals: two weeks before ovulation, when you could not yet be pregnant, then two weeks after ovulation waiting to find out whether conception has occurred. **And each month can bring the disappointment of failure or even mourning** when a menstrual period occurs. In this situation it is hard to feel enthusiastic about planning for a vacation or career advancement. And many couples suffer in isolation, afraid to discuss their problems even with family members or friends. If they did, it is quite likely that they would discover that other couples, too, have had similar experiences and the natural frustration, anger, and anxieties that go along with a fertility struggle.

Often, too, **talking with other couples who are fighting impaired fertility is helpful because of the practical as well as emotional information that is shared.** Resolve is a national organization with chapters in many cities that provides information about

10:8   EARLY PREGNANCY DANGER SIGNS

Possible Ectopic Pregnancy

Sudden intense pain, or persistent pain, or cramping in the lower abdomen, usually localized to one side or the other

Irregular bleeding or spotting with abdominal pain when your period is late or after an abnormally light period

Fainting or dizziness that persists more than a few seconds. These may be signs of internal bleeding. You will not necessarily have bleeding from your vagina if you have internal bleeding.

Possible Miscarriage

Your last period was late, and bleeding is now heavy, possibly with clots or clumps of tissue; cramping is more severe than usual

Your period is prolonged and heavy—5 to 7 days of "heaviest" days

You have abdominal pain and fever

Contact your clinician immediately or go to a hospital emergency room if you develop any of these signs.

fertility treatment and helps establish local couples groups. Participation with a Resolve chapter may be of great value as you cope with the stresses of fertility problems, and in finding out about evaluation and treatment procedures as well.

If stresses are severe, or you are having difficulty making decisions about treatment, then counseling may be a very reasonable step. An experienced psychiatrist, clinical psychologist, or social worker should be able to help you clarify your own feelings and find ways to resolve or negotiate conflicts between you and your partner. Your own physician or fertility specialist can help you find an appropriate counseling referral.

When You Suspect Pregnancy.   At least 50% of couples who seek help for fertility problems are successful in achieving pregnancy. Depending on your specific fertility problem, your success rate may be even higher, so you need to know what to do when you suspect you may be pregnant.

If you have been taking basal body temperatures you should suspect pregnancy if your temperature readings continue to be high for more than 14 or 15 days after ovulation, and you have not begun bleeding. For most women, the first signs of pregnancy are overdue menses and sensitive, tender nipples. Breast tenderness, fatigue, nausea, and unusual sensitivity to food odors are other early signs that may begin approximately two weeks after conception.

As soon as you suspect pregnancy, be extra careful about routine pregnancy precautions. Reread Chapter 9 for specific recommendations about optimal pregnancy, and remember not to take any drugs or over-the-counter medications until you have discussed them with your physician.

Arrange for a pregnancy test and exam right away. Sensitive blood and urine tests can confirm pregnancy as early as about eight days after conception, so there is no reason to delay in scheduling your test. Early pregnancy verification is especially important for women who have fertility problems. The risk of ectopic (tubal) pregnancy is high for any woman who has had previous tubal damage or infection, and early evaluation is key in reducing the risk of serious problems with ectopic pregnancy. It is important to **watch for the danger signs** of problems in early pregnancy (see Illustration 10-8). Your clinician will want to know immediately if you experience any of these symptoms.

When pregnancy occurs, it is natural to feel tremendous excitement and relief. Don't be surprised, however, if you also experience some fear and even misgivings. Also, remember that early pregnancy is a high-risk time for miscarriage. The first 12 weeks or so are a wait-and-see time, because most miscarriages occur early. The likelihood of success with full-term pregnancy increases each week that pregnancy continues.

SUGGESTED READING

Andrews, Lori B.: *New Conceptions—A Consumer's Guide to the Newest Infertility Treatments, Including In Vitro Fertilization, Artificial Insemination and Surrogate Motherhood.* New York: St. Martin's Press, 1984.

Arms, Suzanne: *To Love and Let Go.* New York: Random House, 1984. The experiences of adopting couples and birth mothers with independent adoption.

Bolles, Edmund B.: *The Penguin Adoption Handbook.* New York: Penguin Books, 1984.

Corson, Stephanie L.: *Conquering Infertility.* Norwalk: Appleton-Century-Crofts, 1983.

Glass, Robert H., and Ericsson, Ronald J.: *Getting Pregnant in the 1980's.* Berkeley: University of California Press, 1982.

Harkness, Carla: *The Infertility Book: A Comprehensive Medical and Emotional Guide.* San Francisco: Volcano Press, 1987.

Swanson, Janice M., and Forrest, Katherine A.: *Men's Reproductive Health.* New York: Springer Publishing Co., 1984.

RESOURCES

American Fertility Society
2131 Magnolia Avenue, Suite 201
Birmingham, Alabama 35256
For referral to physician members of the society, and some literature.

March of Dimes Birth Defects Foundation
1275 Mamaroneck Avenue
White Plains, New York 10605
For information on genetic counseling and testing and referral to physicians and genetics centers.

Resolve, Inc.
National Office
P.O. Box 474
Belmont, Massachusetts 02178
Resolve is a nonprofit, national organization with chapters in many cities. The national office can provide a list of fertility specialists and chapter members in your area as well as a bibliography, medical fact sheets, and a national newsletter.

REFERENCES

1. Aral SO, Cates W Jr: The increasing concern with fertility. Journal of the American Medical Association 250:2327–2331, 1983.
2. Speroff L, Glass RH, Kase NG: *Clinical Gynecologic Endocrinology and Infertility* (ed 3). Baltimore: Williams & Wilkins, 1983.
3. Edwards RG: *Conception in the Human Female.* San Francisco: Academic Press, 1980.
4. Menken J, Trussell J, Larsen U: Age and infertility. *Science* 233:1389–1394, 1986.
5. Garcia C-R, Mastroianni L, Amelar RD, et al: *Current Therapy of Infertility 1984–85.* Philadelphia: B.C. Decker, 1984.
6. Amelar RD, Dubin L, Walsh PC: *Male Infertility.* Philadelphia: W.B. Saunders, 1977.
7. Vogt H-J, Heller W-D, Borelli S: Sperm quality of healthy smokers, ex-smokers, and never-smokers. *Fertility and Sterility* 45:106–110, 1986.
8. Council on Scientific Affairs: Effects of toxic chemicals on the reproductive system. *Journal of the American Medical Association* 253:3431–3437, 1985.
9. Whorton MD, Meyer CR: Sperm count results from 861 American chemical/agricultural workers from 14 separate studies. *Fertility and Sterility* 42:82–86, 1984.
10. Becker CE: Male reproductive hazards. *Western Journal of Medicine* 139:212, 1983.
11. Reproductive toxicity of the glycol ethers. *Reproductive Toxicology, a Medical Letter* 4:15–18, 1985.
12. Aafjes JH, van der Vijver JCM: Fertility of men with and without a varicocele. *Fertility and Sterility* 43:901–904, 1985.
13. Holmes KK, Mardh P-A, Sparling PF, et al: *Sexually Transmitted Diseases.* New York: McGraw Hill Book Co., 1984.
14. Daly DC, Soto-Albors C, Walters C, et al: Ultrasonographic assessment of luteinized unruptured follicle syndrome in unexplained infertility. *Fertility and Sterility* 43:62–65, 1985.
15. Ritchie WGM: Ultrasound in the evaluation of normal and induced ovulation. *Fertility and Sterility* 43:167–181, 1985.
16. Ben-David M, Schenker JG: Transient hyperprolactinemia: A correctable cause of idiopathic female infertility. *Journal of Endocrinology and Metabolism* 57:442–444, 1983.
17. Stillman RJ: In utero exposure to diethylstilbestrol: Adverse effects on the reproductive tract and reproductive performance in male and female offspring. *American Journal of Obstetrics and Gynecology* 142:905–921, 1982.
18. Quinn PA, Shewchuk AB, Shuber J, et al: Efficacy of therapy in preventing spontaneous pregnancy loss among couples colonized with genital mycoplasmas. *American Journal of Obstetrics and Gynecology* 145:239–244, 1983.

19. Poland ML, Moghissi KS, Giblin PT, et al: Variation of semen measures within normal men. *Fertility and Sterility* 44:396–400, 1985.

20. Overstreet JW, Price MJ, Blazak WF, et al: Simultaneous assessment of human sperm motility and morphology by videomicrography. *Journal of Urology* 126:357–360, 1981.

21. Keller DW, Strickler RC, Warren JC: *Clinical Infertility.* Norwalk: Appleton-Century-Crofts, 1984.

22. Maathuis JB, Horback JGM, vanHall EV: A comparison of the results of hysterosalpingography and laparoscopy in the diagnosis of fallopian tube dysfunction. *Fertility and Sterility* 23:428–431, 1972.

23. Barnea ER, Holford TR, McInnes DRA: Long-term prognosis of infertile couples with normal basic investigations: A life-table analysis. *Obstetrics and Gynecology* 66:24–26, 1985.

24. Weinerth JL: Long term management of vasovasostomy patients. *Fertility and Sterility* 41:625–628, 1984.

25. Wramsby H, Fredga K, Liedholm P: Chromosome analysis of human oocytes recovered from preovulatory follicles in stimulated cycles. *New England Journal of Medicine* 316:121–124, 1987.

26. Hurley DM, Brian R, Outch K, et al: Induction of ovulation and fertility in amenorrheic women by pulsatile low-dose gonadotropin-releasing hormone. *New England Journal of Medicine* 310:1069–1074, 1984.

27. Boer-Meisel ME, te Velde ER, Habbema JDF, et al: Predicting the pregnancy outcome in patients treated for hydrosalpinx: A prospective study. *Fertility and Sterility* 45:23–29, 1986.

28. Buttram VC, Reiter RC: *Surgical Treatment of the Infertile Female.* Baltimore: Williams & Wilkins, 1985.

29. Weckstein LN: Current perspective on ectopic pregnancy. *Obstetrical and Gynecological Survey* 40:259–272, 1985.

30. Berger T, Marrs RP, Moyer DL: Comparison of techniques for selection of motile spermatozoa. *Fertility and Sterility* 43:268–273, 1985.

31. Nunley WC Jr, Bateman BG, Kitchin JD III: Homologous insemination—revisited. *American Journal of Obstetrics and Gynecology* 153:201–206, 1985.

32. McGuire M, Alexander NJ: Artificial insemination of single women. *Fertility and Sterility* 43:182–184, 1985.

33. Schlaff WD: Transmission of disease during artificial insemination. *New England Journal of Medicine* 315:1289, 1986.

34. Toffle RC, Nagel TC, Tagatz GE, et al: Intrauterine insemination: The University of Minnesota experience. *Fertility and Sterility* 43:743–747, 1985.

35. Wood C, McMaster R, Rennie G, et al: Factors influencing pregnancy rates following in vitro fertilization and embryo transfer. *Fertility and Sterility* 43:245–254, 1985.

36. Wilkes CA, Rosenwaks Z, Jones DL, et al: Pregnancy related to infertility diagnosis, number of attempts, and age in a program of in vitro fertilization. *Obstetrics and Gynecology* 66:350–352, 1985.

37. Asch RH, Balmaceda JP, Ellsworth LR, et al: Preliminary experiences with gamete intrafallopian transfer (GIFT). *Fertility and Sterility* 45:366–371, 1986.

11

❖

Choosing a Method of Birth Control

No woman can call herself free who does not own and control her body. No woman can call herself free until she can choose consciously whether she will or will not be a mother.

—MARGARET SANGER, 1920

If there were a perfect method of birth control, we wouldn't need this chapter. A perfect contraceptive would be 100% effective, totally safe, available to everyone, inexpensive, completely without side effects, instantly reversible, and easy to use. It would not interfere with lovemaking in any way, and would require a minimum of advice and care from a clinician. There is no such method. It doesn't exist today, and according to research experts there are no likely prospects for the near future.

What we do have today is an array of quite good methods, each with advantages and disadvantages. Your task is to discover which method or combination of methods comes closest to meeting your own needs. Your first concerns will probably be safety and reliability, and rightly so. Many other factors also influence how well you do with birth control: your health status, your lifestyle, and the patterns in your sex life.

Choosing a method of birth control is not a totally rational process; romance isn't rational, and sexual feelings may be even less so. Your feelings, your fears, and your unadorned instincts and hunches are valid considerations.

Remember that you can always change your mind about your method, unless you choose sterilization. Most people use several different methods over the years.

It may be that, as one birth control expert said, we will leave this century with fewer methods of birth control than we had at its beginning. Contraceptive manufacturers are not willing to market low-profit, high-liability products in such a litigious age. Savor your choices while you have them, and make the acquaintance of several different methods to hedge your bets.

Basic Birth Control Assumptions

Start with these basic assumptions as you consider your own choices about birth control:

1. There are several methods of birth control that have proved to be extremely effective—2 pregnancies per 100 couples per year or less—in reliable studies of very careful couples who followed instructions exactly. They are:

- Pills (combined estrogen and progestin)
- Minipills (progestin alone)
- IUDs
- Diaphragms
- Condoms (spermicidal)
- Charting skills (with intercourse after ovulation only)
- Sterilization

These are the most effective popular methods. This list does not include methods that fall into a lower average range of effectiveness, such as foams, sponges, creams, gels, suppositories, vaginal contraceptive film, and withdrawal.

Remember that a 2% failure rate is not 0%. No method is perfect. One doctor even gives each woman using contraceptives whom she sees in her practice an emergency supply of morning-after pills (provided there are no health risks present). If you use a method with a 2% failure rate for 25 years, you have a 40% chance for an accidental pregnancy.

2. The effectiveness of your method of birth control depends in large part on how carefully and consistently you use it.

3. Two methods are better than one: you need a primary method and a back-up method. Pills are indeed forgotten, and it is possible to be snowed in with no diaphragm gel. Think of condoms or foam or sponges as your birth control first-aid kit. Some couples use two methods all the time for extra protection. *Using anything* helps. Don't leave your diaphragm in the drawer just because you are out of gel. Use your diaphragm anyway, if you aren't willing to delay intercourse.

4. **If you plan on pregnancy at any point in your future life, choose birth control that also protects your fertility.** Choose Pills and condoms, or sponges and condoms, or a diaphragm and condoms. More than 100,000 women in the United States are involuntarily sterilized each year because of sexual infections. Latex condoms lubricated with spermicide are your best choice for STD protection. Plus good judgment, of course. (Read Chapters 10, 22, and 25 for more details.)

5. **Most women in the United States have all the children they want by their late 20s,** and face 20 to 25 more years of fertility. Sterilization procedures for both men and women can be performed safely without overnight hospital stays and are very close to 100% effective. (See Chapters 19, 20, and 21 for a full discussion of sterilization.)

6. **There is no "best method" of birth control.** The best method for you is the one you and your partner trust and feel most comfortable about using, and will use correctly and consistently.

7. **There are danger times when birth control is often abandoned or forgotten:**

• **At the beginning of a relationship**
• **At the end of a relationship**
• **After a pregnancy scare, abortion, or sexual infection** when a woman says, "Never again. Sex isn't worth it."
• **During major life changes**: a divorce, new job, new school, a move, or serious illness in the family

Basically, it's easier to remember birth control when there isn't a man in your life. A design flaw.

6. **Using birth control is far less risky than having a baby.** Pills are safer than pregnancy for healthy nonsmokers up until age 40 or so. Pills are safer than pregnancy for smokers (15 or more cigarettes a day) until age 35 or so. All other methods of birth control are **safer than** pregnancy for women in all age groups.

Failure Rates:
What Do the Numbers Mean?

I was sitting in my doctor's office flipping through magazines. One article said diaphragms were 98% effective, and another one said 81%.
I asked my doctor which was right, and she said, "Take your pick, they're

both right." That's no way to comfort a woman who still has one in diapers!

—WOMAN, 26

Investigators calculate efficacy rates for methods of birth control by following a group of couples who use the method for a certain length of time and counting the pregnancies that occur. In general, the larger the study group the more reliable the results. For example, you can have more confidence in a Pill study that follows 2,000 users for two years than in a study that follows 500 users for six months, all other factors being equal. You can have more confidence in results reported for a group of women close to you in age, cultural background, and socioeconomic status. If you are a 26-year-old single female, for example, you can't really put a lot of stock in a foam study that investigated only teenage married women in Bora Bora.

Effectiveness rates are calculated in terms of pregnancies per 100 women per year of use. **A failure rate of 3% means 3 pregnancies per 100 women per year studied.**

Health professionals (including at least one of the authors) sometimes turn failure rates around, subtract the failure rate from 100, and describe an effectiveness rate: 98% effectiveness rather than 2% failure, for example. Effectiveness rates have the advantage of being positive and optimistic, and the disadvantage of being intellectually dishonest: **A researcher doing a birth control study can count only failures, not successes.** If 2 out of 100 women in a study become pregnant in 12 months of using method X, that **does not prove** that method X successfully protected the other 98 women! Perhaps they were less fertile. Perhaps their partners were less fertile. Perhaps the couples had intercourse less often than the couples with accidental pregnancies. Researchers do try to assure that they are studying couples with normal fertility and normal frequency of intercourse. Nonetheless, it does make sense to remember the small but valid distinction between a failure rate and an effectiveness rate.

Table 11-1 lists two types of failure rates for each of the common methods of birth control. **The lowest observed failure rate represents a method's absolute top performance, the highest efficacy ever achieved in a reputable clinical trial. The failure rate for typical users is just that, an average rate based on analysis of a range of reputable studies.** Typical failure rates are lower than the best observed failure rates, of course; **how much lower gives you a rough idea what the margin of error is for using that particular method.** Foam, for example, has a best reported failure rate of 3% to 5% and an average failure rate of 18%. Partly these figures tell us that plenty of people found plenty of ways to use foam incorrectly or not at all; other factors as well, however, may account for an abnormally high level of success in a "best reported" study. Perhaps the study participants had lower fertility than "typical" couples because of less frequent intercourse, or higher STD (sexually transmitted disease) rates, for example.

TABLE 11-1
BIRTH CONTROL EFFICACY

METHOD	PERCENT OF WOMEN WHO BECOME PREGNANT DURING FIRST YEAR OF METHOD USE	
	LOWEST REPORTED RATE	RATE FOR TYPICAL USERS
Tubal ligation[a]	0.3	0.4
Vasectomy[a]	0.1	0.15
Birth control Pills[a]	0.1	3
Minipills (progestin only)	1	3
IUD	0.5	6
Condoms		
Plain	4	12
Spermicidal	2	—
Diaphragm with cream or gel	2	18
Sponges		
No previous full-term pregnancy	14	18
Previous full-term birth	28	more than 28
Cervical cap	8	18
Foam, cream, gel, suppository, film[a]	3	21
Withdrawal	7	18
Charting skills[b]	2	20
No method	—	89

[a]Failure rates of zero have been reported for these methods, but the authors believe that rates shown here are the lowest that reasonably can be expected with perfect use.
[b]Charting skills (natural family planning, rhythm method) are most effective when intercourse is limited to days after ovulation only.

SOURCE: Adapted from Trussell J, Kost K: Contraceptive failure in the United States: A critical review of the literature. *Studies in Family Planning* 18(5), September/October 1987.

Using two methods at once will give you an extremely high level of effectiveness. You can figure combined rates for yourself. Simply **multiply** the two failure rates to get an approximate **combined failure rate**. Pills (3% failure) used with condoms (12% failure) gives a combined failure rate of 0.3% (0.03 x 0.10 = 0.003). Obviously, this is a theoretical number. There are no extensive clinical studies to tell us what actually happens when methods are used in combination.

None of us is free of biases. Clinicians tend to quote from the best reported rates column for methods they like and trust and from the average rates column for methods they don't like (1). For example, a Pill-fan clinician might say, "Pills have less than 1% failure, and diaphragms 18%. On the other hand, if your clinician is a diaphragm fan, she/he may say, "Diaphragms can achieve a 2% failure rate, practically as good as Pills." It isn't sound logic to quote a best reported rate for one method and compare it with an *average* rate for another method.

WHAT FAILURE RATES MEAN TO YOU

At best, failure rates can give you a general idea of how successful other couples have been who used your method in the past. Remember that someone else's high degree of efficacy cannot protect you if you are careless; someone else's low success rate need not deter you from using a method if you believe that you can use it correctly.

Age influences the efficacy of birth control methods. In general, older women are much more successful contraceptors than younger women. For example, in one study, women in general achieved about a 2% failure rate with Pills. Married women less than 22 years old experienced a 4.7% failure rate. With the diaphragm the differences are even more dramatic, 19% and 33.1%, respectively, and condoms 10% and 20.6%, respectively (2). Young women may be less effective contraceptors than older women because they are less experienced at careful planning, or because they are more fertile, have intercourse more often, or most likely, some combination of these factors. If you are a young woman who would like to avoid pregnancy, it makes sense to heed these numbers and be doubly careful about contraception.

Older women are often deep into careers, fearful of the increasing risk of chromosome defects such as Down's syndrome, and/or happy to have smaller families (3) so contraception can be profoundly important, but accidental pregnancies do happen, even long after the bassinet has been stored in the attic.

The doctor who told her patient that diaphragms can have failure rates of both 18% and 2% (82% and 98% effective) was right; a 2% rate is about the maximum protection a woman can hope for if she is careful about following instructions each and every time. If she is average, she can expect about a 18% rate. If she has intercourse more often than average, or is more fertile than average, or is not so careful, she must expect a failure rate higher than 18%. Whether she spends the next year at the 2% level or at a level of 18% or more depends on her and her partner: personal fertility factors count and so does diligence. Then add just a touch of luck.

Risks: What Are Your Odds?

If women think first about birth control effectiveness, they think second about risks. "What are the chances I'll have a serious medical problem or be hospitalized? What are the chances I will die?" Morbidity (illness) and mortality (death), the scientists call it. Some risks are truly caused by the birth control method. Pills, for example, do directly cause circulatory disorders that result in some deaths each year. Other birth

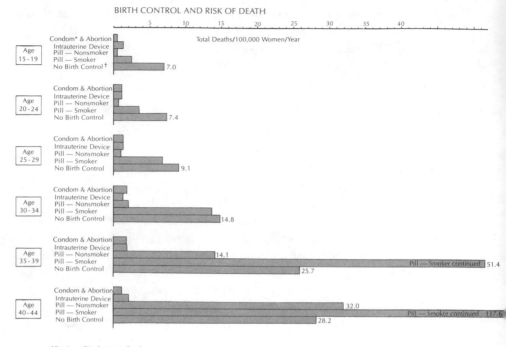

BIRTH CONTROL AND RISK OF DEATH

*Barrier = Diaphragm or Condom
†Deaths in women not using birth control = Deaths from pregnancy complications

ILLUSTRATION 11-1   Birth control is safer than pregnancy except for older Pill users, particularly those who smoke. (Adapted from Ory HW: Mortality associated with fertility and fertility control: 1983. *Family Planning Perspectives* 15:57–63, 1983.) Deaths in women using no birth control are the result of complications of pregnancy.

control risks are indirect; when your method fails, you are vulnerable to the medical risks of full-term pregnancy, miscarriage, or abortion.

Risks vary from method to method and are spelled out in great detail in the following chapters. **Remember that birth control methods offer benefits as well as risks.** Benefits too are spelled out in the chapters that follow. As an example, Pills *protect* users from cancer of the ovary and cancer of the lining of the uterus, and several hundred deaths from these cancers are averted each year among Pill users. Pills and all the barrier methods also offer degrees of protection against sexually transmitted infections.

Birth control risks may be best understood in relation to your overall risk of death during the reproductive years. Overall death risk for women is described in Chapter 7, especially Table 7-1. The risk of death associated with birth control use is described in this chapter in Illustration 11-1 and in greater detail in Table 11-2. For example, if you are a 19-year-old Pill user who does not smoke, your risk of death from Pill complications is 0.5 per 100,000 users per year. If you are 35 years old, use Pills, and

TABLE 11-2
BIRTH CONTROL AND RISK OF DEATH

	DEATHS PER 100,000 USERS PER YEAR, BY AGE GROUP					
	15–19	20–24	25–29	30–34	35–39	40–44
Pill/nonsmoker	0.5	0.7	1.1	2.1	14.1	32.0
Pill/smoker	2.4	3.6	6.8	13.7	51.4	117.6
Condom[a]	1.1	1.6	0.7	0.2	0.3	0.4
Diaphragm[a]	1.9	1.2	1.2	1.3	2.2	2.8
Charting skills[a]	2.5	1.6	1.6	1.7	2.9	3.6
Condom/abortion	0.1	0.1	0.1	<0.1[b]	<0.1	<0.1
IUD	1.3	1.1	1.3	1.3	1.9	2.1
No method[a]	7.0	7.4	9.1	14.8	25.7	28.2

[a]Deaths associated with condom, diaphragm, charting skills, and no method are the result of complications of pregnancy.
[b]The sign $<$ means less than.
SOURCE: Adapted from Ory HW: Mortality associated with fertility and fertility control: 1983. *Family Planning Perspectives* 15:57-63, 1983.

smoke, your risk of death is 51.4 per 100,000 users per year. If you are 30 years old and have an IUD, your risk of death from IUD complications is 1.3 per 100,000 users per year.

Another way to understand contraceptive risk is to compare your risk of death in a year from using birth control with your risk of death from other activities, such as driving a car. Table 11-3 lists these statistical comparisons. **Clearly, it is safer to use Pills for a year than to drive for a year, and safer *by far* to use Pills than to smoke** cigarettes. Even intercourse carries a 1 in 50,000 risk of death!

LONG-TERM RISKS

Condoms and barrier methods such as diaphragms, sponges, and foam are unlikely to carry any long-term risks that we don't yet know about. The chemicals in these products have been studied extensively for many years.

Whether Pills, IUDs, and sterilization have long-term risks is still not completely clear, although recent studies are reassuring. The first U.S. Pill user swallowed her first Pill in 1960, and IUDs have been marketed in the United States since 1959. We cannot yet be absolutely certain what will happen, if anything, to these women in their menopausal years and after.

TABLE 11-3
PUTTING VOLUNTARY RISKS INTO PERSPECTIVE

RISK	CHANCE OF DEATH IN A YEAR (U.S.)
Smoking	1 in 200
Motorcycling	1 in 1,000
Automobile driving	1 in 6,000
Power boating	1 in 6,000
Rock climbing	1 in 7,500
Playing football	1 in 25,000
Canoeing	1 in 100,000
Using tampons (toxic shock)	1 in 350,000
Having sexual intercourse (pelvic infection)	1 in 50,000
PREVENTING PREGNANCY:	
Oral contraception—nonsmoker	1 in 63,000
Oral contraception—smoker	1 in 16,000
Using IUDs	1 in 100,000
Using barrier methods	None
Using charting skills	None
Undergoing sterilization:	
Laparoscopic tubal ligation	1 in 20,000
Hysterectomy	1 in 1,600
Vasectomy	None
DECIDING ABOUT PREGNANCY:	
Continuing pregnancy	1 in 10,000
Terminating pregnancy:	
Nonlegal abortion	1 in 3,000
Legal abortion:	
Before 9 weeks	1 in 400,000
9–12 weeks	1 in 100,000
13–16 weeks	1 in 25,000
After 16 weeks	1 in 10,000

SOURCE: Adapted from Hatcher RA, Guest FJ, Stewart FH, et al: *Contraceptive Technology 1986–1987* (ed 13). New York: Irvington Publishers, 1986.

CONTRAINDICATIONS

Some women are more likely to encounter problems with birth control than others, and contraindications to the methods are an important element to consider as you make your birth control choice. A contraindication is a medical condition that renders a course of treatment inadvisable or unsafe that might otherwise be recommended. For example, a history of thrombophlebitis, blood clots caused by inflammation of the veins, is a contraindication to Pill use; a woman with a history of thrombophlebitis is more likely than average to develop a blood-clotting disorder while taking Pills, and she should **never** use Pills. Knowing—and respecting—the contraindications for your method may be the single most important way to avoid problems.

Clinicians usually rank contraindications on three levels:

• **Absolute** contraindications: **you must not** try to use the method.
• **Strong relative** contraindications: you will be **strongly advised** not to use the method.
• **Relative** contraindications: you **may be able** to try the method if you are willing to be followed very carefully by your clinician so that she/he can watch for early signs of trouble.

Review your own medical history and the contraindications for methods you are considering before you adopt a method. There is nothing to be gained by hiding a contraindication from your clinician; **you may fool her or him, but you won't fool your body.** Be alert to contraindications after you start using your method as well. If you develop a condition that you know is a contraindication, talk to your clinician at once.

Many clinicians ask you to sign a consent form before you begin using a method, and drug manufacturers are now required by the Food and Drug Administration to provide Pill and IUD users with a pamphlet that spells out the risks and benefits to be expected. Risks are serious business to your clinician, and it is important for you to take risks seriously, too. Be sure that you understand any consent form completely before you sign, and remember that you have a right to have all your questions answered.

You **can** put risks and benefits in perspective for yourself and make your own decision about a method. The birth control chapters in this book may be a good place to begin. They are designed to give you a complete picture of what we know about each method, both the comforting facts and the disquieting ones, common problems as well as exceedingly rare ones. If these chapters contain more bad news than you are accustomed to reading, you will know why.

Living in
Harmony with Your Method

Choosing a birth control method that will please you is part politics, part pure instinct, and part predicting the future. Remember that you can always change your mind, so don't bog down in trying to make a ''perfect'' choice. There are no perfect methods, and your needs are likely to change over time anyway. Begin by asking yourself these questions:

When do you want to become pregnant? Never? Sterilization may be an option to consider if you are absolutely positive about no pregnancies, or an IUD might be a reasonable choice. Otherwise you could choose one of the most effective temporary methods, or, better yet, two methods in combination, such as Pills and condoms.

Three years from now? Think about the most effective temporary methods. Pills or a diaphragm plus condoms might be good choices. Remember to safeguard your fertility and protect yourself from sexual infection.

Some time this year? Use anything you like. Remember to stop Pills for at least three cycles before you try to become pregnant.

Planning for pregnancy in your future isn't always as easy as it sounds. For many young women it is excruciatingly tough to decide what life would ideally be like in years to come. Where in the education/working continuum should childbearing come? Should childbearing be a part of life at all? Do you want to hold out for a chance to raise children with a partner, or are you willing and able to go it alone? Do you want an only child? Two? Is it ethical to have three or more on a crowded planet? The only wrong approach to these questions is to ignore them.

How do you feel about abortion? If you would not choose abortion, and an unplanned pregnancy would be a disaster for you, consider a combination of two good methods, such as foam and condoms, Pills and condoms, or a diaphragm and condoms. Think about sterilization if you plan no future childbearing.

How often are you having intercourse? If you have intercourse frequently, you might get tired of foam, sponges, condoms, or a diaphragm. If you have intercourse infrequently, you may feel frustrated about exposing yourself to Pill or IUD risks 30 days a month in order to be protected 2 or 3 days.

How many partners do you have? If you have two or more partners—or your partner has another partner—you need effective contraception and infection protection as well. The more partners you have, the greater your risk of infection. Foam, sponges, or a diaphragm will protect you from infection to some degree, but a condom with a spermicide plus Pills will give you the best protection against sexually transmitted infections, and excellent contraception as well.

How good is your access to medical care? Avoid Pills and IUDs and pregnancy if it would be hard for you to get quick, competent medical care in an emergency.

How old are you? If you are a young teenager and have difficulty getting birth control services, condoms and foam or sponges may be your best choice.

If you are over 35, smoke, and use Pills, your risk of cardiovascular problems such as heart attack and stroke is significant; if you are over 40, your risk is significant, even if you don't smoke.

How much money can you afford to spend for birth control? Good birth control protection can cost less than a dollar for one condom, but doctor visits for prescription methods can be expensive. If money is a factor for you, try to find a family planning clinic that offers supplies free or on a sliding scale based on your income. Keep birth control expenses in perspective: it now costs between $100,000 and $140,000 to raise a child to age 18 and put him or her through a four-year public college (4). Early abortion cost about $250 in 1987, and prenatal care and delivery cost $1,500. Double that figure for a cesarean section delivery.

MATTERS OF THE HEART

Why is it so hard to talk about sex? I am a teacher and I talk for a living, for heaven's sake. I've slept with Roger for three years, and I still don't really know what he thinks about our sex life. We make love under some kind of self-imposed vow of silence that by now is habit more than anything else. Could *you* say, "Well, Roger, tell me what you've thought about me as a lover for the last three years"?

—WOMAN, 29

As you think about a method of birth control, think about the patterns in your sex life. Intimacy flowers in different ways for different couples, and birth control is a less obtrusive visitor to the bedroom (or forest or backseat) when it is compatible with your own particular lovemaking style. Here are some questions to ask yourself:

How much cooperation can you expect from your partner? Methods such as a diaphragm, foam, or condoms are more likely to succeed if contraception is a joint undertaking. If you have a top-notch, stable relationship with plenty of trust, charting skills may be an option.

How do you feel about touching yourself? Using a diaphragm, sponge, or foam calls for an easy familiarity with your vagina. Checking for an IUD string on a regular basis requires putting a finger deep inside your vagina. (Your partner might help with these tasks.)

Are you afraid of any of the methods? You may have a sister who had an IUD-related infection, a friend who was hospitalized with a Pill complication, or a co-worker with two "diaphragm babies." It would be hard to use a method consistently if it scares you. "Life is too short to be scared when you don't have to be," one woman said. Stay away from methods you fear.

What methods have you had difficulties with in the past? If you couldn't remember Pills on time three years ago, or if you found yourself risking unprotected intercourse from time to time after you decided on a diaphragm, foam, or condoms, chances are you might still be vulnerable to the same mistakes.

Do you like a lot of spontaneity in your sex life? Unanticipated sex has enormous appeal for many people, and if you fit into that category, you may not enjoy calling time-out for foam, condoms, or a diaphragm.

Actually, it's close to miraculous that almost 50% of U.S. pregnancies each year *are* planned! It is *very* tough to be practical and careful about birth control when you are madly in love, or when you are very young and sex is a dizzying adventure. Ph.D.'s leave their diaphragms in the drawer, too. **Risk taking is normal human behavior!** We aren't perfect with seatbelts or speed limits or smoking, and we aren't perfect with birth control. The goal is to do the absolute best you can, because you deserve your own best efforts.

MAKING UP YOUR MIND

When the time comes to choose a method, start with a list of all your options. Go through the contraindications first and eliminate methods that are unsafe for you. As the list gets shorter and you discard some methods for concrete, objective reasons, begin to consider **your feelings and your partner's feelings.** Your goal is to choose the safest, most effective method you will feel comfortable about using.

Remember to select two methods, your primary method and a back-up method as well. Unexpected problems happen often enough to warrant a second line of defense for all birth control users, except those who have been sterilized.

You can always change your mind. There is no reason to stay with a method if you don't like it or if your contraceptive needs change. If your clinician is reluctant to have you switch methods, try another clinician or go to a family planning clinic.

Other Forms of Birth Control

This chapter has focused on the most popular and effective forms of birth control in the United States. Other contraceptives deserve mention, and are discussed in this section.

ABSTINENCE AND WITHDRAWAL

Abstinence and withdrawal probably rank at the top of the birth control list from a historical or worldwide perspective. Abstinence, particularly, is a cornerstone, and very strong abstinence rules in most cultures insure that the society's childbearing goals are protected. Cultural values set the proper marriage age and proper abstinence interval after a baby is born. Historians credit withdrawal for the dramatic decline in the birth rate in the United States during the Great Depression, and probably this practice accounted for earlier birth rate declines as well.

These methods certainly are valid approaches to birth control. They are often omitted from the family planning specialist's "recommended list" because each relies heavily on user commitment and significant willpower, and because failure rates for these methods, even among motivated couples, are not consistently as low as rates for other approaches to birth control. Nevertheless, almost everyone relies upon one of these two birth control techniques at some time in her/his life.

Abstinence means no intercourse at all. Many couples who are highly motivated to prevent pregnancy simply don't have intercourse. It is one of the most commonly used forms of birth control, especially among young people. Only about 70% of the women in the United States, for example, have had intercourse by age 20 (5). And abstinence is everybody's first method of birth control.

Willpower is all. Abstinence is 100% effective only if you use it. Many people resolve to use abstinence after a disastrous relationship, a pregnancy scare, or an abortion, but it is easy to underestimate powerful needs for affection; and abstinence, indeed, may make the heart grow fonder.

Remember that abstinence as a form of birth control means only that you abstain from penis-in-vagina intercourse; it doesn't mean abstaining from sex. Many couples use abstinence for birth control by substituting oral sex, mutual masturbation, or any number of other pleasurable activities for intercourse. It's important to know yourself and your partner well enough to be confident that you can resist intercourse when the going gets passionate—and no cheating: no putting the penis in the vagina "just a little," and no penis hovering near the vagina when ejaculation occurs. If you can resist intercourse and still enjoy sex, you have a terrific method of birth control: free, safe, highly effective, and always available.

Many people find, however, that they are not reliable abstainers. If you have decided on abstinence, it may help if you try to minimize temptations. Most people find it extremely hard to resist intercourse when the mood, scene, and opportunity converge.

Tom and I did go all the way one time. We were *panicked* till my period started. We went back to his father's cabin once after that, but it certainly is easier just to go out with a group of other kids. Sex is really hard to resist out there by the lake, even though we both try as hard as we can.

—WOMAN, 16

You remember Onan, of course. He's the biblical family planning hero who "spilled his seed on the ground" in the 38th chapter of Genesis. (Dorothy Parker had a canary named Onan because he spilled his seed on the ground, too.) **Withdrawal or coitus interruptus—interrupting intercourse before the man's ejaculation—**is a method of birth control as old as recorded history. As soon as people figured out that semen had something to do with pregnancy, they figured out withdrawal.

A couple using withdrawal has intercourse until the man feels that ejaculation is imminent. At that point he withdraws his penis, taking care to ejaculate well away from the entrance to his partner's vagina. Since sperm theoretically do not enter the vagina, they cannot travel through the cervix, uterus, and tube to meet an egg, and pregnancy cannot occur.

There are no careful studies of withdrawal to provide information on failure rates that is comparable to rates for other birth control methods. The best reported failure rate for withdrawal is 7%, and among average couples who use withdrawal, 18 women out of 100 can expect to become pregnant in a year's time (see Table 11-1). Withdrawal can fail either because the man is unable to withdraw his penis in time or because some sperm are deposited in his partner's vagina *before* he ejaculates. Using withdrawal in combination with another method increases your protection dramatically.

There are no serious medical risks associated with withdrawal, other than those associated with pregnancy or abortion should withdrawal fail to work and a woman becomes pregnant. The failure rate for withdrawal is fairly high because it is difficult for a man to know precisely when ejaculation will occur, and it is difficult to stop intercourse in the middle.

Like most men, I guess, I think of intercourse as something that isn't over till I come. And coming in midair isn't half as satisfying as coming in my wife's vagina. And the worst part is, when you have to pull out, you really can't get lost in sex; you can't let yourself get blissed out. It must be even worse for women—like having intercourse with a time bomb.

—MAN, 34

Some men, hard as they try, simply can't pull out in time; the momentum toward orgasm is too great. If you and your partner have a failure, use a full dose of birth control foam immediately and call your clinician if you want to discuss "morning-after" options (see Chapter 15).

Withdrawal can fail even if a man pulls out in time. If sperm are deposited near the entrance to the vagina, pregnancy is possible. Even if a man withdraws his penis and ejaculates in the next county, withdrawal can still fail. A drop of clear lubrication fluid normally collects on the tip of the penis during sexual arousal, and this fluid can contain thousands of living sperm. If a man has had a recent ejaculation, the sperm count in that drop of fluid will be even higher. These sperm enter the vagina as soon as the penis does. You can decrease your pregnancy risk by wiping away the fluid just before the man inserts his penis, and by using another method of birth control such as condoms for repeated acts of intercourse.

Most of the problems associated with withdrawal are psychological. Some couples may feel sexually shortchanged, and withdrawal can be rough on the nerves, as well.

It was a weird feeling, lying there having intercourse with a man I've
loved and lived with for years, and suddenly asking myself, "Can I
trust this guy to pull out?" I think using withdrawal causes a lot of
deep-seated doubts, and it gives me the hoo-hahs. Who needs that,
especially when you're making love?

—WOMAN, 28

One aspect of using withdrawal that bothers many sex therapists is that withdrawal
tends to promote sexual "spectatoring," an ungainly word that means shifting your
concentration from pleasure to performance. When both you and your partner
concentrate on his pulling out in time, it is hard to concentrate on bliss. **It is certainly
better than no birth control at all, since it offers a fair degree of protection.**

Part of my luggage got lost in Italy, and it was two weeks before
my Pills caught up with me. Chuck and I used withdrawal that whole
time. I wouldn't want to use it all the time, and I know Chuck
wouldn't, but it worked for us in a pinch.

—WOMAN, 19

Some couples find that withdrawal is an effective, comfortable method for long periods
of time. It can be a reasonable, satisfactory choice as a primary method of birth
control for couples who can live with a moderate pregnancy risk. It is an excellent
back-up along with other methods such as foam; and it is quite handy in emergency
situations. It certainly makes sense for couples to explore the full range of satisfying
sexual communications; there is a lot more to sex than ejaculation in the vagina.

A man may be more comfortable using withdrawal if his partner takes his penis in
her hands and stimulates him to orgasm as soon as he withdraws, so he doesn't feel so
lost in space. Have intercourse in positions from which you can extricate yourself
quickly. Avoid withdrawal when one or both of you might be a little short on
willpower—after drinking, for example. Switch to another mode of sexual pleasuring,
or use a barrier method of birth control.

BREASTFEEDING

Breastfeeding has many health benefits for the infant and also for the mother, and is
important and entirely worthwhile on its own merits. It is unwise, however, to count

on breastfeeding for effective birth control protection. Breastfeeding does delay your return to fertility after giving birth, but it is impossible to predict how long. Since ovulation usually occurs before menstrual periods return, nursing women have no advance warning of their return to fertility. **Begin using reliable birth control as soon as you resume intercourse after delivery.**

One study found that 50% of women who did not breastfeed were ovulating 3 months after delivery; 50% of the women who did nurse were ovulating 4.5 months after delivery. Clearly, breastfeeding does not delay a return to fertility very much. In fact, one investigator found that **more than half of nursing women who did not use birth control conceived within nine months** after delivery, and that can mean two in diapers (6).

While you are breastfeeding, you will want to avoid birth control Pills. They may decrease milk supply, and your baby may be exposed to Pill hormones present in breast milk. Condoms, a diaphragm, or a combination of condoms and spermicide would be reasonable options.

UNRELIABLE FORMS OF BIRTH CONTROL

You may know of birth control methods that haven't been discussed in this chapter. Many less reliable methods do exist, but you would probably be wise to avoid them. These methods are at the low end of the effectiveness scale as far as we can tell.

My cousin's wife used Coca-Cola douches faithfully for years, and she *never* got pregnant. Then when they *wanted* a baby, they found out that both her tubes were blocked from an old infection. I hope she hadn't talked any of her friends into using douching for birth control!

—WOMAN, 35

Birth control techniques that don't work well (or perhaps even at all) are douching; avoiding orgasm; pseudobarriers inserted in the vagina such as lemon slices, plastic wrap, petroleum jelly, and tampons; pseudo-sperm-killers such as Norforms and other hygiene suppositories, hygiene sprays, hot baths for men, and jockey shorts for men; variations of rhythm such as astrological birth control and lunaception; and standing up after intercourse.

A significant problem with the methods on this list is that they have not been thoroughly evaluated. No one has ever determined the exact failure rates for astrological birth control or any of these other methods, because researchers do not have any promising evidence that would encourage them to undertake such studies. It would be unethical (and costly) for them to ask couples to participate in a study without some reasonable expectation that the couples could avoid unplanned pregnancy.

REFERENCES

1. Trussell TJ, Faden R, Hatcher RA: Efficacy information in contraceptive counseling: Those little white lies. *American Journal of Public Health* 66:761–767, 1976.
2. Ory HW, Forrest JD, Lincoln R: *Making Choices: Evaluating the Health Risks and Benefits of Birth Control Methods.* New York: Alan Guttmacher Institute, 1983.
3. Committee on Gynecologic Practice: Contraception for women in their late reproductive years. *American College of Obstetricians and Gynecologists Newsletter* January, 1986.
4. Espenshade TJ: as quoted in the *Wall Street Journal,* October 2, 1980, p. 33; from the Population Reference Bureau.
5. Marsiglio W, Mott FL: The impact of sex education on sexual activity, contraceptive use and premarital pregnancy among American teenages. *Family Planning Perspectives* 18:151–162, 1986.
6. Vorherr H: Contraception after abortion and postpartum. *American Journal of Obstetrics and Gynecology* 117:1002–1025, 1973.

12

❖

Barriers: Condoms, Diaphragms, and Spermicides

*A generation ago, diaphragms and condoms were the front-line contraceptives. In today's high-tech era barriers may seem quaint, but this is also an era of rampant sexually transmitted infection. **Barrier methods protect users from infection.** Chemicals that kill sperm also kill bacteria and viruses, and diaphragms, cervical caps, and condoms literally and mechanically shield one lover's germs from the other's. When the consequences of sexual infection are misery, pelvic inflammatory disease, infertility, ectopic pregnancy, and cervical cancer, the barrier method trade-offs in convenience and efficacy seem less important. The ultimate barrier is probably the condom, with an excellent track record for protection from both pregnancy and infection.*

The barrier trade-offs can be circumvented to some degree. Most vaginal products can be inserted up to an hour before intercourse, and diaphragms and sponges many hours before. Using these products needn't feel so disruptive. Using two barriers together—condoms plus a sponge, a diaphragm plus condoms, any duo you like—vastly improves your chance of avoiding unintended pregnancy. For that matter, Pill and IUD users would do well to add a barrier contraceptive for protection against infection.

Welcome to the barrier renaissance.

Barriers:
What They Are and How They Work

The barrier methods of birth control—condom, diaphragm, cervical cap, sponge, creams, gels, film, and suppositories—are just that, physical or chemical barriers to keep sperm and egg apart. All barrier methods (with the exception of some condoms) add a spermicide or sperm-killing chemical to enhance effectiveness. The spermicidal agent is usually a surfactant that breaks down the cell walls of sperm. Condoms enclose the penis in a protective sheath during intercourse and ejaculation. All other barriers are used **inside** the vagina to cover and block the opening in the cervix that leads to the uterus and to kill sperm in the vagina.

History.   For a long time barriers were *the* modern birth control methods. Venerable. Effective. Simple. Inexpensive. Virtually free of medical risks. The earliest **condoms** were probably linen sheaths, which Fallopius described in Italy as early as 1564. Condoms made from animal intestines soon followed. Today there is an array of latex condoms: transparent or a whole rainbow of colors, plain end or reservoir-tipped, ribbed or smooth, dry or lubricated, spermicide-coated or not. All latex condoms meet U.S. standards for quality control (length between 16 and 22 cm, width unstretched between 4.9 and 5.6 cm, thickness at least 0.08 mm, and weight no more than 1.7 gm), and they are tested for holes, strength, and aging. The dozens of latex condom brands are essentially the same, and no one brand is better than any other. In fact, practically all condoms in this country are manufactured by three companies. "Skin" condoms, made from lamb intestine, are favored by some couples. **STD (sexually transmitted disease) experts, however, recommend latex condoms, especially spermicide-lubricated condoms.** Latex may provide better protection against the organisms that cause AIDS and other STDs, and spermicide kills STD organisms(1). The spermicide coating also can kill sperm and your pregnancy risk may be even lower than it is with plain condoms, which also provide excellent pregnancy protection.

The newest development in condoms is marketing to women. Products and package designs in "feminine" colors are evidence of increasing sales to women. The adhesive rim condom is one example. Unfortunately, this product does not have spermicide, so "masculine" **brands with spermicide may be a better choice.**

The **cervical cap** was invented in 1823 by the German physician Frederic Wilde and the first **diaphragm** was produced 60 years later by another pioneering German physician, W.P.J. Mensigna (pseudonym Karl Hasse). Birth control pioneer Margaret Sanger introduced the diaphragm to the United States, but because of the "Comstock laws" prohibiting the import of contraceptives she was unable to distribute the diaphragm. In the 1920s the Holland-Rantos Company began manufacturing latex diaphragms in the United States, and diaphragms became widely available for the first time.

The cervical cap has never been widely used in the United States, although it is somewhat more popular in England and mainland Europe. The one manufacturer that did make plastic cervical caps in this country stopped, presumably because sales were low. The cervical cap, which looks like a small deep diaphragm, fits snugly over the cervix and stays in place by suction. It is used with spermicidal cream or jelly and works very much like a diaphragm. Caps were developed at the same time as the diaphragm and were originally custom-made of silver or gold. Plastic cervical caps were available in England and the United States 35 years ago but have now been replaced by latex models.

The Today contraceptive **sponge** was first marketed in 1983, and is a modern version of a very old idea. For centuries women have soaked sea sponges in vinegar, lemon juice, or other liquids and used them inside the vagina for birth control. The Today polyurethane sponge contains a spermicide and has a nylon loop for easier retrieval.

Contraceptive film, spermicide contained in a discrete, 2-inch-square, thin sheet of glycerine, is the newest vaginal contraceptive product. Placed over the cervix prior to intercourse, the sheet dissolves and releases spermicide. Its effect is similar to that of contraceptive suppositories.

Several million women in the United States use **foam, cream, gel, film, or suppositories**, and they follow in another tradition as old as time. More than 2,000 years ago, Egyptian women used a recipe of sodium carbonate, honey, and crocodile dung for a contraceptive paste. Aristotle's concoction was probably more savory; he recommended frankincense, oil of cedar, and olive oil. In the Middle Ages, rock salt was popular. The perseverance and inventiveness of these early birth control users were remarkable, and it is comforting to know that their efforts probably did prevent unwanted pregnancy to some degree. Pastes *will* seal off the cervix, and anything very acidic or very alkaline *will* kill some sperm. Modern products have powerful sperm-killing chemicals, are easy to use, aren't abrasive (can you imagine having intercourse with rock salt inside your vagina?), and don't smell like crocodile dung.

Effectiveness

Barrier methods are quite effective for older women and careful users, and are less effective for younger women, for couples who have very frequent intercourse, and for users who aren't diligent about careful use. Table 12-1 shows in summary form what we know from recent studies of barrier method efficacy.

Highest reported success rates for condoms equal those for IUDs and diaphragms. In one study of couples using spermicide-lubricated condoms only 2 out of every 100 women became pregnant in a year's time (2). Even if condoms are used perfectly, however, failures might be caused by defective condoms that rupture or have pinhole faults (no product quality control is perfect).

Studies of average couples who use condoms show that if 100 couples use condoms

TABLE 12-1
EFFECTIVENESS OF BARRIER METHODS:
PREGNANCY RATES FOR FIRST YEAR OF USE
(PER 100 WOMEN)

METHOD	BEST REPORTED FAILURE RATE	TYPICAL FAILURE RATE	FAILURE RATE FOR WOMEN LESS THAN 22 YEARS OLD
Condoms			
Plain	4	12	21
Spermicidal	2	—	—
Diaphragm/spermicide	2	18	33
Cervical cap	8	18	—
Sponges			
No previous term pregnancy	14	18	—
Previous fullterm birth	28	more than 28 —	
Foams, creams, gels, suppositories	3	21	32

SOURCES: Trussel J, Kost K: Contraceptive failure in the United States: A critical review of the literature. *Studies in Family Planning 18*(5), September/October 1987.
For women less than 22 years old: Ory HW, Forrest JD, Lincoln R: *Making Choices: Evaluating the Health Risks and Benefits of Birth Control Methods.* New York: Alan Guttmacher Institute, 1983.

for a year about 12 women might become pregnant (2). Among women less than 22 years old, about 21 women out of 100 might become pregnant (3).

Diaphragm effectiveness depends in part on medical factors such as proper fit, but effectiveness also depends partly on how careful—or how careless—the diaphragm user is.

The largest study of diaphragm effectiveness in the United States followed 2,000 users for two years and reported a 2% failure rate among this group of young, unmarried women with no previous diaphragm experience (4).

A more typical diaphragm failure rate is 18% (2), and women less than 22 years old fare less well, with a 33% failure rate (3).

U.S. studies of the cervical cap report failure rates in the 8% to 18% range. In some of these studies users left the cap in place for several days.

Typical failure rates reported in studies of sponge users show that 18 to 28 pregnancies occur in the first year of use for each 100 sponge users (2). Sponge effectiveness depends in part on a woman's previous pregnancy history. This product is less effective for women who have previously completed a full-term pregnancy and delivery than for women who have not. In a large study that compared sponge users and diaphragm users, the failure rates were identical (about 14 pregnancies per 100 women per year) for sponge and diaphragm users with no previous births, and for diaphragm users who had borne a full-term pregnancy. The failure rate, however, was much higher (28 pregnancies per 100 women per year) for women who had previously delivered a pregnancy and used the sponge (5).

Studies of average couples who use foam, cream, gel, film, or suppositories show that if 100 couples use them for a year, about 21 women might become pregnant (2). Young women have less success with these products, experiencing a 32% failure rate (3). The failures might be caused by the product's inability to kill all the sperm or by its inability to stay on and near the cervix long enough to work, even when placed properly. Failure rates as low as 3% to 5% have been reported for spermicide products in some studies. With consistent use, exactly according to instructions, this is the best any couple can hope for.

What am I supposed to think about a contraceptive that has "2% to 19%" failures? Is it 2 or is it 19? There's quite a difference!

—WOMAN, 25

The substantial gulf between best reported failure rates and typical failure rates for barrier methods is distressing for many women, and understandably so. There is a considerable margin for error with these methods. **You can predict your likelihood of success with barrier methods if you compare yourself with an "ideal" barrier user,** a woman whose success is likely to approach the best reported rates. The ideal user:

- **Is able and willing to use the method** (or remind her partner to use it) each and every time she has intercourse, with no skipping "just this once"
- **Can predict when and where intercourse will happen** so that she can arrange to have supplies with her
- **Has "average" intercourse frequency** (eight or so times a month). Very frequent intercourse may mean that your risk for conception is higher than average, and you may find that using your method conscientiously is burdensome.

Another important factor is probably fertility level. Some couples are more fertile than others, and many factors influence the likelihood of conception. Couples who are young, for example, and couples who have intercourse frequently are more likely to conceive than are older couples or those who have intercourse less often. This is true for couples who are trying to conceive, and it is also true for birth control users. Fertility may be one of the reasons that younger couples have higher failure rates in birth control studies.

If you already have had one or more birth control failure pregnancies, or conceived immediately when you were not using birth control, then you may be at the high end of the normal fertility curve. You will need to think carefully about birth control options, and select a highly effective method. A combination such as diaphragm **plus** condoms, or a barrier **plus** Pills or an IUD, can provide extremely effective protection.

12:1   TOXIC SHOCK SYNDROME DANGER SIGNS

Fever (temperature of 101 degrees F. or more)
Diarrhea
Vomiting
Muscle aches
Rash (like sunburn)

Contact your clinician immediately or go to a hospital emergency
room if these symptoms occur during a menstrual period, or while
you are wearing a diaphragm or sponge for birth control.

Problems and Risks

Barrier methods are extremely safe, and problems and risks tend to be minor.
The only risk of hospitalization or death to which a user is exposed is the risk of
pregnancy-related illness or death in the event of unintended pregnancy and the very
slight risk of toxic shock syndrome (TSS) illness or death with the diaphragm, cap,
and sponge. (Read Chapter 11 for a comparison of the risk of death from birth control,
pregnancy, and activities of daily life.)

Toxic Shock Syndrome.   Toxic shock syndrome can occur with use of tampons
and other vaginal products including the sponge, diaphragm, and possibly the cervical
cap. Whether or not using these methods increases a woman's risk for TSS is not clear.
Researchers in one study found that eight sponge users out of 100,000 developed TSS
each year, and concluded that TSS risk was increased eightfold in comparison to
the risk for all women (6). Other researchers, however, believe that an accurate
estimate of overall risk is not possible with existing data, so the comparison may not
be meaningful. In any case the total number of TSS cases is small. Only a handful of
TSS cases have been reported in association with sponge or diaphragm use. Nevertheless, women using sponges, a diaphragm, or a cervical cap need to be aware of TSS
and its danger signs (see Illustration 12-1).

TSS risk is the reason that experts **no longer recommend** use of a diaphragm,
sponges, or a cervical cap **during a menstrual period or when you have vaginal
bleeding for any reason.** The Centers for Disease Control (CDC) also recommends that
you avoid these contraceptives if you have had TSS. The CDC further recommends that
all diaphragm, sponge, and cervical cap users **avoid using these methods for four to
six weeks after delivering a baby or until postpartum bleeding completely stops.
You may minimize your TSS risk if you are careful not to leave your contraceptive
in the vagina for longer than the recommended time period.** (See Chapter 24 for
more on TSS.)

Allergy.   Allergy to latex is rare, but perhaps 1% to 4% of users develop spermicide allergy. Allergy can cause symptoms of burning, itching, swelling, or even blistering. Changing brands may help, but if you are allergic to the spermicidal chemical itself, you may need to choose another method of birth control.

Urinary Tract Infection.   There is some evidence that diaphragm users develop cystitis (bladder infection) and urethritis (inflammation of the urinary opening) more frequently than women who use other birth control methods. Researchers in one study found a doubled risk for diaphragm users compared to women taking birth control Pills, and also found higher vaginal counts of *E. coli* bacteria in diaphragm users (7). This bacteria can cause urinary infection, and could be spread accidentally during diaphragm insertion to the vagina from the rectal area where it is normally present. It is also possible that in some women the diaphragm rim exerts enough pressure against the lower part of the bladder or urethra to increase susceptibility to infection. If recurrent urinary infection is a problem, and persists despite a change in diaphragm rim type or size, it may be prudent to change to another method of birth control.

Diaphragm Rim Pressure.   Some diaphragm users experience bladder pressure, rectal pressure, or cramps when the diaphragm is left in place six hours after intercourse as recommended. You might talk to your clinician and try a smaller diaphragm or a different rim type.

Vaginal Infection or Injury.   Your diaphragm, sponge, or cap may cause a vaginal bacterial infection if you leave it in place more than 24 hours, just as a forgotten tampon can cause infection. These infections cause a foul-smelling discharge, and merit prompt evaluation by your clinician. Cervical or vaginal trauma has occasionally been reported with diaphragms and cervical caps, and irritation or laceration might predispose you to infection.

Partner Complaints.   Most barrier users and their partners are not even aware of the method during intercourse. Occasionally, however, a diaphragm or cap user's partner may complain about "bumping something" or may have some discomfort during deep penetration. Recheck your diaphragm or cap position to be sure you have inserted it properly. Your partner's penis is likely to bump the rim of a small diaphragm; so you might see your clinician and find out if you can use a larger diaphragm.

Esthetic Concerns.   Some users find barrier methods disruptive or messy to use, and the taste or smell of the spermicide interferes with lovemaking for some people. The sponge and unlubricated condoms sometimes cause unpleasant friction or dryness during intercourse. Try extra lubrication with spermicidal jelly, or use lubricated condoms.

Inability to Insert or Remove Vaginal Methods.   A physically disabled woman who is not able to insert and remove a diaphragm, sponge, or other vaginal contraceptives and cannot rely on her partner to do so will not be able to use these methods.

Sponge users may have trouble grasping the nylon loop for removing the sponge, or find that it breaks into fragments. Try squatting and bearing down as though for a bowel movement to shorten your vagina so you can reach the sponge or its fragments with your fingers. You can also ask your partner to help you.

Spermicide Effects.   There is some evidence that spermicide can be absorbed through the walls of the vagina and into a woman's circulation. So far, however, there have been no reports of serious side effects among spermicide users, nor any evidence in long-term studies that women exposed to spermicide have any higher incidence of cancer, serious illness, or death than do women using no contraception (8).

A recent review of 14 different studies of spermicide use and subsequent reproductive outcomes concluded that **no association has been demonstrated between these products and miscarriages or birth defects** (9), and these conclusions have also been affirmed by the FDA (national Food and Drug Administration) (10). A 1981 study that found an increased risk of birth defects with spermicide use received a great deal of publicity, but is generally considered to be flawed in several important respects; even the authors labeled their findings as tentative. Users can be reassured that large, careful studies have not found any cause for alarm.

Contraindications

A contraindication is a medical problem or other condition that renders inadvisable or unsafe a course of treatment that might otherwise be recommended. There are few contraindications to the use of barrier methods, but some do exist:

- **Allergy to latex:** For diaphragm, cervical cap, and latex condoms only.
- **Allergy to spermicide:** For all barriers except condoms that are not spermicide-coated. Changing brands sometimes solves the problem.
- **Repeated or persistent urinary tract infection:** Using a diaphragm may increase your risk for urinary tract infection.
- **Previous toxic shock syndrome (TSS):** A woman who had had TSS should not use contraceptive sponges; it may be prudent to avoid the diaphragm as well.
- **Physical or intellectual disability:** People with illnesses that impair the use of their hands may have trouble handling any of the barrier methods for proper insertion or removal. Intellectual impairment could interfere with following use instructions with enough care. Neither condition is a contraindication when the partner is able and willing to help use the method properly.
- **Vaginal abnormality:** Defects in vaginal shape or very poor vaginal muscle tone may make it impossible to use a diaphragm or cervical cap.

Advantages

The barrier methods are extremely safe and pose very few health risks. They provide quite effective contraception, particularly for older, careful women who have "average" intercourse frequency—no more than eight or so times a month. With the exception of the diaphragm and cervical cap, barriers are very convenient to buy: they are as accessible as the neighborhood drugstore.

Barriers help protect users from sexually transmitted diseases (STDs), and this advantage is extremely significant in an age of epidemic infections that lead to illness, infertility, ectopic pregnancy, and even death. Both clinical and laboratory studies show that spermicides kill the pathogens that cause gonorrhea, herpes, and trichomonas (11). The risk of gonorrhea, for example, among spermicide users appears to be about half the risk for nonusers (12). STDs often lead to pelvic inflammatory disease (PID), and a large study has found that spermicide users have about 0.6 times the risk of being hospitalized for first episodes of PID (13). The protective effect appears most pronounced for methods that employ both a mechanical **and** a chemical barrier, such as the spermicide-coated condom.

Barrier methods may protect against cervical cancer, a disease that can quite accurately be considered a STD. The virus family that causes genital warts also appears to be responsible for cervical cancer (see Chapter 27 for more details), and herpes virus may be a cofactor in cervical cancer as well. Barrier methods inhibit the transmission of these organisms. British studies have found that diaphragm users were 0.23 times (about one fifth) as likely to develop cervical cancer compared to users of other methods such as the Pill and IUD, and the risk for developing cervical disease **decreased** the longer women used either a condom or a diaphragm, from equal risk initially to 0.2 times the risk in comparison with other women after ten years of barrier method use (11).

Spermicidal chemicals have been shown to kill *Staphylococcus aureus*, the bacterium that causes toxic shock syndrome in some laboratory studies but not in others (11), and it is not yet possible to predict whether this effect is a true advantage of spermicide use.

I like milk in glass bottles, ironed cotton shirts, fountain pens, and my diaphragm. So I'm old-fashioned!

—WOMAN, 29

For many people the primary advantage of barrier methods is the noninvasive nature of these products. Many women simply don't want a foreign body inside the uterus, and don't wish to manipulate the body's hormonal patterns. Newer is not better for many people.

One of the most important advantages of barriers is their **convenience and reliability as a back-up contraceptive.** Many couples who rely on Pills or IUDs as primary contraceptives use barriers on occasion. Pill users can rely on condoms during the initial 14 days when they first begin to use Pills, when the Pill-taking schedule gets interrupted, and for several months after stopping Pills before planning to become pregnant. Couples who choose the IUD often rely on barriers during the first three months after the IUD is inserted when pregnancy risk is highest, when the woman is unable to find her IUD strings, or during the seven or so "fertile" days each month when she is most likely to conceive (see Chapter 6 for detailed instructions on how to predict possible fertile days).

Barriers can be especially appealing to couples who have intercourse infrequently or sporadically, for you use them only when you need them.

Some method-specific advantages: Condoms are extremely portable and disposable. Women whose partners use condoms have little or no postintercourse drippiness. Condoms permit men to take an active role in birth control; and they provide users with instant visible proof—after intercourse—of how well they worked.

Most clinicians recommend that couples use condoms during and after treatment for reproductive tract infections to protect against immediate reinfection.

Sex therapists may recommend condoms as an adjunct to treatment for premature ejaculation, because condoms may reduce sensitivity and help prolong intercourse. Condoms may have esthetic value for those who find penis–vagina contact distasteful or for a woman who dislikes having semen in her vagina. The silicone lubrication on prelubricated condoms can reduce friction during intercourse and reduce the risk of vaginal or penile irritation. Men who are older or have had lower abdominal surgery may have trouble maintaining an erection long enough to achieve orgasm, and the slight tourniquet effect of the condom rim may help them maintain a satisfactory erection.

Diaphragms and cervical caps can be inserted up to six hours before intercourse, so they need not interrupt lovemaking.

The **sponge** is very portable and disposable. It can be inserted up to 24 hours before intercourse, and need not interrupt lovemaking. It is the only barrier that doesn't require a repeat application for a second act of intercourse. The sponge is likely to be less messy than foam, cream, gel, or a suppository.

Foam, cream, and gel work immediately, so they can be used as an emergency measure if a condom ruptures or slips off, your diaphragm seems dislodged, or you have intercourse without any birth control at all. If you insert one of these products immediately after intercourse, you'll kill lots of sperm, but there are no guarantees. Sperm released into an unprotected vagina can enter the cervical canal in seconds, and then they are safely out of harm's way, even if you do add spermicide. (That's why douching isn't effective birth control.) An after-the-fact spermicide may help some, but it's impossible to say how much. All these products add extra lubrication for intercourse, a boon for many users.

Acquiring and Using Barrier Methods

Condoms, sponges, foams, creams, gels, film, and suppositories are available without prescription at your drugstore, and many products now include very helpful and detailed printed instructions. Diaphragms and cervical caps require a clinician's exam, fitting, and prescription.

Store all barrier methods away from moisture, heat, and extreme cold. Room temperature is ideal.

All foams, creams, gels, film, and suppositories have time limits for their effectiveness. See Table 12-2 to get an idea of when to insert your product so it works well for you. Always use an additional application each time intercourse is repeated, and always leave your product in place, with no douching, for at least six hours after the last time you have intercourse.

Try always to follow your method's particular instructions to the letter if you can, but if you feel you have to make a choice between bending the rules and having intercourse without any birth control, bend the rules. For example, if you can leave your diaphragm in place for only three hours after intercourse rather than the recommended six hours, leave it in three hours.

Many products include an expiration date on the package, so be sure to buy fresh products and replace them when the date expires. Specific advice on acquiring and successfully using each of the barrier methods follows.

CONDOMS

Rule 1 is use condoms every time. Commitment and discipline are called for, and it is hard to get out of a cozy bed and hunt around in the bathroom when you're feeling amorous. It helps to keep a supply of condoms in a bedside table drawer, or wherever you're most likely to need them.

Use a spermicide-coated condom brand for most effective birth control protection, or if there is any reason to expect either of you is at risk for a sexually transmitted infection, particularly if you are under 30 and either of you has more than one sex partner. Spermicidal condom brands to look for are Prime, Ramses Extra, and Contracept Plus.

Put the condom on before the penis comes anywhere near the entrance to the vagina. The clear lubricating fluid that collects at the tip of the erect penis may contain living sperm, especially after a recent ejaculation. If you have intercourse for a while and then stop in the middle to put on the condom, you expose the cervix to those sperm (and to possible sexually transmitted infection).

Leave room at the tip of the condom for the semen. Some condoms are made with receptacles at the end to catch semen, but others aren't. If you use condoms

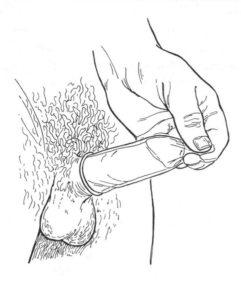

ILLUSTRATION 12-2   When putting on a condom without a reservoir end, pinch the tip to leave a little space for semen.

without a reservoir end, allow for a little space at the end by pinching the very tip of the condom as you roll it on (see Illustration 12-2). A condom stretched very tightly across the head of the penis is more likely to rupture; or semen may be pushed back along the length of the penis and out into freedom (and the vagina). There's no reason a woman can't help her partner put on the condom. It's not difficult, and besides, as one user says, "It makes it more of a treat than a treatment."

Hold on to the rim of the condom as the penis is withdrawn from the vagina. The penis begins to lose its erection soon after ejaculation, and a form-fitting condom will quickly become baggy.

Withdraw the penis before erection completely subsides, and check the condom before you throw it away. A quick look tells you whether it's intact.

Store condoms away from heat. Condoms are good for five years from the date of manufacture if they are stored properly. Most condoms, especially lubricated ones, are sealed in individual packets to keep them from drying out. Heat deteriorates latex and makes it brittle. Don't store condoms near heat vents or radiators, in glove compartments, or in a wallet—even body heat can deteriorate condoms. Purses, on the other hand, are fine for carrying condoms.

Don't lubricate condoms with petroleum jellies such as Vaseline. Lubrication is important because well-lubricated condoms are less likely to tear. But petroleum jelly may weaken latex, and condoms are only 0.08 mm thick to start with. If you need extra lubrication, try contraceptive foam, lubricated condoms, or a sterile water-soluble lubricant such as K-Y Jelly, available in drugstores without a prescription.

Always have a back-up method available. A time may come when you just don't want to use a condom; so be prepared with foam, a sponge, or a diaphragm.

I thought John would *hate* condoms, but he doesn't. We started using them after I had *had it* with four years of spotting on Pills. I got a diaphragm last year in case he changed his mind, but I haven't used it yet.

—WOMAN, 27

Try to talk about your feelings. Problems with condoms can sometimes be solved by talking about what you like and what you don't like. Your partner may not be able to guess how you are feeling. You may find that a special signal for the right time to put on the condom helps, for example. Some couples find that variety makes a big difference—condoms on Monday, Wednesday, and Friday; a diaphragm on Tuesday, Thursday, and Saturday.

Share the responsibility for cost and for keeping the bedside table supplied.

Some men consider natural skin condoms to be exquisitely sensitive. They make up about 2% to 4% of all condom sales in the United States. Skin condoms aren't regulated the way latex condoms are, and size and thickness may vary. No study has ever compared the effectiveness of latex and skin condoms, so we don't know whether skin condoms are as effective as the latex products. Also, latex condoms may be preferable for protection against sexually transmitted disease. Latex is probably less permeable than natural skin.

If a condom breaks or slips off inside the vagina, or you suspect a leak, then think about emergency measures. You can use contraceptive foam, gel, or cream to fill the vagina immediately. If you don't have any one of these contraceptives on hand, then a douche (see Chapter 39) with plain warm water is reasonable. Also, you may want to consider morning-after treatment (see Chapter 15); if so, plan to contact your clinician within 24 hours.

Starting to Use Condoms: The Moment of Truth. The beginning of a new relationship is one of the most risky times for unwanted pregnancy and sexual infection because so many couples find it difficult—or at least uncomfortable—to talk about birth control beforehand. Probably both partners are quietly worried about it. A woman may feel good if a new partner reaches for a condom, even if she does use Pills. He is saying, "I care about us and about you, and I am willing to bear some of the birth control burden; I don't want a pregnancy scare to jeopardize the beginning of our relationship."

For a woman, being prepared with a condom certainly makes as much sense as being prepared with Pills or a diaphragm. He probably won't say a word, but if he does, "Let's do this right, from the very beginning" should do it. As you hand him the condom or put it on him yourself you don't have to say anything, but maybe you could think of something loving and funny: "I know it's your favorite color." "Do you think this will fit?" "I got these on sale at a flea market." "My brother left these here last weekend." It isn't easy, but it does make sense. Mostly it takes courage.

THE DIAPHRAGM

The diaphragm is a dome-shaped latex cup rimmed with a firm, flexible metal band or spring. The diaphragm is first coated with sperm-killing cream or gel and then inserted in the vagina before intercourse. **The latex dome covers the cervix and holds the spermicidal cream or gel directly against the cervix.** The diaphragm is a physical barrier between your partner's penis and your cervix, but it does not remain perfectly stationary or create a tight seal against the walls of your vagina. Sperm can travel around the rim of your diaphragm and come into contact with your cervix, but spermicidal cream or gel inside the diaphragm dome will immobilize sperm before they have a chance to enter your cervical canal. The primary function of the diaphragm is to hold spermicidal gel or cream directly against your cervix.

You will need to see your clinician for an examination and fitting. Fitting is not difficult or painful for you, but it does require training and experience on the part of your clinician. Your local family planning clinic or Planned Parenthood clinic can fit your diaphragm or refer you to clinicians who have the necessary knowledge and experience.

Diaphragm Fitting.   There are three types of diaphragms: flat spring, coil spring, and arcing spring. They differ slightly in rim construction only. The differences are most evident when the diaphragm is folded for insertion: each of the three assumes a slightly different shape. **Most women could use all three types with equal success,** but in certain circumstances one rim type may prove to be better than the others.

Many clinicians recommend the arcing spring as a first choice for most patients; it is well tolerated by most women, and it is difficult to insert incorrectly. Some women find the coil spring more comfortable. The flat spring type is the gentlest spring.

Diaphragm sizes range from 50 to 105—the rim diameter is expressed in millimeters. Your clinician's goal is to select the **largest size that is comfortable for you.** The most common fitting error is selecting too small a size.

Two factors will determine the size of the diaphragm you need: the depth and width of your vagina and the strength of your vaginal muscle tone. Two women with the same vaginal depth in millimeters may need different diaphragm sizes because of a difference in muscle tone. Masters and Johnson have demonstrated that during sexual excitement the vaginal depth increases as much as several inches (14). Using the largest comfortable fit will help insure that your diaphragm remains in position and covers your cervix during sexual excitement.

The most common diaphragm sizes are 70 to 85. The 90 to 100 sizes are fairly common, and 50 to 65 sizes are fairly uncommon.

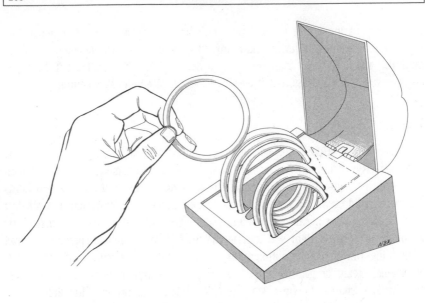

ILLUSTRATION 12-3   Your clinician uses graduated fitting rings or sample diaphragms to determine your correct diaphragm size.

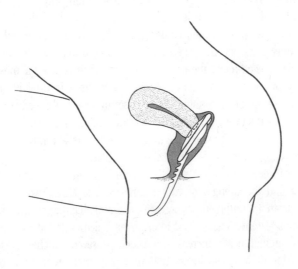

ILLUSTRATION 12-4   Some women prefer to use a plastic introducer for diaphragm insertion.

A variation of the standard diaphragm configuration is Milex's wide-seal diaphragm, which adds an extra inner latex rim designed to hold the spermicide in place more effectively. If you use this diaphragm, be extra careful to dry both sides of the inner rim carefully when you clean the diaphragm, because moisture could promote bacterial growth and possible infection.

Your clinician may fit you with sample diaphragms, or she/he may use fitting rings (see Illustration 12-3). Do not be confused by the rings, which are the latex-covered rims alone, without the latex dome. Your diaphragm will have a dome. It needs a dome to cover your cervix.

Be sure that you have a chance to practice inserting and removing your diaphragm before you leave your doctor's office or clinic. Have your clinician check to be sure you are inserting it correctly. Most women insert the diaphragm with their hands alone, but some women find it easier to use a special diaphragm introducer (see Illustration 12-4). You may want to practice with and without an introducer to decide which you prefer.

Some clinicians ask that you return in a week or two wearing your diaphragm to have your size checked and to make sure you are inserting it properly. Be sure to use another method of birth control, such as condoms or foam, until you have had your size and your insertion technique checked. **Be sure to pick up all the supplies that you will need:**

• A diaphragm in a plastic case
• One or two tubes of spermicidal jelly or cream
• A plastic applicator tube for inserting extra jelly or cream
• An introducer if you choose to use one

Spermicidal gel and cream are equally effective with your diaphragm. You may wish to try both and decide which you prefer. Most women find that gel provides a more lubricating effect. Some women find that cream has a more pleasant smell.

Several different brands of gel and cream are available, and they differ primarily in perfume and price. Table 12-2 lists selected creams and gels designed for use with a diaphragm. **If one brand seems to cause irritation, try a different brand**; the perfume chemical is often the irritant. Although brands do have slightly different sperm-killing chemicals, there is no evidence that any one is more effective than another.

Applying Gel or Cream.

To apply contraceptive gel or cream, hold your diaphragm with the dome down, like a cup. Squeeze the gel or cream from the tube into the dome (see Illustration 12-5). Be sure to use plenty, about a tablespoon, and spread a little around the rim of the diaphragm with your finger. The gel or cream remains active for at least six hours; so you can insert your diaphragm with cream or gel up to six hours before you have intercourse. If you haven't had intercourse within that time, you can remove the diaphragm to use fresh gel or cream. You can insert your diaphragm, of course, just before intercourse, but if you find that inserting it as long

TABLE 12-2   CHARACTERISTICS OF SELECTED VAGINAL CONTRACEPTIVES

ALL PRODUCTS: • Use an *additional* application each time intercourse is repeated.
• Leave in place, with no douching, for at least *6 hours* after last intercourse.

	INTENDED USE	SPERMICIDE	CORRECT TIMING OF INSERTION BEFORE INTERCOURSE	OTHER CHARACTERISTICS
FOAMS				
Delfen (use 2 applicators-full)	Alone	Nonoxynol-9 12.5%	1–60 minutes	
Emko	Alone or with diaphragm	Nonoxynol-9 8.0%	1–60 minutes	Container indicates when supply is low
Emko Because	Alone or with diaphragm	Nonoxynol-9 8.0%	1–60 minutes; up to 6 hours with diaphragm	Portable—contains 6 applications
Emko Pre-Fil	Alone or with diaphragm	Nonoxynol-9 8.0%	1–60 minutes; up to 6 hours with diaphragm	Can be filled ahead of time; container indicates when supply is low
Koromex (use 2 applicators-full)	Alone	Nonoxynol-9 12.5%	1–60 minutes	
CREAMS				
Conceptrol	Alone	Nonoxynol-9 5%	1–60 minutes	
Koromex	With diaphragm	Octoxynol 3%	Up to 6 hours	
Ortho-Creme	With diaphragm	Nonoxynol-9 2%	Up to 6 hours	

GELS

	Use	Active Ingredient	Time	Packaging
Conceptrol Gel	Alone	Nonoxynol-9 4%	1–60 minutes	
Conceptrol Disposable Gel	Alone	Nonoxynol-9 4%	1–60 minutes	Prefilled, disposable packages of 6, 10
Gynol II Jelly	With diaphragm	Nonoxynol-9 2%	Up to 6 hours	
Koromex Crystal Clear Gel	With diaphragm	Nonoxynol-9 2%	Up to 6 hours	
Koromex Jelly	Alone or with diaphragm	Nonoxynol-9 3%	1–60 minutes; up to 6 hours with diaphragm	
Ortho-Gynol-Jelly	With diaphragm	Octoxynol-9 1%	Up to 6 hours	
Ramses Jelly	Alone or with diaphragm	Nonoxynol-9 5%	Just before intercourse; up to 6 hours with diaphragm	
Shur-Seal Jelly	With diaphragm	Nonoxynol-9 2%	Up to 6 hours	Portable 1-dose packages

SUPPOSITORIES

	Use	Active Ingredient	Time	Packaging
Encare	Alone or as repeat (not first) application with diaphragm	Nonoxynol-9 2.27%	10–60 minutes	Boxes of 12, 24
Intercept	Alone	Nonoxynol-9 100 mg	10–60 minutes	Boxes of 12 with applicator
Semicid	Alone	Nonoxynol-9 100 mg	15–60 minutes	Packets of 3, 10, 20

FILM

	Use	Active Ingredient	Time	Packaging
VCF (Vaginal Contraceptive Film)	Alone	Nonoxynol-9 28%	15–90 minutes	Box of 12 thin sheets of film (2-inch square)

SOURCES: *Physicians' Desk Reference for Nonprescription Drugs* (ed 6). Oradell, N.J.: Medical Economics Co., 1986, and package inserts.

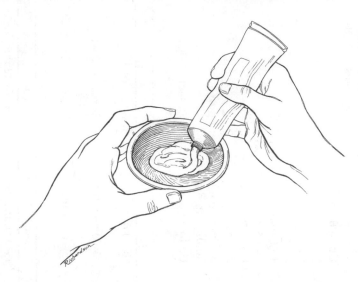

ILLUSTRATION 12-5   Sperm-killing cream or gel goes inside the dome of the diaphragm.

as four, five, or six hours beforehand helps you to use it consistently, then by all means do so.

If you don't have an opportunity to remove your diaphragm, or have already had intercourse in the last six hours, you can insert extra gel or cream into your vagina with an applicator. To use the plastic applicator, just attach the tube of gel or cream to the open end of the applicator and squeeze the tube to force cream or gel up into the applicator barrel. Insert the open end of the applicator into your vagina in front of your diaphragm, much as you would insert a tampon. Push the applicator plunger to release the gel or cream (see Illustration 12-6).

If you have intercourse more than once, use an additional applicator full of spermicide each time, no matter how short a time your diaphragm has been in place. **Do not remove or dislodge your diaphragm to add cream or gel if you have already had intercourse.**

Some women find that extra applications of jelly or cream are messy. Use condoms for a second or third act of intercourse instead of more spermicide if you prefer.

Inserting the Diaphragm.   You can insert your diaphragm while you are standing with one foot propped up, or while you are squatting or lying down. To insert your diaphragm, hold it dome down (with spermicide inside the dome) in one hand and press the opposite sides of the rim together so that the diaphragm folds (see Illustration 12-7). Spread the lips of your vagina with your other hand and insert the folded diaphragm into your vagina. Push the diaphragm inward and along the back wall of your vagina toward the small of your back as far as it will go (see Illustration

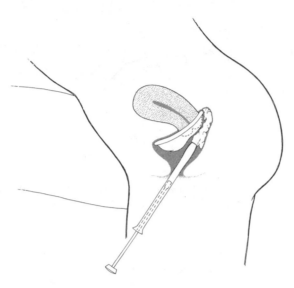

ILLUSTRATION 12-6   Insert more cream or gel for repeat intercourse *without* removing or dislodging your diaphragm.

12-8). Then tuck the nearest rim up behind the firm bulge in the roof of your vagina that covers the pubic bone. Once your diaphragm is in proper place, you should not be able to feel it except with your fingers. If it is uncomfortable, it may be incorrectly placed; so take it out and insert it again.

You can use a plastic introducer with a coil spring diaphragm if you prefer (see Illustration 12-4). Some women find insertion easier with an introducer, but all types of diaphragms can be inserted by hand. To use the introducer, put 1 tablespoon of spermicidal gel or cream into the cup of the diaphragm and, with the cup up, place it on the introducer. Do this by squeezing opposite sides of the rim together, slipping one end into the notched end of the introducer and the other end over the notch corresponding to your diaphragm's size. With the cup still up, gently push the introducer and diaphragm into the deepest part of your vagina and gently twist the introducer to release the diaphragm in place. With your finger, tuck the near end of the diaphragm up behind the pubic bone and check the placement of the diaphragm.

Double-checking the Position of the Diaphragm.   Always check the position of your diaphragm before you have intercourse. The back rim should be below and behind your cervix, and the front (nearest) rim tucked up behind your pubic bone. Often it is impossible to feel the back rim with your finger. Check to be sure that you can feel your cervix through the soft rubber dome of the diaphragm (see Illustration 12-9), and check to be sure that the front rim is snugly in place behind the pubic bone. The gel or cream should be on the **inside**, in contact with your cervix.

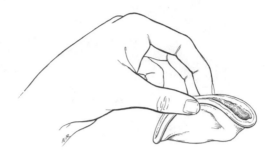

ILLUSTRATION 12-7   Once you've covered the inside of the dome with cream or gel, fold your diaphragm for insertion. This woman is using an arcing spring diaphragm.

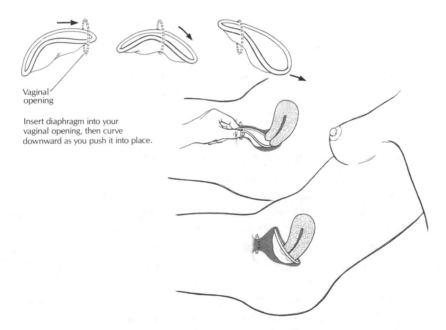

Vaginal opening

Insert diaphragm into your vaginal opening, then curve downward as you push it into place.

ILLUSTRATION 12-8   Use your fingers to guide the diaphragm along the back wall of your vagina.

Finding your cervix often takes practice. You might try to find it first without your diaphragm. Use two fingers rather than one, and try a squatting position. Your cervix will feel like a firm, round bump, somewhat like the tip of your nose.

Check your diaphragm again after intercourse. If it seems to be dislodged, add more gel or cream with your applicator and talk to your clinician if you want to consider morning-after emergency birth control (see Chapter 15). You might also want to see your clinician to check for proper fitting and insertion techniques.

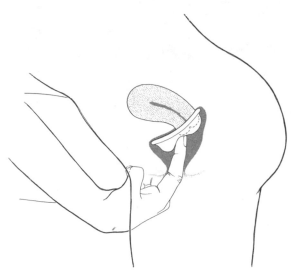

ILLUSTRATION 12-9   Check for proper diaphragm placement. You should be able to feel your cervix *through* the dome of your diaphragm.

The position of your diaphragm should not be affected by either urination or bowel movement, but you can check afterward to be sure. Urination will not wash away the cream or gel. An ordinary shower or tub bath won't interfere with your diaphragm either—but douching might wash away gel or cream.

When to Remove the Diaphragm.   Leave the diaphragm in place for six hours after intercourse, and do not douche during that time. You can remove your diaphragm any time after the six-hour minimum. If you anticipate intercourse again, simply wash and dry it, add more gel or cream, and reinsert it. **Remove and wash your diaphragm after 24 hours to avoid infection and an unpleasant odor,** and toxic shock syndrome (see "Problems and Risks" earlier in this chapter), but **stick to the six-hour minimum** after intercourse for leaving your diaphragm in place. It may take six hours for spermicidal chemicals to immobilize and kill all the sperm.

To remove your diaphragm, reach inside with your index finger or thumb, hook your finger behind the front rim of the diaphragm, and pull down and out (see Illustration 12-10). Be careful not to tear your diaphragm with a fingernail. If you find it hard to hook your finger behind the rim, try a squatting position and push downward with your abdominal muscles. You can also remove the diaphragm with the hook end of your introducer.

Caring for the Diaphragm.   Wash your diaphragm with plain soap and water, rinse it thoroughly, and dry it with a towel. Store it in its plastic container, well away from radiators and other heat sources. Do not powder your diaphragm.

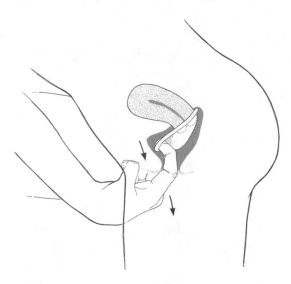

ILLUSTRATION 12-10   To remove your diaphragm, hook a finger underneath the rim and pull downward.

Inspect your diaphragm for defects or holes each time you use it. **Do not use petroleum jelly such as Vaseline with your diaphragm,** because it can cause deterioration of the latex. If you use extra lubrication, try a water-soluble lubricant such as K-Y Jelly, which you can buy in a drugstore without a prescription.

The latex part of your diaphragm will discolor and turn darker brown or mottled brown in time, but even so, your diaphragm will last for about two years if you care for it properly.

If you have had a vaginal infection of any kind, be especially thorough as you wash your diaphragm. Wash and dry your plastic storage case, introducer, and plastic spermicide applicator carefully as well. Common infection organisms will be killed by thorough washing and drying.

When to See Your Clinician.   Your diaphragm size may not always remain the same. Vaginal depth and muscle tone are usually altered by full-term pregnancy, and they can also change after you first begin to have intercourse regularly. Have your diaphragm fit checked as part of your routine annual examination. Be sure to take your diaphragm with you when you visit your clinician.

Be sure to see your clinician promptly for a check on your diaphragm fit:

• Any time you believe for any reason that your diaphragm is not fitting properly or if you have any doubt about whether you are inserting it correctly
• If you have discomfort, pain, or recurring bladder infections
• After you have been pregnant

• After you have had surgery involving your reproductive organs
• If your partner finds the diaphragm uncomfortable during intercourse

Tips for Success.   Practice inserting your diaphragm by yourself several times when you first get it until you are confident about your technique. If you have intercourse before you feel sure that you are inserting it correctly, protect yourself with a back-up method such as condoms or foam.

Some women find it convenient to have two diaphragms, one for home and one for travel or to permit each one to dry thoroughly after use. Be sure to keep an extra tube of gel or cream on hand.

Check the fit of your diaphragm yourself. The diaphragm rim should be a snug fit. When it is in its proper place, there should be only a small gap between the front edge of the rim and your pubic bone, about half an inch or so. If the gap is so large that you can insert more than one fingertip between the bone and the rim, then you may need a larger diaphragm size.

Pay attention to the position of your diaphragm in case it should slip during intercourse, for it is occasionally possible for the diaphragm to be dislodged. Masters and Johnson found that the diaphragm could be dislodged during initial penetration of the penis, but was most likely to be dislodged with rapid, repeated penetration. You may want to help guide your partner's penis along the back vaginal wall during entry. Masters and Johnson found that the woman-on-top position was especially risky for dislodging the diaphragm at the time of penis entry. When you use this position be especially careful to guide your partner's penis away from the front diaphragm rim (14).

Your diaphragm will not interfere with your own natural lubrication during lovemaking. The normal lubrication response to arousal is secreted or "sweated" directly from the walls of the vagina and is not blocked by the diaphragm.

Any substance containing petroleum such as Vaseline and certain medications may deteriorate the latex of your diaphragm. Read the medication label, or check with your clinician or pharmacist to determine whether your medication does contain petroleum. Ask your clinician whether to abstain from intercourse during treatment for infection. Some kinds of vaginal infection are contagious; and in some cases intercourse might interfere with your own recovery.

I don't know if Allen worries about pregnancy as much as I do or not; why would he? He isn't going to get pregnant! But he acts as if he cares as much as I do. He never complains about my diaphragm, and is as conscientious about using it right as I am. That kind of empathy means more to me than I could ever tell him. He's a prince.

—WOMAN, 30

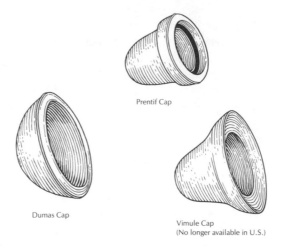

Prentif Cap

Dumas Cap

Vimule Cap
(No longer available in U.S.)

ILLUSTRATION 12-11   Three cap styles are available at centers participating in cap research. Most women use the Prentif cavity rim model.

CERVICAL CAP

The cervical cap works much like the diaphragm except that it fits just over the cervix and stays in place partly by suction. It is made of latex and is used with a spermicidal cream or gel. There are three types of cervical caps that differ in size and configuration: the Prentif cavity rim, Vimule, and Dumas (see Illustration 12-11).

As of 1987, none of the three caps was approved by the Food and Drug Administration (FDA) for use in the United States. Caps are presently available in a limited number of U.S. clinics that are participating in clinical trials, however. Caps are manufactured in England, and are available also in some other countries.

A custom-fitted cap called the ContraCap was tested in several centers. The ContraCap was custom-made to a mold of the woman's cervix and included a valve to release cervical secretions and menstrual blood. Recent studies on ContraCap were stopped because of high rates of cap dislodgement and pregnancy.

Fitting.   The length and diameter of your cervix determine the cap size and type that will fit you best. A woman with an average cervix is likely to do well with the Prentif cap; the Dumas cap is sometimes better for women with a short cervix (11). Each cap type is available in several sizes, expressed as a rim diameter measurement in millimeters.

Some women find cap insertion and removal distinctly tricky, **so be sure you have ample time to practice before you leave your clinician's office.**

Spermicidal Gel or Cream.   Always use your cap in conjunction with a spermicidal gel or cream that is intended for use with a diaphragm. Instructions prepared by the cap manufacturer require spermicide, and research on cap effectiveness has included spermicide use in most cases. Selected brands are described in Table 12-2. Fill the dome of your cap about one-third full of spermicide each time you use it.

Insertion and Removal.   Wash your hands and locate your cervix with a finger first. You can shorten your vagina and make your cervix more accessible by squatting and bearing down as though for a bowel movement. Add spermicide to your cap, and slide the cap onto your cervix with your fingers, then check to be sure you can feel your cervix **through** the latex dome of your cap. This may take some practice. **Check your cap to be sure it is in place again after intercourse**, because caps occasionally get dislodged during intercourse. To remove your cap, tilt it with your fingers to break the suction, then hook a fingertip under the rim and pull it out.

Some women use the cap constantly for several days or even weeks. The latex caps now available, however, are not intended for prolonged use, and the advantage of fresh spermicide in providing optimal birth control protection is probably important for the latex cap just as it is for the diaphragm. **The authors recommend that your cap be inserted up to six hours before intercourse.** You do need to leave your cap in place (with no douching) a full six hours after intercourse to allow the spermicide plenty of time to kill all sperm. If you **minimize** the amount of time your cap is in place—respecting always the six-hour postintercourse waiting period—you can probably minimize your risk for toxic shock syndrome, laceration or irritation from the cap, and foul-smelling bacterial growth on the cap.

Caring for Your Cervical Cap.   When you remove your cap, wash it thoroughly in plain soap and water, dry it completely, and store it in a cool, dry, dark place. Don't powder your cap.

Problems.   Research on possible complications of cap use is limited. Prolonged or frequent cap wear, however, does expose the surface of the cervix to a pool of cervical secretions, spermicide, and microorganisms trapped within the cap. There is some evidence that abnormal, precancerous Pap smear changes occur more often among cap users than among comparable diaphragm users (15), and cervical and pelvic infections have also been reported among cap users. Whether or not cap use caused or contributed to these problems, however, remains to be determined.

The Vimule cap has a thin tapered rim unlike the blunt rims of the other cap styles. Vaginal injuries in the precise area of contact with a Vimule rim have been reported, so this cap may be less desirable than the other styles available, and the national Food and Drug Administration (FDA) has stopped its use in clinical research trials in the United States (16).

When to See Your Clinician.   Have your cap fit checked as part of your routine annual examination. See your clinician promptly:

• Any time your cap becomes **dislodged, or seems too large or too small**. The size of the cervix changes slightly during the menstrual cycle, and some women even use two different cap sizes for different cyclic phases.
• Any time you have pain during intercourse, unusual odor, discharge, bleeding, or spotting, or any other signs of **injury or infection**
• Any time you develop signs of **toxic shock syndrome**: fever (temperature of 101 degrees Fahrenheit or more), diarrhea, vomiting, muscle aches, or sunburn-like rash
• After you have been pregnant

Tips for Success.   Remember that not everyone who wants to use a cap can use one. One experienced clinician reported that only about half the women he saw who wanted to use the cap could be fitted or could master insertion and removal techniques (9). Be prepared to switch methods of birth control if you aren't successful, rather than risking pregnancy.

Keep a container of contraceptive foam on hand, and **add an application of foam immediately** if you find that your cap has become dislodged during lovemaking. You may also want to talk to your clinician about morning-after birth control (see Chapter 15).

SPONGE

The contraceptive sponge acts both as a cervical barrier and as a source of sperm-killing chemical. It is made of polyurethane and is impregnated (sorry) with the spermicide nonoxynol-9. It comes in one size; as one woman put it, "sort of a one-size-fits-all tube socks style diaphragm." One side of the sponge has a dimple to fit against your cervix, and the other side has a loop of nylon to grasp for removal. It is available without prescription in drugstores, and is also sold in some family planning clinics. There is one brand of sponge available, the Today sponge manufactured by VLI Corporation.

Insertion.   Remove the sponge from its wrapping, moisten it with about 2 table-spoons of tap water to enhance spermicide release, and squeeze it once. Insert it in your vagina with your fingers so that the dimple (see Illustration 12-12) fits against your cervix and the nylon loop is away from your cervix. Check with a finger to be sure you can feel your cervix through the sponge. You can have intercourse immediately or any time within the next 24 hours. You do not have to add more spermicide for repeated intercourse within the 24-hour time period.

Removal.   The sponge is designed for 24 hours of use, and should remain in place for six hours after the last act of intercourse, so the maximum amount of time to leave in your sponge is **30 hours**. If you don't anticipate repeated intercourse within the 24-hour use period, go ahead and remove the sponge after six hours. **Be careful that**

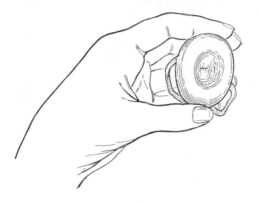

ILLUSTRATION 12-12   The dimple in the sponge should be placed directly *against* your cervix, and the nylon loop should be *away* from your cervix.

you don't leave the sponge in your vagina longer than you need to, so that you don't increase your risk for toxic shock syndrome. Read the "Problems and Risks" section earlier in this chapter for more details.

Before you throw away the used sponge, check to make sure it is intact, then simply throw it away. (Don't try to flush it in your toilet, because it floats and could also clog your plumbing.)

If you find your sponge has crumbled, search your vagina carefully to remove all the fragments. If you have trouble removing your sponge or sponge fragments, remember that squatting and bearing down as though for a bowel movement will shorten your vagina. If you can't remove your sponge, ask your partner to help, or see your clinician promptly.

When to See Your Clinician.   See your clinician any time you have pain during intercourse or unusual bleeding, spotting, discharge, or odor so you can be checked for infection. If you or your partner notice burning or itching when you use the sponge, you may be allergic to the spermicide. You will need to switch to another method of birth control because there is only one brand of sponge to try. See your clinician any time you have fever (higher than 101 degrees Fahrenheit), diarrhea, vomiting, muscle aches, or sunburn-like rash. These are symptoms of toxic shock syndrome.

Tips for Success.   When you moisten the sponge prior to insertion, be careful that you don't wet it or squeeze it excessively and squeeze out some of the spermicide.

The sponge can absorb vaginal lubrication, so if you feel too dry during intercourse, try adding spermicidal jelly or a water-soluble lubricant such as K-Y Jelly **after** your sponge is in place.

Research suggests that the sponge may be less effective for women who have delivered babies than for women who have not (5), possibly because the vagina gets longer after childbirth and the sponge doesn't fit as snugly. **If you have delivered one**

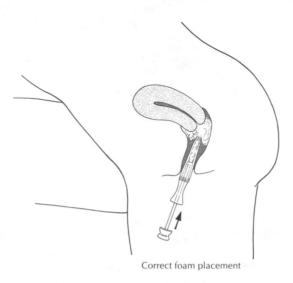

Correct foam placement

ILLUSTRATION 12-13   Insert the applicator deep in your vagina so that foam will cover your cervix.

or more babies, it would be prudent to use condoms along with your sponge, particularly during your fertile days each cycle. Read Chapter 6 to learn how to identify your fertile days.

FOAMS, CREAMS, GELS, FILM, AND SUPPOSITORIES

When you insert a dose of foam, cream, gel, film, or a suppository deep inside your vagina, two contraceptive actions are ready to work for you. First, the product spreads over the surface of your cervix and vagina and serves as a mechanical barrier between your cervical opening and sperm. Second, the spermicidal chemical coats and breaks down the surface of sperm cells on contact. The sperm-killing action is a more important contraceptive effect than the mechanical barrier.

Insertion.   To use these methods effectively, **timing** must be right and **placement** must be right. After the recommended time interval, the contraceptive will begin to drip out of your vagina, away from the cervix where it is needed. And if it isn't inserted deep enough to begin with, it may not reach the cervix and may not be effective. Masters and Johnson studied the dispersal characteristics of several types of vaginal spermicides, and foam won out over gels and suppositories. They found that foam dispersed rapidly and formed an effective barrier (17). (How do they know? you may well be asking yourself. Women volunteers had simulated intercourse with a see-through plastic penis. The penis had a little camera inside it. Honest.)

Read Table 12-2 carefully and **follow the timing instructions for your product** as precisely as possible. Always read the printed instructions that come in your package, too. Remember with foam that comes in aerosol cans you must **shake the can vigorously 20 to 30 times** to make sure plenty of spermicide gets mixed in with the bubbles. Always check to see if the recommended dosage is **one or two** applicators, because products vary.

Insert the spermicide applicator, suppository, or film the same way you insert a tampon, and take care to place it as deep inside your vagina as possible. If you don't have any experience using tampons, practice insertion a few times before you use it with a partner. Illustration 12-13 shows correct placement, deep in the vagina.

Foam, gels, and creams are ready to work within seconds after insertion. An adequate interval for melting or foaming and dispersal, however, is essential for suppositories and for the newest spermicide option, VCF film. Film contains spermicide in a thin glycerine sheet, 2-inches square. The glycerine melts quickly on contact with moisture and body heat, releasing spermicide wherever the film was placed. Accurate positioning on or very near the cervix is essential, and may require a little practice. Be sure to wash your hands before inserting a suppository or film, and dry them thoroughly before touching a film sheet. Then allow the full 10 to 15 minutes required for your product before beginning intercourse. If you use suppositories you can check with your finger for complete melting before intercourse.

I decided to quit using suppositories the morning I got up and one fell out *intact* that I inserted the night before. It's a good thing Larry fell asleep watching David Letterman!

—WOMAN, 20

You are protected for an hour. If more time elapses, insert another dose before you have intercourse. Use another full dose beforehand each time you have intercourse, even if it means more every 15 minutes. (There are new legions of sperm.) Do not douche until at least six hours after the last time you have intercourse. Give your spermicide plenty of time to work. (Generally, clinicians say douching is not necessary except in the treatment of certain infections.)

Rinse the applicator in warm water after each use, and store it in a dry place so that the inside has a chance to dry out. Applicators need no special soaps or disinfectants. Foam, cream, and gel are no good without an applicator, so keep them together at all times.

When to See Your Clinician. Talk to your clinician any time you have burning or itching, or unusual pain, bleeding, spotting, odor, or discharge, so you can be checked for irritation and infection. Try changing brands as a first step to eliminate burning or itching unless you suspect that infection may be the culprit.

Tips for Success. Keep your supplies handy so that you can reach them without getting up.

Some cans of foam have indicators that show when your supply is running low, and others don't. If you use a brand without an indicator, keep at least two cans on hand at all times. (It's almost impossible to shake and jiggle a can and tell how much you have left. They're all deceptively heavy.) Store products away from heat. One nice thing about prefilled single-dose applicators is that you always know exactly how much you have, but they are more expensive.

If you are bothered by dripping after intercourse, you can use a pad or panty shield.

Don't be misled by deodorants, hygiene sprays, or fancy shaving creams. Make sure the box you select (except for some suppositories and film) has a plastic applicator tube enclosed.

Most clinicians recommend foam over creams, gels, or suppositories, because the effectiveness rates with foam are generally higher than those with other vaginal spermicides.

On the other hand, it is one of the eternal verities of birth control practice that couples are likely to be successful with the methods they like to use, and many people use cream, gels, and suppositories very effectively. It is unlikely that a clinician would try to convince a happy and successful cream user to switch to foam.

OTHER PRODUCTS

Spermicidal products come and go, and researchers are constantly looking for better ways to package chemicals to kill sperm. In the United States, and especially if you are traveling to other countries, you may find spermicides that are unfamiliar to you. If possible, use the well-tested products described in detail in this chapter. A word of warning: mercury-based spermicides were sold in the past and may still be marketed in other countries. Mercury may be harmful, so avoid products that contain phenylmercuric acetate or other mercury compounds.

REFERENCES

1. Goldsmith MF: Sex in the age of AIDS calls for common sense and 'condom sense.' *Journal of the American Medical Association* 257:2261-2266, 1987.
2. Hatcher RA, Guest FJ, Stewart FH, et al: *Contraceptive Technology 1988–1989* (ed. 14). New York: Irvington Publishers, in press.

3. Ory HW, Forrest JD, Lincoln R: *Making Choices: Evaluating the Health Risks and Benefits of Birth Control Methods.* New York: Alan Guttmacher Institute, 1983.
4. Lane ME, Arceo R, Sobrero AJ: Successful use of the diaphragm and jelly by a young population: Report of a clinical study. *Family Planning Perspectives* 8:81–86, 1976.
5. McIntyre SL, Higgins JE: Parity and use-effectiveness with the contraceptive sponge. *American Journal of Obstetrics and Gynecology* 155:796–801, 1986.
6. Faich G, Pearson K, Fleming D, et al: Toxic shock syndrome and the vaginal contraceptive sponge. *Journal of the American Medical Association* 255:216–218, 1986.
7. Fihn SD, Latham RH, Roberts P, et al: Association between diaphragm use and urinary tract infection. *Journal of the American Medical Association* 254:240–245, 1985.
8. Coleman S, Piotrow PT: Spermicides—simplicity and safety are major assets. *Population Reports,* Ser H, No 5, September 1979. Baltimore: Johns Hopkins University.
9. Bracken MB: Spermicidal contraceptives and poor reproductive outcomes: The epidemiologic evidence against an association. *American Journal of Obstetrics and Gynecology* 151:552–556, 1984.
10. Data do not support association between spermicides, birth defects. *FDA Drug Bulletin* November, 1986.
11. Sherris JD: New developments in vaginal contraception. *Population Reports,* Ser H, No 7, January–February 1984. Baltimore: Johns Hopkins University.
12. Austin H, Louv WC, Alexander J: A case-control study of spermicides and gonorrhea. *Journal of the American Medical Association* 251:2822–2824, 1984.
13. Kelaghan J, Rubin GL, Ory HW, et al: Barrier-method contraceptives and pelvic inflammatory disease. *Journal of the American Medical Association* 248:184–187, 1982.
14. Johnson VE, Masters WH: Intravaginal contraceptive study Phase I: Anatomy. *Western Journal of Surgical Obstetrics and Gynecology* 70:202–207, 1962.
15. Potik R: Use, risk and effectiveness of the cervical cap. Presented at Cervical Cap symposium, June 1983, Los Angeles.
16. Bernstein GS, Kilzer LH, Coulson AH, et al: Studies of cervical caps: I. Vaginal lesions associated with use of the Vimule cap. *Contraception* 5:443–446, 1983.
17. Johnson VE, Masters WH, Lewis KC: The physiology of intravaginal contraceptive failure, in Calderone MS (ed): *Manual of Family Planning and Contraceptive Practice* (ed 2). Baltimore: Williams & Wilkins, 1970.

13

Birth Control Pills and Implants

The earliest Pill package insert decades ago was about 2 by 4 inches in size and briefly listed a handful of circulatory disease risk factors. Today's insert is likely to be 18 by 24 inches in size and absolutely covered front and back with tiny print about every possible Pill risk and benefit. The Pill is the most thoroughly studied drug in history.

In the 1960s Pills were a wonder drug. In the 1970s the honeymoon ended. We learned about cardiovascular risks, and discovered that sequential Pills (discontinued in 1970) could cause cancer of the uterus. In the 1980s Pills look fairly good again. **Dosages have dropped dramatically, and so have serious complications and side effects.** Patterns are beginning to emerge that will help us answer the Pills and cancer questions. Research has shown that today's Pills reduce a woman's risk for uterine cancer and ovary cancer. Pill users may, however, have a somewhat higher risk for cervical cancer and for a very rare form of liver cancer. The breast cancer question has not yet been entirely resolved. The increased cervical cancer risk may be a Pill effect, although other factors like frequency of Pap smear testing and the number of sexual partners may also explain the differences found in research studies. In the last edition of this book there were not yet good data on the cancer question. Now that the picture is a bit clearer, you will notice, if you compare editions, that we are now more confident and optimistic about Pill safety.

We still can't predict the future, however. We can only tell today's version of the truth. We will all continue to learn more about Pills, so do your best to stay current. You will find, as we do, that to be intellectually honest, you may have to throw out some of your old, cherished ideas about oral contraceptives.

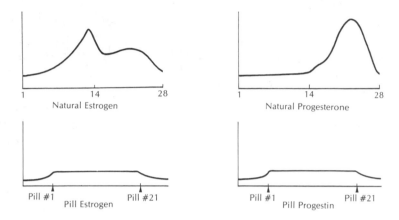

ILLUSTRATION 13-1   **Pill users have low, steady hormone levels throughout the cycle.**

The Pill era began in April 1956, in San Juan, Puerto Rico, with the first large clinical trial of combined estrogen and progestin oral contraceptives. Four years later, the Food and Drug Administration approved birth control Pills* for use in the United States. Pills achieved worldwide popularity almost immediately. About 39 million U.S. women have used Pills, and some 10 million used them in the mid 80s (1).

The first Pills contained 150 micrograms (mcg) of estrogen and 10 milligrams (mg) of progestin. Today's Pills contain one third or less that amount of estrogen and one tenth as much progestin as the earliest products, for many studies have shown that lower doses are just as effective and are less likely to cause side effects and serious complications.

How Pills Work

Both estrogen and progestin contribute to the Pill's birth control effects. The synthetic Pill hormones mimic the effects of natural estrogen and progesterone that your ovaries ordinarily produce, and your brain does not distinguish these synthetic hormones from natural ones. Because there is a steady synthetic hormone level day after day, your pituitary gland does not produce its normal cyclic pattern of FSH and LH, the hormones that stimulate your ovaries (see Chapter 2). Your ovaries, therefore, do not produce their cyclic pattern of estrogen and progesterone. As long as you take Pills, your own reproductive hormone cycle is suppressed and the Pills' synthetic estrogen

*The authors use the term "birth control Pills" and "Pills" for regular, *combined* estrogen and progestin oral contraceptives, no matter what the dose level. The term does not encompass progestin-only pills, which we consistently call "Minipills" or "progestin-only pills."

and progestin take the place of natural hormones produced by your ovary. **You do not have your own cycles. Instead, you have a Pill cycle** (see Illustration 13-1).

Without your brain's signal for cyclic FSH and LH release, the **ovary egg follicle cannot mature and ovulation will not occur.** Suppression of ovulation is a primary reason Pills work as a contraceptive.

A steady level of estrogen is extremely effective in suppressing ovulation. A steady level of progestin also blocks ovulation, but somewhat less reliably. In case ovulation does occur, which can happen once in a while on Pills, several additonal contraceptive effects of Pills nevertheless help to prevent pregnancy.

Other Effects.   Cervical mucus remains thick, sticky, and scant throughout the Pill cycle. The profuse, slippery mucus of ovulation does not occur. Thick cervical mucus impedes sperm travel through the cervical canal and inhibits chemical changes in sperm cells that would allow the sperm to penetrate the egg's outer covering.

In a natural cycle, the uterine lining thickens under the influence of estrogen during the first part of the cycle, and then matures under the influence of both progesterone and estrogen after ovulation. This development sequence is not possible during a Pill cycle because both progestin and estrogen are present throughout the cycle. Even if ovulation and conception did occur, successful implantation would be unlikely.

Estrogen and progestin may also alter the pattern of muscle contractions in the tubes and uterus. This effect may interfere with implantation by altering the fertilized egg's travel time so that it reaches the uterus at the wrong time to implant.

CHANGES YOU MAY NOTICE WHILE TAKING BIRTH CONTROL PILLS

Pills have many effects that are unrelated to birth control. These changes are called "side effects" because they have nothing to do with birth control, the primary reason for using Pills. Some of the changes occur in every woman who uses Pills; others occur only in a small number of Pill users; some side effects are beneficial; others can cause serious medical problems or even death. You are almost certain to notice at least some of the minor Pill side effects that have no known serious health consequences. They are described in the next few pages.

Your menstrual periods will probably be short and light. The cyclic growth of your uterine lining is governed by Pill hormones, and the overall lining is almost always thinner during a Pill cycle than it is during a natural cycle. Because you have less lining to be shed, your periods are shorter. These changes do not mean that something is wrong with your uterus or that blood is building up inside. (If you do miss a period altogether, read the section on using Pills later in this chapter to decide whether you need to call your clinician.)

Your menstrual cramps will probably diminish or disappear. Cramps seem to be linked to ovulation in some way, and it is rare for a woman who is not ovulating to have cramps. Pill users almost never ovulate; therefore, they are very unlikely to have cramps (or midcycle pain of ovulation).

Some women notice mood changes when they take Pills. Pill hormones may have a direct chemical effect on emotions in some women; other women may be affected indirectly because of their own psychological reaction to taking Pills. For example, when you have no worries about unwanted pregnancy, you may be less anxious, and that can cause an increased sex drive (libido). Other Pill users experience a decreased sex drive. Some women also report depression, irritability, or mood swings when they use Pills. These mood changes may be directly caused by the Pill hormones or perhaps by hormone-induced alterations in your vitamin levels. One study has shown that vitamin B_6 (20 mg daily) may counteract Pill-related depression in some cases (2).

Pill-related depression can be insidious, and it isn't unusual for a woman to say, "I had no idea how low I really felt until I stopped Pills! I feel so much better!" Life causes more depression than Pills do, but if you believe your depression is caused by Pills, it may be worthwhile to stop them and use condoms or a diaphragm for a few months and look for improvement. Remember, though, that unplanned pregnancy can also aggravate depression; using a good birth control alternative is essential.

Your premenstrual symptoms may be diminished. Although some women do experience breast tenderness, fluid retention, or irritability on Pills, these problems tend to be milder and more uniform throughout a Pill cycle and can sometimes be improved by changing to a different Pill. While you are taking Pills you don't really have a "premenstrual" phase because you don't have a cyclic hormone pattern. For some women, however, symptoms typical of premenstrual syndrome are worse with Pills than in natural cycles.

You may have spotting or bleeding between periods. A low or dropping estrogen level may trigger uterine bleeding, and the level of synthetic estrogen during a Pill cycle is often lower than the level of natural estrogen that your ovaries produce during a natural cycle. Your clinician may call this breakthrough bleeding: uterine bleeding that breaks through (occurs despite) the hormones in Pills. If you forget a Pill or are late taking a Pill, you may find that even this short interruption in your estrogen supply is enough to start an episode of spotting. Breakthrough bleeding is not harmful in and of itself. It can be annoying, and it can cause confusion, because irregular bleeding can also be a danger sign for serious problems such as infection or uterine cancer. Contact your clinician if you have an irregular bleeding pattern; you may need evaluation to be certain that your irregular bleeding is not caused by an unrelated problem. If your clinician finds that Pills are probably responsible for your bleeding, she/he may be able to correct the problem by giving you a different type of Pill.

Today's Pills contain only a small amount of estrogen, and nausea is quite uncommon. Nausea is not medically hazardous, but it can be very unpleasant. If you have nausea, try taking your Pill in the evening with dinner. You may find that nausea subsides after the first cycle or two. Changing your Pill brand sometimes eliminates this problem.

Pills can influence weight. Some Pill users add pounds and others lose pounds, and although most of the time a weight change is unrelated to Pills, weight gain for some women is definitely caused by the oral contraceptives. There are several possible ways in which Pills could cause weight gain:

You may notice a gain each month while you take hormone Pills, followed by a loss during the seven days you are not taking active hormone pills. This weight gain is caused by fluid retention and rarely amounts to more than five pounds. Limiting salt intake and drinking plenty of water should help. Pill estrogen may also affect fat distribution, weight, and body shape. Breast and hip size, for example, may be increased. You may find that taking Pills influences your appetite. Some women have a decreased appetite on Pills and lose weight, but others have an increased appetite and gain weight. The synthetic progestin in some Pills has male (androgen) hormone effects to some degree, and male hormone effects may influence appetite. Steady weight gain on Pills could also be caused by increased blood insulin or overeating associated with depression. Your clinician may be able to help with Pill-related weight gain by switching Pills to modify the estrogen or progestin that seems to be causing your problem. Remember that weight gain almost always responds to decreased calorie intake and increased exercise. A familiar story.

Most women who have acne notice significant improvement when they take Pills. Less frequently, Pills may make acne worse. It is often helpful to change to a different type of Pill.

Pills may cause chloasma, darkening of skin pigment on the upper lip, under the eyes, and on the forehead (see Illustration 13-2). Chloasma is fairly common, and affects perhaps 5% of Pill users. It is not hazardous and will usually fade after you stop Pills. It can be permanent in some cases. **Loss of scalp hair** (alopecia) can occur as a result of Pill use. It can begin while you are taking Pills or after you stop them. Do not despair if regrowth seems slow; hair grows slowly.

Women occasionally notice **increased hair growth** or the appearance of darker hair on the body and face, which can be a result of male hormone effects that some progestins cause, and may improve if you change to a Pill with a different progestin.

One small British study found that Pill progestins may cause **fatigue.** Seven British athletes were tested before, during, and after Pill use, and Pill use was associated with shortness of breath and inability to use oxygen efficiently. Although the evidence is scanty, many athletes do choose to avoid the Pill and use another method of birth control during times of intense training and competition.

Pills cause many **changes in body chemistry** that you will probably not detect. Levels of vitamins B_2 (riboflavin), B_6 (pyridoxine), B_{12} (cyanocobalamin), and C (ascorbic acid), and of folic acid are lower in Pill users than in women who do not take Pills; vitamin A (retinol) levels are elevated, as are iron and copper levels (3).

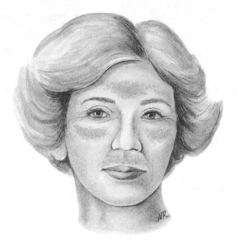

ILLUSTRATION 13-2   Chloasma usually fades away once you stop taking Pills.

Folic acid deficiency and resulting anemia have been reported among Pill users who have low folic acid intake. Vitamin B_6 (pyridoxine) deficiency may lead to depression (2). It is not known whether the other vitamin and mineral alterations can lead to medical problems, and Pills do not cause any genuine vitamin deficiency for the great majority of users. **Most clinicians do not recommend routine vitamin or mineral supplements for Pill users.**

Some of the common lab tests that Pills may alter include thyroid level, liver chemistry, iron level, blood cholesterol and fat levels, glucose tolerance, blood sugar level, and white blood cell count. In most cases, the test results—even though elevated or depressed compared to your own **normal** values—do remain within the normal range. It is important for your clinician to know that you are taking Pills, however, so that your results can be interpreted correctly.

Effectiveness

All the brands of Pills containing combined estrogen and progestin are extremely effective if you take them properly. Studies of women who take Pills consistently and correctly have shown first-year failure rates of less than 1% (4). Failure rates of about 3% are more typical (4), and failure rates as high as 4.7% have been reported for women less than 22 years old (1).

No matter which Pill brand is prescribed, you can expect effectiveness of 99% or better if you take them correctly. Pills containing 50 mcg of estrogen or more are no more effective than the brands containing 30 or 35 mcg.

Pills are not perfect. Women can and do become pregnant even when taking Pills on schedule every day. If all 10 million U.S. Pill users used Pills perfectly and achieved a .5% failure rate there would still be 50,000 accidental pregnancies a year (10,000,000 x 0.005 = 50,000).

Consistent use is important because Pills have their contraceptive effect not day by day, but cycle by cycle. Ovulation is suppressed because of the prolonged, steady level of synthetic hormone you have when you take Pills. When you miss a Pill or two, the level drops, and if you miss Pills, **especially in the first two weeks of a cycle,** you may ovulate. Clearly, taking Pills for a few days, or once in a while, or even several Pills a day once in a while, does not provide reliable contraception.

Also, **it is essential to have a back-up method on hand.** You may need it if you decide to stop Pills for some reason, or accidentally find yourself without them. Turning immediately to condoms, a diaphragm, sponges, or foam any time your Pill schedule is interrupted is the best way to protect yourself from unwanted pregnancy.

Occasionally we see a pregnant woman who is sure she has not missed any Pills—and I believe her.

One of the most common situations, though, is a woman who stopped taking Pills—maybe because her doctor told her to—and didn't get started right away with something else.

—ABORTION CLINIC COUNSELOR

Pill Risks and Complications

Hundreds (perhaps thousands) of clinical studies on Pill risks and complications have been published since 1960. Many different groups of women have been studied, and no two studies find exactly the same rate for Pill complications. This discussion relies on rates that seem to be representative, or are from the best, most careful studies.

A very large number of women must be studied for a long period of time in order to determine whether rare health risks are truly increased by Pills or whether the same number of problems would have occurred among Pill users anyway because of random chance. For example, researchers estimate that they would have to study 125,000 women for a full year in order to document a 100% increase in the risk of lung blood clots. Rare problems can only be evaluated accurately in very large studies.

Most of the statistics used in this chapter are taken directly from the FDA-approved Pill product labeling (5), which includes complete reference citations, and these statistics appear without any reference citation here. In some cases, when we felt that additional information would be helpful, statistics from other sources are cited.

*Pills are extremely safe for healthy, nonsmoking women under age 35. It is safer to use Pills than to deliver a baby, unless you are older than 35 and smoke more than 15 cigarettes a day. Of course, both Pill use and pregnancy are **extremely** safe, compared to driving a car or smoking cigarettes.*

*If you were to draw a line 700 feet high—the height of a 70-story building—to represent 100,000 young nonsmoking Pill users, and then draw a line beside it to represent the number of Pill users who die each year of Pill complications, **that line would be less than a quarter-inch high**. Your line representing the number of women who die from pregnancy complications would be just under 1 inch high.*

Of the 10 million or so current U.S. Pill users, about 200 to 500 die each year from a Pill complication. During that same year, some 800 to 1,100 deaths are prevented by Pill use. (Read the "Advantages of Pills" section later in this chapter.) Deaths related to Pill use are almost all from embolisms, heart attacks, and strokes among older Pill users who smoke. If no one older than 35 used Pills, and if no one who smoked cigarettes used Pills, then total Pill deaths would fall to about 70 (1).

Your age, smoking status, and medical history determine how safe or unsafe Pills are likely to be for you. The medical community does everything in its power to get smoking Pill users to give up smoking. She who has ears, let her hear.

CIRCULATORY DISORDERS

Circulatory disorders are the most important cause of serious and fatal Pill complications.

Estrogen hormone in Pills can alter the body chemicals that are responsible for blood clotting, and in some women these alterations may increase abnormal, inappropriate clotting, so clots occur more readily. Abnormal blood clot formation can occur in any blood vessel in the body. A clot is especially serious if a vital organ such as the brain, heart, or lungs is involved, or if a large clot forms in the veins of the leg or abdomen and then travels to the lung where it can block blood circulation through the lung.

Pills may also alter blood lipid levels. Blood lipids such as cholesterol also affect heart attack risk because high lipid levels or an undesirable balance between the different types of lipids can cause fatty deposits on the inner lining of arteries. This is called atherosclerosis or hardening of the arteries. Arteries in the heart are narrow, and may become completely blocked so that a heart attack results.

Cholesterol in your bloodstream combines with proteins to form high-density

TABLE 13-1
HEART AND BLOOD VESSEL DISORDERS

MEDICAL NAME	LOCATION OF CLOT OR BLOCKAGE	SYMPTOMS
Thrombophlebitis	Lower leg	Calf pain, swelling, heat, or tenderness
Thrombophlebitis	Thigh	Pain, heat, or redness
Pulmonary embolism	Lung	Chest pain, cough, shortness of breath
Myocardial infarction (heart attack)	Heart	Chest pain, left arm and shoulder pain, difficulty breathing, weakness
Cerebral infarction (stroke)	Brain	Headache, weakness, or numbness, visual problems, sudden intellectual impairment
Retinal vein thrombosis	Eye	Complete or partial loss of vision, headache
Mesenteric vein thrombosis	Intestine	Abdominal pain, vomiting, weakness
Pelvic vein thrombosis	Pelvis	Lower abdominal pain, cramps

lipoproteins (HDLs) and low-density lipoproteins (LDLs), molecules that are essential for the transport of cholesterol into and out of cells. Elevated levels of LDL, or depressed levels of HDL, are associated with circulatory diseases such as coronary artery disease, or hardening of the arteries. Estrogens tend to increase HDL levels, which means protection against artery deposits, and progestins tend to decrease HDL levels, an adverse effect (6,7). Progestins may also adversely alter the balance of various lipid components.

Table 13-1 shows the technical names for important circulatory disorders. All these disorders can occur in women who do not use Pills, and in men, and they are strongly associated with the following risk factors:

• Smoking
• Age over 35 (risk increases dramatically after menopause)
• High blood pressure
• Diabetes or family history of diabetes
• Heart or blood vessel disease
• Heart attack in a close relative under 50, particularly a mother or sister

TABLE 13-2
RISK OF DEATH FROM PILL-RELATED PROBLEMS

	DEATHS PER 100,000 USERS PER YEAR	
AGE	PILL USERS WHO SMOKE	PILL USERS WHO DON'T SMOKE
15–19	2.4	0.5
20–24	3.6	0.7
25–29	6.8	1.1
30–34	13.7	2.1
35–39	51.4	14.1
40–44	117.6	32.0

SOURCE: Ory HW: Mortality associated with fertility and fertility control: 1983. *Family Planning Perspectives* 15:57–63, 1983.

- Obesity
- High blood lipid levels
- Inadequate physical activity
- Being immobilized (after a serious injury or surgery, for example)

Having more than one risk factor multiplies your risk. Heart and blood disorders are very rare in young people, but many careful research studies clearly show that using Pills increases your risk. Women with A, B, or AB blood types appear to have a greater risk for abnormal clot problems with Pills than do type O women (8). The increased risk is higher if your Pill contains more than 50 mcg of estrogen, if you smoke, and if you are over 35 years old. Your increased risk for stroke and heart attack may extend even after you stop Pills (8). Table 13-2 shows your risk of death from Pills.

By about age 35, the death risk of Pills for smokers is higher than the death risk of full-term pregnancy, so **Pills are not a good birth control method for women over 35 who smoke. More significantly, smoking isn't good for anyone.** Many clinicians discourage Pill use even for 30-year-old smokers. Plan to stop Pills by about age 40 even if you don't smoke if you have any other risk factors for cardiovascular disease.

A woman who has already had a stroke, thrombophlebitis, a heart attack, or clots in her legs, lungs, or any part of her body should never take Pills. Her risk of a circulatory disorder with Pills is high.

For women who do not have other cardiovascular disease risk factors, the overall risk with Pills is low. Since the hormone dose in Pills does affect risk, though, it is very important to use **Pills with the very least potent estrogen and progestin that will prevent pregnancy.** A high estrogen level is undesirable because estrogen increases blood clotting risks and a high progestin level has undesirable effects on blood lipids.

PROGESTIN (mg)   ESTROGEN (mcg)

PROGESTIN (mg)	Progestin	Brand	Estrogen	ESTROGEN (mcg)
0.3	Norethindrone 0.35	Micronor Nor-QD		
2.2	Norgestrel 0.075	Ovrette		
2.0	Norethindrone Acetate 1.0	Loestrin 1/20	Ethinyl Estradiol 20	0.7-0.8
1.0	Norethindrone 1.0	Norinyl 1/50 Ortho-Novum 1/50	Mestranol 50	1.0
3.0-7.5	L-Norgestrel 0.05/0.075/0.125	Triphasil Tri-Levlen	Ethinyl Estradiol 30/40	1.0-1.2
9.0	L-Norgestrel 0.15	Nordette Levlen	Ethinyl Estradiol 30	1.0-1.2
9.0	Norgestrel 0.3	Lo/Ovral	Ethinyl Estradiol 30	1.0-1.2
3.0	Norethindrone Acetate 1.5	Loestrin 1.5/30	Ethinyl Estradiol 30	1.0-1.2
0.4	Norethindrone 0.4	Ovcon 35	Ethinyl Estradiol 35	1.2-1.4
0.5	Norethindrone 0.5	Brevicon Modicon	Ethinyl Estradiol 35	1.2-1.4
0.5-1.0	Norethindrone 0.5/1.0	Ortho 10/11	Ethinyl Estradiol 35	1.2-1.4
0.5-1.0	Norethindrone 0.5/0.75/1.0	Ortho 7/7/7	Ethinyl Estradiol 35	1.2-1.4
0.5-1.0	Norethindrone 0.5/1.0/0.5	Tri-Norinyl	Ethinyl Estradiol 35	1.2-1.4
1.0	Norethindrone 1.0	Norinyl 1/35 Ortho Novum 1/35	Ethinyl Estradiol 35	1.2-1.4
15	Ethynodiol Diacetate 1.0	Demulen 1/35	Ethinyl Estradiol 35	1.2-1.4
1.0	Norethindrone 1.0	Norinyl 1/80 Ortho Novum 1/80	Mestranol 80	1.6
1.0	Norethindrone 1.0	Ovcon 50	Ethinyl Estradiol 50	1.7-2.0
2.0	Norethindrone Acetate 1.0	Norlestrin 1	Ethinyl Estradiol 50	1.7-2.0
2.0	Norethindrone 2.0	Norinyl 2 Ortho Novum 2	Mestranol 100	2.0
2.7	Norethynodrel 2.5	Enovid-E	Mestranol 100	2.0
5.0	Norethindrone Acetate 2.5	Norlestrin 2.5	Ethinyl Estradiol 50	1.7-2.0
15	Norgestrel 0.5	Ovral	Ethinyl Estradiol 50	1.7-2.0
15	Ethynodiol Diacetate 1.0	Demulen 1/50	Ethinyl Estradiol 50	1.7-2.0
15	Ethynodiol Diacetate 1.0	Ovulen	Mestranol 100	2.0

15 10 5   0   0   1.0 2.0
Potency Units   Potency Units

ILLUSTRATION 13-3   Hormone potency of the various Pill brands.

Illustration 13-3 shows approximate relative potencies for the hormones in oral contraceptives now available. The National Medical Committee of the Planned Parenthood Federation of America recommends these dosages of the currently available estrogens and progestins (6):

Ethinyl estradiol: 35 mcg or less

Norethindrone: 1.0 mg or less

Norethindrone acetate: 0.5 mg or less

Ethynodiol diacetate: 1.0 mg or less

Norgestrel: 0.3 mg or less

Levonorgestrel: 0.15 mg or less

A 1985 study of progestin potency found that norethindrone, norethindrone acetate, and ethynodiol diacetate are all about equal in potency, while norgestrel is about 5 to 10 times as potent and levonorgestrel 10 to 20 times as potent (9).

LIVER PROBLEMS

Pills can cause jaundice, a liver problem that leads to the accumulation of pigments that give the skin and eyes a yellow tinge. Jaundice is probably related to the progestin in Pills and is quite rare: about 1 Pill user in 10,000 (10). Jaundice is serious enough that you should stop Pills. Women who have had jaundice during pregnancy should not take Pills because the problem may recur.

Other liver problems such as hepatitis and mononucleosis can also cause jaundice. **Don't use Pills if blood tests show any evidence of liver damage**: your liver's ability to deactivate and break down estrogen may be impaired and high levels of estrogen could accumulate in your body.

Pill users also have an increased risk of developing a liver tumor called hepatocellular adenoma (HCA). These tumors are extremely rare. HCA is not cancer, but nevertheless can cause serious or even fatal problems because of internal bleeding. The risk of liver tumors among long-term Pill users is about 3 to 4 per 100,000 per year (11). Use of Pills may also increase a woman's risk for malignant liver tumors. This form of cancer is exceedingly rare, however, and accounts for 1 to 8 deaths per million women (12). Also, it is strongly linked to hepatitis B infection and alcoholic liver damage so the specific contribution of Pill use to its risk is extremely difficult for researchers to assess. Symptoms of liver tumor or cancer might include severe abdominal pain, swelling in the upper right abdomen, and dizziness and weakness from internal bleeding.

CHLAMYDIAL CERVICITIS

Pills can cause changes in the surface of the cervix that may make the Pill user more **vulnerable to sexually transmitted diseases (STDs) of the cervix, particularly Chlamydia** infections (13). The viruses that cause herpes and genital warts and the bacteria that cause gonorrhea and chlamydia readily attack the delicate tissue that lines the cervical canal, but are less likely to attack the smooth, tough outer surface of the cervix. Pill users, and also very young women, tend to have a larger area near the opening of the cervical canal where delicate cervical lining tissue extends out from the canal onto the surface of the cervix. Having this condition, called **cervical ectropion** (see Chapter 40), means that viruses or bacteria from your sexual partner's penis are more likely to touch tissues in which they can live and multiply. **Many clinicians now recommend that you use Pills for birth control along with condoms for STDs routinely, particularly if you are younger than 25 and/or have more than one sexual partner.**

Despite increased susceptibility to cervix infection, Pills **protect users against**

infection in the uterus and tubes. Infection on the cervix is somewhat less likely to spread upward into a Pill user's uterus and tubes, so rates for pelvic infection (pelvic inflammatory disease, PID) are lower for Pill users than for women who are not using birth control (14). See "Advantages of Pills" later in this chapter.

GALLBLADDER DISEASE

Although Pills seem not to affect a woman's overall long-term risk of developing gallbladder disease, they may accelerate gallbladder problems for women who are already susceptible to the disease so that gallbladder problems become evident earlier than they would have without Pills (15). Early studies seemed to show that a woman who used (earlier, higher dose) Pills for two years or more had twice the risk of gallbladder disease as a woman who didn't use Pills. The progestin in Pills probably impairs the gallbladder's ability to fill and empty properly (16). Gallbladder disease is fairly common among Pill users (2 in 1,000 users per year) and among other women (1 in 1,000), and usually is not life-threatening, although surgery may be required to remove the gallbladder. The risk of gallbladder disease is increased by obesity, previous pregnancies, and older age for Pill users and other women alike.

HIGH BLOOD PRESSURE (HYPERTENSION)

About 1% to 5% of Pill users develop elevated blood pressure (8). Hypertension is three times as likely after five years on Pills as it is after one year, and your risk increases with age. Pill-related hypertension usually is not severe and is unlikely to be life-threatening. High blood pressure is a contributing cause in heart disease and stroke; so you should stop Pills and get your pressure down in any event, even if it isn't seriously elevated. Consistent blood pressure readings of 140/90 or higher (either number) mean that you need to stop taking Pills. Pill-related high blood pressure usually subsides within a few weeks after you stop Pills.

Pills may or may not influence your blood pressure if it is already high. Your risks for extreme blood pressure elevation are higher, however, and most clinicians would advise you not to try Pills. Women who have previously experienced hormone-related blood pressure elevation, during pregnancy, for example, are more likely to develop hypertension with Pills. **All women who use Pills should have a blood pressure check at least once every 12 months, as long as they use Pills.** Checks every six months may be needed if you have a history of blood pressure problems or one of the other cardiovascular disease risk factors listed at the beginning of this section.

PROLONGED HORMONE SUPPRESSION AND FUTURE FERTILITY

For about 1% to 2% of Pill users, there is a significant delay in the return of normal cycles and normal ovulatory hormone patterns after they stop Pills. Your clinician may call this "post-Pill amenorrhea." A delay is more likely if you had irregular periods or long intervals between periods before you took Pills than if your periods were fairly regular. Prolonged hormone suppression may be more likely to occur among very young Pill users who began Pills before their natural cyclic patterns were well established.

When a woman has "post-Pill amenorrhea," her hormones remain suppressed, as they were on Pills: ovary follicles fail to mature, ovulation does not occur, and menstrual periods may be light, infrequent, or entirely absent. As long as your natural hormone cycle is suppressed, it is extremely unlikely that you would be able to conceive. Hormone suppression can continue for months or even years, but **in most cases menstrual periods return spontaneously within three months.** If your periods have not resumed within six months, evaluation probably will be recommended by your clinician (see Chapter 33 for a discussion of amenorrhea). You may have some other problem altogether that is causing hormone suppression. Hormone suppression can definitely cause temporary infertility, and it may also be responsible for a slight decrease in overall fertility for women who use Pills until late in their reproductive years and do not start trying to conceive until age 30 or later. Women who stopped Pills at age 30 to 34 to conceive were compared to women the same age who stopped other methods in a large British study (17). Researchers found that 83% of former Pill users had completed a full-term pregnancy within 48 months compared to 89% of the women who stopped other methods. At the end of 72 months the rates were closer, 87% of former Pill users and 90% of other method users, but the small difference of 3% did persist. Researchers concluded that the difference was not due to statistical effects, and that Pill use was responsible for the lower fertility documented.

For younger women, less than 30 when they began trying to conceive, or women who have had one or more full-term pregnancies already, previous Pill use may cause a delay, but overall pregnancy rates are the same as rates for other method users at the end of 36 to 48 months.

These research findings mean that future pregnancy plans deserve consideration as decisions about using Pills are made. **If future pregnancy success is a high priority for you, then starting to try for pregnancy before age 30 is a reasonable precaution** no matter what method you have been using. If you are using Pills, you may want to stop them and **use some other method when you get close to 30.** If you do have hormone suppression, this may allow time for your body to resume normal cycles before you reach your mid to late 30s, when overall fertility may be declining.

Also, if you have a precise timetable for pregnancy, and definitely want to conceive at a specific time, it may be reasonable to stop Pills and switch to another method well before that time. Using a barrier method such as condoms or a diaphragm for the last 12 to 24 months before pregnancy will allow your hormone system time to return to normal, and you will have time for evaluation and treatment if you are one of the rare women who has prolonged suppression after stopping Pills.

Remember, though, that hormone suppression is not common. **Most women conceive soon after they stop using any method** of birth control, including Pills. So if you don't yet want to be pregnant, you definitely need to begin using another method such as condoms or a diaphragm as soon as you stop your Pills.

PILLS AND CANCER

Does the Pill cause cancer? That's all I want to know, and I'm not going to take Pills until I feel like I have a straight answer. My boyfriend says yes. My best friend says no. The family planning clinic says maybe. Frustrating!

—WOMAN, 20

Most of the recent research about Pills and cancer brings very good news. Combined Pills **protect users from cancer of the ovary and cancer of the uterus,** and the benefit has been shown in numerous excellent studies (18,19). Pill users have about **half** the rate of these cancers that would normally be expected. The protective effect occurs after about a year of Pill use and persists even after Pills are stopped; protection may last as long as ten years or more. This effect saves the lives of 100 women who would otherwise die from endometrial cancer and 1,000 women who would die from ovarian cancer each year.

Researchers suspect that the protective effect is related to the continuous progestin exposure that Pills provide along with their steady, but lower-than-natural, level of estrogen. Uterine cancer occurs naturally when estrogen levels are higher than average and are not balanced by cyclic progesterone release from the ovary. Progestin treatment can protect against uterine cancer.

Ovarian cancer rates are higher among women who have few or no breaks from ovulation during their reproductive years: women who have few or no pregnancies. One theory is that the incessant cyclic bombardment of the ovaries by pituitary hormones and/or the regular, cyclic disruption of ovulation may somehow prompt cancer. Pill users do not ovulate and do not produce pituitary hormones. Their ovaries are at rest.

Of all the Pill and cancer risk questions, however, breast cancer is almost certainly the most important because breast cancer is so very common. And **the breast cancer question is not yet settled.** A large study conducted by the U.S. Centers for Disease Control (CDC), and several other major studies as well, have found that **Pills neither increase nor decrease a woman's breast cancer risk** (20). Even women with strong family histories of breast cancer or with fibrocystic breast disease were not at increased risk. On the other hand, a small study in 1983 found higher breast cancer rates among young Pill users who took Pills with high levels of progestin (21) and a 1986

Scandinavian study also found that women who used Pills 12 years or more, or who used Pills 8 years before delivering their first baby, had an elevated risk of breast cancer (22); Swedish women who were long-term Pill users had approximately a doubled risk for breast cancer. Meanwhile, re-analysis of data from several other large United States studies to look specifically for risk with higher progestin Pills or with Pill use very early in the reproductive years has not confirmed the risk reported in the 1983 study (23).

How can the thoughtful reader—not blessed with a crystal ball—guess whether the few disquieting reports are important, ominous, seminal studies, or an aberration in a basically reassuring pattern of research? As these early studies of Pills and breast cancer come in, it is difficult to know what to make of them. It is probably too soon to know with complete certainty just how Pills affect breast cancer risk, because there are not yet large numbers of women who have taken Pills and then reached their 40s, the decade when breast cancer risk becomes significant. One thing is sure, be wary of anyone claiming to have incontrovertible evidence to answer the Pill and breast cancer question! As with so much else, your own instincts, your own careful breast exams, your medical history, and your clinician's instincts must suffice.

Early concern about an increased risk for malignant melanoma, a serious form of skin cancer, has not appeared in recent careful studies and so concern has quieted. Sun exposure is a powerful risk factor for melanoma, and it may be that Pill users in early studies sunbathed more than other women.

Pill users are at somewhat higher risk for developing a rare form of liver cancer and also for premalignant or malignant cell changes of the cervix (24,25). Liver tumors and cancer are discussed in the "Liver Problems" section earlier in this chapter. The cervical cancer issue is much more significant, however, because cervical cancer is a much more common disease. **Cervical cancer appears to be about 1.5 to 2 times more common among Pill users than it is among nonusers,** and its incidence may be increased with long-term Pill use. In one study, the rate of precancerous and cancerous disease was 0.9 per 1,000 women each year for women who used the Pill less than two years and 2.2 per 1,000 for women who used the Pill more than eight years. The rate for IUD users, the comparison group in this study, was 1 per 1,000 (26). Some researchers believe that Pills may somehow increase a woman's susceptibility for developing cervical abnormalities and cancer as well. It is impossible to tell how much of this finding is a true pharmacologic effect of Pills, and how much is because Pill users tend to have intercourse more often with more partners than other women: cervical cancer is essentially a sexually transmitted disease. Pill users also have more frequent Pap tests on the average than do other women, so it may be that the higher rate for precancerous abnormalities among Pill users is partly explained by better detection. Some of the "other" women may have similar problems but remain uncounted because of less frequent Pap tests. A **causal** relationship between Pills and cervical cancer has not been established, and may never be; clinicians (appropriately) intervene early when cervical cell changes begin to occur. Treatment for precancerous abnormalities is so effective that true cervical cancer should almost never have a chance to occur.

Be faithful about annual Pap smears during and after the time you use Pills, so any cell changes can be found and cured well before they become cancerous. Abnormal Pap smears are discussed in detail in Chapter 35.

No one can predict what researchers will learn about Pills and cancer in the years to come, but the findings of the early 80s are fairly reassuring. **Good news probably outweighs bad news.** Most clinicians now prescribe Pills with some measure of peace of mind about the cancer issue. If you are afraid of cancer anyway, you probably will be happier with another method. No one is very successful for very long with a contraceptive that engenders fear and worry.

The FDA-approved labeling (5) for Pills includes a discussion of the cancer issue and stresses the importance of careful routine exams, including breast examination, liver examination, and Pap tests for all Pill users. **It is clearly essential that an abnormal Pap smear, a breast lump, abnormal vaginal bleeding, or other cancer danger signs be thoroughly investigated.** The FDA-approved labeling further recommends that a woman who has had previous breast lumps, hyperplastic fibrocystic breast problems, abnormal mammograms, or diethylstilbestrol (DES) exposure, or has a strong family history of breast cancer, be followed with special care if she chooses to use Pills.

EYE PROBLEMS

On rare occasions, Pills may cause inflammation of the optic nerve, with loss of vision, double vision, swelling, or pain in one or both eyes.

Women who wear contact lenses may find that lenses don't fit well when they take Pills. Pill-related fluid retention can steepen your cornea contour, and you may need a new lens fitting. Some Pill users find that they can't wear contact lenses at all.

HEADACHE

Some women develop severe, recurrent, or persistent headaches while taking Pills, and others notice an increase in the frequency or severity of migraine headaches. Headaches may be a direct Pill effect, or they may be caused by Pill-related fluid retention. Severe headaches may be a danger sign of stroke or other serious circulatory disorders. Pay particular attention to headaches that have any of these characteristics:

• A new or different headache pattern that you did not have before using Pills
• Pain that lasts an hour or longer
• Dizziness, nausea, or vomiting accompanying the headache
• Blurred vision, tearing, spots before your eyes, or complete or partial loss of vision
• Pain localized to just one side of your head

• Headache that persists despite over-the-counter pain relievers
• Throbbing pain

These can be symptoms of serious vascular headache, so see your clinician as soon as you can. **Stop your Pills** and use condoms, foam, or sponges until your headaches are evaluated.

BLADDER, KIDNEY, AND OTHER INFECTIONS

Women who use Pills have a slightly higher incidence of bladder and kidney infections, bronchitis, viral illness, cervical ectropion, and vaginal discharges. The cause of these increased rates is not known. Progestin causes mild relaxation of bladder muscles and the tubes (ureters) that carry urine from the kidney to the bladder, and this effect might delay urine transport and allow more time for bacteria to multiply. Pills also decrease the level of infection-fighting gamma globulin protein in the blood, so susceptibility to infection could be generally increased. Women who use Pills tend to have intercourse more frequently than do women who use other methods, and this increased intimate contact may be the reason urinary tract infection, upper respiratory illness, flu, and other viral illness rates are higher. Pill users may simply be exposed to more germs more often than are other women.

FETAL DEVELOPMENT

Women who stop Pills and then become pregnant appear to have no increased risk for birth defects. Some studies have shown that babies of women who accidentally took Pills **during** early pregnancy may have an increased risk of heart or limb defects of as much as 1 in 1,000 (1). Remember that in all pregnancies, regardless of contraceptive history, the risk of having a baby with a birth defect is about 30 per 1,000. That means that the excess risk of birth defects from inadvertently using Pills in early pregnancy is quite small, increasing from roughly 30 per 1,000 to 31 per 1,000. Other researchers have found no excess birth defect risk at all, and see no reason for worry.

It is not known whether Pill use prior to pregnancy affects the rate of miscarriage. There is some evidence that severe fetal chromosome abnormalities leading to miscarriage may occur more frequently when pregnancy begins immediately after Pill use.

Never use Pills during pregnancy or when you think you might be pregnant. When you want to stop Pills and become pregnant, **plan on switching to a diaphragm, condoms, foam, or sponges for several cycles first,** and keep a careful record of your menstrual periods. This practice eliminates the risk of fetal exposure to Pills, and makes it easier for you and your obstetrician to date your pregnancy accurately.

Read the "Using Pills" section later in this chapter for instructions on what to do if you miss one or more periods on Pills and suspect you could be pregnant.

BREASTFEEDING AND ALTERED MILK PRODUCTION

Pills may cause a significant decrease in the amount and quality of milk you produce while you are breastfeeding. Pill hormones do appear in breast milk in minute quantities. It is not known whether or how exposure to Pill hormones might affect a breastfed infant. The FDA-approved Pill labeling recommends that Pill use begin only after your infant has been weaned if at all possible.

Women occasionally develop breast milk while they are using Pills and are neither pregnant nor breastfeeding (27). Abnormal milk production is called **galactorrhea. Get in touch with your clinician if you develop breast milk when you are not nursing.** Breast milk is not directly harmful but can occasionally be a symptom of a pituitary gland tumor. Your clinician will probably suggest laboratory tests to be sure that Pills are actually responsible for the breast milk. Galactorrhea is discussed further in Chapter 37.

MEDICAL PROBLEMS THAT MAY BE AGGRAVATED BY PILLS

Pills alter insulin and blood sugar balance. Women with **diabetes** may find that they must adjust their medication and diet if they use Pills.

Pills can stimulate (or retard) the growth of uterine **fibroid tumors**. If you have fibroids and choose Pills, be sure to have frequent pelvic examinations so that your clinician can determine if your fibroids are increasing in size. (Read more about managing fibroids in Chapter 40.)

Pills can cause **depression** or aggravate preexisting depression. (Some women find that Pills actually improve depression.) If you have been seriously depressed or have attempted suicide in the past, your clinician will want to follow you carefully if you choose to use Pills. Read more about depression in "Changes You May Notice While Taking Birth Control Pills" earlier in this chapter.

Migraine headaches, asthma, heart disease, and kidney disease can all worsen under the influence of Pill-related fluid retention. You must be careful to see your clinician regularly if you choose Pills.

Women exposed to **diethylstilbestrol (DES)** during fetal life or pregnancy will need to be followed with special care if they use Pills. See Chapter 42 for recommendations on routine health screening for DES-exposed women.

True allergy to Pills is very rare but could cause skin rash, redness, or itchiness. Painful red bumps or blotches (erythema nodosum) have occasionally been reported. Several rare problems that have been reported among Pill users but that have not yet been definitely linked to Pills include chorea (abnormal movements of the trunk and limbs), dizziness, and porphyria (abnormal pigments in the urine).

PILL INTERACTION WITH OTHER DRUGS

Two drugs can interact with each other if you take them at the same time, and some interactions can be harmful. Pill/medication interactions could result in decreased effectiveness of the medication, decreased effectiveness of the birth control Pill, or sometimes even an undesirable increase in the action of your medication. **Tell every clinician who cares for you that you are taking Pills even if your medical problem has no apparent relationship to birth control.**

The effectiveness of birth control Pills may be **decreased** by drugs that alter liver function such as barbiturates, ampicillin, Dilantin (diphenylhydantoin), rifampin (for tuberculosis), tetracycline, and phenylbutazone (for arthritis). Consider using a different method of birth control if you routinely use any of these medications, or at least use a back-up method such as condoms, a diaphragm, sponges, or foam. Accidental pregnancies have also been reported with a number of other drugs, including antihistamines.

The likelihood of accidental pregnancy with temporary, short-term treatment is not high, and you are not likely to be advised about a back-up method if you are treated for bladder infection, a vaginal infection, or a temporary allergy problem that requires an antihistamine. If accidental pregnancy would be disastrous for you and you want to be extra cautious, however, **there is no harm in using a back-up method along with your Pills.** To do so, continue your birth control Pills on your normal Pill schedule and simply begin using condoms, a diaphragm, sponges, or foam when you begin your medication prescription. Continue using your back-up along with Pills until at least two weeks after you finish your medication.

Spotting could be your first or only indication that a drug interaction is decreasing the effectiveness of your birth control Pills, so notify your clinician right away if you think there is a connection between medication, Pills, and spotting in your case.

Table 13-3 lists drug interactions in detail, along with possible corrective actions to consider. Talk to your clinician or pharmacist if you want to check your medications against the generic drug names in this table.

MAJOR PILL RISKS IN PERSPECTIVE

Would a rational woman choose Pills? The list of possible Pill complications and risks is long and overwhelming. The reason that so many well-informed women do choose Pills and that responsible and knowledgeable clinicians continue to prescribe Pills for patients who want them is that Pill risks are acceptable to many women, especially when they compare Pill risks with the risks of pregnancy and many other common, accepted activities of daily living. (See Chapter 11 for a comparison of death risks of various birth control methods and death rates for common accidents and illnesses and other causes of death in the childbearing years.)

TABLE 13-3
PILL INTERACTIONS WITH OTHER DRUGS

INTERACTING DRUGS	ADVERSE EFFECTS (PROBABLE MECHANISM)	COMMENTS AND RECOMMENDATIONS
Acetaminophen (Tylenol and others)	Possible decreased pain-relieving effect (increased metabolism)	Monitor pain-relieving response
Alcohol	Possible increased effect of alcohol	Use with caution
Anticoagulants (oral)	Decreased anticoagulant effect	Use alternative contraceptive
Antidepressants (Elavil, Norpramin, Tofranil, and others)	Possible increased antidepressant effect	Monitor antidepressant concentration
Barbiturates (phenobarbital and others)	Decreased contraceptive effect	Avoid simultaneous use; use alternative contraceptive for epileptics
Benzodiazepine Tranquilizers (Ativan, Librium, Serax, Tranxene, Valium, Xanax, and others)	Possible increased or decreased tranquilizer effects including psychomotor impairment	Use with caution. Greatest impairment during menstrual pause in oral contraceptive dosage
Beta-blockers (Corgard, Inderal, Lopressor, Tenormin)	Possible increased blocker effect	Monitor cardiovascular status
Carbamazepine (Tegretol)	Possible decreased contraceptive effect	Use alternative contraceptive
Corticosteroids (cortisone)	Possible increased corticosteroid toxicity	Clinical significance not established
Griseofulvin (Fulvicin, Grifulvin V, and others)	Decreased contraceptive effect	Use alternative contraceptive

Drug	Effect	Recommendation
Guanethidine (Esimil, Ismelin)	Decreased guanethidine effect (mechanism not established)	Avoid simultaneous use
Hypoglycemics (tolbutamide, Diabinese, Orinase, Tolinase)	Possible decreased hypoglycemic effect	Monitor blood glucose
Methyldopa (Aldoclor, Aldomet, and others)	Decreased antihypertensive effect	Avoid simultaneous use
Penicillin	Decreased contraceptive effect with ampicillin	Low but unpredictable incidence; use alternative contraceptive
Phenytoin (Dilantin)	Decreased contraceptive effect Possible increased phenytoin effect	Use alternative contraceptive Monitor phenytoin concentration
Primidone (Mysoline)	Decreased contraceptive effect	Use alternative contraceptive
Rifampin	Decreased contraceptive effect	Use alternative contraceptive
Tetracycline	Decreased contraceptive effect	Use alternative contraceptive
Theophylline (Bronkotabs, Marax, Primatene, Quibron, Tedral, Theor-Dur, and others)	Increased theophylline effect	Monitor theophylline concentration
Troleandomycin (TAO)	Jaundice (additive)	Avoid simultaneous use
Vitamin C	Increased serum concentration and possible increased adverse effects of estrogens with 1 g or more per day of vitamin C	Decrease vitamin C to 100 mg per day

SOURCE: Adapted from Rizack MA, Hillman CDM: *The Medical Letter Handbook of Adverse Drug Interactions*. New Rochelle, N.Y.: The Medical Letter, 1985.

There are many different kinds of Pill complications, but in total the serious complications are **rare**. Circulatory disorders account for nearly all the deaths and serious complications.

If you take into consideration the known Pill risks, statistics show that Pills are not as safe as a diaphragm, foam, or condoms backed up by abortion in the event of pregnancy. Safety, however, is not the only valid factor to consider as you choose a birth control method. Effectiveness is uppermost for many women, especially those for whom abortion is not an acceptable option. When Pill risks are weighed against risks of (unplanned) full-term pregnancy associated with less effective methods, Pills may be safer than less effective methods.

Pills aren't really natural, and I don't like that. But I hate condoms, hate diaphragms, hate all those vaginal methods, and I know I wouldn't use them! I don't want to get pregnant. So I use Pills.

—WOMAN, 26

Minimizing Your Risks of Pill Complications

Serious Pill complications sometimes occur suddenly with no warning, but many times complications have danger signs—early warnings of potential trouble.

Always pay attention to Pill danger signs. Read the list of danger signs in Illustration 13-4. Memorizing the list would be even better. Don't ignore these symptoms or wait to see if they go away. Stop taking Pills, use another method of birth control, and see your clinician immediately.

13:4   PILL DANGER SIGNS

A   Abdominal pain (severe)
C   Chest pain, shortness of breath, cough
H   Headache (severe), dizziness, weakness, numbness
E   Eye problems (vision loss or blurring), speech problems
S   Severe leg pain (calf or thigh)

Stop taking Pills and see your clinician at once if you have any of these problems, or if you develop depression, jaundice, or a breast lump.

❖

Early symptoms of circulatory disorders are not necessarily dramatic. If you have mild chest pain, your clinician will ask about coughing and breathing difficulty. Even an examination and a chest x-ray may not reveal a lung clot. Your clinician may have to arrange for a heart tracing (electrocardiogram) and a lung scan to be certain. Be sure you have a thorough evaluation, and don't be content with superficial reassurance.

About three weeks after I started taking Pills I noticed a little dull ache in my chest. It didn't hurt much, and stayed in one spot. It kept on for a couple of days; so I called my doctor, because she told me to if I had chest pain.

She examined me that same afternoon but couldn't tell whether anything was the matter. When she asked me about it, I remembered I had been coughing more than usual. She had my chest x-rayed, and the x-ray doctor thought I had a little pneumonia.

My doctor was surprised; she said I should have a fever and feel sick if I had pneumonia; so she sent me to the hospital for more tests. When they did the lung scan and electrocardiogram, they found out I had blood clots in my lung. I had to stay in the hospital for about a week for blood-thinning medicine, and I took medicine for another month after I went home. I didn't have any more trouble after that. They never did find out where the blood clots started.

—FORMER PILL USER, age 15

The following paragraphs summarize the authors' suggestions for using Pills as safely as possible. Don't be surprised if your clinician doesn't mention these suggestions to you: these are not all routine instructions. You may or may not decide to pay attention to all these recommendations; but you can use them to help keep your Pill risks at a minimum.

Stop your Pills and use another method of birth control if you develop a contraindication. Read the FDA-required Pill pamphlet or leaflet each time you receive your Pill refill to double-check the list of contraindications. Ask your clinician if you are not certain about any illnesses or problems you have had. (Read more about Pill contraindications in the following section.)

Be faithful about routine checkups as long as you take Pills. Have your blood pressure checked every 12 months, and make sure your exam includes your breasts, abdomen (for enlarged liver), a pelvic exam, and Pap smear. At about age 35, be sure your annual exam includes blood tests for lipids and glucose (sugar). Be sure to examine your breasts yourself once a month. See your clinician promptly if you have any question about your own exams.

Avoid using Pills that contain more than 35 micrograms (mcg) of estrogen. Look up your Pill in Illustration 13-3, or look on your package insert. The estrogen will be either mestranol or ethinyl estradiol. The lowest mestranol dose available in Pills is 50 mcg and is probably similar to an ethinyl estradiol dose of 35 mcg, but many clinicians now advise their patients to switch to a 35 mcg product even if they are having no side effects at all. All the 35 mcg Pills contain ethinyl estradiol; the amount can be written 0.035 mg, or 35 mcg. Older women who have used Pills for several years are especially likely to still be using Pills with 50 mcg or more of estrogen, so read your label and talk to your clinician about a dose reduction.

Keeping the **progestin dose low is also important.** All the 35-mcg estrogen Pills meet the progestin dose recommendations given earlier in this chapter.

Don't think of Pills as your permanent answer to birth control. Pills are probably best for women in the early reproductive years. If you are planning for future pregnancy, stop your Pills well ahead of time (see the section titled "Prolonged Hormone Suppression and Future Fertility" earlier in this chapter). Otherwise, follow these guidelines for when to stop Pills:

• **At age 35** if you smoke more than 15 cigarettes a day
• **At age 40** if you have any risk factors for cardiovascular disease
• **At age 45** if you have absolutely no risk factors for cardiovascular disease

Be sure that any clinician who takes care of you for any problem is aware that you are taking Pills. If your clinician prescribes other drugs, ask if the other drugs will interact with Pills.

Stop Pills if you have a serious injury such as a broken leg, or if you stay in bed at complete rest longer than a day or two at home or in a hospital. **Stop Pills one month before any major elective surgery.** Talk to your clinician and be sure to use an effective birth control alternative such as condoms or a diaphragm in the meantime.

Remember that smoking increases Pill risks: one more good reason to stop smoking.

Assess your own risks by comparing yourself with this hypothetical woman who has the lowest possible risk for Pill complications:

AGE: 15 to 35
WEIGHT: Normal
SMOKING: None
BLOOD PRESSURE: Normal or low, and remained normal during pregnancy
VARICOSE VEINS: None
CONTRAINDICATIONS: None
DANGER SIGNS: None

Contraindications

A contraindication is a medical condition that renders inadvisable or unsafe a treatment or procedure that might otherwise be recommended. **Respecting contraindications is extremely important for safe Pill use.** The list of contraindications for Pills is long, but most of the medical conditions on the list are rare, especially among young women. Nevertheless, this list means that there are many women who should never use Pills, even if they would like to very much.

CONTRAINDICATIONS DILEMMAS

The following section includes some arbitrary age cutoffs for safe Pill use. Basically these arbitrary cutoffs are designed roughly to reflect the ages at which increasing cardiovascular risks become significant.

If you have been reading about Pills for long, you've probably noticed that these arbitrary ages wander around from time to time, based on what the latest research shows. You may also have noticed that healthy women stop taking estrogen and progestin at age 45 because it isn't safe, then may start taking estrogen and progestin again at age 50 or thereabouts as postmenopausal hormone replacement! It probably seems a little strange that there are only five years in your whole life (if you are a healthy woman) when it is dangerous to take hormones.

It is strange. Although the estrogens and progestins in Pills and in hormone replacement therapy are significantly different from each other, they are indeed both estrogens and progestins, and it would make more sense if we could come to think of hormones as drugs along a continuum, with varying risks and benefits throughout life, waiting to be weighed and evaluated one woman at a time, one year at a time, in the light of the best research available. For now we must put up with arbitrary age cutoffs, because medicine changes its collective mind quite slowly.

Smoking is another contraindications dilemma. If you are a smoker, you may have had the puzzling experience of being told by your clinician or a counselor that you must stop Pills because you are 35. Smoking is thousands of times more likely to kill you than Pills are, so **stopping Pills at 35 while you keep on smoking does not protect your health!** What protects your health is getting off cigarettes.

ABSOLUTE CONTRAINDICATIONS

A woman with any of the following conditions **must not take Pills under any circumstances, with no exception.** If you develop any of these conditions while taking Pills, you must stop your Pills at once.

• Circulatory disorder now or in the past, such as thrombophlebitis (clots in the legs), pulmonary embolism (clots in the lung), heart attack or stroke, coronary artery disease, or angina (heart pain)
• Impaired liver function, including active or recent hepatitis, alcohol liver damage, severe mononucleosis, or jaundice with pregnancy or Pill use in the past, or liver tumor now or in the past

- Known or suspected cancer of the breast, or other known or suspected estrogen-dependent cancer such as uterine or ovary cancer
- Current pregnancy or suspected pregnancy
- Abnormal vaginal bleeding whose cause has not yet been determined.

STRONG RELATIVE CONTRAINDICATIONS

The following conditions mean that your clinician will **strongly advise you not to use Pills**. You may be vulnerable to serious health risks.

- High blood pressure now or in the past, even if your blood pressure is controlled with medication
- Severe headaches, particularly vascular or migraine types*
- Diabetes
- Gallbladder disease
- Precancerous cervical abnormalities (dysplasia, cervical intraepithelial neoplasia, CIN)
- Mononucleosis now or in the recent past
- Sickle cell anemia or other hemoglobin disease
- Leg cast, body cast, or serious leg injury
- Major surgery scheduled within the next month
- Age 35 and a heavy smoker (more than 15 cigarettes a day)*
- Age 40 or older with a second risk factor for cardiovascular disease such as obesity, high blood pressure, high lipid levels*

RELATIVE CONTRAINDICATIONS

The following conditions mean that you **may be able to use Pills** if you are willing to be **followed very carefully** by your clinician so that she/he can watch for early signs of trouble.

- Serious heart or kidney disease*
- Serious depression or suicidal feelings now or in the past (depression may worsen or improve on Pills)*
- Severe asthma*
- Severe varicose veins*
- History of chloasma (darkening of facial skin) or hair loss during pregnancy or during previous Pill use*
- Uterine fibroid tumors (may worsen or improve on Pills)*
- Menstrual periods recently begun and not yet regular (young teens)

A star (*) at the end of a contraindication means that the authors believe the contraindication is *more significant* for combined birth control Pill use than for Minipill use, and in some cases might not be considered a Minipill contraindication at all.

- Breastfeeding*
- Strong family history of diabetes
- Congenital hyperbilirubinemia (Gilbert's disease)
- Age 45 or older*
- Impaired liver function within the past year
- Delivery of term pregnancy within past 10 to 14 days*
- Weight gain of 10 or more pounds while on the Pill*
- Use of epilepsy or tuberculosis medication that may reduce Pill effectiveness or other medication that can interact with Pills in a dangerous way (see Table 13-3)*
- Family history of death of a parent or sibling (particularly mother or sister) by heart attack before age 50. (Have blood lipids checked first for hereditary blood lipid elevation.)
- Family history of hereditary blood lipid elevation
- Compromised ability to use Pills safely (no access to emergency care for Pill problems; emotional or intellectual impairment that would make it difficult to follow Pill schedule or recognize danger signs)

Some clinicians do not agree that all these conditions should be treated as relative contraindications, and some would add others to the list.

Advantages of Pills

Pills provide the best contraceptive protection possible with a temporary birth control method—99% or better—when you use them consistently and correctly. They do not interrupt lovemaking and require minimal paraphernalia. Pills provide continuous protection throughout the Pill cycle and during the one-week interval when you are off hormones, no matter how frequently you have intercourse.

Many women use Pills less for the contraceptive protection than for incidental advantages that are associated with Pills. In one study, about 12% of Pill users used them strictly for noncontraceptive reasons, while another 27% used them for contraceptive **and** noncontraceptive reasons together.

For many women the greatest advantage of Pills is freedom from debilitating cramps and heavy bleeding.

I never would have made it through my medical training without Pills. I couldn't have endured 48 hours on call with cramps like the ones I used to have every month! I also needed really good contraceptive protection, because when you're pushed to your physical and emotional limit all the time, you don't want pregnancy scares or the stress of an unplanned pregnancy.

—WOMAN PHYSICIAN, 29

TABLE 13-4
HEALTH BENEFITS OF PILLS

Hospitalizations and illnesses are prevented each year by the use of Pills. These totals and rates are based on estimates for 8.5 million Pill users in 1981; overall totals today would be somewhat higher because more women are using Pills.

DISEASE	HOSPITALIZATIONS AND/OR ILLNESSES PREVENTED PER 100,000 PILL USERS	TOTAL NUMBER OF HOSPITALIZATIONS OR ILLNESSES PREVENTED	NUMBER OF DEATHS PREVENTED
Benign breast disease	235	20,000	—
Ovarian retention cysts	35	3,000	—
Iron deficiency anemia	320	27,000	—
Pelvic inflammatory disease (first episodes)			
Total episodes	600	51,000	100
Hospitalizations	156	13,300	—
Ectopic pregnancy	117	9,900	10
Endometrial cancer	5	2,000	100
Ovarian cancer	4	1,700	1,000

SOURCE: Adapted from Ory HW: The noncontraceptive health benefits from oral contraceptive use. *Family Planning Perspectives* 14:182–184, 1982.

Your periods are almost always regular, predictable, light, and painless. Your clinician can help you reschedule your periods to avoid having periods during important events. Pill users are less likely to have premenstrual symptoms than are other women.

Perhaps the most exciting news about Pills in recent years is the finding that **Pills protect women from a number of health problems** (28). Table 13-4 lists illnesses, hospitalizations, and deaths that are prevented because of Pill use.

Iron deficiency anemia is less common among Pill users than among women who do not use Pills because the amount of blood you lose during a period on Pills is about half the amount you would normally lose, so your body's iron supply is less likely to become depleted.

The steady-state hormonal pattern on Pills protects users from developing **benign breast disease**, and from hospitalization (and anxiety) for benign breast lump biopsy (see Chapter 37). About 20,000 breast biopsy hospitalizations are prevented each year.

Because Pills suppress ovulation, **ovarian retention cysts** are far less likely to occur. These cysts either arise from the developing egg follicle itself or from the corpus luteum, the postovulatory transformed follicle (see Chapter 2). Pill users' ovaries are inactive throughout the cycle.

First episodes of **pelvic inflammatory disease** (PID) are far less common among Pill users, with some 50,000 cases prevented each year. Researchers suspect that Pills make it less likely that bacteria growing on the cervix will ascend to the uterus and tubes, because:

• There is less blood in the uterus and vagina for fewer days each cycle, and blood is an excellent nutrient medium for bacteria
• A thick plug of mucus remains in the cervical canal throughout most of the cycle, which serves as a mechanical barrier to the ascent of pathogens

Pill users do have a higher rate for chlamydial infection of the cervix, and chlamydia is a very important culprit in causing pelvic infection (see the section entitled "Chlamydial Cervicitis" earlier in this chapter). Nevertheless, Pills still protect against infection in the uterus and fallopian tubes (pelvic infection).

A 1985 study found that chlamydial tubal infections were four times as likely among women who use barrier methods of birth control or no birth control as among Pill users (29). PID is a major cause of infertility in women, and any level of protective effect is a boon for Pill users. Be careful, however, that you don't depend on Pills to protect you from sexual infection.

The Pill's substantial protective effects against **ovarian and endometrial cancer** are discussed in "Pills and Cancer" earlier in this chapter.

Because Pills so effectively prevent ovulation and pregnancy, they prevent literally thousands of hospitalizations each year for complications of pregnancy such as **miscarriage, ectopic pregnancy** (see Chapter 8), and **cesarean section delivery.**

Studies published in 1978 and 1982 appeared to show that Pills prevent **rheumatoid arthritis** that otherwise would occur among Pill users. The reason for a protective effect, if one exists, is not understood. However, a 1985 Mayo Clinic study found that Pill users and never users have very comparable rates for rheumatoid arthritis (30).

Pills may protect women from **toxic shock syndrome (TSS)**. Toxic shock syndrome is caused by bacterial toxin from staphylococcus bacteria in the vagina. Using tampons increases a woman's risk for this rare problem (see Chapter 24). Rates of TSS are lower for all contraceptors, including Pill users. In limited studies researchers have estimated that Pill users have 25% the rate of TSS as do women who use no birth control method (31).

Pills offer a number of protective effects that can be especially important to women who plan **future childbearing**. Protection against acute pelvic inflammatory disease, ovarian cysts, and ectopic pregnancy helps safeguard fertility, and Pills may also slow the development of potential fertility-impairing conditions such as endometriosis and uterine fibroid tumors.

Other Uses of Pills.   Pills have been used in the past to treat severe cramps or acne, and to regulate periods for women who have irregular menstrual cycles. Most clinicians no longer recommend Pills in such situations, unless a woman also wants the birth control effect of Pills. Other effective treatments are available for cramps and acne. If your natural cycle is irregular, you will almost surely have regular periods on Pills, but Pills do not correct your underlying problem. In some instances Pills can even cause prolonged hormone suppression after you stop taking them, and you may have a delay in resuming fertility when you want to become pregnant.

Pills are sometimes used as hormone replacement for women with premature menopause, a chromosomal sexual abnormality, or surgically removed ovaries.

Clinicians occasionally prescribe Pills for women with medical problems such as endometriosis, polycystic ovaries (Stein-Leventhal syndrome), and deficient blood-clotting factors (idiopathic thrombocytopenic purpura or ITP), and to control extremely heavy menstrual bleeding.

Short-term treatment with higher-dose birth control Pills can also be used for morning-after treatment (see Chapter 15). If morning-after hormone treatment is started within 24 to 72 hours after unprotected intercourse, it has a failure rate of only 2%, so call your clinician immediately if you have a birth control emergency and want to consider morning-after hormones.

Using Pills

Your clinician will review your medical history for any factors that might increase the risk of Pills for you and will perform a physical examination. Your exam will include blood pressure and weight, a breast exam, an abdominal exam, inspection of your cervix, a Pap test, and a bimanual exam to be sure your uterus, tubes, and ovaries feel normal. Some clinicians also include a gonorrhea test, routine blood count, and urine test as part of your initial exam.

How Young Is Too Young.   Ideally, a young woman should wait until she has 6 to 12 normal menstrual periods before she begins to use Pills. **Physiologic maturity is a more important factor than chronological age**, so even a quite young girl can safely begin Pills—if her periods are already under way. (Whether other aspects of sexual activity are wise for very young girls is another matter.) Beginning to use Pills before menstrual periods are well established, however, could cause a delay in identifying abnormal hormone patterns. Abnormal hormones are most often diagnosed because of the abnormal menstrual bleeding patterns they cause. A young woman taking Pills could have apparently normal periods as a result of Pills, and thus remain unaware of an underlying hormone disorder. This risk has to be weighed against the risks of accidental pregnancy very early in life, and most clinicians see pregnancy as a far greater health threat to young women than Pills. There is no evidence that Pills will stunt the growth of young teens.

CHOOSING WHICH PILL TO USE

There are about 40 different Pill brands. In some cases, different brands are identical except for packaging; in other cases, brands have different hormones in slightly differing amounts.

Each of the synthetic Pill hormones has unique properties. The two synthetic estrogens used in the United States are **mestranol** and **ethinyl estradiol**. Ethinyl estradiol is somewhat more potent—more estrogen effect per gram—than mestranol. Progestins, too, vary in potency and also in the degree to which they cause additional estrogen-like or androgen-like effects. Illustration 13-3 ranks Pills in rough order of potency.

Generic Pills, available in the United States for the first time in 1987, are identical in composition to brand name products containing 35 mcg of ethinyl estradiol and either 0.5 mg or 1.0 mg of norethindrone (Brevicon, Modicon, Norinyl 1 + 35, and Ortho-Novum 1/35). These products are monophasic—each cycle provides 21 identical hormone-containing pills.

In the early 1980s Pill manufacturers began marketing biphasic and triphasic brands of Pills. In contrast to earlier brands, the biphasic (two-phase) and triphasic (three-phase) Pills **alter the daily hormone dosage within a single cycle.** Triphasic brands commonly used now (Ortho-Novum 7/7/7, Tri-Norinyl, Tri-Levlen, Triphasil) have three different progestin doses for different parts of each Pill cycle. Triphasil and Tri-Levlen also have three different estrogen doses.

The main advantage of triphasic Pills is that the overall amount of progestin in a Pill cycle is lower than it is with regular, identical-dose Pills. Experts hope that the lower progestin dose will reduce possible adverse blood lipid effects and thus reduce risks for serious Pill complications. This potential benefit, however, has not yet been documented in research, so there is no clear, established advantage for triphasic products compared to older low-dose Pills also available (32). Manufacturers also promote phasic Pills as products that more closely resemble natural hormone patterns. Phasic pills appear to be just as effective as other combined Pills (32). Spotting may occur slightly more often than with older Pill types.

Clearly, staying on a careful Pill schedule becomes crucial when your pack is made up of three or even four different colors of Pills! Making up missed Pills or altering schedules to avoid a period during special events can be especially confusing.

Most clinicians consider estrogen dose the single most important factor in choosing a Pill. The risk of serious Pill complications is higher among women who take more than 50 mcg of estrogen, and most clinicians now recommend that patients stick to Pills containing 35 mcg or less if at all possible. Higher progestin potency, as well as higher estrogen potency, may increase your risk for complications. It makes sense to

TABLE 13-5
COMMON PILL SIDE EFFECTS AND POSSIBLE SOLUTIONS

SIDE EFFECT	POSSIBLE SOLUTION
Nausea	Reduce estrogen
Spotting	Increase progestin and/or increase estrogen
Missed menstrual periods	Increase estrogen and/or use progestin with estrogenic effect and/or reduce or increase progestin
Fluid retention, breast tenderness	Reduce estrogen and/or reduce progestin
Contact lenses don't fit	Reduce estrogen
Breast enlargement	Reduce progestin and/or reduce estrogen
Weight gain	Reduce estrogen and/or reduce progestin
Irritability, depression	Reduce or increase estrogen and/or reduce progestin
Decreased sex drive	Reduce progestin and/or increase estrogen or use progestin with androgenic effect
Heavy menstrual periods	Increase progestin
Excessive vaginal discharge	Reduce estrogen and/or reduce progestin

try to choose a Pill with the **lowest estrogen and progestin potency that will be effective in preventing pregnancy.** Most clinicians start women on a Pill containing 30 to 35 mcg of estrogen and a low progestin dose.

Chances are good that you will be able to use any of the available brands with no difficulty. If side effects do occur, your clinician may recommend another brand. Some common Pill side effects and possible solutions are listed in Table 13-5. Remember that your estrogen dose should not be increased above 50 mcg without discussion and a very good reason.

GETTING STARTED ON PILLS

Pills are set up in packs to allow for a period of bleeding once every four weeks—the "normal" pattern in Western cultures. This Pill schedule is completely arbitrary. You can take the first Pill in your first Pill pack any time during the first seven days of a natural cycle. Counting the first day of a normal menstrual period as day 1, you can take your first Pill any day from day 1 through day 7. If you start Pills before day 8, chances are good that you will not ovulate during your very first Pill cycle; most clinicians recommend, however, that you rely on another method of birth control, such as foam, condoms, sponges, or a diaphragm, for the first 10 to 14 days you use Pills. **Be sure to use another birth control method while you are waiting to start your first pack.** Many, many pregnancies are conceived during the "waiting to start Pills" interval.

Do not start Pills if you think there is any chance you might be already pregnant. For example, if your last menstrual period did not seem entirely normal (too light, early, or late), then consult your clinician to decide whether it would be safe for you to begin Pills.

One easy Pill-taking scheme is the **Start-on-Sunday** method. Begin your first pack of Pills on the first Sunday after a normal menstrual period begins. You will begin a new pack of Pills every fourth Sunday, and you can avoid having menstrual periods on weekends.

Once you have started your first Pill pack, your Pill cycle is set and you will always follow the same Pill schedule.

Two different types of Pill packs are available: 21-day packs and 28-day packs.

The 21-day pack contains 21 hormone Pills. Your schedule will be 21 days of Pills, 7 days off, 21 days of Pills, 7 days off, and so on. Swallow one Pill a day for three weeks until the pack is empty. Wait one full week; then begin your next pack. If you are using the Start-on-Sunday method, your calendar will look like Illustration 13-5.

The 28-day pack contains two different kinds of tablets: 21 hormone Pills and 7 **tablets that contain no hormone** (the blank tablets contain inert powder or inert powder plus iron). Take the 21 hormone Pills first, and then the 7 blank tablets. When you have taken all the tablets in your pack, you **begin your next pack immediately,** with no days off, starting with the 21 hormone Pills. On the 28-day schedule the 7 blank tablets are your 7 days without hormones.

No matter which type of pack you use, **you can expect your menstrual period during the seven no-hormone days;** bleeding usually begins about 48 hours after your last hormone Pill.

USING PILLS CORRECTLY

I used to think my older sisters were real dopes because they never could remember their Pills. Pam would jump up in the middle of the night to see if she forgot a Pill. Gwen had to double up on Pills on just about every pack.

Now I understand. It *is* hard to remember! Finally I just started marking my calendar every time I took a Pill. But sometimes I forget to mark the calendar . . .

—WOMAN, 17

Try to take your Pill at about the same time each day. Remembering Pills may be easier if you link your Pill to some other routine activity such as brushing your teeth or dinner or setting your alarm clock. You may find it helpful to keep a calendar and mark off each day as you take your Pill.

Have a back-up method of birth control on hand, such as a diaphragm, condoms, foam, or sponges. You will need your back-up method until you have taken the first 14 Pills in your first pack, or if you stop Pills for any reason, or if you miss more than one Pill. The generally prescribed directions for taking the Pill are:

If you miss one Pill, take two the next day. Take a missed pill as soon as you remember, and take your regular Pill for that day at the regular time. You do not need to call your clinician or use back-up birth control.

If you miss two Pills in a row, take two each day for two days until you catch up. Take the first missed Pill as soon as you remember and the regular Pill for that day at the regular time. Take the second missed Pill along with your regular Pill the following day. You may have some spotting. Use your back-up method until you have your next period.

If you miss three Pills or more in a row, stop your Pills and wait until you have some bleeding. Then start a new pack of Pills as you normally would after your period starts. Begin using your back-up method as soon as you realize you have missed Pills, and continue using it until you have taken 14 Pills in your new pack. Call your clinician if you do not have a menstrual period.

If you do not have a menstrual period during your seven no-hormone days and are sure that you have taken all your Pills on schedule, you can begin a new pack on schedule. There is only a very small chance that you could be pregnant.

If you miss a period and are not sure you have taken all your Pills correctly, do not start a new pack. Stop Pills, begin using your back-up method, and arrange for a pregnancy test and exam as soon as you can.

If you miss two periods in a row, even if you are sure that you have taken all your Pills on schedule, stop Pills. Begin using your back-up method, and arrange to see your clinician for a pregnancy test.

If you have spotting or bleeding while you are taking Pills, stay on your regular Pill schedule. Bleeding usually subsides after a few days and is most likely during the first month or two on Pills. If your bleeding is heavier than on the heavy days of a natural period, if you soak more than three pads or tampons in an hour, or if spotting continues through more than one cycle, call your clinician. You may need evaluation to be certain that Pills are the cause of your unusual bleeding. **If you have cramps or fever along with bleeding, you need to see your clinician at once. You may have an infection.**

If you have nausea, try taking your Pill along with dinner or in the evening. If you vomit within an hour after taking a Pill, take an extra Pill from a separate pack to replace the Pill vomited up. If you have moderate or severe **diarrhea**, double up your

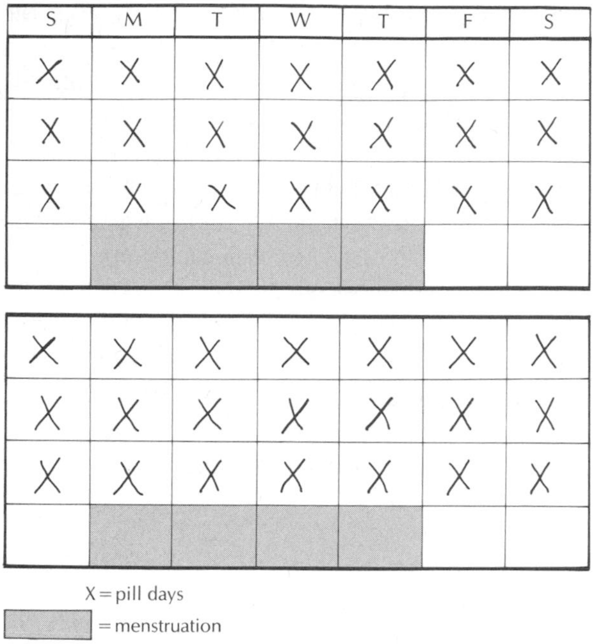

S	M	T	W	T	F	S
X	X	X	X	X	X	X
X	X	X	X	X	X	X
X	X	X	X	X	X	X

S	M	T	W	T	F	S
X	X	X	X	X	X	X
X	X	X	X	X	X	X
X	X	X	X	X	X	X

X = pill days

= menstruation

ILLUSTRATION 13-5   The 21-day Pill schedule using the Start-on-Sunday method.

Pills on that day. If you have diarrhea for several days in a row, use a back-up method until your next period.

If you accidentally damage or lose your Pills or run out of Pills, call your clinician. An immediate telephone refill can almost always be arranged so that you won't have to interrupt your Pill schedule. Many family planning clinics are able to provide emergency refills for their own patients or for other women in emergency situations.

If you want to alter your Pill schedule and avoid having your menstrual period during final exams or a trip, for example, you will need to talk to your clinician and do a little advance planning. You can change your cycle length by taking as many as seven additional Pills added on to your regular pack or by starting a new pack one or two days earlier than you normally would. If you take some extra Pills, your menstrual bleeding will begin about 48 hours after your last hormone Pill—up to seven days later than usual. Set aside the pack you used; you may need extra pills again.

PILL EMERGENCIES

It is essential that you learn how to recognize a true Pill emergency. If you develop any of the Pill danger signs (see Illustration 13-5), stop the Pills, contact your clinician at once, and use a back-up method of birth control. Do not wait to see if the symptoms go away. If you can't see your clinician or get to your clinic, go to an emergency room.

STOPPING PILLS

You can stop Pills after you finish a Pill pack or any time in the middle. Nothing bad happens when you stop Pills, but you do need to begin using another method of birth control immediately. **There is no carry-over birth control protection once you stop taking Pills.** Many Pill users ovulate within two to three weeks after their last Pill, and almost all ovulate within three months. Whether you stop in the middle of a pack or at the end, your body quickly begins to reestablish its own cyclic patterns. You will probably have a menstrual period a day or two after your last Pill. Your first natural menstrual period will usually come four, five, or six weeks after that. Then you can expect natural cycles to be as regular—or as irregular—as they were before you started Pills.

"VACATIONS" FROM PILLS

In the earliest days of Pill use in this country, the FDA-approved pill labeling recommended that Pill users go off Pills for a cycle or two every year or so. However, so many women became pregnant during their "Pill vacations" that most clinicians stopped recommending a rest from Pills. Today there is absolutely **no evidence** that there is anything to be gained by Pill vacations.

PLANNING PREGNANCY AFTER PILLS

You need to plan ahead for pregnancy if you use Pills. Stop taking Pills at least three months before you would like to conceive, switch to another method of birth control—condoms, foam, sponges, or a diaphragm—and begin to keep careful records of your periods, and perhaps even your basal body temperature (see Chapter 6). This Pill-free interval allows your natural cycle a chance to reestablish itself.

If you have a very precise time schedule for pregnancy, or you are already reaching your late twenties, **you may want to allow a longer interval off Pills.** Using a barrier method such as condoms or a diaphragm for the last year or two before pregnancy may help you avoid fertility problems caused by hormone suppression (see the section entitled "Prolonged Hormone Suppression and Future Fertility" earlier in this chapter). If you are one of the uncommon former Pill users who does have suppression, it will be evident and you will have time to arrange for evaluation and treatment before you actually want to begin trying to conceive.

If you conceive before you have your first natural period, it may be difficult for you and your clinician to determine exactly when you became pregnant. It is important to be able to estimate the beginning of your pregnancy accurately in case you should need a cesarean section delivery or should need to have labor induced. Your clinician decides when to perform these procedures on the basis of your estimated length of pregnancy. If her/his estimate is wrong because pregnancy began when you weren't having normal periods, your baby could be born prematurely.

Studies have shown a slightly increased risk of birth defects in infants conceived during Pill use, and abnormalities were seen in miscarried pregnancies that were conceived during or immediately after Pill use. (See the previous section on risks and complications.) **There is no evidence of increased risk of abnormality among full-term infants conceived immediately after Pill use.**

Minipills

Minipills are estrogen-free contraceptive tablets that provide a continuous, low dose of progestin. They were approved for use in the United States in 1972 and 1973, 12 years after the approval of regular combined Pills containing both estrogen and progestin. The idea behind Minipills, however, is not new. The original research on hormone contraception started with progestin as the primary ingredient. Estrogen was added later to insure a more regular pattern of bleeding.

Commercial marketing policies may explain the limited acceptance of Minipills, which have not been advertised or promoted aggressively by their manufacturers. All three brands sold in the United States are produced by companies that also produce successful, widely advertised combined Pills.

Another explanation may be the Minipill's shortcomings. **Minipills are slightly less effective than regular Pills and often cause irregular menstrual patterns.** Also, long-term research on Minipills is not extensive. Studies of very large numbers of Minipill users would be necessary to determine what, if any, safety advantages Minipills have. Their use is so limited that such data may never be available.

Minipills can be an excellent contraceptive choice for a woman who would like to use an oral contraceptive but should not use estrogen. Minipills may be a good choice for women who develop estrogen-related side effects such as headaches on regular combined Pills, and for older or breastfeeding women.

HOW MINIPILLS WORK

A low dose of progestin taken by mouth every day alters several different components of fertility. Contraceptive effectiveness may result from the sum of all these effects, or it may be that one specific effect is most important. Minipills cause the following changes:

The steady, continuous level of progestin from Minipills in the bloodstream distorts the normal pattern of pituitary hormone production. The pituitary hormone is not fully suppressed, as is the case with combined Pills, but the LH (luteinizing hormone, see Chapter 2) trigger for ovulation is blunted or absent, so that in **15% to 40% of the Minipill user's cycles the ovaries do not release an egg.**

Cervical mucus remains scant, thick, and sticky throughout the cycle under the influence of the progestin in Minipills. Thick mucus decreases the likelihood that sperm will be able to penetrate the cervical canal and enter the uterus and tubes. Thick mucus may also inhibit chemical changes within sperm cells that permit them to fertilize an egg. Furthermore, the thick mucus decreases sperm swimming capacity (motility), and may not provide the nutrients that sperm require for optimal survival.

Continuous progestin may **interfere with normal development of the corpus luteum** from an egg follicle after ovulation (see Chapter 2). The high levels of progesterone normally produced by the corpus luteum are necessary for establishing and maintaining a healthy pregnancy.

Normal development of the uterine lining (endometrium) requires an initial estrogen phase followed by a combined estrogen and progesterone phase after ovulation. Minipills provide progestin continuously throughout the cycle and thus interfere with endometrial development, so it is less likely that a fertilized egg could implant in the uterine lining.

Safe passage of a fertilized egg through the fallopian tube down to the uterus depends in part on rhythmic contractions of the tube itself. Minipill progestin may alter fallopian tube contractions, causing the fertilized ovum to reach the uterus at the wrong time to implant properly.

Despite all these alterations in the normal fertility cycle, Minipills do not totally suppress hormone production. Your normal hormone pattern is altered, but you will nevertheless have natural estrogen and progesterone production that is usually sufficient to trigger menstrual periods. **Your own internal cycle will determine when your menstrual periods will occur,** not the Minipill. In this respect, Minipills are completely different from regular combined Pills.

EFFECTIVENESS

Studies of women who used Minipills consistently and correctly have documented a failure rate as low as 1%. Most studies, however, have reported rates of about 3% (4). As with almost all studies of contraceptive efficacy, younger women have more accidental pregnancies than older women—3.1 per 100 woman/years for women in their 20s and 0.3 for women 40 or older in one large British study (33).

Like regular birth control Pills, Minipills have their contraceptive effect because of a continuous, steady level of hormone intake. Obviously, they are effective only if they are taken consistently.

One major difference between progestin-only pills and regular Pills is that there is little margin for error with Minipills. The likelihood of pregnancy increases substantially if you miss only one or two tablets, and contraceptive protection is almost entirely lost if you forget more than three consecutive pills. **It is essential to take your Minipill every day without fail.**

To protect yourself against pregnancy, be sure that you and your partner have a back-up method on hand. Begin using a diaphragm, condoms, sponges, or foam whenever you forget to take two or more Minipills, and continue using your back-up until your next period starts. Use your back-up method immediately if you stop Minipills for any reason.

COMMON MINIPILL SIDE EFFECTS

Side effects of Minipills—effects unrelated to birth control—seem to be less numerous than side effects of regular Pills. But since experience with Minipills is much less extensive than experience with regular Pills, it is entirely possible that new side effects will be discovered in the future. Common side effects that are not believed to be dangerous are discussed in this section. Potentially harmful side effects are discussed in the section on Minipill risks and complications.

Most women who use Minipills find that they have **fewer premenstrual symptoms** than they do during a natural cycle. Your menstrual bleeding may be lighter and shorter, and you will probably have very mild cramps, or none at all.

The interval between your periods may remain the same, but it may become longer or shorter, and it may vary from cycle to cycle. **Menstrual periods tend to be less predictable when you use Minipills.** It is also common to have episodes of spotting or light bleeding between periods.

Some of the common side effects associated with regular combined Pills may also occur with Minipills, but they are somewhat less likely. Nausea, headache, breast tenderness, vaginal discharge, and depression have been reported but seem to be less common with Minipills than during a natural hormone cycle. Acne problems, increased appetite, and weight gain also can occur but are not common with Minipills, perhaps because Minipills contain 10% to 70% less progestin than do regular combined Pills. Other possible side effects as yet not definitely linked with Minipills include dark patches on the skin of the face (chloasma) and changes in sex drive (libido).

Minipills probably do not decrease the amount of breast milk produced or alter milk content the way regular Pills do. Progestin from Minipills does appear in the breast milk, however; about 0.1% of the amount in the woman's blood. Whether or not this trace of hormone has any harmful effect on the nursing infant is not known. Minipills would probably be a better birth control choice than regular Pills if you are nursing and you choose not to use a diaphragm, condoms, foam, or sponges.

Studies of Minipill effects on vitamin levels, the body's chemical processes, and lab test results so far do not show the alterations that occur with regular combined Pills.

RISKS AND COMPLICATIONS

Even though Minipills contain only a low dose of one of the two hormones in regular combined Pills, **the official FDA-approved Minipill labeling provides the same risk warnings for Minipills as for regular Pills.** Minipills have been used by a relatively small number of women; hence, the kind of long-term research involving tens of thousands of users that would be necessary to determine whether or not Minipill risks are the same as combined Pill risks is simply not available. In the absence of good information, the FDA has decided that the safest course is to presume that Minipill risks and combined Pill risks are the same. These risks are described in detail earlier in the chapter.

Although official information brochures must be identical, **most family planning experts believe that Minipills are safer than combined Pills.** Estrogen is probably responsible for many serious Pill-related risks. Estrogen is known to cause major alterations in blood-clotting factors. The progestin in regular birth control Pills does affect lipids—blood cholesterol—and fat balance. Progestin, along with estrogen, may play a role in causing circulatory problems, especially when Pills with a high dose of progestin are used. The total dose of progestin in Minipills, however, is lower than the dose of progestin in regular birth control Pills and it is not known whether the lower dose in Minipills has any adverse effect on users. A large 1985 Minipill study suggests that overall, Minipills are likely to be safer than combined Pills (33). **The lower hormone dose in Minipills, however, may also mean that possible health benefits are reduced** for Minipill users compared to women who take regular birth control Pills.

Unpredictable bleeding is the single most common reason women stop taking Minipills. In the 1985 British study, menstrual disturbance was the overwhelming reason for stopping Minipills (33). Menstrual problems are not in themselves medically harmful. Irregular bleeding can be a hazard, however, if it is **falsely** attributed to Minipills and there is a delay in recognizing a serious medical problem such as infection or uterine or cervical tumors. About 40% of Minipill users ovulate regularly, 40% don't ovulate at all, and 20% sometimes ovulate. Absence of ovulation is more likely to be associated with unpredictable bleeding.

Another important Minipill problem is **ectopic pregnancy**: pregnancy that implants in one of the fallopian tubes rather than in the uterus. If a woman using Minipills becomes pregnant, her risk of ectopic pregnancy is higher than her risk of regular uterine pregnancy, because the Minipill probably protects a woman more effectively against a uterine than a tubal pregnancy. This risk is more important for Minipill users than for regular Pill users, because the overall pregnancy rate is a little higher with Minipills and ovulation is suppressed less dependably, so the ectopic pregnancy risk is higher as well. See Chapter 8 for danger signs of ectopic pregnancy.

CONTRAINDICATIONS

A contraindication is a medical condition that renders a treatment or procedure unsafe or inadvisable that might otherwise be recommended. The official FDA-approved labeling information for Minipills lists exactly the same contraindications for Minipills as it does for regular combined Pills. There is no evidence that Minipills will aggravate all the problems on the list of contraindications, but neither is there evidence that Minipills would be safe. Because some of these problems are so serious, even potentially fatal, it seems prudent to respect these contraindications until further research clarifies Minipill safety. Pill contraindications are listed earlier in this chapter, and several contraindications are starred to show that the authors believe these may not be significant factors for Minipill users.

ADVANTAGES OF MINIPILLS

Minipills offer **protection** about equal to that of combined Pills and other effective contraceptives when used carefully and correctly. Minipills do not interrupt lovemaking and require minimal paraphernalia. They are easy to take, one pill every day, and you do not have to remember a cyclic pattern. Minipills provide continuous protection, no matter how frequently you have intercourse.

Although menstrual periods may be less regular than during natural cycles, bleeding is often lighter, premenstrual symptoms are often less severe, and menstrual cramps are usually mild or absent.

The primary advantage of Minipills compared to regular combined Pills is **probably** safety. The word "probably" is stressed because there is as yet no research evidence that proves this advantage. Theoretical factors that make it seem likely that a safety advantage will someday be documented include the following: Minipills contain no estrogen, Minipills contain a lower dose of progestin than regular combined Pills, and Minipills do not totally suppress the pituitary hormone cycle, as combined Pills do.

Whether Minipills confer such important combined Pill health benefits as protection from ovarian and endometrial cancer is not known.

USING MINIPILLS

Evaluation and examination procedures for starting Minipills are the same as those necessary for regular Pills, so you will need to see your clinician.

Choosing which Minipill to use is fairly easy because only three brands are now available in the United States and two of them are identical in hormone content. They are:

• Micronor (0.35 mg norethindrone in each tablet)
• Nor-Q.D. (0.35 mg norethindrone in each tablet)
• Ovrette (0.075 mg norgestrel in each tablet)

The norgestrel in Ovrette is a more potent progestin than the norethindrone in Micronor and Nor-Q.D., so the progestin effect and the efficacy of Ovrette is probably higher than that of Micronor or Nor-Q.D. even though the milligram dose is lower. Norgestrel is a synthetic progestin that has almost no estrogen effects, whereas norethindrone does have some estrogen effect in addition to the primary progestin effect.

There is no clear-cut way to choose a Minipill brand. You may find, however, that you are able to tolerate one better than another. If you do have problems such as irregular menstrual patterns, it may be worthwhile to try a Minipill with a different progestin.

Most clinicians (and the FDA-approved Minipill labeling information) recommend that you begin Minipills on day 1 of a natural cycle; that is, on the first day of a normal menstrual period. **If you begin Minipills on the first day of bleeding**, the pills will probably protect you from pregnancy in your very first cycle, but you should use foams, condoms, sponges, or a diaphragm along with your Minipills for the first two weeks. Using an additional method for the first two or three days on Minipills is especially important. **Do not start taking Minipills if there is any chance you might be pregnant already.**

Once you have started taking Minipills, simply swallow one tablet each day for as long as you wish to avoid pregnancy. **Do not stop taking Minipills during your period. There are no breaks** and no placebo pills at all for Minipill users. Take your Minipill at about the same time each day, with no interruptions whatsoever. Some clinicians recommend late afternoon as the best time for your daily Minipill since the peak effect on cervical mucus will occur four to six hours after you take a Minipill, and most couples have intercourse in the evening.

Have a back-up method of birth control on hand. You will need it if you forget more than one Minipill or if you stop taking them for any reason.

If you miss one Minipill, take it as soon as you remember, and take your next Minipill at the regular time. For extra protection, you can use a back-up method until your next period starts.

If you miss two Minipills, take one of the missed Minipills as soon as you remember, and take your regular Minipill for that day on schedule. Take the second forgotten Minipill plus the regular Minipill the next day. Use a back-up method until your next period starts.

If you miss more than two Minipills, stop taking Minipills and use your back-up method until your next menstrual period starts. You can safely begin taking Minipills again on the first day of your period. Use your back-up method for the first two weeks of your new pack.

If you do not start a menstrual period within 45 days of starting your last period, stop taking Minipills and see your clinician promptly to determine whether you are pregnant.

If you have repeated spotting or frequent, irregular menstrual periods, discuss this problem with your clinician. She/he may decide that you need further evaluation to be certain that Minipills are truly the cause of your problem. Some clinicians prescribe two Minipills a day—one in the morning and one in the late afternoon—for persistent spotting. **If you have cramps or fever associated with bleeding, see your clinician at once, because you could have a pelvic infection.**

Anticipate some change in your menstrual cycle length. Changes may be more likely during the first few months that you use Minipills. You may want to keep a tampon in your purse in case you have unexpected spotting or begin a period.

If you have nausea, try taking your Minipill with dinner or in the evening. If you vomit for any reason within an hour after you have taken a Minipill, take an extra Minipill immediately to replace the one vomited up. If you have diarrhea, take an extra Minipill that day. If you have diarrhea for several days in a row, use a back-up method until your next period.

If you accidentally damage, lose, or run out of Minipills, call your clinician. An immediate telephone refill can almost always be arranged so that you don't have to miss any Minipills. If you are traveling, you may be able to get an emergency refill from a local Planned Parenthood clinic.

Some Minipill users are able to identify their own cycles well enough to recognize signs of ovulation (see Chapter 6 for details). If you can tell when you ovulate, consider improving your protection by adding a back-up method for several days before and after ovulation.

Knowing when to **stop** taking Minipills and when to see your clinician could be important for your safety. Read the section on stopping Pills earlier in this chapter; all these rules also apply to Minipill users. Remember that you also need to see your clinician if you go more than 45 days without a menstrual period. The overall chance of pregnancy and the chance of ectopic pregnancy are higher with Minipills than with regular combined Pills; you must be alert to the early signs of pregnancy and ectopic pregnancy (see Chapter 8).

If you want to stop Minipills because you have decided to use another birth control method, **you can stop any time during your cycle.** If you are not bleeding when you stop Minipills, you can expect a menstrual period to begin within a few days after your last Minipill. After that you can expect your own natural cycle to resume.

As with regular combined Pills, most clinicians recommend that you plan ahead for pregnancy. **Ideally, this means stopping Minipills at least three months before you would like to become pregnant,** and using another birth control method—a diaphragm, condoms, sponges, or foam—during the three-month interval. Reasons for this recommendation are explained earlier in "Planning Pregnancy After Pills."

Hormonal Implants

Many Pill users say they love everything about Pills except having to remember to take one every day. Researchers recognize this drawback and are developing improved ways to deliver hormonal contraceptives to a woman's body with less bother. One of the most promising advances is the subdermal implant.

Implants are 1- to 2-inch rods of Silastic, a blend of plastic and silicone. The rods are filled with the hormonal contraceptive drug and implanted (with local anesthesia) just under a woman's skin, usually on the upper arm, through a 1/4-inch incision. The incision is closed with a stitch or just a Band-Aid. The contraceptive hormone then gradually leaches out through the walls of the rods and enters the bloodstream. The rods can be quickly removed in the event of a complication or problem, or at the end of the device's period of effectiveness.

One subdermal implant system that has been extensively tested in clinical trials is Norplant, developed by the Population Council. This system contains no estrogen and the progestin is levonorgestrel. It is designed to remain in place and prevent pregnancy for at least five years.

In one Finnish study (34), 124 women used Norplant for five years. There were no accidental pregnancies, and 45% of the women who began the study chose to keep the implant for the full five years. Some left the study to become pregnant and others because of menstrual irregularity and other problems. Some 76% of the women who had Norplant removed to plan pregnancy did become pregnant within a year.

The Norplant system works in much the same way as the Minipill (35), and has the same risks and contraindications. In essence, the mechanism of drug delivery differs.

The Norplant system could be approved for general use in the United States in the late 1980s; in the meantime, it is available only to women participating in research programs that are evaluating the method.

REFERENCES

1. Ory HW, Forrest JD, Lincoln R: *Making Choices: Evaluating the Health Risks and Benefits of Birth Control Methods.* New York: Alan Guttmacher Institute, 1983.
2. Adams PW, Rose DP, Folkard J, et al: Effect of pyridoxine hydrochloride (vitamin B6) upon depression associated with oral contraception. *Lancet* 1:897–904, 1973.
3. Wynn V: Vitamins and oral contraceptive use. *Lancet* 1:561–564, 1975.
4. Hatcher RA, Guest FJ, Stewart FH, et al: *Contraceptive Technology 1988–1989* (ed. 14). New York: Irvington Publishers, in press. Failure rate studies are extensively referenced in this manual.
5. FDA-approved labeling for oral contraceptives. Manufacturers of oral contraceptives are required to provide a booklet or leaflet explaining the benefits, risks, and possible complications of Pills for each woman who fills a Pill prescription. You will be able to get

a copy from your clinician or pharmacist. The manufacturer's information for physicians and the text of the patient booklet or leaflet appear in *Physicians' Desk Reference* (ed 40). Oradell, N.J.: Medical Economics Co., 1986. The *Physicians' Desk Reference* is updated annually.

6. Knopp RH: Oral contraceptives and lipoproteins. *Outlook* 2:2–5, 1984.

7. Powell MG, Hedlin AM, Cerskus I, et al: Effects of oral contraceptives on lipoprotein lipids: A prospective study. *Obstetrics and Gynecology* 63:764–769, 1984.

8. Connell EB: Oral contraceptives: The current risk-benefit ratio. *Journal of Reproductive Medicine* 29:513–521, 1984.

9. Dorflinger LJ: Relative potency of progestins used in oral contraceptives. *Contraception* 31:557–570, 1985.

10. Metreau JM, Dhumeaux D, Perthelot P: Oral contraceptives and the liver. *Digestion* 7:318–335, 1972.

11. Rooks JB, Ory HW, Ishak KG, et al: Epidemiology of hepatocellular adenoma: The role of oral contraceptive use. *Journal of the American Medical Association* 242:644–648, 1979.

12. Neuberger J, Forman D, Doll R, et al: Oral contraceptives and hepatocellular carcinoma. *British Medical Journal* 292:1355–1357, 1986.

13. Cates W Jr, Washington AE, Rubin GL, et al: The pill, *Chlamydia*, and PID. *Family Planning Perspectives* 17:175–176, 1985.

14. Wolner-Hannsen P, Svensson L, Mardh P-A, et al: Laparoscopic findings and contraceptive use in women with signs and symptoms suggestive of acute salpingitis. *Obstetrics and Gynecology* 66:233–238, 1985.

15. Royal College of General Practitioners' Oral Contraception Study: Oral contraceptives and gallbladder disease. *Lancet* 2:957–959, 1982.

16. Shaffer EA, Taylor PJ, Logan K, et al: The effect of a progestin on gallbladder function in young women. *American Journal of Obstetrics and Gynecology* 148:504–507, 1984.

17. Vessey MP, Smith MA, Yeates D: Return of fertility after discontinuation of oral contraceptives: Influence of age and parity. *British Journal of Family Planning* 11:120–124, 1986.

18. Division of Reproductive Health, Centers for Disease Control, Atlanta: Oral contraceptive use and the risk of ovarian cancer. *Journal of the American Medical Association* 249:1596–1599, 1983.

19. Division of Reproductive Health, Centers for Disease Control, Atlanta: The reduction in risk of ovarian cancer associated with oral contraceptive use. *New England Journal of Medicine* 316:650–655, 1987.

20. Division of Reproductive Health, Centers for Disease Control, Atlanta: Oral-contraceptive use and the risk of breast cancer: The Cancer and Steroid Hormone Study of the Centers for Disease Control and the National Institute of Child Health and Human Development. *New England Journal of Medicine* 315:405–411, 1986.

21. Pike MC, Henderson BE, Krailo MD, et al: Breast cancer in young women and use of oral contraceptives: Possible modifying effect of formulation and age at use. *Lancet* 2:926–930, 1983.

22. Meirik O, Adami H-O, Christoffersen T, et al: Oral contraceptive use and breast cancer in young women: A joint national case-control study in Sweden and Norway. *Lancet* 2:650–653, 1986.

23. Stadel BV, Rubin GL, Webster LA, et al: Oral contraceptives and breast cancer in young women. *Lancet* 2:970–973, 1985.

24. Clarke EA, Hatcher J, McKeown-Eyssen GE, et al: Cervical dysplasia: Association with sexual behavior, smoking, and oral contraceptive use? *American Journal of Obstetrics and Gynecology* 151:612–616, 1985.

25. Oral contraceptives and cancer. *FDA Drug Bulletin* 14:2–3, 1984.

26. Lincoln R: The pill, breast and cervical cancer, and the role of progestogens in arterial disease. *Family Planning Perspectives* 16:55–63, 1984.

27. Taler SJ, Coulam CB, Annegers JF, et al: Case-control study of galactorrhea and its relationship to the use of oral contraceptives. *Obstetrics and Gynecology* 65:665–668, 1985.

28. Ory HW: The noncontraceptive health benefits from oral contraceptive use. *Family Planning Perspectives* 14:182–184, 1982.

29. Risk of tubal infection from chlamydial PID reduced by pills. *Family Planning Perspectives* 17:269–270, 1985.

30. Del Junco DJ, Annegers JF, Luthra HS, et al: Do oral contraceptives prevent rheumatoid arthritis? *Journal of the American Medical Association* 254:1938–1941, 1985.

31. Kols A, Rinehart W, Piotrow P, et al: Oral contraceptives in the 1980s. *Population Reports,* Ser A, No 6, May–June 1982. Baltimore: Johns Hopkins University.

32. Tri-Norinyl and Ortho-Novum 7/7/7—two triphasic oral contraceptives. *Medical Letter on Drugs and Therapeutics* 26:93–94, 1984.

33. Vessey MP, Lawless M, Yeates D, et al: Progestogen-only oral contraception. Findings in a large prospective study with special reference to effectiveness. *British Journal of Family Planning* 10:117–121, 1985.

34. Holma P: Long-term experience with Norplant contraceptive implants in Finland. *Contraception* 31:231–241, 1985.

35. Brache V, Faundes A, Johansson E, et al: Anovulation, inadequate luteal phase and poor sperm penetration in cervical mucus during prolonged use of Norplant implants. *Contraception* 31:261–273, 1985.

14

Intrauterine Devices (IUDs)

Worldwide the IUD has been, and still is, a very important birth control option. In the United States its popularity peaked in the 1970s when it was worn by as many as 2 to 3 million American women. Then problems with pelvic infection linked to IUD use were recognized and its popularity waned. Medical problems were followed by lawsuits against IUD manufacturers, and the possible financial impact of future legal cases led most IUD makers to stop sales of their products in the United States.

1975	*Dalkon Shield is withdrawn from sale by A.H. Robins Company because of severe pelvic infection*
1980	*A.H. Robins recommends that all remaining Dalkon Shields be removed from women still wearing them*
1983	*Schmid discontinues sales of its IUD, the Saf-T-Coil*
August, 1985	*A.H. Robins declares bankruptcy. Approximately 10,000 lawsuits settled by that date cost 480 million dollars.*
September, 1985	*Ortho Pharmaceuticals discontinues U.S. sales of its IUD, the Lippes Loop*
January, 1986	*Searle discontinues U.S. sales of its two IUDs, the Cu-7 (Copper-7) and Tatum T (Copper-T)*

So as of 1987, U.S. women had only one remaining IUD option, the Progestasert, and women still wearing IUDs are certain to have questions and concerns.

If You Have a Discontinued IUD

The legal and financial decisions by the IUD companies, obviously, do not alter your IUD risks one way or the other. Your risks are the same now as they would have been if the companies were still selling their devices. Your future options, however, may be affected and this may be a good time to reassess the pros and cons of the IUD for your own personal situation.

Making sure what kind of IUD you have may take some investigating. If you have a copper IUD or Progestasert, you should remember being told about a replacement date. Plain plastic IUDs such as the Lippes Loop and Saf-T-Coil do not have to be replaced. Your clinician may have a record of your IUD insertion or may be able to identify the type by the appearance of your IUD string(s). The Dalkon Shield string is particularly easy to recognize: it is the only IUD with a thick string, and the string has a knot.

COPPER-7 (Cu-7) AND COPPER-T (TATUM T)

If you have a copper IUD now, and want to continue wearing it, you have the option to do so. The company has not recommended removal, and there is no startling new research evidence to suggest that you should have it removed unless you develop problems or wish to change to another method or become pregnant.

The effectiveness of your IUD in preventing pregnancy depends on its copper, and as the copper is gradually released the IUD's effectiveness will decline. The FDA-approved instructions for copper IUDs set the time limit at three years. There is some research evidence to show that good effectiveness is maintained for as long as four years (1), but leaving your copper IUD in place for longer than three years means that you and your clinician are stepping outside the FDA (national Food and Drug Administration) guidelines.

When you have your copper IUD removed, you can change to another birth control method or you can have a Progestasert IUD inserted. The Progestasert has some advantage compared to copper IUDs. Its infection risk may be somewhat lower, and it is less likely to cause problems with menstrual cramps. The main disadvantage of the Progestasert is that it must be replaced once a year as its progesterone supply is used up.

LIPPES LOOP AND SAF-T-COIL

If you have a Lippes Loop or Saf-T-Coil, you can continue wearing it as long as you wish unless you develop problems. Manufacturers of these IUDs have not recommended removal, and their effectiveness does not deteriorate over time.

14:1   IUD DANGER SIGNS

P   Period late (possible pregnancy), abnormal spotting or bleeding
A   Abdominal pain, pain with intercourse
I   Infection exposure (such as gonorrhea or chlamydia), abnormal
      vaginal discharge
N   Not feeling well, fever, chills
S   String missing, shorter or longer

See your clinician right away if you develop a danger sign.

DALKON SHIELD

The Dalkon Shield has not been marketed since 1974, but there may be many thousands of women still using the device (some 2.8 million were inserted). Research shows that infection risk with the Dalkon Shield is significantly higher than the risk with other IUDs, and removal is strongly recommended by its manufacturer and by the FDA.

If you have a Dalkon Shield, ask your clinician to remove it without delay even if you feel perfectly well. If you don't know what kind of device you have, ask your clinician to examine you. A.H. Robins Company, manufacturer of the Dalkon Shield, will reimburse your clinician for the cost of examining you and removing an IUD, even if it turns out you didn't have a Dalkon Shield after all.

SHOULD YOUR IUD BE REMOVED?

If you have a plain plastic IUD such as the Lippes Loop or Saf-T-Coil, or a copper IUD that was inserted within the past three or four years, you may be wondering whether you should continue wearing it. This is a good time to reassess your own personal risk factors. If you are similar to the ideal IUD candidate described in the next section, your risks with the IUD are low. If your life exposes you to the infection risk factors listed in the contraindication section later in this chapter, you may be facing higher risks than you realize.

In the meantime, you also need to be aware of the danger signs of possible IUD problems shown in Illustration 14-1. These are the symptoms that can alert you to possible infection or pregnancy with an IUD. If you become pregnant with your IUD in place or develop symptoms of possible infection, you will need to see your clinician immediately. You will need treatment and your IUD will almost certainly need to be removed.

Deciding About an IUD

The intrauterine device (IUD) is wonderful for some women and disastrous for others. Risk of infection is the determining factor, because IUD-related infection can lead to illness, infertility, and, in rare instances, death. The IUD can be an excellent contraceptive choice for a woman who has finished her childbearing and whose risk of infection is extremely low. **The IUD should not be used by any woman who might want a future pregnancy, or has more than one sexual partner, or will have more than one partner during the time she is wearing her IUD.**

With the IUD, you yourself play the major role in determining how safe and effective the IUD is for you. Statistics on IUD-related infection in this chapter are for average women, and you may be able to minimize risks for yourself dramatically. From a risk and safety perspective, the ideal IUD user is a woman who:

• Has one permanent partner (who is himself strictly monogamous)
• Has no risk of exposure to sexually transmitted infections
• Has had one or more previous pregnancies
• Does not plan any future pregnancies
• Would be able to recognize accidental pregnancy early and consult her clinician promptly
• Is comfortable using foam, condoms, sponges, or a diaphragm during the first three months after IUD insertion and perhaps during her fertile days each cycle thereafter
• Has a clinician who is experienced with the IUD and who is readily available should any problem occur
• Is over age 25 to 30
• Does not have severe menstrual cramps or heavy periods

If you choose the IUD, remember that early danger signs of IUD-related infection can be subtle. If you have any problems at all, **medical evaluation must be your first priority.** Don't let other obligations delay you in seeing your clinician. Early treatment for IUD problems can prevent really serious complications.

The types of IUDs that have been commonly used in the United States are shown in Illustration 14-2. All are made of inert plastic that is infused with a small amount of barium to make the IUD visible in an x-ray. All the IUDs have nylon strings that trail out of the uterus through the cervix and into the vagina so that an IUD user can check to be sure that her device is in place.

HOW THE IUD WORKS

The presence of an IUD inside the uterus alters a number of factors necessary for pregnancy, but most experts believe that the primary birth control effect is the **uterine inflammatory response** its presence causes—the same kind of foreign body reaction

COMMON IUD's

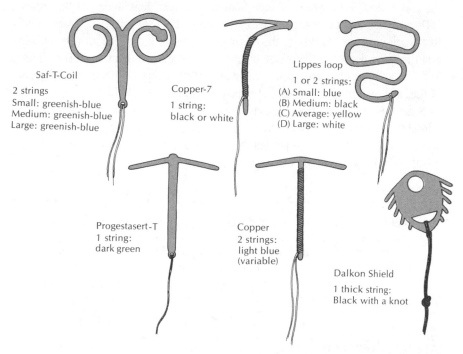

Saf-T-Coil

2 strings
Small: greenish-blue
Medium: greenish-blue
Large: greenish-blue

Copper-7

1 string:
black or white

Lippes loop

1 or 2 strings:
(A) Small: blue
(B) Medium: black
(C) Average: yellow
(D) Large: white

Progestasert-T
1 string:
dark green

Copper
2 strings:
light blue
(variable)

Dalkon Shield

1 thick string:
Black with a knot

ILLUSTRATION 14-2   IUDs used in the United States in recent years.

your body produces when you get a splinter in your finger, for example. Infection-fighting white blood cells and inflammatory cells (macrophages) gather in the lining of the uterus and disrupt the normal structure of the uterine lining with the result that implantation of a fertilized egg is unlikely to occur (1). The copper on the copper-bearing devices appears to enhance the inflammatory effect. The inflammatory response may also destroy sperm inside the uterus so the sperm never reach the egg at all.

Copper and progesterone IUDs provide a continuous release of copper or progesterone into the uterine cavity. These substances add to the contraceptive effects of the IUD because they are at least partially absorbed by the uterine lining cells. Copper may alter chemical processes within uterine lining cells and low-dose progesterone absorbed from a Progestasert causes thick cervical mucus and makes the uterine lining unsuitable for implantation of an embryo.

EFFECTIVENESS

IUDs are among the most effective methods of birth control. First-year failure rates as low as 0.5% have been documented for some IUD users, but are generally around 6%. Among women less than 22, about 9% of IUD users become pregnant in the first year of use (2).

Pregnancies are most common in the first few months after an IUD is inserted, and the effectiveness rate improves steadily from year to year. Effectiveness of the copper IUDs and the Progestasert depends partly on the effect of the copper or progesterone that is released from the IUD, so the effectiveness rates for these IUDs improve initially and then later decline as the release of copper or progesterone from the IUD declines. The FDA and manufacturers recommend replacement of copper IUDs after three years of use, and the Progestasert must be replaced once every 12 months.

Some pregnancies occur because a woman expels her IUD and isn't aware of it. Partial or complete expulsion can cause cramps or unusual bleeding that would alert you to check for your IUD strings, but expulsion can also occur with no symptoms at all. If your IUD is not inside your uterus, it cannot work.

After my IUD was inserted I had some cramps for the first day, but not a twinge after that. I was astounded when my clinician checked me two weeks later and told me it was coming out. I hadn't checked it my-self for a few days because I wasn't having sex . . . thank goodness.

—WOMAN, 22

ADVANTAGES OF THE IUD

The IUD is an extremely effective method of birth control. Using an IUD does not interrupt lovemaking and requires no extra equipment or supplies (except on the days you use a back-up method). There is nothing to remember except paying attention to danger signs and being diligent about your routine string check. The IUD provides continuous protection as long as it remains in place. The IUD does not affect your normal cyclic hormone patterns.

I decided to get an IUD after my second daughter was born. Bob and I really didn't think we wanted a third child, but neither of us felt ready for a permanent decision yet. I didn't want to use Pills again because I was close to 35; and we had tried the diaphragm before, but frankly, I just didn't like it. My doctor explained about infections with an IUD, but I felt that for me the risk would be small. Bob and I have an old-fashioned relationship; so there isn't much chance I am going to get chlamydia or anything, and we feel okay about using condoms once or twice a month when we have sex during my fertile days. Overall I have liked my IUD. I certainly don't worry about getting pregnant, and the only thing I really have had to get used to is long periods.

—WOMAN, 39

An IUD can help reestablish normal menstrual periods that have stopped because of uterine scar tissue (Asherman's syndrome). The IUD physically separates the two walls of your uterus so that uterine lining tissue can grow and develop normally. The Progestasert may actually diminish menstrual cramps and bleeding for some women.

DISADVANTAGES

Overall health risks with the IUD are low compared to other birth control options. Only vasectomy and barrier methods are safer. Health risks, especially the risk of serious pelvic infection, are nevertheless the IUD's main disadvantage. Pelvic infection is unlikely to be fatal but it can cause permanent damage and infertility, and can be a serious illness. Before you decide to have an IUD inserted, be sure to read about risks in the next section, and check the list of contraindications carefully. A contraindication is a medical factor that makes inadvisable or unsafe a treatment or procedure that might otherwise be recommended. If you have one or more contraindications, then using an IUD may be unwise.

Problems and Risks

Infection, pregnancy, ectopic pregnancy, and perforation are the most serious complications that can occur with an IUD. IUD complications are serious enough to require hospitalization for 1 out of every 100 to 300 IUD users each year. The rate of hospitalization for IUD-related problems is probably higher than the hospitalization rate for Pill-related problems, but the likelihood of death is lower. See Chapter 11 for a comparison of overall death risks for the common methods of birth control.

INFECTION

The presence of an IUD may cause an infection, may make an existing infection worse, or may interfere with your body's infection-fighting defenses and increase your susceptibility to pelvic infection. A woman who uses an IUD has a risk of pelvic infection that is significantly higher than the risk for a woman who uses another birth control method (3,4).

Risk of infection is higher among IUD users who have never been pregnant than among users who have delivered babies, and the risk **increases** with the number of sex partners the user has. Most researchers find that risk of infection is highest in the first few months of IUD use, suggesting that the IUD insertion procedure itself may contaminate the uterus with bacteria (5).

Recent studies have confirmed what has long been suspected: not only do IUD users have an increased risk for pelvic inflammatory disease (PID), they also have an

TABLE 14-1
RISK OF INFERTILITY BY TYPE OF IUD AMONG
NEVER-PREGNANT WOMEN

TYPE OF IUD	RELATIVE RISK OF TUBAL INFERTILITY IN COMPARISON TO NON IUD USERS (NON IUD USERS RISK = 1.0)	
	CRAMER, ET AL	DALING, ET AL
Dalkon Shield	3.3	6.8
Lippes Loop, Saf-T-Coil	2.9	3.2
Copper-bearing IUD	1.6	1.9

SOURCES: Cramer DW, Schiff I, Schoenbaum SC, et al: Tubal infertility and the intrauterine device. *New England Journal of Medicine* 312:941–947, 1985.
Daling JR, Weiss NS, Metch BJ, et al: Primary tubal infertility in relation to the use of an intra-uterine device. *New England Journal of Medicine* 312:937–941, 1985.

increased risk of infertility from infection-damaged fallopian tubes (6,7). An important finding of these studies is that the type of IUD influences the risk of infection and infection-related infertility. The Dalkon Shield IUD poses the highest risk, plain plastic IUDs pose an intermediate risk, and copper-bearing IUDs pose the lowest risk. Unfortunately, the number of Progestasert users in these studies was too small to provide a risk comparison for the progesterone IUD. Table 14-1 summarizes these infection findings.

Many IUD-related infections are diagnosed and treated at an early stage when they are not life-threatening and can be cured with antibiotic pills and rest at home. Infection can be severe, however, and can have a serious impact on a woman's health and future fertility. (Read Chapter 25 for a full description of pelvic infection treatment and consequences.) Severe infection can spread to the entire abdomen (peritonitis), or to the liver and cause liver damage and jaundice. You may need surgery to drain an abscess or even to remove your uterus, tubes, and ovaries. Spread of infectious bacteria through the bloodstream can even be fatal.

Obviously, it is important to see your clinician immediately if you have any of the IUD danger signs shown in Illustration 14-1. Starting treatment for infection promptly is essential.

If you have an infection, your clinician will almost certainly recommend that your IUD be removed—especially if you plan to become pregnant in the future—for the presence of the IUD may hinder the healing process. If you are not concerned about future pregnancy, your infection is mild, and you want to keep your IUD, your clinician may believe that it is safe to leave your IUD in place, begin treatment with antibiotics, and evaluate your progress after 24 to 36 hours. If your infection is improving satisfactorily, you may be able to keep your IUD. If your infection isn't improving after 24 to 36 hours, your clinician will definitely remove your IUD, and you may need to be hospitalized for intensive antibiotic treatment.

Treatment for IUD-related infection includes antibiotics, bed rest, and tests to determine, if possible, what kind of bacteria is causing your infection. Chlamydia and gonorrhea organisms are a frequent cause of IUD-related infection, but other kinds of bacteria can cause infection as well. Do not assume that pain, bleeding, or discharge in the days or weeks following insertion (or reinsertion) is normal. See your clinician promptly.

Infection During Pregnancy. **The combination of infection and pregnancy is potentially fatal for an IUD user.** The likelihood that you will become pregnant with your IUD in place is small, about 5% per year; but when pregnancy does occur and infection follows, the presence of an IUD can result in an extremely serious, life-threatening illness. You are more likely to have a miscarriage (spontaneous abortion) with an IUD than you would ordinarily be, and a uterus that contains remnants of a miscarried pregnancy is a perfect growth site for bacteria. As a result, **a massive infection can develop in a very short period of time.** You might feel entirely well one morning and have an infection so severe that you are gravely ill 12 hours later.

Your symptoms may be subtle as infection begins. You may suspect that you have flu because of headache, muscle aches, chills, and fever. Even your clinician may fail to recognize that you have an IUD-related infection. If you have an IUD and you ever have any signs of early pregnancy such as a menstrual period that is late, too short, or too light, breast tenderness, nausea, or fatigue, **be sure to let your clinician know that you think you could be pregnant.** If you have signs of early pregnancy combined with infection danger signs, **run, don't walk,** to your clinician.

If you are pregnant, your clinician will want to remove your IUD in order to decrease your infection risk. Your risk of death from infected spontaneous abortion is about 50 times higher if you have an IUD than it would be during a normal pregnancy (8).

Actinomycosis and IUDs. Pelvic infection with the bacterium *Actinomyces* occurs occasionally in long-term IUD users (9). Although this is a very uncommon organism, it can cause pelvic inflammatory disease, often acting in concert with other bacteria. The actinomyces organism occasionally appears on the IUD user's Pap smear even when no symptoms are present. In this case you and your clinician can decide together whether or not to remove your IUD and whether or not to treat the actinomyces infection with antibiotics. You will be guided by your future pregnancy plans, any previous history of pelvic infection, and your willingness and ability to use other kinds of birth control. The best approach for protecting your future fertility if you have *Actinomyces* on your Pap smear is to remove your IUD and take appropriate antibiotics.

PREGNANCY

Pregnancy itself can sometimes cause serious problems for an IUD user even without infection. If you become pregnant with an IUD in place, your likelihood of miscarriage (spontaneous abortion) is high. Miscarriage most often occurs during the first three months of pregnancy, but with an IUD in place late miscarriage can also occur even after six or more months of pregnancy. **About 50% of IUD pregnancies end in spontaneous abortion**, compared with about 15% of other pregnancies. The risk of miscarriage is slightly lower, about 30%, if your IUD is removed as soon as you are aware of the pregnancy (10).

A miscarriage very early in pregnancy may involve little more than an extra-heavy period with stronger than average cramps. Later in pregnancy, spontaneous abortion can cause prolonged, severe cramps and considerable bleeding. You need to see your clinician in either case. She/he will test your blood Rh type to determine whether you need Rh protection (see Chapter 18) and will examine you carefully to be certain that all the fetal and placental tissue has been expelled. Retained tissue or clots will increase your risk of infection, so if there is any question, your clinician will recommend a vacuum procedure (see Chapter 18) or a D&C (see Chapter 47) to be sure that your uterus is empty.

If you are pregnant but have no evidence of infection or miscarriage, you will want to consider several factors as you decide whether to continue the pregnancy or to have an abortion. Unless you are absolutely certain that you will have an abortion, your clinician will try to remove your IUD when she/he first confirms that you are pregnant.

If you are certain that you will have an abortion, your IUD can be removed during your abortion procedure. Remember that abortion is safest when done early in pregnancy, so decide what you want to do as quickly as you can.

Removing the IUD decreases your risk of infection and miscarriage if you continue the pregnancy. It may be impossible, however, for your clinician to remove your IUD without disturbing the pregnancy if your IUD strings have drawn up inside your enlarging uterus. If the IUD cannot be removed, your risk of serious infection is high enough that your clinician will probably advise that you at least consider abortion.

Many women have delivered babies with an IUD in place. With plain plastic IUDs or with copper IUDs there is no documented increase in fetal deformities (11). Whether or not fetal exposure to progesterone from a Progestasert can cause adverse effects is not known.

ECTOPIC PREGNANCY

An ectopic pregnancy is a pregnancy that develops anywhere outside the uterus. Ectopic pregnancy most often develops in one of the fallopian tubes. It is an extremely dangerous problem because growth of the pregnancy can cause the tube to rupture, and massive internal bleeding or even death can result. An IUD user who becomes

14:3   EARLY PREGNANCY DANGER SIGNS

Possible Ectopic Pregnancy

Sudden intense pain, or persistent pain, or cramping in the lower abdomen, usually localized to one side or the other

Irregular bleeding or spotting with abdominal pain when your period is late or after an abnormally light period

Fainting or dizziness that persists more than a few seconds. These may be signs of internal bleeding. You will not necessarily have bleeding from your vagina if you have internal bleeding.

Possible Miscarriage

Your last period was late, and bleeding is now heavy, possibly with clots or clumps of tissue; cramping is more severe than usual

Your period is prolonged and heavy—5 to 7 days of "heaviest" days

You have abdominal pain and fever

Contact your clinician immediately or go to a hospital emergency room if you develop any of these signs.

pregnant is more likely to have an ectopic pregnancy than is a woman who becomes pregnant using foam, condoms, a sponge, Pills, or a diaphragm. Ectopic pregnancies account for about 1 out of every 5 pregnancies that occur with a Progestasert in place; with the plain plastic IUDs the proportion is lower: 1 out of 20; with the copper IUDs the proportion is 1 out of 60 (12). The percentage of ectopic pregnancies is higher for IUD users because the IUD protects against uterine pregnancy more effectively than it protects against ectopic pregnancy. Researchers estimate that about one or two ectopic pregnancies occur among every 1,000 IUD users each year (13).

Read Chapter 8 for a description of ectopic pregnancy, and watch for the danger signs shown in Illustration 14-3. If you have an IUD in place and these signs occur, **see your clinician immediately or go to an emergency room.** Be sure to explain that you think you might be pregnant and that you have an IUD.

PERFORATION OF THE UTERUS

The muscle wall of the uterus is about 1/2 inch thick, and it is possible for an IUD to puncture (perforate) the uterine wall partially or completely. This rare complication is most likely to occur during IUD insertion and is probably more likely if your clinician is not experienced with IUD insertion techniques. Reported rates for perforation vary from less than 1 to about 9 in 1,000 IUD users (11). Perforation may not be immediately apparent. You might not find out about perforation until several days or weeks later when your IUD strings disappear and your clinician discovers that your IUD is not inside your uterus as she/he attempts to retrieve the strings. If you do not routinely check for your strings, pregnancy may be what tips you off to perforation; an IUD cannot work if it isn't in your uterus. Perforation rates also may be increased for women who are breastfeeding at the time of insertion.

Spontaneous puncture or gradual migration of an IUD through the uterine wall long after insertion is uncommon but has been documented. Muscular contractions of the uterus may also push the IUD through the wall of the cervix itself. Partial perforation or embedding of an IUD within the muscle wall of the uterus also occasionally occurs.

Perforation may cause pain when it occurs, but unless infection develops or the IUD entangles a loop of intestines, you are apt to have few symptoms. The all-plastic IUDs may not cause any problems even if they stay inside your abdomen. However, the presence of an IUD in your abdomen, especially a copper device, can cause an inflammation response and can trigger scar tissue formation. **Most clinicians recommend that any lost IUD be removed.**

Removal of an IUD that has perforated the uterus is done in a hospital or surgical center, and will require general anesthesia. The clinician may be able to use a laparoscope, a lighted tube inserted through a 1-inch incision below your navel, or you may need a full 5-inch incision across your lower abdomen.

SPONTANEOUS EXPULSION

Between 5% and 20% of IUD users spontaneously expel the device within the first year of IUD use (11). The likelihood of expulsion is higher for women who have never been pregnant, women who have a relatively small uterus, and women who are using small IUDs. Clinician skill may also be a factor. Expulsion may cause cramping and bleeding, or it may be completely painless. You can expel your IUD without even knowing it; it could fall into the toilet and get flushed away unnoticed, for example. Expulsion is most likely to occur during a menstrual period within the first few weeks after insertion but can also occur after months or years of problem-free IUD use. Signs that would alert you to the possibility of expulsion are:

- Unusual vaginal discharge
- Bleeding or spotting
- Cramps or abdominal pain
- Your IUD strings seem longer. (The Copper-7 IUD was packaged with a loop of string bending upward so the string may seem to get longer simply because this loop of string inside the uterus straightens itself out. In this case, a longer string does not necessarily mean you are having a spontaneous expulsion.)
- Your IUD strings disappear
- You feel the IUD itself protruding from your cervix
- Your partner feels the IUD with his finger or during intercourse
- Your menstrual period is overdue, or other symptoms indicate pregnancy

If you expel an IUD, your clinician will probably be willing to insert another IUD if you want her/him to do so. Some clinicians prefer to wait a month before inserting another IUD. If you expel an IUD more than once, it may mean that your uterus does not tolerate the IUD for some reason; your uterine cavity may have an abnormal shape, for example.

INCREASED BLEEDING AND CRAMPING

You are likely to notice at least some change in your menstrual periods after you get an IUD. Many women find that the total amount of menstrual blood loss increases and also that the number of days of bleeding increases. You might have light bleeding or spotting for a day or two before your period begins in earnest, and then spotting for several additional days at the end of a regular period. Menstrual problems tend to improve with time; so it may be worthwhile to see how your second and third periods go before you decide whether to have your IUD removed. Read Chapter 31 for a discussion of medications that are effective for menstrual pain. Unlike other IUD types, the Progestasert may reduce cramping during menstrual periods because of the effect of progesterone hormone on the uterine lining.

It may be hard for you to distinguish between abnormal bleeding and cramps due to infection and those due simply to a typically heavy menstrual period. Menstrual cramps are almost always intermittent, with episodes of real pain lasting only a few hours, then subsiding, and possibly returning again. **If you have cramps or pain that is continuous and persists for longer than 12 to 24 hours, think seriously about the possibility of infection.** Remember that infection is most likely to develop within the first few weeks of IUD use and that it often begins with menstrual bleeding or causes abnormal bleeding. If your pain is severe or persistent or if you have other symptoms of infection, see your clinician promptly.

Overall blood loss because of heavy menstrual periods is usually not a serious medical problem unless you are anemic in the first place or your nutritional iron intake is inadequate. Some clinicians recommend iron supplements for IUD users, such as nonprescription ferrous sulfate tablets once or twice a day. Your clinician can check your blood count to determine whether you are anemic if there is any doubt.

It is common for IUD users to have bleeding or spotting between periods. You may notice spotting especially around the time of ovulation, or you may have some spotting throughout your cycle. Be sure to discuss this problem with your clinician, for you may need further evaluation to be sure that the bleeding is not caused by infection, tumor, or another serious problem. Your clinician may also recommend that you try vitamin C for spotting. One study showed significant improvement in heavy spotting after treatment with 200 mg of vitamin C (ascorbic acid) three times a day (14).

An episode of sudden, heavy bleeding is a problem some IUD users encounter. The IUD may rub against the uterine wall, erode a spot, and trigger sudden, massive bleeding. Your clinician will probably remove the IUD, and you will probably find that the bleeding stops promptly.

Cramps, pain, and backache are common during the first 24 hours after IUD insertion. Pain that is severe, that is not relieved by aspirin, or that persists longer than 24 hours merits a call to your clinician.

Many IUD users notice cramps or pelvic pain whenever uterine contractions are stimulated, such as during intercourse, during orgasm, or during breastfeeding. Backache, leg pain, and soreness can also be associated with contraction cramps. You may also find that ovulation pain is more noticeable after you get an IUD. Remember that pain can be a sign of serious problems. See your clinician promptly if you have any questions.

VAGINITIS AND CERVICITIS

Vaginitis, infection on the surface of the cervix, and infection in the cervical canal are more frequent among IUD users than among women who use other birth control methods. Persistent discharge with a strong fishy odor occurs in up to 20% of IUD users (15). The presence of the IUD string inside the cervical canal may cause irritation and predispose the user to infection in some way, or may decrease the cervix's normal resistance to bacterial invasion. The organisms responsible for bacterial vaginosis seem to be present in most cases, so read Chapter 23 for a full description of the symptoms, diagnosis, and treatment of this condition. Treatment with oral antibiotics is usually effective. It is common for this problem to recur. Remember that abnormal discharge can also mean **serious uterine infection**. An examination is essential to determine what treatment you need and whether it is safe to leave your IUD in place. **You and your clinician will want to take discharge very seriously. You must assume that it is pelvic inflammatory disease until you can prove otherwise.**

INSERTION AND REMOVAL PROBLEMS

Some women become quite weak and faint immediately after IUD insertion. Stimulation of nerves in your cervix during insertion can trigger a drop in blood pressure and marked slowing of your heart rate so that you feel dizzy, faint, nauseated, and extremely weak. Convulsions or even heart arrest is possible. Most reactions are fairly mild and subside spontaneously within 15 to 30 minutes. If you do have a severe reaction, your clinician may try using a local anesthetic or another drug called atropine after insertion to stop the reaction, or she/he may recommend that your IUD be removed immediately. Symptoms are likely to subside promptly once your IUD is removed.

IUD removal is usually quick, uncomplicated, and less painful than insertion, but in some cases removal is difficult. If your IUD strings are not visible, if the IUD has become embedded, if it has been in your uterus for several years, if the IUD strings break off, or if the IUD has become fragmented, then removal may be tricky. Your clinician may need to use special grasping instruments to retrieve the IUD and may need to dilate your cervical opening slightly to make removal easier. Occasionally, removal requires local anesthesia or even general anesthesia in a hospital or surgery center.

STRING DISAPPEARANCE

IUD strings can spontaneously draw up inside your cervix or uterus, and when this happens, you have no way to be sure that your IUD is in its proper position. This problem has been especially common for the Copper-7 device; the Copper-7 string bends upward when it is stored in its inserter, and the string seems to retain an upward-bend tendency even after it is in the uterus. Your clinician will first try to retrieve your strings with a narrow clamp or special IUD thread retriever. If this is not successful, she/he may have to remove the IUD entirely. A new IUD can be inserted immediately if you wish, but some clinicians recommend waiting one month before inserting a new device to minimize infection risk.

ALLERGIC REACTIONS

Allergy to copper is rare, but if you are allergic to copper, you may develop a skin rash or other allergic reaction with a copper IUD. The potential for allergic reaction also exists with the Progestasert IUD. Women who have Wilson's disease, a very rare condition that causes abnormal retention of copper in body tissues, may react adversely to a copper IUD. The actual amount of copper released by the copper IUDs is very small, however: about 1/30 of the normal adult requirement for copper in the daily diet (11).

OTHER PROBLEMS

Partners of IUD users occasionally report discomfort during intercourse or irritation of the penis after intercourse. Check to be sure your IUD has not been completely or partially expelled. Most often, penile irritation is caused by a short, bristly IUD string protruding from the cervix: thrusting during intercourse pushes the penis against the end of the string. Trimming the string so that none of it protrudes at all into the vagina may help, but it also precludes periodic string checks. Occasionally, penile irritation is caused by a knot in the string or by a clump of hair or tampon fibers adhering to the string. You may be able to reposition the end of your string so that the string tip is pointing toward the back of your vagina, or your clinician may be able to help you with these problems by searing the tip of the string with cautery so that a smooth ball forms on the tip.

Many women and their clinicians have expressed concern that the mechanical irritation and the uterine inflammatory response that the IUD causes might increase the risk of uterine or cervical cancer. Exposure of the uterus to copper or progesterone in the medicated IUDs raises similar concerns. So far, there is no evidence that IUD use increases your risk for any type of cancer. It is possible that a cancer association might not become apparent until many years after IUD exposure, but after 25 years of evaluation there are no worrisome research findings.

CONTRAINDICATIONS

A woman who is **pregnant** or has **active pelvic infection** must not have an IUD inserted under any circumstances. Active pelvic infection involving your tubes (salpingitis) or uterus (endometritis) can become much worse if you have an IUD inserted. If you have **chlamydia, gonorrhea, or any other sexually transmitted disease**, or even suspect that you **may have been exposed** to any sexually transmitted disease, have an exam and testing before you decide about an IUD. IUD insertion during pregnancy can lead to miscarriage or to the very dangerous problem of infection in pregnancy.

Many clinicians believe that **your future fertility should be a primary consideration as you evaluate the pros and cons of IUDs.** If you intend to become pregnant in the future, you need to consider infection risk very carefully. A contraindication is a medical condition that renders inadvisable or unsafe a treatment or procedure that might otherwise be recommended. If you have one or more of the following contraindications, your clinician will advise you not to use an IUD. You may be vulnerable to serious health or fertility risks.

- Pregnancy or suspected pregnancy
- An ectopic (tubal) pregnancy in the past
- One or more episodes of pelvic infection in the past
- One or more sexually transmitted infections in the past including gonorrhea, syphilis, or chlamydia
- Previous pelvic surgery
- One or more episodes of infection after pregnancy or abortion in the past
- Abnormal uterus size or shape
- Uterine cancer or cervical cancer, known or suspected
- Abnormal Pap smear results not yet resolved
- Abnormal vaginal bleeding that has not been definitely diagnosed
- Multiple sex partners
- Desire for future pregnancy
- Active cervical infection (cervicitis). Infection should be treated before an IUD is inserted.

Many additional factors may affect your potential success with an IUD. Some of the factors listed below affect infection risk, and the significance of infection, and some relate to other less common problem situations. Despite some of the following conditions you may be able to use the IUD if you are willing to be **followed very carefully** by your clinician so that she/he can watch for early signs of trouble. Other conditions mean that your clinician may not be able to insert an IUD at all.

• Diabetes or other diseases or medications that result in lowered resistance to infection, such as cortisone therapy for asthma or arthritis
• Abnormal blood clotting due to blood-thinning (anticoagulant) drugs or blood disorders. Diminished clotting may cause very heavy bleeding with an IUD.
• Lack of access to emergency care. Immediate attention from a clinician who could remove your IUD and initiate proper treatment for infection could save your life or your future fertility if you develop a serious complication.
• Abnormal thickening of uterine lining (endometrial hyperplasia)
• Rheumatic heart disease or other heart valve abnormalities. An IUD-related infection could spread through your bloodstream to the heart valves and could be potentially catastrophic.
• Copper intolerance (Wilson's disease) or copper allergy. You should not wear a copper IUD.
• Previous problems with IUD expulsion
• Severe menstrual problems, such as heavy bleeding or severe cramps during natural cycles or when you had an IUD in the past
• Severe anemia
• Active vaginal infection or abnormal vaginal discharge. You may have an increased infection risk.
• Abnormal vaginal bleeding, spotting, or bleeding between periods. Bleeding from any cause may be aggravated by an IUD.
• Recent pregnancy (abortion, miscarriage, or full term delivery). Infection risk may be increased.
• Frequent fainting attacks. You may be more likely to have a severe reaction to IUD insertion.
• Fibroid tumors, polyps, or endometriosis. An IUD may aggravate bleeding problems that can occur with these conditions.
• Inability to check for IUD strings or to recognize danger signs

MINIMIZING YOUR RISKS OF IUD COMPLICATIONS

Serious IUD infections sometimes develop gradually and have warning signs that you will notice if you are alert. Prompt treatment can often make the difference between a fairly simple problem and a serious problem.

The following are suggestions for using the IUD as safely as possible based on what is known about IUDs so far. Don't be surprised if your clinician doesn't mention these suggestions to you: **these are not routine instructions**. You may or may not decide to pay attention to all these recommendations; you can use them to help you keep your IUD risks at a minimum.

- Do everything you can to avoid exposure to chlamydia, gonorrhea, or any sexually transmitted disease. If you can't talk to your partner about your concerns, leave quietly by the back door or do anything you have to. Avoid intercourse if your partner has a discharge from his penis, and pay attention to your intuitions. See Chapters 22 through 29 for more information on infections.
- Memorize the IUD danger signs, and get treatment immediately, even if your symptoms are not severe (see Illustration 14-1)
- Rely on condoms routinely for the first few months with a new sexual partner, or any time you (or your partner) have more than one partner, or if you ever suspect that your partner has an infection
- Use foam, condoms, a sponge, or a diaphragm for the first three months you have your IUD and during your fertile days in the middle of each cycle (see Chapter 6 for information on determining your fertile days). Using a back-up method along with your IUD means that your chance of pregnancy is extremely low. Infection complications during pregnancy with an IUD in place are responsible for most of the IUD-related deaths, and if you avoid pregnancy by using a back-up method during your fertile days, you can reduce this risk to almost zero.
- Consider delaying IUD insertion if you have recently been pregnant. After abortion or miscarriage, wait two weeks. After full term delivery, wait 8 to 12 weeks. After cesarean section delivery, wait 12 weeks. Use another method of birth control in the meantime.
- Consider waiting one month after your IUD is removed before you have a new one inserted
- If you move, find a new clinician immediately so that you can minimize any delay in getting care if you develop a danger sign
- Check your strings regularly. Frequent string checks may help you to prevent pregnancy that can occur if your IUD is partially or completely expelled.
- Be sure that you know what kind of IUD you have. If you have a copper or progesterone IUD, know when you will need to have it removed and make your appointment on schedule.
- Choose a clinician who is experienced with IUDs. Some clinicians do not insert IUDs very frequently and do not have extensive experience with recognizing and treating IUD problems.

Getting an IUD

If you want to use an IUD, you will need to see your clinician or go to a family planning clinic. Your clinician will review your medical history for any factors that might increase the risks of an IUD for you, and perform a routine physical examination and Pap test. Make sure that you are examined and tested for sexually transmitted infections. Some clinicians strongly recommend that the IUD insertion itself be delayed at least a few days after your exam so that your clinician will know the results of your tests beforehand.

PREPARING FOR INSERTION

An IUD can be inserted safely at any time early in your menstrual cycle before implantation of a new pregnancy could have occurred. For a woman whose normal cycle is 28 days long, this means any time during the first 16 to 20 days, counting the first day of a normal period as day 1. This policy protects you from IUD insertion during early pregnancy. Some clinicians prefer to schedule insertion during menstrual bleeding to be certain you are not pregnant. A careful study of 9,000 copper IUD insertions found, however, that insertions later in the cycle (after day 11) were somewhat preferable. In the study, medical problems after insertion were similar enough throughout the cycle that the authors concluded there was no reason to place strict limits on the timing of insertion (16).

Arrange for someone to accompany you to the office or clinic when you go for your IUD insertion. If you feel queasy, shaky, or weak after the insertion, you will be glad you don't have to travel home alone.

I've been using my Loop for two years now. I haven't had any real problems, but it sure hurt the first 24 hours. I stayed home from work and took aspirin and a good stiff drink. Every woman getting an IUD should have a friend come along with her to the doctor's office. Driving home was miserable, and I would love to have had my husband do that for me.

—WOMAN, 26

Many clinicians recommend that their patients take aspirin or ibuprofen (Motrin, Advil, or Nuprin) about an hour before insertion. These medications block release of prostaglandin hormone and may decrease uterine contractions and cramps after insertion.

INSERTION

IUD insertion usually takes about five minutes. Most women say that insertion does hurt, but that the pain isn't unbearable. Some women have no pain at all. If you have frequent fainting spells or vagal episodes, be sure to alert your clinician before IUD insertion begins.

After a pelvic exam to confirm the position of your uterus, your clinician will place a speculum in your vagina and wash your cervix with disinfectant. You will probably have fairly intense but brief cramps when your clinician grasps your cervix with a clamp (tenaculum) to hold it steady during insertion, and more cramping as she/he

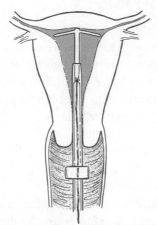

ILLUSTRATION 14-4   IUD insertion usually takes less than five minutes.

inserts a blunt rod through your cervical canal all the way to the top of your uterus to measure your uterine depth. An accurate measurement is important because the size of your uterus may affect the success of an IUD for you. If your uterus is quite small, with a depth of less than 2 3/4 inches (7 cm), your likelihood of spontaneous expulsion will be higher than average. If your uterus is less than 2 1/4 inches deep (6 cm), you may not be able to use an IUD.

Next your clinician will gently push the IUD inserter through the cervical canal into your uterus. The IUD inserter is a hollow plastic tube with the IUD folded inside. The IUD is released once the inserter is inside your uterus (see Illustration 14-4). It is common to have cramping as the IUD is released, because the procedure stimulates uterine contractions; contractions may continue off and on for the first 12 to 24 hours after the insertion. Adverse reactions to IUD insertion (see the "Problems and Risks" section) do occasionally occur and may cause faintness, nausea, vomiting, weakness, and a cold, clammy sensation.

Some clinicians use local anesthesia to decrease discomfort during the insertion. Injection of the local anesthetic into your cervix is unlikely to cause much discomfort, and you may not even be able to tell when it is being done. Some women do find the anesthetic injection fairly painful, however.

AFTER INSERTION

You may have cramps and/or bleeding for several days, or even several weeks, after IUD insertion. Be sure to read the "Problems and Risks" section to assess whether your cramps might be caused by infection. If you have any doubt about your cramps, pain, or bleeding symptoms, don't hesitate to call your clinician. Do not assume pain, bleeding, or discharge is normal.

Your risk for IUD infection is highest in the first few weeks after insertion. **You can minimize infection** risk if you:

• Avoid intercourse for the first two to four weeks
• Use condoms for the first three months
• Be alert for infection signs such as persistent cramps or pelvic pain, pain during intercourse, abnormal vaginal discharge, general aches and pains, fever, or chills
• Have a follow-up examination two to four weeks after insertion so that your clinician can check for uterine tenderness that might indicate infection. She/he will also check for partial or complete IUD expulsion.

You can expect your next period at about its regular time, or perhaps a few days early. You will probably find that your first IUD period is heavier and longer than average. Your periods may return to normal after a couple of cycles, or you may have heavy periods the entire time you have your IUD.

Contraceptive protection with the IUD begins immediately after insertion, but most clinicians recommend that you use a back-up method for the first three months when expulsion is most likely to occur. You do not need to worry about dislodging your IUD during intercourse or when you use tampons, even immediately after insertion. Be sure that you don't pull on your IUD string as you remove a tampon.

CHECKING YOUR IUD STRINGS

Your IUD can fall out unnoticed (hard as that is to believe after what insertion feels like); so check regularly for your strings. Insert one or two fingers into your vagina and locate your cervix. It will feel round, smooth, and firm, like the tip of your nose. Your IUD strings will feel like nylon fishing line extending from your cervix about 2 inches or so. Press your fingertip against the opening in the middle of your cervix to be sure that you don't feel any firm plastic in the opening. Your cervical opening should feel like a dimple or indentation at the center of your cervix.

If you have difficulty locating your strings or your cervix, you can use two fingers (index and third finger) in your vagina to reach deeper inside. Move your finger in a circular motion around the top of your cervix several times. The IUD string is thin and may not be obvious until you feel your finger pass over it as it curves out of your cervical canal over the rim of your cervix. It is sometimes helpful to change your position as you check for IUD strings. Try squatting down, then bear down with your abdominal muscles (just as you would for a bowel movement) to bring your cervix closer to your vaginal opening; or try lying on your back with your knees bent. You can also ask your partner to check for you.

Check for your strings before intercourse, after a menstrual period, and any time you have abdominal pain or cramps.

Instructions for IUD Users

Reread the section "Minimizing Your Risks of IUD Complications" to assess which suggestions make sense for you and your particular lifestyle. There is very little that you will have to do to use your IUD, but **there is a great deal you can do to use it as safely as possible.** Instructions that are essential for safe IUD use are:

- Be sure that you know what kind of IUD you have. If it is a medicated IUD, you will be responsible for arranging to replace it at the proper time. The Copper-7 and Copper-T should be replaced after three or four years; and the Progestasert must be replaced after one year.
- Check your strings regularly. Many women routinely check for their IUD strings beforehand each time they have intercourse. At a minimum, you need to check your IUD strings once a week for the first three months and then at least once a month after each menstrual period and after any episode of bleeding or cramping. If you cannot feel your strings, if you do feel firm plastic, or the string length seems to be changing, or if you have any questions about proper placement, see your clinician as soon as you can and rely on foam, condoms, a sponge, or a diaphragm until she/he can examine you.
- Use a back-up method for the first three months you have your IUD
- If you have any IUD danger signs, see your clinician immediately. Watch for prolonged or abnormal vaginal bleeding, pain, discharge, or signs of pregnancy.
- If you become pregnant while you have your IUD, have it removed as soon as possible, preferably before seven weeks of pregnancy
- See your clinician for regular checkups once every 12 months, or more often if you are having any problems
- Do not try to remove your IUD yourself, and do not let your partner try. See your clinician to have your IUD removed because she/he is able to see what she/he is doing and will be able to deal effectively with any removal problems that might occur.

HAVING YOUR IUD REMOVED

It is possible for your clinician to remove your IUD at any time, but many clinicians prefer to schedule IUD removal during the first ten days or so of your cycle. If your IUD is to be removed during the middle of your cycle, avoid intercourse or use a back-up method for at least seven days before removal. **Removing the IUD after conception but before implantation could lead to pregnancy.** Some clinicians believe that removal is easiest during menstrual bleeding.

Your clinician will first examine you to determine the position of your uterus and cervix and the angle of your cervical canal. Next a speculum will be placed in your vagina so that she/he can see your cervix and IUD string. Your clinician will grasp the string with a clamp and remove the IUD by pulling on it with steady, gentle traction.

You will probably have brief cramps as the IUD travels through the cervical canal, but removal is usually faster and less painful than insertion.

If your IUD is difficult to remove, your clinician may use local anesthesia to block pain nerves in your cervix. She/he can then widen your cervical canal slightly or use other instruments to make removal easier. See the "Problems and Risks" section for further discussion of difficulties with removal.

PLANNING PREGNANCY AFTER AN IUD

The birth control effect of your IUD stops as soon as it is removed. For optimal pregnancy planning, however, it makes sense to use condoms, foam, sponges, or a diaphragm for one to three months after your IUD is removed to allow some time for your uterine lining to return to normal.

REFERENCES

1. Wilcox AJ, Weinberg CR, Armstrong EG, et al: Urinary human chorionic gonadotropin among intrauterine device users: Detection with a highly specific and sensitive assay. *Fertility and Sterility* 47:265–269, 1987.
2. Ory HW, Forrest JD, Lincoln R: *Making Choices: Evaluating the Health Risks and Benefits of Birth Control Methods.* New York: Alan Guttmacher Institute, 1983.
3. Lee NC, Rubin GL, Ory HW, et al: Type of intrauterine device and the risk of pelvic inflammatory disease. *Obstetrics and Gynecology* 62:1–6, 1983.
4. Kaufman DW, Watson J, Rosenberg L, et al: The effect of different types of intrauterine devices on the risk of pelvic inflammatory disease. *Journal of the American Medical Association* 250:759–762, 1983.
5. Mishell DR Jr: Current status of intrauterine devices. *New England Journal of Medicine* 312:984–985, 1985.
6. Daling JR, Weiss NS, Metch BJ, et al: Primary tubal infertility in relation to the use of an intrauterine device. *New England Journal of Medicine* 312:937–941, 1985.
7. Cramer DW, Schiff I, Schoenbaum SC, et al: Tubal infertility and the intrauterine device. *New England Journal of Medicine* 312:941–947, 1985.
8. Cates W Jr, Ory HW, Rochat R, et al: The intrauterine device and deaths from spontaneous abortion. *New England Journal of Medicine* 295:1155–1159, 1976.
9. Yoonessi M, Crickard K, Cellino IS, et al: Association of *Actinomyces* and intrauterine contraceptive devices. *Journal of Reproductive Medicine* 30:48–52, 1985.
10. Lewit S: Outcome of pregnancy with intrauterine devices. *Contraception* 2:47–57, 1970.
11. Huber SC: IUDs reassessed—a decade of experience. *Population Reports,* Ser B, No 2, January 1975. Washington D.C.: George Washington University Medical Center.
12. Food and Drug Administration: The Progestasert IUD and ectopic pregnancy. *FDA Drug Bulletin* 8:6, December 1978–January 1979.
13. Vessey MP, Yeates D, Flavel R: Risk of ectopic pregnancy and duration of use of an intrauterine device. *Lancet* 2:501–502, 1979.

14. Margolis AJ, Jones GF, Doyle LL: Control of intermenstrual bleeding after IUCD insertion. *Excerpta Medica*, International Congress Ser No 86. Proceedings of the Second International Conference on Intrauterine Contraception, New York, October 1964.
15. Kivijarvi A, Jarvinen H, Gronroos M: Microbiology of vaginitis associated with the intrauterine contraceptive device. *British Journal of Obstetrics and Gynecology* 91:917–923, 1984.
16. White MK, Ory HW, Rooks JB, et al: Intrauterine device termination rates and the menstrual cycle day of insertion. *Obstetrics and Gynecology* 55:220–224, 1980.

15

Morning-After Birth Control

"Morning-after" emergencies happen to almost everyone, and it is natural to have a heart-sinking, panicky feeling the next morning when you think about the possibility of unwanted pregnancy. You may have had intercourse when you didn't expect to, or your diaphragm moved out of position, or a condom broke. It's amazing how many things can go wrong.

If you know within the first few minutes after intercourse that you are unprotected, **try to repair the damage.** Use a full applicator of birth control foam, cream, or jelly immediately if a condom breaks or if your diaphragm seems out of position. If you don't have any foam or spermicidal cream or jelly close at hand, douche at once with warm water and vinegar, 2 tablespoons of vinegar per quart of water.

Next, try to relax a little. The chance of pregnancy after intercourse just once without birth control is not as great as you might think. The likelihood of pregnancy depends on your age, your fertility and that of your partner, and where you are in your cycle. The chance of pregnancy may be as little as 2% if you have intercourse without birth control only once during a cycle, and is probably no more than 30% even if you have intercourse without birth control during your most fertile 24 hours (1).

You can choose from three basic approaches to an emergency birth control situation:

1. Wait and see whether you have conceived. Have a pregnancy test and decide between abortion and continuing the pregnancy if you are pregnant.
2. Take morning-after hormone treatment.
3. Have an IUD inserted.

If you are considering morning-after treatment with an IUD or hormones, you need to see your clinician within 48 hours if at all possible. Morning-after hormones should be started as soon as possible to be most effective, within 24 to 72 hours at most, and an IUD must be inserted within five to seven days.

Your clinician probably will not recommend any kind of morning-after treatment unless you had unprotected intercourse within a few days on either side of your estimated ovulation time. The likelihood of conception is quite small during the rest of your cycle. Use your menstrual period calendar to calculate your fertile days yourself by following the directions in Chapter 6.

Your clinician is also unlikely to recommend morning-after treatment if you had unprotected intercourse more than once; if you are already pregnant, morning-after treatment is not likely to be effective and could be dangerous for you or a developing fetus.

WAIT AND SEE

If you are really anxious, you can arrange for a highly sensitive blood pregnancy test in about ten days. If you are not so anxious, you can wait to see whether your next period arrives on time and is normal, and then arrange for a pregnancy test if your period is overdue. (Pregnancy tests are discussed in detail in Chapter 8.) In the meantime, try to decide whether you would continue the pregnancy or whether you would have an abortion. If abortion is your choice, make your arrangements promptly. Abortions are safest when they are performed early in pregnancy. (Abortion is covered in Chapters 16, 17, and 18.)

HORMONE TREATMENT

Hormone treatment alters the uterine lining so that it is unfavorable for implantation, and may temporarily interfere with hormone production by the ovary to induce a menstrual period earlier than it normally would occur (2).

Treatment with high-dose estrogen for five days after unprotected intercourse was the first effective morning-after hormone method developed. A variety of estrogen medications appear to be equally effective, including conjugated estrogens (Premarin) and ethinyl estradiol, but DES (diethylstilbestrol) is the only one for which official approval by the Food and Drug Administration has been requested (and granted). High-dose estrogen treatment of any kind is likely to cause nausea and vomiting, and DES use is an unattractive option because of possible risks with fetal exposure (see Chapter 42), so this approach has been replaced with a new hormone method that involves combined estrogen and progestin.

The combined hormone approach uses a regular birth control Pill (Ovral) containing ethinyl estradiol and norgestrel. This method is particularly appealing because it is so simple, and because the total hormone dose—two pills immediately and two more

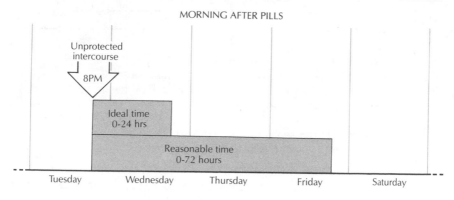

ILLUSTRATION 15-1   Ideally morning-after hormone treatment should be started within 24 hours after unprotected intercourse; 72 hours is the maximum.

pills 12 hours later—is quite low. Timing is critical for combined hormone treatment (see Illustration 15-1). Hormones started within the first 24 hours have the best chance for success and treatment must be started within no more than 72 hours after intercourse.

Reported rates for pregnancy despite morning-after hormone treatment average about 1% or 2% (2).

There are several important factors to consider as you weigh the risks and benefits of morning-after hormone treatment. The most serious immediate risk with hormone treatment is abnormal blood clotting. **If you have had clotting problems in the past, such as pulmonary embolism, stroke, heart attack, or thrombophlebitis, you must not take** hormones for morning-after treatment. Hormones are also unwise if you have a breast lump or unusual vaginal bleeding whose cause is not yet known, a serious liver problem, active gallbladder disease, or high blood pressure. Other medical problems may also affect hormone risks (see Chapter 13); your clinician can help you evaluate the pros and cons in your particular situation.

Nausea is the most common adverse effect with combined hormone treatment. Nausea is not nearly as common with birth control Pills as it was with high-dose estrogen, but taking two pills at a time is enough to cause nausea for about one third of the women who do (3).

Overall, serious problems with hormones are extremely rare, and safety is an important advantage of this morning-after option. Hormone treatment also is simple and inexpensive.

What to Expect After Hormone Treatment.   Taking morning-after hormone treatment may alter the timing of your next period. For 50% to 70% of women the next period is at least six days earlier than expected, but it may be as much as six days late (3). You need to pay careful attention, though; if your period is more than 14 days late you will need a pregnancy test and an exam.

15:2   PILL DANGER SIGNS

A   Abdominal pain (severe)
C   Chest pain, shortness of breath, cough
H   Headache (severe), dizziness, weakness, numbness
E   Eye problems (vision loss or blurring), speech problems
S   Severe leg pain (calf or thigh)

Stop taking Pills and see your clinician at once if you have any of these problems, or if you develop depression, jaundice, or a breast lump.

While you take hormone treatment, and during the first two weeks afterward, you should also watch for the danger signs of possible birth control Pill complications shown in Illustration 15-2.

IUD INSERTION

Excellent morning-after effectiveness has been reported with copper IUDs inserted within five to seven days after unprotected intercourse. Research reports include more than 1,300 patients with only 1 pregnancy resulting from morning-after treatment failure (2). The IUD probably interferes with implantation of the embryo in the uterine lining. If inserted just after implantation, which occurs about five to six days after conception, an IUD may disrupt the implantation process or the reaction of the uterine lining to the new IUD may be unfavorable for the embryo.

Since copper IUDs are no longer available in the United States, it is no longer possible to use the precise approach for which research data are available. The only IUD option now available is the progesterone IUD. There is no particular reason to fear that the progesterone IUD would not work, but there is no research reported as yet on its use as a morning-after treatment.

The main disadvantage of morning-after IUD treatment is the possible risk of pelvic infection that occurs with insertion of an IUD at any time. The IUD is not an attractive birth control option for any woman who may wish to be pregnant in the future. Infection can cause permanent damage and infertility. Infection risks are highest for very young women who are statistically at greatest risk for infection with or without an IUD.

The main advantages of an IUD for morning-after treatment are extremely high effectiveness and the wide time interval for emergency treatment. Evaluation of effectiveness for morning-after treatment is based on calculations of how many pregnancies would be expected. Most studies have evaluated IUD use within five days after intercourse. In a study of copper IUDs inserted up to seven days after intercourse, researchers calculated that 14 pregnancies would have been expected for the 102 women treated, but none occurred (4). Results reported by other researchers for IUD

15:3   IUD DANGER SIGNS

P   Period late (possible pregnancy), abnormal spotting or bleeding
A   Abdominal pain, pain with intercourse
I   Infection exposure (such as gonorrhea or chlamydia), abnormal
    vaginal discharge
N   Not feeling well, fever, chills
S   String missing, shorter or longer

See your clinician right away if you develop a danger sign.

---

use within five days have been similar, and IUD treatment is probably somewhat more effective than hormone treatment for morning-after use. Also, to be effective hormone treatment must be started within 72 hours (three days) after intercourse and preferably sooner. IUD treatment is effective up to five or even seven days.

IUD treatment is not a common choice for morning-after use; most women choose hormone treatment. It may be a very reasonable choice, though, if you are considering the IUD for ongoing birth control protection anyway. Advantages and risks for the IUD are described in more detail in Chapter 14.

What to Expect After IUD Insertion.   You may have light spotting or bleeding for the first few days after your IUD is inserted. The IUD, however, should not affect the timing of your next period. If you do not have a normal period at the normal time, you will need to see your clinician for a pregnancy test and exam to be sure you are not pregnant. Also, be sure to watch for the danger signs of possible IUD complications shown in Illustration 15-3.

ARRANGING MORNING-AFTER TREATMENT

Aggressive action on your part is essential. If you want to try hormone treatment, call your clinician as soon as possible (9:00 A.M. the morning after). It may be possible for her/him to provide a prescription by telephone if you have had a recent exam and you don't have any medical problems that would make hormone treatment risky in your case. Otherwise you will need an emergency appointment that very day.

Arranging for morning-after IUD insertion may be a little harder; insertion will require an office visit. Also, you may have to circumvent routine policies your clinician or clinic has about IUD insertion timing. Routine policies are likely to include an initial exam with tests for possible sexually transmitted infections, and a later visit during or just after a normal menstrual period for the IUD insertion. You will need immediate insertion. If your clinician or clinic is experienced with morning-after treatment, this should not be a problem. If not, you may have to be quite assertive to get it arranged. There are risks with IUD insertion any time, but research evidence shows that overall risks are about the same whether an IUD is inserted during a period, just after, or late in the cycle (5).

If you do not have your own clinician, or cannot arrange morning-after treatment with her/him, your local Planned Parenthood agency or health department may be able to refer you to a gynecologist who does provide morning-after treatment.

Morning-after treatment is not commonly used in the United States. It is not available at some clinics including those affiliated with Planned Parenthood because the best treatments available have not been specifically approved by the United States Food and Drug Administration (2). Lack of approval is a Catch-22 situation: the pharmaceutical companies have not requested approval and the FDA has no mechanism to grant approval unless it is requested! Lack of approval for this specific use does not make morning-after treatment illegal; it just means that the pharmaceutical company cannot promote or advertise the drug or IUD for this purpose. Your clinician can prescribe any approved drug for uses not included in the official labeling if she/he feels it is appropriate (6).

EVALUATING YOUR OPTIONS

It may be hard for you to decide whether morning-after treatment is a good choice or not. If your own health and safety are your main concerns and you would have an early abortion if you did conceive, then the "wait and see" option is certainly reasonable. The likelihood of pregnancy is not high and your health risks with early abortion are quite low.

Your own health and safety, however, may not be the only factors you are considering. If abortion is not an option for you, then morning-after IUD or hormone treatment may well be a good choice and may be your safest option. You may decide that preserving your peace of mind justifies the possible risks of morning-after treatment.

REFERENCES

1. Tietze C: Probability of pregnancy resulting from a single unprotected coitus. *Fertility and Sterility* 11:485–488, 1960.
2. Johnson JH: Contraception—the morning after. *Family Planning Perspectives* 16:266–270, 1984.
3. Van Santen MR, Haspels AA: A comparison of high-dose estrogens versus low-dose ethinyl estradiol and norgestrel combination in postcoital interception: A study in 493 women. *Fertility and Sterility* 43:206–213, 1985.
4. Luerti M, Tonta P, Ferla R, et al: Post-coital contraception by estrogen/progestogen combination or IUD insertion. *Contraception* 33:61–68, 1986.
5. White MK, Ory HW, Rooks JB, et al: Intrauterine device termination rates and the menstrual cycle day of insertion. *Obstetrics and Gynecology* 55:220–224, 1980.
6. Food and Drug Administration: Use of approved drugs for unlabeled indications. *FDA Drug Bulletin* 12:4–5, 1982.

16

Personal Decision Making About Unplanned Pregnancy

*"Your pregnancy test was positive. You **are** pregnant."*

These words can make you feel jubilant, or they can make you feel devastated; but if you are like many women, you won't immediately be sure exactly how you do feel. Most women have a powerful emotional reaction to a new pregnancy, and if the pregnancy is unplanned, the emotional reaction can be extremely complex and ambivalent. Within a very short time, a pregnant woman must sort out her feelings and decide whether or not to continue the pregnancy.

Some women are able to decide in advance which option they would choose in the event of accidental pregnancy. Other women may not give the choices any serious thought before accidental pregnancy happens. Many women who choose abortion, for example, say that they never imagined themselves having an abortion before they became pregnant.

If you have an unplanned pregnancy, it makes sense to consider your options carefully before you make a decision. There are only three possibilities as you face an unplanned pregnancy:

• Continue the pregnancy and assume parenthood of the child
• Continue the pregnancy and relinquish the child for adoption
• Have an abortion

The choice may not be easy when pregnancy is unplanned, but since you are the person who will live with the decision, be sure to make it for yourself. You may never feel absolutely great about what you decide, but you will feel better if you are sure that you made the best choice you could at the time. Hardly anyone gets through life without confronting some hard choices, and you may even learn valuable lessons about yourself and your life. The right decision about your unplanned pregnancy is the decision that you yourself believe is right.

TIME PRESSURE

If you think you may be pregnant, find out promptly whether you really are. Have a pregnancy test and a pelvic examination to determine how many weeks pregnant you are. (Pregnancy testing is discussed in Chapter 8.) If your clinician is not certain about your pregnancy dates, an ultrasound test (see Chapter 4) is a good idea, because with ultrasound, the size of your uterus and the pregnancy inside it can be measured quite precisely by recording sound wave echos. It is a safe and painless test, and is an essential test if you are considering abortion and your pregnancy has already passed the 12th week.

Don't wait and worry trying to decide what to do about the pregnancy. **Find out first and then decide.** Only an examination will tell you how long a "thinking" time you have. Be sure to **tell the appointment clerk that you need a pregnancy test and an exam** to verify pregnancy so that she/he will recognize that it is important for you to be seen without delay. **If you find that you have to wait more than a week for a pregnancy test appointment, look for another clinician who can see you sooner.**

GETTING TO A DECISION

Time pressure is one factor that makes resolving an accidental pregnancy such a difficult decision. Prenatal care should begin early in pregnancy, or abortion should be performed during the first 12 weeks when health risks are lowest. In most cases, this means no more than **one month** for decision making, since most women are already at least six weeks pregnant by the time they suspect and confirm pregnancy. Very long delays can lead to decision by default, for legal abortion is limited to the first 24 weeks of pregnancy.

No one is really prepared for an unplanned pregnancy, and faithful birth control users are often totally surprised and dismayed.

We wanted two children. When Sheryl was 6 and Peter was 3, I got pregnant, even though I was a *very* careful diaphragm user. My husband and I discussed it some, but basically we decided very quickly that three children would be fine; no big problem.

I got an IUD after Erica was born, and I got pregnant *again* when she was 2 1/2. We didn't have enough room for another child; we were spending all kinds of money fixing up the house, and neither of us wanted a fourth child *at all*. I was 36 years old, and it was the first time I had ever considered abortion in my life. I thought I'd never get pregnant if I was careful about birth control, but I was wrong.

—WOMAN, 38

Other women have taken chances—consciously or unconsciously—with unprotected intercourse.

I didn't use anything. Dumb, right?

—WOMAN, 19

You may find your choice difficult and discover that you have ambivalent feelings. Even if you have thought about the issue and have already made up your mind, ambivalent feelings can be more intense and distressing than you imagined. It is common for a woman to change her mind repeatedly as she assesses the pros and cons of continuing a pregnancy; she decides that continuing her pregnancy is the best option one day, and the next day she goes over the same facts and arrives at the opposite conclusion. In this situation counseling makes sense. Talking to an experienced counselor who is not involved in your life situation may help you gain the perspective you need, free of the natural biases that your partner, friends, and members of your family inevitably have one way or the other.

Assessing Your Life Situation.   Another important factor is the meaning of pregnancy to a woman's life situation. An accidental pregnancy can force a woman to reassess her basic feelings about a current relationship: if it is a good relationship, why does pregnancy seem undesirable? If this is not an optimal time or if financial considerations are unfavorable, when, if ever, will the situation be ideal for pregnancy? If the relationship is not good, what can be done to improve it? Should the relationship be continued, or should it be ended, in the hope of finding a better one?

Deciding about an unplanned pregnancy often raises questions about overall life goals: Is childbearing desirable at all? How does parenthood fit into education and career goals? What priorities should be assigned to each of these aspects of life?

Counseling.   The decision-making process about pregnancy is intimately related to major, life-changing issues that most people find difficult to assess, and that certainly deserve more than a few days or weeks of thought. Decision making can be difficult and stressful, and women, couples, and families often find that counseling is beneficial. Many agencies such as Planned Parenthood associations, local health departments, and family service agencies offer pregnancy counseling services. Counseling usually involves one or two sessions with a counselor especially trained in pregnancy decision making; often the counselor is a psychiatric social worker, psychologist, or trained medical worker. The goal of counseling is to help the individual(s) clarify feelings about pregnancy and come to a decision. **Counselors at reputable agencies do not attempt to influence your decision in any way.** The counselor should be able to provide information about abortion services in your community as well as prenatal care and adoption. No one, including counselors at an abortion clinic or Planned Parenthood, should want to pressure you toward abortion. You may find, however, that there are antiabortion counseling agencies in your community whose purpose is to pressure women toward continuing pregnancy to term. This is not reputable counseling. Coercion is not helpful, one way or the other, for a woman who is unsure, and may make her decision even more painful.

Ethical and moral issues are important to almost every woman. **Your counselor's goal should be to help you clarify your own beliefs and values.** You may also find it helpful to read the official religious statements about abortion ethics in Chapter 17. Religious groups do not all agree about this issue, so it is not surprising that the ethical meaning of the pregnancy decision can be such a thorny problem for an individual woman.

You may want to work with your counselor alone, or it may be reasonable to include your partner or another trusted person. If you are unsure, plan to talk to your counselor by yourself initially and allow time to discuss the pros and cons of involving someone else. Other guidelines that experienced counselors recommend are:

- **Be sure of the facts.** Don't rely on secondhand information about questions such as welfare support, adoption alternatives, or medical costs, and don't assume that your experience will be the same as that of a friend. Get the facts directly from an expert.
- **Be sure that you are making your own decision.** Even the wisest and most sympathetic clinician, religious advisor, parent, or close friend may not weigh all the factors as you would. You are the one who will live with the decision.
- **Try to consider all three options**—raising a child, abortion, and adoption—realistically and fully. It may be helpful to list each option and your own pros and cons for each, especially the practical and emotional impact for yourself, your family, and your close friends.

Depending on the issues that are significant for you, your decision-making process may require a little research. For example, it may help you to find out about the resources in your community for day care or school programs for mothers with young children. If you are considering adoption, you will want to find out about public agencies that handle adoption and also about private arrangements for independent adoption. Independent adoption is completely legal, and may have some advantages. You may, for example, wish to be involved in selecting the adopting family. Knowing in advance that your baby will not be placed in foster care, but will go directly from the hospital to a home you have chosen, may help your peace of mind. Adoption is a choice that requires great love and strength, but it can be a right choice.

TEENAGERS AND PREGNANCY

I never thought a lot about what I would do after graduation till I got pregnant. Then I felt like I had to figure out what to do about the pregnancy, *and* Kevin. *And* college. *And* a career. I felt like I had about 15 minutes to plan my whole life!

—WOMAN, 16

Many pregnant teenagers wonder whether or not to involve their parents or other trusted adults in the decision. They are reluctant to upset their parents, and they worry that their parents will disapprove or even reject them. Despite these natural fears, however, most young women find that their parents are supportive and helpful. Often the family has already sensed that something is wrong; an unspoken problem this significant may create tension and block communication, which both the young woman and her parents find very distressing. Parents often express relief when the truth is finally open for discussion. For many young women, the choice about an unplanned pregnancy is the very first major decision they ever make, and the support of concerned parents can mean a great deal, and may be especially important for finding good medical care and arranging the finances for care. Some teens, however, decide to handle the whole pregnancy experience on their own.

It can be difficult for a teenager to find a good way to bring up "The Problem." Sometimes it is easier to approach one parent first. You might ask a parent to help you find a doctor, to open the door just enough to begin a real discussion. Your clinician or pregnancy counselor may also be able to help you discuss the pregnancy with one or both parents if you wish.

No matter how hard it is to face the problem, do whatever you can to avoid delay. Waiting just makes the risks higher and limits your options. Have a pregnancy test as soon as possible. **If your period is more than three or four days late, it is time to make arrangements for your test.** Don't wait for nausea or obvious signs: you may not have them!

HEALTH RISKS AND FUTURE FERTILITY

Health risks are low no matter which decision you make. Deaths and serious complications with full term pregnancy are rare, and abortion is even safer. About 5 deaths occur for every 1 million abortion procedures and 80 deaths for every 1 million full term pregnancies (1,2).

Future fertility is likely to be the health issue that worries you most, and this is a reasonable concern. **Complications** with abortion can definitely impair fertility or even make future pregnancy impossible, and so can **complications** of full term pregnancy. Severe problems with either choice could necessitate hysterectomy, or a pelvic infection could develop afterward and cause infertility. Fortunately, such serious complications are very rare. Hysterectomy, following an abortion for example, might be necessary for 1 woman out of 20,000 (3).

Many researchers have studied fertility rates for women who have had abortions, and early reports from Europe and Japan did cause worry about reduced fertility and higher miscarriage rates, especially for women who had had several abortions. More recent studies, however, have not found these problems (3). Researchers suspect that **vacuum** abortion, which has replaced the earlier techniques, is less traumatic, so permanent damage is almost always avoided. Experts reviewing available research have concluded that **overall fertility risks with vacuum abortion, if there are any, must be very small indeed (4), or research data would already have found these risks.**

Severe health and fertility problems after abortion with other techniques, or after several abortions, have not been reported, but research studies are not extensive enough to allow firm conclusions or clear reassurance about fertility effects in these cases (4).

AGE

The ideal physiological age for childbearing is 20 to 35, when risks of maternal and infant complications are lowest. Problems such as prematurity, birth defects, infant deaths, high blood pressure, hemorrhage after delivery, and anemia are, at least to some extent, related to the pregnant woman's age.

The risk of death for a woman during pregnancy is low no matter what her age (about 8 deaths for every 100,000 births), but death rates are highest for very young women and for older women. Overall national statistics show that pregnancy death rates for women 15 to 19 years old are about 10% higher than they are for women 20 to 24, and women 35 years old and older have rates that are four to seven times higher (see Chapter 9).

For many women considering parenthood, the national risk statistics may not really be a valid way to assess personal risks, because variables other than age influence these statistics heavily. Many of the very young women and the women over 35 in the statistics were also economically disadvantaged, perhaps facing a fourth or fifth pregnancy if they were older, and did not receive adequate medical care. A teenager who begins prenatal care early in pregnancy, has a healthy diet, and is able to follow through with any medical care needed may face no greater health risks than a woman in her 20s. Similarly, a woman who is considering a first pregnancy at 35, and who has some of the advantages that later parenthood can confer—enough money, access to good medical care, and good knowledge about her body and health needs—almost certainly has a lower death risk than overall statistics would suggest.

More and more couples are delaying parenthood, and they—and their clinicians— can certainly face a late pregnancy without overwhelming fear. When good prenatal care is begun early, ideally even before conception, medical risks can often be minimized (see Chapter 9 for recommendations on optimal pregnancy planning).

GENETIC FACTORS

Fear of birth defects such as Down's syndrome (mongolism) leads some women to consider abortion, and this is a real concern for older women who have an accidental pregnancy. The risk of Down's syndrome is low in the early reproductive years (about 1 in 1,700 births at age 20) but rises sharply after the mid 30s to about 1 in 90 births at age 40 (5).

It is possible to detect the chromosome defects that cause Down's syndrome and certain other genetic disorders with tests during early pregnancy (see Chapter 9). Counseling to determine whether testing would be advisable in your case and to assess the statistical likelihood of genetic disorders is available through federally supported genetics centers. **Consider genetic counseling in any of these situations:**

• You are 35 or older
• You have already had a child with an inheritable birth defect such as Down's syndrome, Tay-Sachs disease, or spina bifida
• You or your partner has a birth defect or genetic disorder or a family history of birth defects or genetic disorders
• You have had three or more miscarriages, or your partner has fathered several pregnancies ending in miscarriage

With genetic testing and access to abortion, a woman 35 to 45 can reduce her risk of bearing a child with serious birth defects to about the same risk level she would have faced when she was 25 years old (6).

REPEAT ABORTION

I screwed up again, and I'm not 16 this time. What's wrong with me?

—WOMAN, 21

If this is not your first unplanned pregnancy, you may be feeling especially torn. The need for a second or third abortion may give you a sense of failure, and you may find that it is also viewed with dismay by the important people in your life and your health care providers as well. Dismay is understandable in view of the physical and emotional stress, inconvenience, and cost, but **there is no need to feel that you are any less worthy a person.** It may be that you conceived because you were not using effective birth control, or perhaps you conceived despite conscientious efforts. In either case it is safe to say that one of the main reasons you did conceive is that you are fertile—perhaps more fertile than average. So you had (and will continue to have) a greater than average risk for another accidental pregnancy, whether or not you use effective birth control. **There is a quite significant likelihood of another unwanted pregnancy, even when a woman faithfully uses very effective birth control.** If 100 women rely on a method that provides a 1% to 5% failure rate, such as Pills, after a first abortion, about 10 to 50 of them will probably have at least one more unplanned pregnancy within ten years. If 100 women rely on foam (10% failure), approximately 100 unplanned pregnancies will occur within ten years. Even within the first year, a significant number of repeat unwanted pregnancies can be expected (7).

"Average" fertility includes people who are less fertile or completely infertile, many of whom don't know it, and it also includes people who take risks. Some of those risk takers become pregnant, and they are probably among the most fertile portion of "average." The women who have a first abortion are at significantly greater risk than average for another pregnancy, and so also are at risk for repeat abortion, even if they use their birth control method exactly as carefully (or carelessly) as other women the same age.

Studies comparing women having a repeat abortion to those with a first abortion show that there is no difference between them in personality adjustment, or in contraceptive use (8). It doesn't make sense to judge yourself harshly, or view repeat abortion as proof of a deep-seated psychological disorder. Repeat unwanted pregnancy is common, and in most cases reflects nothing more than statistical odds, a normal event in an imperfect world.

Nevertheless, it does make sense to learn from the experience. You may need to be extra careful, more compulsive than the average woman, in order to avoid pregnancy in the future. **For you, choosing an extremely effective birth control method is essential,** with no room for risk taking. You may even want to consider a combination of two methods to improve your odds (see Chapter 11).

REFERENCES

1. Centers for Disease Control: *Abortion Surveillance 1981.* U.S. Department of Health and Human Services, Public Health Service. Issued November 1985.
2. National Center for Health Statistics: Advance report of final mortality statistics, 1982.

3. Stubblefield, PG, Monson RR, Schoenbaum SC, et al: Fertility after induced abortion: a prospective follow-up study. *Obstetrics and Gynecology* 63:186–193, 1984.
4. Castadot RG: Pregnancy termination: Techniques, risks, and complications and their management. *Fertility and Sterility* 45:5–17, 1986.
5. Hook EB: Rates of chromosome abnormalities at different maternal ages. *Obstetrics and Gynecology* 58:282–284, 1981.
6. Goldberg MF, Edmonds LD, Oakley GP: Reducing birth defect risk in advanced maternal age. *Journal of the American Medical Association* 242:2292–2294, 1979.
7. Tietze C, Bongaarts J: Repeat abortion in the United States: New insights. *Studies in Family Planning* 13:373–379, 1982.
8. Berger C, Gold D, Andres D, et al: Repeat abortion: Is it a problem? *Family Planning Perspectives* 16:70–74, 1984.

17

Abortion: Legal and Ethical Issues

It is obvious that the values of women differ very often from the values which have been made by the other sex . . . it is the masculine values that prevail.

—VIRGINIA WOOLF

On January 22, 1973, the United States Supreme Court announced two decisions—*Roe v. Wade* and *Doe v. Bolton*—that made abortion legal throughout the country. These decisions also set a limit for abortion at approximately 24 weeks of pregnancy and eliminated requirements for "justifying" abortion on medical or psychiatric grounds. The Supreme Court stated in part (1):

For the stage prior to approximately the end of the first trimester, the abortion decision and its effectuation must be left to the medical judgment of the pregnant woman's attending physician.

Thus, during the first 12 weeks of pregnancy, state and federal law may not impose any restriction, qualification, or prerequisites on how, when, or where an abortion is performed except to require that abortion be performed by a physician.

For the stage subsequent to approximately the end of the first trimester, the state, in promoting its interest in the health of the mother [sic], may, if it chooses, regulate the abortion procedure in ways that are reasonably related to maternal health.

During the second 12 weeks of pregnancy, the states may impose requirements intended to protect a woman's health. For example, a state may, if it chooses, require that all second trimester abortions be performed in a licensed hospital.

For the stage subsequent to viability a state, in promoting its interest in the potentiality of human life, may, if it chooses, regulate, and even proscribe, abortion except where it is necessary, in appropriate medical judgment, for the preservation of the life or health of the mother [sic].

Once pregnancy has reached the third trimester (after about 24 weeks), the possibility that the fetus could survive outside the uterus increases with each subsequent week. During this portion of pregnancy, a state may prohibit abortion if it chooses except when it is necessary to preserve the woman's life or health.

Federal regulations enacted by Congress since the 1973 Supreme Court decision have **prohibited the expenditure of federal funds** for abortion except in the case of rape or incest or when pregnancy endangers a woman's life. These regulations mean that health payments or insurance plans provided by the federal government to federal employees (including military personnel) do not provide financial coverage for abortion, and federal health programs to aid the poor also exclude abortion services. **These regulations do not make abortion illegal.** Unless the Supreme Court reverses its 1973 position or an amendment to the Constitution is passed, abortion will remain legal throughout the United States.

Since 1973 many states have also enacted laws to **regulate** abortion. You can learn which laws may apply in your state by calling Planned Parenthood, your state attorney general's office, a local abortion provider, or your state representative. Some examples of state regulations are (2):

• Public funds (state and federal) cannot be used to provide abortion for Medicaid recipients except to save a woman's life (or, in one state, to prevent severe and long-lasting physical health damage): 28 states
• Public funds cannot be used for abortion except to save a woman's life or when pregnancy resulted from rape or incest (or, in one state, when pregnancy is likely to result in birth of an infant with severe deformities): five states
• Parents must be informed before abortion if the woman is an unemancipated minor: nine states
• Parental consent or court authorization must be obtained if the woman is an unemancipated minor: seven states
• Coverage under health insurance plans (usually for public employees only) is limited to abortions necessary to prevent a woman's death: eight states
• A married woman's husband must be notified or give consent before abortion: five states
• Abortion is prohibited in public health facilities unless necessary to prevent a woman's death: two states

In most cases, a woman seeking abortion will be required to sign an informed consent document beforehand. The clinician or hospital may request that her spouse or parent also sign the consent form and may make this a prerequisite for care, even though court decisions have upheld a woman's legal right to abortion without a spouse's consent. If this request is unacceptable to the pregnant woman, her alternative is to choose another clinician and/or hospital willing to perform the abortion without spousal consent.

The Medical Impact of Legal and Illegal Abortion

The decision between continuing a pregnancy and electing abortion is sometimes portrayed as a mere matter of convenience, but it is seldom such a simple choice. For most people, the primary factors that influence a decision about unplanned pregnancy are personal, but it is reasonable at least to be aware of the medical impact of each option as well. In terms of health consequences, it is not a choice of mere convenience. The decision involves a choice between substantially different health risks. Neither full term pregnancy nor legal abortion is very dangerous. Pregnancy complications cause about 80 deaths for every 1 million live births; abortion causes about 5 deaths for every 1 million procedures. These statistics mean, however, that **full term pregnancy incurs a risk of death that is 15 times higher than the death risk of abortion**. Full term pregnancy is also more likely than abortion to result in major surgery; approximately 1 in 10 full term deliveries requires cesarean section surgery. The likelihood that abortion complications will necessitate major surgery is less than 1 in 500 (3).

Abortion has always been with us. In many diverse cultures worldwide, women seek and find illegal abortions when no legal services exist. About 70% of the legal abortions performed in New York City replaced what would have been illegal procedures, according to one study of the first two years of legal abortion in that city (4). Investigators have documented the same pattern in other countries following legalization of abortion.

Before 1973, complications of illegal abortions were leading causes of illness and death for pregnant women in the United States. Since legalization of abortion, there has been a significant decline in the number of hospital admissions for complications of abortion (5). Total maternal deaths due to abortion also decrease when abortion is legalized. **The current annual U.S. death rate from abortion is less than one tenth of what it was when abortion was illegal** (see Table 17-1).

Overall data for the United States so far indicate that since legalization of abortion there has been a significant decrease in **prematurity** rates and **infant mortality** rates, as well as **maternal mortality** rates (6). It is not possible to prove what has caused

TABLE 17-1

DEATHS FROM ILLEGAL AND LEGAL ABORTION IN THE UNITED STATES

YEAR	TOTAL NUMBER OF ABORTION DEATHS	ANNUAL DEATH RATE PER MILLION WOMEN AGED 15 TO 44 YEARS
1934	900	90.0
1960	100	7.6
1975	29	0.5
1980	9	0.3

Deaths for 1934 and 1960 are the estimated number of illegal abortion deaths. Deaths for 1975 and 1980 are the number of legal abortion deaths (illegal abortion deaths are excluded) identified by the National Abortion Surveillance Program coordinated by the Centers for Disease Control.

SOURCES: Tietze C, Bongaarts J: The demographic effect of induced abortion. *Obstetrical and Gynecological Survey* 31:699–709, 1976.
Centers for Disease Control: *Abortion Surveillance 1981.* U.S. Department of Health and Human Services, Public Health Service. Issued November 1985.
Tietze C, Henshaw SK: *Induced Abortion: A World Review, 1986* (ed 6). New York: The Alan Guttmacher Institute, 1986.

the decline in infant mortality. It may be that "high-risk" pregnancies are now being aborted more often than "low-risk" pregnancies are; or it may be that a completely unrelated factor such as better nutrition is entirely responsible for the decline in mortality rates.

Abortion is probably a necessary part of family planning for any population group that seeks a stable size. Population stability is achieved at a fertility rate of about 2,100 full term pregnancies per 1,000 women. Even if couples with two children use extremely good methods of birth control (2% failure level, such as Pills or condoms used exactly according to instructions all the time) for all the years of their remaining fertility, as many as 500 couples out of 1,000 (50%) may experience one or more additional unwanted pregnancies because of birth control failure. Average couples have about 25 more years of fertility after the second child is born. Two percent annual failure risk times 25 years means about a 50% risk of method failure. Even for a conscientious population group the fertility rate will probably exceed the no-growth level because of birth control failure alone unless both permanent sterilization and abortion are available options for couples who do not desire further childbearing.

ABORTION STATISTICS

From a worldwide perspective, the current pattern of abortion in the United States is fairly typical (6). About 24 abortions are performed each year for every 1,000

TABLE 17-2
LEGAL ABORTION IN SELECTED COUNTRIES, 1983

COUNTRY	NUMBER OF ABORTIONS PER YEAR FOR EVERY 1,000 WOMEN AGED 15 TO 44
Canada	10.2
China	61.5
Czechoslovakia	33.1
Denmark	18.6
England and Wales	12.1
Hungary	35.5
India (1981)	2.7
Japan	21.5
Sweden	17.9
United States of America	27.4
USSR (1982)	181

SOURCE: Tietze C, Henshaw SK: *Induced Abortion: A World Review, 1986* (ed 6). New York: The Alan Guttmacher Institute, 1986.

women aged 15 to 44. Factors such as contraceptive availability and general fertility probably account for the differences from country to country (see Table 17-2). Most people in the world do have access to legal abortion at least in some circumstances (see Table 17-3). Abortion is one of the most widely used methods of fertility control in the world today. It is also the most common surgical procedure performed on women 15 to 44 years old in the United States.

The total number of abortions performed each year in the United States increased between 1973 and 1980 and then stabilized at about 1.5 million. The increase was partly explained by a parallel increase in population and by wider availability of services; part of the increase occurred because of a shift away from use of birth control Pills to less effective methods of contraception (7).

Most women who have abortions in the United States are young and 75% are unmarried. Women 19 years old or younger account for 28% of all abortions; 10,000 abortions each year involve women (children) 14 years old or younger (8).

About half of all abortion procedures are performed during the first 8 weeks of pregnancy, and 90% during the first 12 weeks. Less than 1% involve pregnancies beyond the 20th week (8).

TABLE 17-3
WORLDWIDE ACCESS TO LEGAL ABORTION

LEGAL STATUS OF ABORTION	% OF WORLD POPULATION
Legal on request	39
Legal for social reasons	24
Legal for medical reasons	13
Legal only to save a woman's life	24

SOURCE: Tietze C, Henshaw SK: *Induced Abortion: A World Review, 1986* (ed 6). New York: The Alan Guttmacher Institute, 1986.

Ethical and Religious
Dimensions of the Abortion Issue

Whether or not legal abortion should be allowed to remain as a possible choice for couples is an issue that sharply divides religious communities in the United States. Several religious groups believe that abortion should not be legal in any circumstances. Some believe that the law should permit abortion only in very limited situations. Others believe that abortion can be a sound moral choice, and that the law should respect the diversity of beliefs in our society about the question of life's beginnings.

The following statements are official national resolutions or policies adopted by some of the major religious organizations in the United States.

American Baptist Churches, U.S.A., General Board, 1981
Abortion presents us with a dilemma. It places in tension several of our historic commitments:

Our commitment to the sanctity of human life;
Our commitment to freedom of conscience and self-determination;
Our commitment to the First Amendment guarantee of the free exercise of religion;

. . . Public law, enacted by human reason and enforced by state power, can never fully express the moral sensitivity of Christian love. We are therefore grateful for the Constitutional protection of religious freedom which guarantees our right to make personal moral decisions based on religious principles. The First Amendment affords each citizen freedom from the religious scruples of others and freedom to follow the religious dictates of conscience.

. . . We recognize that a human embryo is the physical beginning of a life which through a God-given process of development becomes a person. Choosing to terminate this developmental process is a crucial decision to be made only when all other possible alternatives will lead to greater destruction of human life and spirit.

. . . We recognize that Christian persons of sensitive and informed conscience find themselves on differing sides of the abortion issue. In our Baptist tradition the integrity of each person's conscience must be respected; therefore, we believe that abortion must be a matter of responsible, personal decision.

American Friends Service Committee, 1970
On religious, moral, and humanitarian grounds, therefore, we arrived at the view that it is far better to end an unwanted pregnancy than to encourage the evils resulting from forced pregnancy and childbirth. At the center of our position is a profound respect and reverence for human life, not only that of the potential human being who should never have been conceived, but that of the parent and the other children in the human community.

Believing that abortion should be subject to the same regulations and safeguards as those governing other medical and surgical procedures, we urge the repeal of all laws limiting either the circumstances under which a woman may have an abortion or the physician's freedom to use his or her best professional judgment in performing it.

American Humanist Association, Annual Conference, 1977
We affirm the moral right of women to become pregnant by choice and to become mothers by choice. We affirm the moral right of women to freely choose a termination of unwanted pregnancies. We oppose actions by individuals, organizations and governmental bodies that attempt to restrict and limit the woman's moral right and obligation of responsible parenthood.

American Jewish Congress, Biennial Convention, 1982
The American Jewish Congress has long recognized that reproductive freedom is a fundamental right, grounded in the most basic notions of personal privacy, individual integrity and religious liberty. Jewish religious traditions hold that a woman must be left to her own conscience and God to decide for herself what is morally correct. The fundamental right to privacy applies to contraception to avoid unintended pregnancy as well as to freedom of choice on abortion to prevent an unwanted birth.

Catholic Church, Encyclical Letter of Pope Paul VI: Of Human Life, July 25, 1968
. . . Each and every marriage act must remain open to the transmission of life.
. . . Just as man does not have unlimited dominion over his body in

general, so also, with particular reason, he has no such dominion over his generative faculties as such, because of their intrinsic ordination towards raising up life, of which God is the principle. "Human life is sacred," Pope John XXIII recalled; "from its very inception it reveals the creating hand of God."

. . . The direct interruption of the generative process already begun, and, above all, directly willed and procured abortion, even if for therapeutic reasons, are to be absolutely excluded as licit means of regulating birth.

. . . Equally to be excluded, as the teaching authority of the Church has frequently declared, is direct sterilization, whether perpetual or temporary, whether of the man or of the woman. Similarly excluded is every action which, either in anticipation of the conjugal act, or in its accomplishment, or in the development of its natural consequences, proposes, whether as an end or as a means, to render procreation impossible.

Episcopal Church, General Convention, 1982
RESOLVED:

The beginning of new human life, because it is a gift of the power of God's love for his people, and thereby sacred, should not and must not be undertaken unadvisedly or lightly but in full accordance of the understanding for which this power to conceive and give birth is bestowed by God.

Such understanding includes the responsibilty for Christians to limit the size of their families and to practice responsible birth control. Such means for moral limitations do not include abortion for convenience.

The position of this Church, stated at the 62nd General Convention of the Church in Seattle in 1967, which declared support for the "termination of pregnancy" particularly in those cases where "the physical or mental health of the mother is threatened seriously, or where there is substantial reason to believe that the child would be born badly deformed in mind or body, or where the pregnancy has resulted from rape or incest" is reaffirmed. Termination of pregnancy for these reasons is permissible.

In those cases where it is firmly and deeply believed by the person or persons concerned that pregnancy should be terminated for causes other than the above, members of this Church are urged to seek the advice and counsel of a Priest of this Church, and where appropriate, penance.

Whenever members of this Church are consulted with regard to proposed termination of pregnancy, they are to explore, with the person or persons seeking advice and counsel, other preferable courses of action.

The Episcopal Church expresses its unequivocal opposition to any legislation on the part of the national or state governments which would abridge or deny the right of individuals to reach informed decisions in this matter and to act upon them.

Church of Jesus Christ of Latter-day Saints, Priesthood Bulletin, February, 1973.

In view of a recent decision of the United States Supreme Court, we feel it necessary to restate the position of the Church on abortion in order that there will be no misunderstanding of our attitude.

The Church opposes abortion and counsels its members not to submit or to perform an abortion except in the rare cases where, in the opinion of competent medical counsel, the life or good health of the mother is seriously endangered or where the pregnancy was caused by rape and produces serious emotional trauma in the mother. Even then it should be done only after counseling with the local presiding priesthood authority and after receiving divine confirmation through prayer.

Abortion must be considered one of the most revolting and sinful practices in this day, when we are witnessing the frightening evidence of permissiveness leading to sexual immorality.

Members of the Church guilty of being parties to the sin of abortion must be subjected to the disciplinary action of the councils of the church as circumstances warrant. In dealing with this serious matter, it would be well to keep in mind the word of the Lord stated in the 59th Section of the *Doctrine of Covenants,* verse 6. "Thou shalt not steal; neither commit adultery, nor kill, nor do anything like unto it."

Lutheran Church in America, Biennial Convention, 1970 (reaffirmed 1978)

In the consideration of induced abortion the key issue is the status of the unborn fetus. Since the fetus is the organic beginning of human life, the termination of its development is always a serious matter. Nevertheless, a qualitative distinction must be made between its claims and the rights of a responsible person made in God's image who is in living relationships with God and other human beings. This understanding of responsible personhood is congruent with the historical Lutheran teaching and practice whereby only living persons are baptized.

On the basis of the evangelical ethic, a woman or couple may decide responsibly to seek an abortion. Earnest consideration should be given to the life and total health of the mother, her responsibilities to others in her family, the stage of development of the fetus, the economic and psychological stability of the home, the laws of the land, and the consequences for society as a whole.

The Lutheran Church—Missouri Synod, National Convention, 1983

. . . RESOLVED, That the Synod reaffirm its position that "(a) the living but unborn are persons in the sight of God from the time of conception; (b) as persons the unborn stand under the full protection of God's own prohibition against murder; and (c) since abortion takes a human life, abortion is not a moral option, except as a tragically unavoidable byproduct of medical procedures necessary to prevent the death of another human being, viz., the mother."

Presbyterian Church, U.S.A., General Assembly, 1983

Any decision for an abortion should be made as early as possible, generally within the first trimester of pregnancy, for reasons of the woman's health and safety. Abortions later in pregnancy are an option particularly in the case of women of menopausal age who do not discover they are pregnant until the second trimester, women who discover through fetal diagnosis that they are carrying a fetus with a grave genetic disorder, or women who did not seek or have access to medical care during the first trimester. At the point of fetal viability the responsibilities set before us in regard to the fetus begin to shift. Prior to viability, human responsibility is stewardship of life-in-development under the guidance of the Holy Spirit. Once the fetus is viable, its potential for physically autonomous human life means that the principle of inviolability can be applied.

. . . It is a tragic sign of the church's sinfulness that our propensity to judge rather than stand with persons making such decisions too often means that persons in need must bear the additional burden of isolation. It would be far better if the person concerned could experience the strength that comes from shared sensitivity and caring. The church is called to be the loving and supportive community within whose life persons can best make decisions in conformity with God's purposes revealed in Jesus Christ.

. . . The church's position on public policy concerning abortion should reflect respect for other religious traditions and advocacy for full exercise of religious liberty. The Presbyterian church exists within a very pluralistic environment. Its own members hold a variety of views. It is exactly this pluralism of beliefs which lead us to the conviction that the decision regarding abortion must remain with the individual, to be made on the basis of conscience and personal religious principles, and free from governmental interference.

Reorganized Church of Jesus Christ of Latter-day Saints, 1974 (reaffirmed 1980)

We affirm that parenthood is partnership with God in the creative processes of the universe.

We affirm the necessity for parents to make responsible decisions regarding the conception and nurture of their children.

We affirm a profound regard for the personhood of the woman in her emotional, mental, and physical health; we also affirm a profound regard and concern for the potential of the unborn fetus.

We affirm the inadequacy of simplistic answers that regard all abortions as murder, or, on the other hand, regard abortion only as a medical procedure without moral significance.

We affirm the right of the woman to make her own decision regarding the continuation or termination of problem pregnancies.

Southern Baptist Church, Annual Convention, 1984
The Southern Baptist Convention, meeting in New Orleans in June 1982, clearly stated its opposition to abortion and called upon Southern Baptists to work for appropriate legislation and/or constitutional amendment which will prohibit abortions except to save the physical life of the mother.

    . . . In addition to legislative remedies for this national sin, it is incumbent that we encourage the woman who is considering abortion to think seriously about the grave significance of such action by presenting information to her about the unborn child in her womb, who is a living individual human being, and encourage her to consider alternatives to abortion.

Union of American Hebrew Congregations, Biennial Convention, 1975 (reaffirmed 1981)
The UAHC reaffirms its strong support for the right of a woman to obtain a legal abortion on the Constitutional grounds enunciated by the Supreme Court in its 1973 decision. . . . This rule is a sound and enlightened position on this sensitive and difficult issue, and we express our confidence in the ability of the woman to exercise her ethical and religious judgment in making her decision.

    The Supreme Court held that the question of when life begins is a matter of religious belief and not medical or legal fact. While recognizing the right of religious groups whose beliefs differ from ours to follow the dictates of their faith in this matter, we vigorously oppose the attempts to legislate particular beliefs of those groups into the law which governs us all. This is a clear violation of the First Amendment. Furthermore, it may undermine the development of interfaith activities. Mutual respect and tolerance must remain the foundation of interreligious relations.

Unitarian Universalist Association, General Assembly, 1978
WHEREAS, religious freedom under the Bill of Rights is a cherished American right; and

    WHEREAS, right to choice on contraception and abortion are important aspects to the right of privacy, respect for human life and freedom of conscience of women and their families; and

    WHEREAS, there is increasing religious and political pressure in the United States to deny the foregoing right;

    BE IT RESOLVED:

    That the 1978 General Assembly of the Unitarian Universalist Association once again affirms the 1973 decision of the Supreme Court of the United States on abortion and urges the Association and the member societies and individual members of member societies to continue and to intensify efforts to insure that every woman, whatever her financial means, shall have the right to choose to terminate a pregnancy legally and with all possible safeguards.

United Church of Christ, General Synod, 1981

The question of when life (personhood) begins is basic to the abortion debate. It is primarily a theological question, on which denominations or religious groups must be permitted to establish and follow their own teachings.

Every woman must have the freedom of choice to follow her personal religious and moral convictions concerning the completion or termination of her pregnancy. The church as a caring community should provide counseling services and support for those women with both wanted and unwanted pregnancies to assist them in exploring all alternatives.

Freedom of Choice legislation must be passed at both the federal and state levels to provide the funds necessary to insure that all women, including the poor, have access to family planning assistance and safe, legal abortions performed by licensed physicians.

United Methodist Church, General Conference, 1976, 1984

The beginning of life and the ending of life are the God-given boundaries of human existence. While individuals have always had some degree of control over when they would die, they now have the awesome power to determine when, and even whether, new individuals will be born. Our belief in the sanctity of unborn human life makes us reluctant to approve abortion. But we are equally bound to respect the sacredness of life and well-being of the mother for whom devastating damage may result from an unacceptable pregnancy. In continuity with past Christian teaching, we recognize tragic conflicts of life with life that may justify abortion, and in such cases support the legal option of abortion under proper medical procedures. We call all Christians to a searching and prayerful inquiry into the sorts of conditions that may warrant abortion. Governmental laws and regulations do not provide all the guidance required by the informed Christian conscience. Therefore a decision concerning abortion should be made only after thoughtful and prayerful consideration by the parties involved, with medical, pastoral, and other appropriate counsel.—*Social Principles, 1984.*

When an unacceptable pregnancy occurs, a family, and most of all the pregnant woman, is confronted with the need to make a difficult decision. We believe that continuance of a pregnancy which endangers the life or health of the mother, or poses other serious problems concerning the life, health, or mental capability of the child to be, is not a moral necessity. In such a case, we believe the path of mature Christian judgment may indicate the advisability of abortion. We support the legal right to abortion as established by the 1973 Supreme Court decisions. We encourage women in counsel with husbands, doctors, and pastors to make their own responsible decisions concerning the personal or moral questions surrounding the issue of abortion.
—*Resolution on Responsible Parenthood, 1976.*

SUGGESTED READING

Batchelor, Edward, Jr. (editor): *Abortion: The Moral Issues.* New York: Pilgrim Press, 1982. A collection of writings by leading religious ethicists. An excellent resource and overview of the major ethical and religious themes that are intertwined with the abortion issue.

Callahan, Sidney, and Callahan, Daniel (editors): *Abortion: Understanding Differences.* New York: Plenum Press, 1984. A collection of outstanding essays, most written by women, including the perspective of Dr. Daniel Callahan, Director of the Hastings Center, Institute of Society, Ethics and the Life Sciences, and a most articulate spokesperson for those who support a pro-choice conclusion despite Roman Catholic background and/or beliefs.

Harrison, Beverly Wildung: *Our Right to Choose.* Boston: Beacon Press, 1983. Profoundly thoughtful and detailed exploration of ethical and moral dimensions of the abortion issue. The author describes herself as a practicing Christian woman, and is a professor of Christian Ethics at Union Theological Seminary in New York.

Luker, Kristin: *Abortion and the Politics of Motherhood.* Berkeley: University of California Press, 1984. A lucid and fascinating sociological perspective on why and how abortion has emerged in our society as the focus of such passionate debate.

Maguire, Marjorie R., and Maguire, Daniel C.: *Abortion, A Guide to Making Ethical Choices.* Published by Catholics for a Free Choice, 2008 Seventeenth Street Northwest, Washington, D.C. 20009. A concise and detailed guide written specifically for Catholic women and men who are grappling with the abortion issue.

REFERENCES

1. Supreme Court of the United States, Number 70–18. *Jane Roe, et al, Appellants, versus Henry Wade.* January 22, 1973. On appeal from the United States District Court for the Northern District of Texas.

2. Ory HW, Forrest JD, Lincoln R: *Making Choices: Evaluating the Health Risks and Benefits of Birth Control.* New York: Alan Guttmacher Institute, 1983.

3. Centers for Disease Control: *Abortion Surveillance, 1974.* U.S. Department of Health, Education and Welfare, Public Health Service, HEW Publication No (CDC) 76–8276, 1976.

4. Tietze C: Two years' experience with a liberal abortion law: Its impact on fertility trends in New York City. *Family Planning Perspectives* 5:36–41, 1973.

5. Stewart G, Hance F: Legal abortion: Influences upon mortality, morbidity, and population growth. *Advances in Planned Parenthood* 9:1–7, 1976.

6. Tietze C, Henshaw SK: *Induced Abortion: A World Review, 1986* (ed 6). New York: Alan Guttmacher Institute, 1986.

7. Castadot RG: Pregnancy termination: Techniques, risks, and complications and their management. *Fertility and Sterility* 45:5–17, 1986.

8. Centers for Disease Control: *Abortion Surveillance, 1981.* U.S. Department of Health and Human Services, Public Health Service. Issued November 1985.

Abortion Procedures

Be careful that you **don't rush your decision** about an abortion. Take time to consider all your choices for unplanned pregnancy: abortion, continuing the pregnancy and raising the child, continuing the pregnancy and relinquishing the child for adoption. The right decision about your unplanned pregnancy is the decision that you believe is right. Once you decide to have an abortion, however, **make your arrangements as quickly as you can.** Delay can significantly increase your risk of abortion-related medical complications.

Perhaps the most important factor to check as you choose a doctor or clinic to perform your abortion is the arrangement for around-the-clock emergency care. All reputable physicians who perform abortions have 24-hour phone numbers for you to call, and they have immediate access to a hospital emergency room in case you develop a problem of any kind after your abortion. Infection, bleeding, and other abortion complications can almost always be treated successfully if treatment begins promptly. Don't hesitate to call your clinician if you have a problem after your abortion, even in the middle of the night.

Think carefully about why you had an unplanned pregnancy, and determine whether there is anything you can do differently in the future to help prevent another unplanned pregnancy. You may need a better birth control method, or you may need to pay closer attention to your cyclic fertility signs, for example.

Hundreds of thousands of American women (including doctors) have abortions each year. You are certainly not alone if you risked intercourse without birth control or if your birth control method let you down; no one goes through life without taking chances, and birth control technology is far from perfect. There is no reason to think of yourself as anything but a normal person in a less than perfect world.

If you don't already have a gynecologist or family physician you can rely on for abortion, selecting a physician or clinic for your abortion may take a little research on your part. Remember that **when you choose a specific physician or clinic you may be limiting medical choices** about anesthesia and about which particular procedure will be used. Many abortion facilities offer only a limited range of services. It is perfectly reasonable to ask about these details before making a final decision.

Planned Parenthood and other local family planning clinics are good resources for information and referral in your area. The National Abortion Federation, a professional organization for public and private clinics that provide abortion services, can also provide reliable information on services available in your community or nearby. Both the National Abortion Federation and Planned Parenthood have nationally approved guidelines for abortion services, and clinics that are affiliated with either of these organizations must subscribe to standards of care set by the guidelines. See the "Resources" section at the end of this chapter for a list of Planned Parenthood Regional Offices and the National Abortion Federation toll-free telephone service. If you are considering an independent clinic, it may be wise to inquire ahead of time whether the clinic has been medically reviewed, by whom, and whether there are any other clinics you might consider.

Many reputable clinics offer pregnancy testing free or at low cost, and may also provide counseling and referral. Free pregnancy testing is also offered in some areas by antiabortion groups who hope to persuade women not to have an abortion, and this bias may not be obvious from information in the telephone book. Watch carefully for biased counseling: Is the counselor familiar with all your different alternatives? Do you feel pressured to choose one particular clinic, doctor, or procedure? Does the counselor seem to be urging you to continue the pregnancy? To terminate the pregnancy?

The choices are yours, and no one has the right to influence you against your will. If you feel pressured, find another source for counseling and information even if it means long distance phone calls or a trip out of town. In any case, do not be discouraged, and do not delay once you have decided to have an abortion. Abortion surgery is safest at about seven to nine weeks of pregnancy, counting from the beginning of your last normal period. After that, **risks increase with each week of delay.**

MINIMIZING YOUR OWN RISKS

Overall risks with abortion are low, but there are several precautions you can take that may reduce your risks:

- Have a pregnancy test and an exam as early in pregnancy as you can. This will insure that your pregnancy dates are known as accurately as possible.
- Ask your clinician to **check for STDs** (sexually transmitted diseases) when you have your exam. Tests for gonorrhea and chlamydial infection, just to make sure, are reasonable. If you have an infection, it can be treated and cured before your surgery.

- Take special precautions to be sure you are not exposed to a new STD just before, or just after, your abortion. STD exposure risks are very high if either you or your partner has had intercourse with any other partners in the past month or so. Use condoms or avoid intercourse if you have any doubt.
- Schedule your abortion procedure at about seven weeks of pregnancy, counting from the beginning of your last menstrual period. Risks increase somewhat with each week of pregnancy after that, and the possibility of missing part or all of the pregnancy tissue is somewhat higher for abortion before six weeks.
- Be sure the surgeon who performs your abortion is well-trained and experienced
- Be sure to understand your postoperative instructions. Follow your instructions to the letter, including the ban on intercourse, tampons, and douching, and take your temperature **with a thermometer** faithfully, several times daily for the first week.
- If you have a problem after your abortion, **make medical care your first priority.** Don't delay in contacting your clinician and don't delay any care she/he may recommend.

Your medical care for an abortion should include (at a minimum):

- A thorough explanation of the procedure you will have, and a consent form or consent explanation detailing possible risks and complications
- Conscientious review of your medical history, and of any drug allergies you may have
- A pregnancy test
- Tests to detect anemia and determine your blood Rh type
- A careful exam to assess the size of your uterus
- Thorough inspection of the tissue removed by the surgeon immediately after your abortion, and arrangements for laboratory tissue analysis if needed
- Treatment with Rh immune globulin if you are Rh-negative
- Treatment with antibiotics if you have medical history factors such as previous pelvic infection or heart damage
- Reasonable arrangements with a nearby hospital for immediate care if an emergency occurs during surgery
- Reliable arrangements for managing any problems you may have during the first few weeks after surgery. A 24-hour telephone service is essential.

Factors to Consider as You Choose an Abortion Clinic or Physician

Quality and cost are likely to be high on the list of factors you consider in deciding where to go for abortion services. In addition you will also need to think about anesthesia options, the specific type of abortion procedure that seems best for your situation, and your own personal preferences about services from a private physician or a clinic.

ASSESSING QUALITY OF CARE

Assessing the quality of care you can expect from a physician or clinic is difficult, but at a minimum it is perfectly all right to ask what kind of training and specialty certification the physician has and how much experience she/he has had with your particular procedure. It may be helpful to call a physician you trust or perhaps another health agency to inquire about the reputation of the clinic or physician you are considering. You can call your local hospital to verify that the physician is a member in good standing of the hospital staff. The "Suggested Reading" section at the end of this chapter may help you prepare for your quality assessment task.

It is also important to use your own judgment. Your own assessment, based on what you see and hear, is likely to be sound. Does the staff seem sympathetic and competent? Does the facility appear clean and well equipped? If not, you have the absolute right, in fact, a responsibility, to decline treatment. If you don't want to explain your decision, you can simply leave.

It is crucial that the clinic or physician you choose be able to provide immediate access to a hospital, because true medical emergencies do occur with abortion in rare cases. Geographical proximity to a hospital is important, but it is even more important that the physician performing your abortion have staff privileges at the hospital.

Most important of all is the ability of your clinic or doctor to handle any emergency problems after your abortion. The most common serious complications are likely to develop in the first three or four days after your abortion. Competent care 24 hours a day for complications is absolutely essential. **Make sure you know a 24-hour emergency phone number for problems.**

CHOICE OF PROCEDURES

There are several different types of abortion procedures, and detailed descriptions of each technique follow later in this chapter. In choosing your source of care you may also be choosing among these techniques, because the clinic or physician you choose may not offer all of them.

First Trimester Abortion. First trimester means the first 12 weeks of pregnancy, counting from the first day of your last menstrual period. Vacuum aspiration abortion is almost certain to be the procedure recommended, unless you are participating in a research study evaluating new techniques. This is the safest, most widely available technique for abortion, and you should have little difficulty in finding a clinic or physician to perform it. Either local or general anesthesia can be used.

Some physicians and clinics use laminaria or dilating rods for first trimester abortion and some do not. Laminaria are slender rods of dried seaweed that can be inserted into the cervical canal to dilate it gradually as the rods absorb water and swell. Dilating rods are made of synthetic polyacrylate material that also swells as water is absorbed. Laminaria or dilating rods must be inserted several hours before surgery. Dilation with rods occurs more rapidly than with laminaria, and rods must be removed within four hours after insertion, whereas laminaria are often left in place overnight. Used before vacuum aspiration abortion, laminaria or dilating rods may reduce risks for damage to the cervix during surgery, and may reduce discomfort for you as well (1). Their use, however, will mean two visits instead of one, and possibly a slightly higher cost. Laminaria are shown in Illustration 18-9.

Second Trimester Abortion.   The choice among second trimester procedures is complex. To assess your options you need to know **exactly** how many weeks pregnant you are, and an ultrasound test, using sonar to identify and precisely measure the size of your pregnancy, is likely to be recommended. The two basic options are:

• D&E (dilation and evacuation): a technique similar to vacuum aspiration abortion. The pregnancy is removed with instruments and vacuum.
• Induction of labor, or amniocentesis abortion: a solution containing a chemical (saline or urea) or hormone (prostaglandin) is injected into the amniotic fluid surrounding the fetus. Uterine contractions are triggered and the uterus expels the pregnancy within the following 8 to 24 hours or so.

Laminaria or dilating rods will be essential prior to D&E abortion, and are likely to be used in conjunction with amniocentesis abortion as well. General anesthesia is possible with D&E abortion, although it is more risky than local anesthesia; general anesthesia is not used for amniocentesis.

If you are between 13 and 16 weeks pregnant, it makes sense to try to find a physician or clinic able to use the dilation and evacuation (D&E) method. The national Centers for Disease Control have carefully studied complications of D&E and complications of saline and prostaglandin procedures, and have shown that D&E performed between 13 and 16 weeks is definitely safer than saline or prostaglandin procedures during that time period (1). The overall risk of death with D&E is about half as high as the risk with saline or prostaglandin. The D&E procedure is also much quicker, can often be performed without an overnight hospital stay, does not involve labor contractions, is cheaper, and avoids the two- or three-week delay that you would face at 13 weeks waiting for a saline or prostaglandin procedure (2).

If you are between 16 and 24 weeks pregnant, the D&E procedure may still be your safest alternative, but the choice is somewhat less clear-cut. D&E is not available in all areas so it may not be easy for you to arrange. You may even have to travel to another city. If you do go to another city for your abortion procedure, be sure to make good arrangements for emergency and follow-up care in your hometown.

COST

The range of costs for abortion is wide. An early vacuum abortion in a physician's office or clinic is likely to cost $150 to $250. A D&E procedure will be significantly more expensive, as will any procedure performed in a hospital. Your fees for an amniocentesis abortion or a D&E may total $1,500 or more.

ANESTHESIA

Your wishes about anesthesia may dictate your selection from among your abortion options. If you want to be entirely asleep during your surgery, general anesthesia will be needed, and **general anesthesia is likely to require a hospital or surgical center setting.**

General and local anesthesia each have pros and cons, and both techniques carry low risks for young, healthy women. A small number of women have died as a result of abortion anesthesia complications with both local anesthesia and general anesthesia. The risk of death with general anesthesia for abortion early in pregnancy is about two to four times higher than the risk with local anesthesia, and serious complication risks are four to eight times higher (3,4). Rates for severe complications and death are so low, however, that very few catastrophic outcomes would be expected with either anesthesia choice. For abortion before 12 weeks, using general anesthesia might increase the risk of death from about 1 in 200,000 to about 2 to 4 in 200,000.

For local anesthesia abortion you are awake and your cervix and uterus are partially numb. Local anesthesia significantly reduces the overall cost of abortion because you do not use hospital facilities, do not have an anesthesiologist, do not need to undergo more extensive preoperative tests, and you can expect a briefer recovery period. After general anesthesia abortion, you may not feel like yourself for a full day or even longer. After local anesthesia abortion, you will require only two or three hours for recovery.

For the average woman the additional risk and expense of general anesthesia may not be worthwhile, but in some situations general anesthesia is especially reasonable. A woman who is extremely anxious, for example, may find it difficult to remain calm and hold still during surgery; in that case, general anesthesia might be safer and make more sense.

SPECIAL CLINICS

I don't know exactly what I was expecting, but I do remember this Natalie Wood movie where she got an abortion in a sleazy hotel room. The clinic I went to was absolutely regular. It could have been any doctor's office, any dentist's office.

—WOMAN, 33

Many cities have specialized abortion clinics. In most areas, such clinics offer high-quality abortion care at a significantly lower cost than a hospital can offer. The relatively anonymous atmosphere in a large clinic appeals to some women. Clinics are usually staffed by helpful and sympathetic counselors who assist you through the preoperative and postoperative tests and discussions and often remain with you during the abortion procedure itself. The physician plays a relatively less prominent role; you will probably be with her/him for only about ten minutes if you have an early vacuum abortion.

Abortion clinic physicians are likely to have more than average experience with the procedure, and that can be a significant safety advantage. Because of the specialized nature of most abortion clinics, your care is usually limited to the abortion procedure itself and a follow-up examination two weeks later, so you may need another source for your routine care or problems other than unwanted pregnancy.

PRIVATE PHYSICIANS

Most private gynecologists and some family physicians perform in-hospital abortion procedures. Some physicians perform early vacuum abortion in their offices. This service is commonly available in some areas and quite uncommon in other parts of the country. The cost of abortion in an office setting is about the same as or even less than abortion clinic costs. You have the advantages of individualized care and continuity for other kinds of health needs in the future.

Preparing for Abortion

Your clinician will review your general medical history before your abortion. Serious medical problems such as heart disease, bleeding or clotting disorders, or epilepsy may influence the choice of setting for your abortion, and you may need special care during and after surgery. For example, a woman who has had rheumatic heart disease may be treated with penicillin before her abortion to reduce the risk of infection that could spread to her damaged heart valves.

Your clinician will want to know about any adverse drug reactions you may have had, especially if they involved general anesthesia, local anesthetic drugs such as dental Novocain, or disinfectants such as iodine.

Your clinician will carefully review your menstrual history. It is important for you to know precisely when your last normal period started, because **pregnancy length is calculated in weeks, starting from the first day of your last normal period.** Your clinician relies on your menstrual period dates and on the size of your uterus to determine how long you have been pregnant. Since pregnancy length is the key factor in choosing the best and safest abortion method, it is essential to be as accurate and honest as possible about your menstrual dates.

You will need a pregnancy test, a blood count for anemia, and a determination of Rh type. Additional tests may be recommended if you are having general anesthesia.

Your clinician will want to be sure that you understand the abortion procedure and its possible complications and that you feel certain about your decision to have an abortion. You will probably be asked to sign an informed consent document.

You will be given specific instructions about how to prepare for your abortion. Be sure that you understand them, and be sure to arrive on time. Many clinics and hospitals have strict rules requiring that your appointment be canceled if you do not check in on time. Plan to have someone accompany you home after your abortion.

If you will be having general anesthesia, an empty stomach is essential to decrease the likelihood of vomiting and inhaling fluid into your lungs. Don't eat or drink anything for at least eight hours before your abortion. If you are having local anesthesia, your clinic or physician will recommend either a light breakfast or no breakfast at all.

Abortion Procedures

I ran out of Pills. Planned Parenthood closed at five, and I didn't get off work till four. I couldn't get a ride, and I would have been too late on the bus. Anyway, they said I had to have an exam before I could get more Pills.

So here I am. My sister came here, and she told me about it. I only got scared when I heard them turn on the machine in the next room. It wasn't as bad as I thought, though.

—ABORTION CLINIC PATIENT, 18

EARLY VACUUM ABORTION: 4 TO 12 WEEKS OF PREGNANCY

Early vacuum abortions account for 90% of all the abortion procedures in the United States. The vacuum procedure is the accepted technique for terminating pregnancy from 4 to 12 weeks in length. Vacuum abortions are usually done using local paracervical block anesthesia, but general anesthesia can also be used. In the case of general anesthesia, the procedure is identical except that anesthetic drugs are given intravenously to induce sleep and maintain anesthesia. Recovery time is somewhat longer, because you must rest until the anesthetic effect wears off.

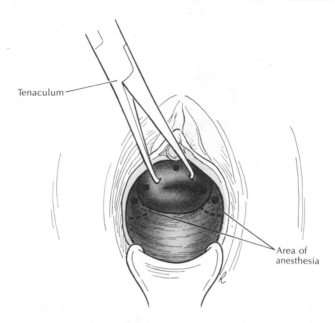

ILLUSTRATION 18-1   The tenaculum steadies the cervix during the abortion procedure. Local anesthesia is injected to block pain sensation from the cervix, and, to some extent, from the uterus as well.

The first step is pelvic examination to confirm the size and position of your uterus (see Chapter 3 for a complete description of the pelvic exam), and to remove laminaria or Dilapan rods if these have been inserted prior to your surgery. Next your surgeon inserts a speculum in your vagina so that she/he can see your cervix, and then cleans your cervix and vagina with iodine solution or another disinfectant. Next, your surgeon will probably inject anesthetic at the top of your cervix where the clamp (tenaculum) will be placed, and then steady your cervix with the clamp and inject more anesthetic into your cervix and uterine ligaments (see Illustration 18-1). The anesthetic begins to take effect within seconds. Since the cervix has few nerve receptors sensitive to pinprick you may not even be aware of getting the injections, but you may have some cramping during this process. Local anesthesia can cause a sensation of numbness in your mouth or fingertips, or dizziness and ringing in your ears. The anesthetic is rapidly absorbed by the many blood vessels near the cervix and small amounts quickly travel through your circulation throughout your body. These effects subside within a couple of minutes.

After the anesthesia takes effect, your physician gently pulls on the tenaculum to straighten out your cervical canal and then widens (dilates) your canal with a series of metal dilating rods (see Illustration 18-2) until the opening is big enough for the appropriate vacuum tube (see Illustration 18-3). The vacuum tube size your surgeon will choose depends upon the length of your pregnancy in weeks. If laminaria or

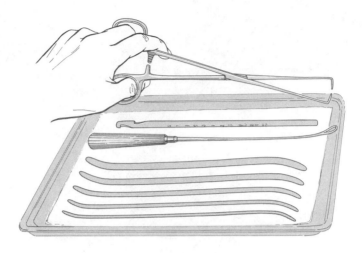

ILLUSTRATION 18-2   The physician is holding a tenaculum, a clamp to steady
the cervix. The tray holds (from the bottom) five graduated dilating rods, a
curet, and a vacuum tube.

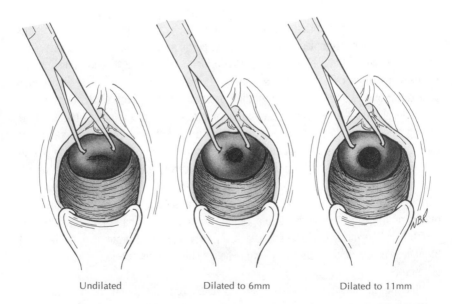

Undilated   Dilated to 6mm   Dilated to 11mm

ILLUSTRATION 18-3   Metal dilating rods, or laminaria or Dilapan rods inserted
several hours beforehand, may be used to widen the cervical canal for
abortion. For early abortion, dilation to 6 mm diameter may be sufficient.

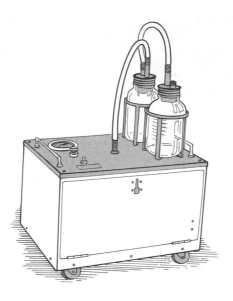

ILLUSTRATION 18-4   **A commonly used vacuum machine for abortion.**

dilating rods have been inserted prior to your surgery, little or no additional dilation will be needed, so metal dilation rods may not be necessary.

Once the vacuum tube is in place inside your uterus, the tube is connected to an electric vacuum pump machine (see Illustration 18-4). The vacuum pump motor often has a loud rumble, so don't be startled when it is turned on. (Some physicians use a large plastic syringe, rather than an electric pump, to create the vacuum when the pregnancy is less than about nine weeks.)

The vacuum procedure usually takes three to five minutes. The vacuum tube is rotated inside your uterus and moved back and forth to remove the pregnancy sac and part of the thick uterine lining that is formed during pregnancy (see Illustration 18-5). The total amount of tissue and blood removed depends on the length of pregnancy. If you are 5 to 6 weeks pregnant, there may be only 1 or 2 ounces (15 to 20 grams); at 11 to 12 weeks, there may be as much as 12 to 16 ounces (100 to 150 grams).

Many surgeons use a sharp, spoon-shaped instrument (curet, see Illustration 18-6) to explore your uterine cavity after using vacuum to make certain that all the tissue has been removed.

When your surgeon is sure that your uterus is empty, she/he removes the tenaculum and speculum. Your total time on the table for the procedure itself is likely to be about ten minutes.

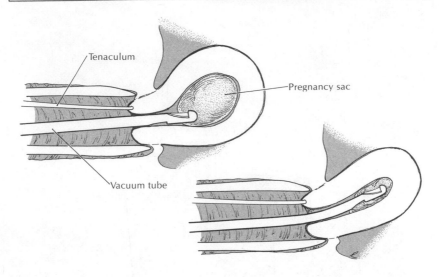

ILLUSTRATION 18-5.   The vacuum tube draws the pregnancy sac out of the uterus. Near the end of the abortion procedure, the uterus begins to contract.

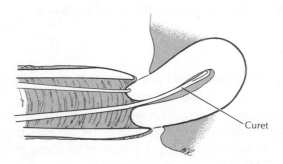

ILLUSTRATION 18-6   The surgeon may explore the uterus with a curet once the vacuuming procedure is completed.

The vacuum part itself wasn't really painful, but it felt very peculiar: a sensation deep inside my abdomen. I did have strong cramps during the last part, maybe 30 seconds or a minute before the machine was turned off. After that the cramps just gradually went away, and I was okay.

—ABORTION CLINIC PATIENT, 20

It is natural to be concerned about how much pain you should expect during a vacuum abortion, especially if you will be having local anesthesia. You may have a reassuring friend who tells you that she had no real pain at all. Some women do have only the most minimal discomfort. **Most women say the vaccum abortion hurts, but that the pain is tolerable.**

During the dilating and also during the vacuum part, I had cramps that were really bad, like my absolutely worst menstrual cramps, but they didn't last very long.

—ABORTION CLINIC PATIENT, 23

As the vacuuming begins, most women notice a tugging sensation in the lower abdomen. Toward the end of the procedure, when most of the tissue has been removed, the uterus itself contracts. You will probably find that this causes a strong cramping sensation that lasts for 2 to 20 minutes or so after your procedure is completed.

Most women are able to get up soon after abortion, and in many clinics patients routinely walk from the procedure room to a recovery lounge. Your surgeon will probably ask you to remain at the office or clinic for about half an hour after the procedure. During the first 10 to 30 minutes it is common to experience cramps and sometimes nausea, but you will almost certainly feel ready to leave within an hour or less.

DILATION AND EVACUATION ABORTION (D&E): 13 TO 24 WEEKS OF PREGNANCY

The dilation and evacuation (D&E) procedure is similar to the vacuum procedure except that cervical dilation is significantly greater (12 to 14 mm—about half an inch—or more). About 7% of all abortions are done with the D&E procedure. **It is the preferred technique for abortion between 13 and 16 weeks of pregnancy, and is also possible for later pregnancies as well.** Risks with D&E even for pregnancy greater than 16 weeks are probably lower than risks with amniocentesis abortion.

Both surgical instruments and the vacuum tube are required for removing the large volume of fetal and placental tissue. The procedure takes about 20 to 30 minutes. Dilating rods placed 4 hours before surgery or laminaria rods 6 to 12 hours before a D&E procedure, or overnight, will be necessary to dilate the cervical canal, and drugs to promote uterine contraction at the conclusion of surgery are usually required.

From the patient's point of view a D&E procedure is very similar to vacuum abortion. Sensations and discomfort during the procedure are similar when local anesthesia is used. When general anesthesia is used, of course, there is no discomfort during the procedure. Recovery after a D&E procedure is also similar to that after a vacuum abortion.

AMNIOCENTESIS ABORTION (SALINE, PROSTAGLANDIN, OR UREA): 15 TO 24 WEEKS OF PREGNANCY

Amniocentesis is the insertion of a hollow needle into the fluid-filled amniotic sac surrounding the fetus in order to remove amniotic fluid or introduce medicine. About 3% of all abortions in the United States use the amniocentesis procedure. It is very difficult to perform amniocentesis before about 15 weeks of pregnancy because the amniotic sac is so small. Some clinicians advise a woman who is 13 weeks pregnant to wait two or three weeks so an amniocentesis abortion can be scheduled, but statistics on abortion complications compiled by the national Centers for Disease Control indicate that **D&E abortion (see above) without waiting is a safer option than amniocentesis in this situation.** Amniocentesis abortion is almost always performed in a hospital.

Your surgeon uses the amniocentesis procedure to insert saline, prostaglandin, or urea into the amniotic sac surrounding the fetus. Saline is a concentrated salt solution. Prostaglandins are a family of hormone drugs. Urea is a concentrated solution of a nitrogen compound that is normally produced by the kidneys. Each of these drugs will induce premature labor. **You will be fully awake and alert during amniocentesis,** because your surgeon relies on you to report any unusual sensations that might mean you are having a drug reaction.

The first step in the amniocentesis procedure is examination of your abdomen. Your surgeon locates the top of your uterus, and a small area on your lower abdomen may be shaved. Next a small amount of local anesthetic is injected to anesthetize a 1-inch circle of skin, muscle, and connective tissue (see Illustration 18-7). Most women experience a brief stinging sensation as the anesthetic is injected.

Next your surgeon inserts a slender hollow needle or plastic tube through the anesthetized area into the amniotic sac (see Illustration 18-8). Most women feel pressure and a short twinge of discomfort as the tube is inserted, but once the tube is in place, you are likely to feel no discomfort. Either saline, urea, or prostaglandin is inserted through the tube into the amniotic sac. You may notice a subtle sense of fullness or pressure in your uterus; **if you have any pain or a sensation of warmth, tell your surgeon at once.** After the saline, urea, or prostaglandin is in place, your physician withdraws the tube and the injection site is covered with a Band-Aid.

Laminaria or dilating rods inserted into the cervical canal either before or immediately after amniocentesis may be used in order to dilate the canal gently before strong labor contractions begin.

Most women have a quiet period of several hours after amniocentesis before labor contractions begin. You may be given a drug called oxytocin through an intravenous (IV) tube in your arm to encourage or strengthen contractions. Oxytocin sometimes

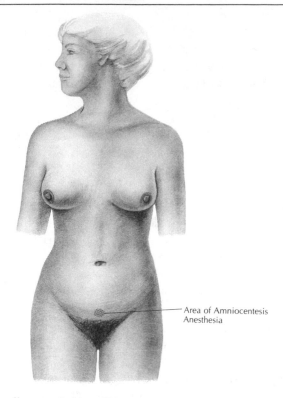

ILLUSTRATION 18-7   A small area of skin will be anesthetized for amniocentesis abortion.

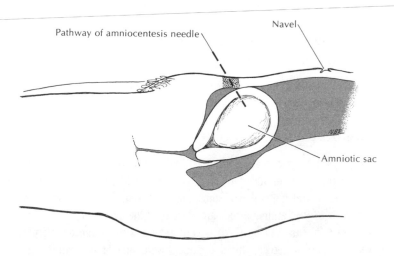

ILLUSTRATION 18-8   The slender amniocentesis needle enters the amniotic sac.

causes increased fluid retention so you and the hospital staff must keep careful records of your urine output and all fluids you are given by mouth and by IV. Keep your records accurately so that excessive fluid retention can be recognized and corrected promptly; untreated fluid retention can cause serious complications, including coma and convulsions.

Uterine contractions cause expulsion of the pregnancy through the vagina in amniocentesis abortion. There is wide variation in the length of time that abortion labor lasts and in the amount of discomfort women have. You can have pain medications if you need them.

As the time for abortion approaches, you are likely to feel a sense of fullness and pressure in your vagina, similar to the pressure and urge for a bowel movement. In most cases, the fetus is expelled first, followed a short time later by the placenta. Because the fetus is relatively small, expulsion is usually not painful, usually does not cause tearing, and does not require the incision in the vaginal opening (episiotomy) that is often used with full term pregnancy.

The hospital nursing staff will plan to assist you during expulsion. In case expulsion occurs before a nurse arrives, it is important that you be prepared for the fact that the fetus is recognizable at this stage of pregnancy.

In about one out of four cases expulsion of the placenta is delayed, and it may be necessary for the physician to remove the placenta. She/he will first try to pull the placenta free with a blunt grasping instrument; if this technique fails, you may need general anesthesia and a D&C procedure (see Chapter 47).

You will be encouraged to remain in the hospital for observation for at least three to four hours after amniocentesis abortion. During this time you are likely to feel well and should be able to shower and prepare to go home.

The total time in the hospital for amniocentesis abortion varies widely and is not predictable. On the average, saline and prostaglandin abortions require about a 24-hour stay. Abortion may occur quite a bit earlier (6 to 8 hours) or later (36 to 48 hours). You must be prepared to remain in the hospital for 48 hours or even longer.

LAMINARIA AND DILATING RODS

Laminaria are slender rods made of seaweed that has been processed and sterilized for medical use. One, two, or more dry laminaria rods are inserted into your cervical canal, and over several hours they absorb moisture, swell, and gently widen the canal (see Illustration 18-9). Laminaria rods are often used the day before a vacuum or D&E abortion, and they can also be used in conjunction with amniocentesis procedures. When wide dilation is needed, initial treatment with one or two laminaria may be followed by insertion of a second batch of several rods six to eight hours later or the next day.

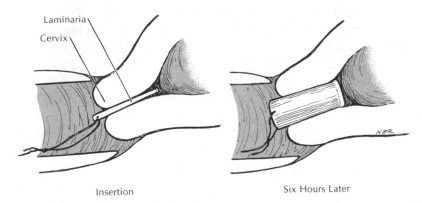

Laminaria
Cervix

Insertion   Six Hours Later

ILLUSTRATION 18-9 **The surgeon may insert a laminaria rod in the cervical canal. The rod will absorb moisture, swell, and gradually widen the canal in about six hours. Synthetic dilating rods are similar in appearance but require about four hours for maximal effect.**

Dilapan or Lamicel rods are a synthetic alternative to laminaria. They are made of a chemical that swells as it absorbs moisture. Dry, the rods are similar in appearance to slender tapered laminaria rods. Dilation with dilating rods, however, is more rapid than it is with laminaria. Dilation sufficient for early vacuum abortion occurs within about two hours, and maximal dilation is reached in 4 to 12 hours.

For laminaria or dilating rod insertion you will be positioned as for a standard pelvic examination. You may feel some cramping during insertion, and your clinician may use a local anesthetic for the insertion procedure. After insertion, a folded gauze square is placed against your cervix to hold the rod(s) in place. As the rod(s) dilate your cervix, you may experience some cramping. If pain is severe, call your physician. It is likely to be mild, however, and some women have no discomfort at all. You may also notice some spotting or light bleeding after insertion. Spotting is not a cause for alarm, but heavy bleeding should be reported to your physician.

One or more laminaria or dilating rods may come out spontaneously before or during your abortion. Watch for this—rods look like small brown tampons—when you go to the bathroom. **Your surgeon will want to know that one or more rods have already been expelled, so save them in a plastic bag.**

As an alternative to laminaria or dilating rods your physician may use prostaglandin hormone vaginal suppositories (see next section) to promote softening and dilation of the cervix.

THE Rh-NEGATIVE WOMAN AND ABORTION

Rh disease of the newborn infant was a common cause of severe newborn jaundice and fetal or infant death until the late 60s. This problem arises when **a woman who is**

Rh-negative herself becomes pregnant with an **Rh-positive fetus.** At the time of delivery, miscarriage, or abortion, Rh-positive cells from the infant or fetus can enter the woman's bloodstream and cause her body to build antibodies, special proteins that attach to the "foreign" Rh-positive cells. This antibody buildup is a normal defense against invasion by foreign chemical structures.

Usually, antibodies are not a problem during a first Rh-positive pregnancy. If the same woman becomes pregnant again with another Rh-positive fetus, the antibody response that was established during her first pregnancy is stimulated and antibody levels in her blood rise. These antibodies are able to cross the placenta into the blood circulation of the fetus, where they can attack **fetal** Rh-positive cells. Breakdown of fetal blood cells can cause severe anemia and jaundice in the fetus, called Rh hemolytic disease. It tends to be worse with each succeeding Rh-positive pregnancy.

Today, Rh hemolytic disease can almost always be prevented. In 1968 the Food and Drug Administration approved the first Rh immune globulin drug. An injection of Rh immune globulin, given to the Rh-negative woman at the time of delivery, miscarriage, or abortion, prevents her from initiating an antibody response. The globulin in the drug acts by coating any Rh-positive cells that do enter the woman's circulation; consequently, her own body does not perceive that a foreign chemical has entered her bloodstream, and she does not build antibodies. This drug must be administered if possible within 36 to 72 hours after delivery, miscarriage, or abortion. **Every woman who has an abortion must have a blood test to determine whether she is Rh-positive or Rh-negative.**

Without treatment, about 4% of Rh-negative women develop antibodies after an early vacuum abortion. The percentage is somewhat higher for women undergoing second trimester abortion (5). Fewer than 1% of the Rh-negative women treated with Rh immune globulin shots develop antibodies (5).

It is wise to have Rh treatment even if you don't plan any future pregnancies. You could change your mind, for one thing; and also, you may protect yourself against future problems with blood transfusions.

In 1978 the FDA approved a smaller dose of Rh immune globulin specifically for women undergoing abortion in the first 12 weeks of pregnancy, when a smaller dose can provide effective protection (6) at a lower cost.

Other Abortion Techniques

MENSTRUAL EXTRACTION

Terms such as "menstrual induction," "menstrual extraction," and "aspiration without dilation" have been used in the past to refer to vacuum procedures performed very early in pregnancy before a routine urine pregnancy test could confirm pregnancy.

The technique for menstrual induction or extraction is identical to that for early vacuum abortion.

Since it is now possible to confirm pregnancy as early as one week after conception, these terms are no longer meaningful. (Read more about early pregnancy tests in Chapter 8). In other words, a woman who requests "menstrual induction" because her period is a few days late can now find out for certain whether or not she is pregnant. If the pregnancy test is positive, her vacuum procedure should properly be called an abortion. **If her pregnancy test is negative, she is not pregnant, and there is no justification for performing a procedure at all.**

If a vacuum procedure is performed before the sixth week of pregnancy, there is a higher risk of retained fetal and placental tissue and failure to terminate the pregnancy compared to abortions performed after six weeks (3). This risk is especially a problem if your physician does not know for certain whether you are pregnant. **Be certain you have a positive pregnancy test before you have any abortion procedure.**

DRUGS FOR ABORTION

Prostaglandin Vaginal Tablet.   The newest abortion method is a prostaglandin vaginal tablet, approved in 1977 by the Food and Drug Administration. Prostaglandins are a family of closely related hormones normally present in many body tissues. One of the prominent prostaglandin effects is stimulation of smooth muscle contraction, including that of uterine muscle. A prostaglandin vaginal tablet is inserted into the vagina, and the drug is absorbed through the vaginal walls. The tablet causes labor contractions similar to those caused by saline or prostaglandin injected into the amniotic sac itself. Compared to amniocentesis techniques, vaginal prostaglandin tablets have the advantage that the amniocentesis injection is eliminated, and the hormone tablet can be quickly removed if you develop an adverse reaction to the drug. Prostaglandin vaginal tablets have also been investigated as an alternative for first trimester abortion, and are being used in some experimental programs (7). The dose of hormone needed to induce abortion is high enough that side effects such as nausea, vomiting, and diarrhea are common, so further research will be needed to find a form of prostaglandin that has fewer side effects. Also, experience with prostaglandin is limited, and there are no extensive data to provide a safety estimate for this method. The risk of serious or fatal reactions with the vaginal tablets is not known.

RU 486.   This experimental drug, developed by a French pharmaceutical company, is similar in structure to natural hormones, but instead of mimicking hormone effects, it blocks the uterine lining cells from receiving natural progesterone. With no progesterone support, uterine lining cells shed just as they would during a regular menstrual period.

Prostaglandin vaginal tablets and RU 486 are both being tried on an experimental basis by research programs in the United States and elsewhere. The idea of a medication for abortion has some merit, but medication is not likely to replace current abortion procedures because early vacuum abortion has such a good safety record. Even commonly accepted and widely used drugs usually carry higher risks: the death rate associated with a penicillin shot, for example, is 1.5 to 2.0 per 100,000 people. The comparable risk for abortion during the first eight weeks of pregnancy is less than 0.5 per 100,000 procedures (8). It is unlikely that any potent drug will prove to have a comparable safety record.

Special Warning. At least three cases of poisoning caused by **pennyroyal oil** (*Mentha pulegium,* also called squaw mint or mosquito plant) have been reported to the Centers for Disease Control (9). In one case, a young woman who drank an ounce of pennyroyal oil died six days later despite intensive treatment for massive liver destruction apparently caused by the poison. Pennyroyal is clearly not a safe abortion option.

Herbal remedies, like conventional drugs, can have serious side effects. Any preparation that has active ingredients potent enough to have beneficial effects is likely also to have detrimental effects for at least some individuals. A major problem in using herbal remedies is that the identity of the active ingredient is, in many cases, unknown and there is no good way to determine an effective, but safe, dose.

Hysterotomy and Hysterectomy. Abortion methods that are very rarely used today are hysterotomy and hysterectomy. Hysterotomy, a miniature cesarean section, was more common in the first few years after abortion was legalized in the United States. These procedures are now reserved for women with specific, serious medical problems that make it dangerous to use saline, prostaglandin, or urea, or for cases in which other abortion methods have failed.

Complications and Risks

Serious complications and deaths from legal abortion are rare. The national Centers for Disease Control monitors abortion deaths in the United States, and the risk of death from legal abortion has declined quite steadily since the early 70s. In 1972, there were 4 deaths reported for every 100,000 legal abortions; in 1981 the rate was 1 death in 200,000. About seven women die each year in the United States as a result of legal abortion (1).

The very small number of deaths makes safety comparisons between different stages of pregnancy and types of procedures impossible on a one-year basis, so the comparisons shown in Table 18-1 are based on cumulative statistics. As you look at these statistics remember that the totals for cumulative years used to calculate these

TABLE 18-1
DEATHS FROM ABORTION BY TYPE OF PROCEDURE (1977–1982)

ABORTION PROCEDURE	DEATHS PER 100,000 PROCEDURES
Vacuum	0.6
D&E	3.2
Amniocentesis	
Prostaglandin	3.2
Saline	5.1
Hysterotomy/hysterectomy	58.5

SOURCE: Atrash HK, MacKay HT, Binkin NJ, et al: Legal abortion mortality in the United States: 1972-1982. *American Journal of Obstetrics and Gynecology* 156:605-612, 1987.

numbers are somewhat higher than the numbers would be today. Abortion has gradually become safer over time.

By far the most important factor that determines abortion safety is how early in pregnancy you have your procedure. The risk of complications and death increases with each week of delay (see Illustration 18-10). Risks are lowest for early vacuum procedures.

Most abortion complications are mild and respond promptly to treatment. Problems can occasionally be serious and can cause permanent damage to your reproductive organs or even require surgical removal of your uterus, tubes, and ovaries. Infection and incomplete abortion are the most common complications.

INFECTION

Infection in the uterus and/or fallopian tubes usually causes persistent cramps and abdominal pain that become worse over time. Fever, vaginal discharge, and general fatigue can also be symptoms of infection. Signs of infection most often begin 24 to 36 hours after abortion or even later. Rapidly developing infections with symptoms in the first 24 hours occasionally occur as well.

You are the single most important factor in minimizing the seriousness of infection. Be alert to the early signs of infection, take your temperature regularly, and seek immediate care as soon as you suspect infection; chances are good the infection can be stopped before it becomes a serious threat if it is treated early. Infection can usually be controlled with antibiotic pills and rest at home if it is confined to your uterus. Serious infection may require treatment with intravenous antibiotics in the hospital. Even if infection subsides with antibiotic treatment, it can cause permanent scarring or obstruction of your fallopian tubes, and you may find it difficult or impossible to become pregnant in the future.

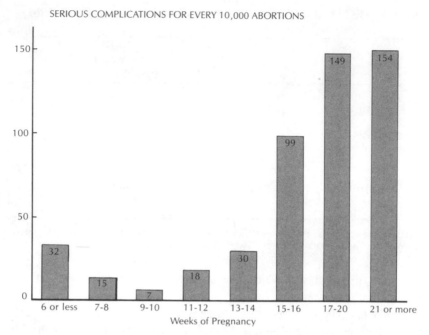

SERIOUS COMPLICATIONS FOR EVERY 10,000 ABORTIONS

Weeks of Pregnancy

ILLUSTRATION 18-10 The risk of serious complications with abortion is lowest at about seven to nine weeks of pregnancy; thereafter the *risk increases with each week surgery is delayed.* Serious complications shown here include severe infection, bleeding heavy enough to require transfusion, or problems that require further surgery. Risks are quite low for healthy women: overall, at least 99.6% of women who have abortion procedures have no serious complications. (*Induced Abortion, A World Review, 1983* (ed 5). New York: The Population Council, 1983.)

The risk of infection is increased if all fetal and placental tissues are not completely removed during abortion. If your surgeon suspects that you have retained tissue or if your infection does not respond promptly to antibiotics, you may need to have a repeat vacuum aspiration procedure to be sure that your uterus is empty.

Infection risk is also increased if you have gonorrhea or a cervical infection caused by chlamydia or other bacteria. **If you suspect that you may have been exposed to a sexually transmitted infection, get the tests and treatment you need before your abortion.** Be careful to avoid exposure to infection after your abortion, especially for the first four weeks.

INCOMPLETE ABORTION

Incomplete abortion means that you have retained fetal or placental tissue in your uterus.

Bleeding and strong cramping can alert you to incomplete abortion. The absence of fever and malaise distinguish this problem from infection; however, your risk of infection is increased if you have retained pregnancy tissue.

Incomplete abortion can also mean that your pregnancy is not terminated. You may continue to have symptoms of pregnancy such as fatigue, nausea, and breast soreness. You may have less postabortion bleeding than would be expected. Other women with continuing pregnancy have no symptoms at all.

Your most important assurance that your abortion was complete is a normal uterus at the time of your follow-up examination, so be sure to keep your follow-up appointment. If your abortion is incomplete, your surgeon probably failed to empty your uterus completely. Since she/he cannot see inside your uterus during abortion, this is an understandable possibility. Occasionally, incomplete abortion means that you have an ectopic pregnancy, twin pregnancy, or an abnormal uterine shape.

Your surgeon will repeat your vacuum procedure or perform a D&C under general anesthesia (see Chapter 47).

About 1 in 1,000 women who have early vacuum procedures experience another more immediate form of incomplete abortion: accumulation of blood clots in the uterus during the first few hours after abortion. This complication, called "re-do" syndrome, causes severe, progressive cramps that begin within the first few hours after an abortion procedure and subside as soon as the clots are removed by a repeat vacuum procedure.

HEMORRHAGE

Excessive bleeding during or after abortion can occur with any of the abortion procedures, but hemorrhage is minimized when your surgeon uses local anesthesia for early abortion; general anesthesia can decrease the strength of normal uterine contractions, which help stop bleeding.

Hemorrhage is a more frequent complication of late abortion procedures with prostaglandin, urea, or saline. Saline can temporarily alter blood coagulation factors. Bleeding is most likely to occur during the actual abortion process while you are in the hospital, so immediate removal of remaining pregnancy tissue, uterine scraping, and uterine massage can usually stop the bleeding effectively. Blood transfusions are sometimes necessary to replace the blood that you have lost.

Hemorrhage risk is increased if you have a bleeding disorder or take medication that alters blood coagulation. Large doses of aspirin for a long period of time can cause excessive bleeding, and blood-thinning medications (anticoagulants) have a similar effect.

Excessive bleeding after abortion is rare. Heavy or prolonged bleeding may indicate incomplete abortion, a tear in your cervix or uterus, or inadequate uterine contraction. Your surgeon needs to investigate and treat your excessive bleeding at once.

INJURY TO THE CERVIX, UTERUS, OR OTHER ABDOMINAL ORGANS

Actual uterine perforation is very rare, but damage to the cervix, uterus, and lower abdominal organs can occur any time instruments are inserted into the uterine cavity. A puncture wound in your uterus caused by an abortion instrument is likely to close spontaneously and heal without treatment. If nearby organs such as the bladder, rectum, intestines, or major arteries or veins are injured by the puncture, however, emergency surgery to repair the damage will be necessary. Even if you have no evidence of internal damage, your surgeon may want you to be hospitalized for observation if she/he suspects that you have a perforation.

Injury to the cervix is a more common problem than perforation and can occur with both early vacuum and later procedures. The cervical clamp used in vacuum abortion and D&E can tear your cervix, and you may need stitches to control bleeding. Tearing of the cervix can also occur as a result of forceful labor contractions with saline, urea, or prostaglandin abortion. Cervical injury may be a cause of miscarriage (spontaneous abortion) and premature delivery in future pregnancies.

ADVERSE REACTIONS TO DRUGS

Rash, hives, difficulty in breathing, heart arrest, or even death can be caused by drug reactions, but allergy to the drugs used in abortion procedures is rare.

Local Anesthetics. Be sure to inform your physician if you have ever had a reaction to local anesthetics such as dental Novocain. You may be able to have a different type of local anesthetic, or general anesthesia may be recommended. Heart rhythm changes and seizures can occur when drug reactions are severe.

Tetracycline. For some people, taking tetracycline can trigger severe skin rash on areas of the body exposed to sunlight. Avoid sunbathing or sunburn when you are taking this drug. Severe allergy reactions are rare.

Ampicillin or Amoxicillin. These antibiotics are chemically similar to penicillin. If you are allergic to penicillin you should avoid them as well. Be sure your physician is aware of your allergy so an alternative antibiotic can be prescribed.

Methergine. This drug is sometimes prescribed after abortion to stimulate contraction of the uterus. Some women find that it causes excessive cramping. Consult your physician if cramps are severe. Methergine can also cause a rise in blood pressure that would be especially dangerous for a person who already had high blood pressure.

Saline. Saline does not cause allergic reactions, but an adverse reaction can occur if it is absorbed too rapidly or is injected accidentally into the bloodstream or uterine muscle. Excessive levels of saline in the bloodstream can cause rapid absorption of fluid; in severe cases this can cause coma or death. Retention of extra fluid in the lungs or circulation can also cause heart strain that would be hazardous for a woman with preexisting heart disease. Concentrated saline can destroy muscle tissue if it is accidentally injected directly into the muscle itself.

Prostaglandin. If prostaglandin is absorbed too rapidly into the bloodstream, it can cause difficulty in breathing (much like an asthma attack), rapid heart rate, change in blood pressure, and immediate strong contractions of the uterus, intestine, and stomach. These symptoms usually subside within a few minutes and usually do not require treatment. Prostaglandin commonly causes nausea, vomiting, and diarrhea. Many surgeons routinely prescribe additional medications to counteract these effects.

Oxytocin. In addition to causing strong uterine contractions, this hormone causes the kidneys to retain fluid. Large amounts of oxytocin over a period of many hours can cause serious brain swelling, coma, and convulsions.

EFFECTS OF ABORTION ON FUTURE FERTILITY

Abortion **complications** can clearly jeopardize your future fertility. Infection can scar and block your fallopian tubes, or an injured cervix can be the cause of miscarriage (spontaneous abortion) and premature delivery in future pregnancies. This problem, called incompetent cervix, can be treated by placing a temporary tie (cerclage) on the cervix to hold it closed during pregnancy. The tie is removed when pregnancy reaches full term or when labor begins.

Complications like these are rare, however, and it may be that the statistics on overall long-term effects will never be able to measure the impact of such problems on overall future fertility, even though the impact is clear for an individual woman who has had a serious complication.

Overall fertility rates for women who have had abortions in the past have been studied by many researchers. Statistics from Europe and Japan reported in the 1960s caused worry about reduced future fertility and problems like miscarriage, especially for women who had had multiple abortions. More recent studies, however, have not found these problems, and reports from the United States have been quite reassuring. One study of 5,003 pregnancy records showed that women who reported one previous induced abortion had no higher rates for prematurity, low birth weight, placenta problems, or newborn abnormalities than women who had never had an abortion (10). Another study of 3,100 women followed for 3 1/2 years found that subsequent pregnancy rates for women who began the study after an induced abortion were no lower than pregnancy rates for women who began the study after full term pregnancy or after attending a gynecology clinic (11). A detailed 1982 review of U.S. and international research in this area identified 7 major studies of fertility after abortion, and only one of the studies found a link between abortion and subsequent fertility problems (12).

Research on patients with fertility problems also provides some reassurance. One 1985 U.S. study compared previous abortion rates among patients with damaged tubes to previous abortion rates for women who conceived successfully and found that both groups reported similar numbers of previous abortions (13). Researchers studying miscarriage rates for 31,900 women in California, however, found that women with one or more previous induced abortions had higher rates of miscarriage late in pregnancy than did other women. They also showed that the excess risk had decreased over time and concluded that improvements in abortion techniques, with more gentle dilation, for example, might explain the drop in risk (14). It may be that significant differences in techniques used for abortion explain why research results 20 years ago from other countries found fertility effects that are no longer evident.

Overall, the effects of one or even multiple abortions on future fertility are probably small except for the very rare woman who has severe complications. Research is not entirely clear-cut, but if abortion did cause a significant overall decrease in fertility, the research already completed should have been able to detect it.

Contraindications

A contraindication is a medical condition that renders inadvisable or unsafe a procedure that might otherwise be recommended. **There are no true contraindications to abortion.** Any medical problem that might make abortion risky would make continuing pregnancy even more dangerous.

Your surgeon will consider certain medical issues as she/he advises you about the safest abortion procedure for you, and decides whether you need to be hospitalized for your procedure.

• If you are allergic to local anesthesia, then general anesthesia may be recommended
• If you have severe anemia, a bleeding disorder, asthma, heart disease, diabetes, epilepsy that is not well controlled, or an orthopedic problem, a hospital may be safer
• If you have an emotional disorder that might interfere with your ability to be calm and cooperative during a local anesthesia procedure, you and your surgeon may prefer general anesthesia
• If your surgeon is unable to determine exact dates for your pregnancy because of obesity or tense muscles during your exam, she/he may want you to have a sonogram (a test to measure your pregnancy size; see Chapter 4) or may suggest general anesthesia for your procedure. General anesthesia permits her/him to examine you when your muscles are completely relaxed and may make it easier to perform a vacuum or D&E abortion.

- If you have serious heart or kidney disease, your surgeon will probably avoid saline, because you could have serious complications if the saline caused abnormal fluid retention
- If you have an active pelvic infection, your surgeon will probably recommend that abortion be temporarily delayed while your infection is treated
- Your surgeon will avoid prostaglandin if you have a known allergy to the drug or if you have medical problems that may be aggravated by prostaglandin such as high blood pressure, asthma, heart disease, lung disease, epilepsy, or glaucoma

Caring for Yourself After Abortion

You may eat or drink anything you like and return to most of your normal activities as soon as you feel like it. Most women find it best to avoid especially strenuous exercise for a few days. Be guided by how you feel.

Most women have some cramps and vaginal bleeding during the first couple of weeks. If your bleeding is heavier than on the heaviest day of a normal menstrual period and persists more than a day or two, call your clinician. It is not unusual to have spotting as long as four weeks after abortion. Spotting may stop completely and then start up again several days later. As your hormone levels drop after abortion, you may find that your bleeding becomes heavier after the first three or four days. Some women have no bleeding at all, or only a brown-tinged discharge.

Severe cramps are not normal. Arrange to see your clinician if your cramps are persistent or if you have pain that becomes progressively more severe.

Your first normal period should begin in four to six weeks. If you are taking birth control Pills, your first period will come at the end of your first pack. **It is possible to become pregnant again even before your first period begins.** If you want to avoid another pregnancy, begin using a method of birth control as soon as you begin having intercourse again.

No one will be able to tell for sure that you have had an abortion. In the rare event that your cervix is damaged during the procedure, it may have scar tissue after it heals. A clinician who examines you in the future might see the scar and surmise that you have had an abortion.

DO'S AND DON'TS

- Be sure that you have a 24-hour emergency telephone number to call in case you have problems
- Take your temperature carefully each morning and late afternoon for a full week, and any time you feel warm or have chills. If you are taking aspirin or an aspirin substitute, record your temperature **before** you take each dose. Call your physician if your temperature is 100.4 degrees (Fahrenheit) by mouth, or higher.

• Do not have intercourse for the first two weeks
• Do not douche for two weeks
• Use sanitary pads only. No tampons for the first two weeks.
• Baths, showers, and shampoos are fine
• If you develop breast milk after abortion, wear a snug bra day and night for two or three days and avoid any stimulation of your nipples. Squeezing milk from your breast will result in increased milk flow.
• Keep your appointment for your follow-up exam in two weeks

ANTIBIOTICS

Some clinics and surgeons provide antibiotic treatment with abortion as a routine part of care and some do not. If you have had previous pelvic infection involving your uterus and fallopian tubes, antibiotic treatment is especially reasonable. It is also advised if you have damaged heart valves or an artificial heart valve; you should take antibiotics before and after any surgery including dental work.

Research on routine antibiotics for healthy women undergoing abortion is somewhat contradictory. Reviewing the research evidence available, however, experts at the Centers for Disease Control have concluded that short-term treatment with an antibiotic such as tetracycline is probably desirable (15). Tetracycline causes few serious side effects, and may help reduce infection rates after abortion. Ideally this type of prophylactic antibiotic treatment should begin a few hours before surgery (or immediately after surgery if earlier treatment isn't feasible), and should be stopped after 24 hours or so.

Antibiotic treatment before and immediately after abortion also may be recommended for women who have serious heart valve disorders to prevent heart valve infection (endocarditis). The risk of endocarditis after abortion is probably lower than the risk after dental procedures, but antibiotic treatment may be reasonable if your heart problem is serious or if there is any question about active infection involving your cervix or uterus when the abortion is performed (16). If you have had endocarditis in the past or have rheumatic heart disease, congenital heart abnormalities, an artificial heart valve, or mitral valve prolapse, discuss the pros and cons of antibiotic treatment with your heart specialist and with your surgeon before your abortion is scheduled.

MEDICATION INSTRUCTIONS

Make sure you have written instructions for any medications you will take at home, and be sure to take your medication on schedule.

Methergine.   This drug, a preparation of methylergonovine, is sometimes prescribed for the first 24 to 48 hours after surgery to maintain firm uterine contractions. If you

---

18:11   DANGER SIGNS AFTER ABORTION

Fever (temperature over 100.4 degrees F.)

Chills or malaise (fatigue, aching)

Cramping or persistent abdominal pain that is progressively more severe

Abdominal tenderness with pressure or activity such as walking, coughing, or jumping

Prolonged or heavy bleeding that lasts more than 3 weeks, or is heavier than a heavy menstrual flow for 3 days or more

Unusual or foul-smelling vaginal discharge

Allergy symptoms such as rash, hives, asthma, or difficulty in breathing

Your first menstrual period does not begin within 6 weeks

Contact your clinician at once or go to a hospital emergency room if you develop any of these symptoms after surgery.

have severe cramps or pain radiating down to your thighs, call your clinician. She/he may want you to stop Methergine to reduce your cramping.

Tetracycline.   While you are taking this antibiotic, avoid antacids, milk, and milk products for two hours before and after each dose, and do not sunbathe. Tetracycline can cause skin rash with sun exposure.

Pain Medications.   If your cramps are so severe that aspirin or an aspirin substitute does not relieve your pain, call your clinician. Usually, two or three aspirin tablets every three to four hours will provide good pain relief.

DANGER SIGNS

Be alert to the danger signs of serious trouble shown in Illustration 18-11. Prompt medical attention can mean that a minor problem never becomes a major problem. Call your clinician at once if you develop any of the danger signs.

BIRTH CONTROL

I don't like taking the Pill. But I don't want to do this again either (patting her stomach).

—ABORTION CLINIC PATIENT, 27

Most surgeons or clinic counselors discuss contraception with abortion patients and can prescribe a method of birth control at the time of abortion. If you choose a diaphragm, sponges, condoms, or foam, be sure to use them as soon as you begin having intercourse. If you choose birth control Pills, you can take your first Pill the first Sunday after your abortion. A Pill pack started any time within the first seven days after your abortion should provide good birth control protection even during your first cycle.

Plan for and be prepared to use birth control immediately after an abortion. Ovulation usually returns two or three weeks after abortion, but some women may ovulate within a week or ten days and another pregnancy is entirely possible.

YOUR EMOTIONS

It is normal to have strong emotional feelings after abortion.

I still think it's—unnatural—to just erase it like that. I feel all washed out. I had intercourse just one time without protection.

—WOMAN, 22

You may be sad; angry at your partner; angry at yourself; uncertain that you did the right thing. It will probably comfort you to remember that you made the best decision you could at the time.

You may be feeling particularly dismayed if this is not your first abortion. Be sure to read the section entitled "Repeat Abortion" in Chapter 16. The need for repeat abortion is not at all uncommon, so you are not alone. Having one pregnancy means that a woman is more fertile than average, and has a greater risk than average for having another unplanned pregnancy in the future (17). This is true if she takes the same precautions and "chances" with intercourse that an average woman takes. Repeat abortion does not prove that the woman has deep psychological problems, or is unusually careless.

Many women express a sense of relief after an abortion, and the overall emotional impact of abortion can be positive.

It was such a relief to have the whole thing over with, the worrying and tension, and dreading the surgery. The abortion did hurt, but it wasn't as bad as I had expected. I did feel sad as well, but mostly just relieved.

—WOMAN, 28

From in-depth psychological interviews with vacuum abortion patients, researchers found that six months later about half felt that the experience had had positive effects, such as personal growth or improvement in family relations; about 10% had negative reactions, such as guilt or fear of men; and about 25% had no change in their feelings at all (18). Another study compared women who had vacuum abortion with women who completed pregnancy and found no significant psychological differences between the groups one year later (19).

SUGGESTED READING

Benderly, Beryl Lieff: *Thinking About Abortion—An Essential Handbook for the Woman Who Wants to Come to Terms with What Abortion Means in Her Life.* Garden City: Dial Press, 1984. A thoughtful and probing book with special emphasis on ethical and moral issues that are painful for many women.

Consaro, Maria, and Korzeniowski, Carole: *A Woman's Guide to Safe Abortion.* New York: Holt, Rinehart & Winston, 1983. Slightly less detailed and easier to read information, in a less academic style.

Dornblaser, Carole, and Landy, Uta: *The Abortion Guide: A Handbook for Women and Men.* New York: Playboy Paperbacks, 1982. Clear and detailed information on all aspects of abortion; an invaluable resource in selecting a clinic or physician. Personal, ethical, and legal issues are included.

RESOURCES

National Abortion Federation
900 Pennsylvania Avenue, SE
Washington, D.C. 20003
Office: 1-202-546-9060 Hotline: 1-800-772-9100
The NAF Hotline can provide information on services in your area, 9:30 A.M. to 5:30 P.M. EST.

Planned Parenthood Regional Offices
Western Region
333 Broadway, 3rd Floor
San Francisco, California 94133 (1-415-956-8856)

Southern Region
3030 Peachtree Road, NW, Room 303
Atlanta, Georgia 30305 (1-404-262-1128)

Washington Office
2010 Massachusetts Avenue, NW, Suite 500
Washington, D.C. 20036 (1-202-785-3351)

Northern Region
2625 Butterfield Road
Oakbrook, Illinois 60521 (1-312-986-9270)

National Office
810 Seventh Avenue
New York, New York 10019 (1-212-541-7800)

REFERENCES

1. Centers for Disease Control: *Abortion Surveillance 1981.* U.S. Department of Health and Human Services, Public Health Service. Issued November 1985.
2. Cates W Jr, Schulz KF, Grimes DA, et al: The effect of delay and method choice on the risk of abortion morbidity. *Family Planning Perspectives* 9:266–273, 1977.
3. Hern WM: *Abortion Practice.* Philadelphia: J.B. Lippincott Co., 1984.
4. MacKay HT, Schulz KF, Grimes DA: Safety of local versus general anesthesia for second-trimester dilatation and evacuation abortion. *Obstetrics and Gynecology* 66:661–665, 1985.
5. Prevention of Rh sensitizations, report of a World Health Organization group. *WHO Technical Report* Ser No 468, 1971.
6. Stewart F, Burnhill MS, Bozorgi N: Reduced dose of Rh immunoglobulin following first trimester pregnancy termination. *Obstetrics and Gynecology* 51:318–322, 1978.
7. Foster HW Jr, Smith M, McGruder CE, et al: Postconception menses induction using prostaglandin vaginal suppositories. *Obstetrics and Gynecology* 65:682–685, 1985.
8. Atrash HK, MacKay HT, Binkin NJ, et al: Legal abortion mortality in the United States: 1972 to 1982. *American Journal of Obstetrics and Gynecology* 156:605–612, 1987.
9. Centers for Disease Control: Fatality and illness associated with consumption of pennyroyal oil—Colorado. *Morbidity and Mortality Weekly Report* 27:511–512, 1978.
10. Schoenbaum SC, Monson RR, Stubblefield PG, et al: Outcome of the delivery following an induced or spontaneous abortion. *American Journal of Obstetrics and Gynecology* 136:19–24, 1980.
11. Stubblefield PG, Monson RR, Schoenbaum SC: Fertility after induced abortion: A prospective follow-up study. *Obstetrics and Gynecology* 63:186–193, 1984.
12. Hogue CJ, Cates W Jr, Tietze C: The effects of induced abortion on subsequent reproduction. *Epidemiologic Reviews* 4:66–94, 1982.
13. Daling JR, Weiss NS, Voigt L, et al: Tubal infertility in relation to prior induced abortion. *Fertility and Sterility* 43:389–394, 1985.
14. Harlap S, Shiono PH, Ramcharan S, et al: A prospective study of spontaneous fetal losses after induced abortions. *New England Journal of Medicine* 301:677–681, 1979.
15. Grimes DA, Schulz KF, Cates W Jr: Prophylactic antibiotics for curettage abortion. *American Journal of Obstetrics and Gynecology* 150:689–694, 1984.
16. Seaworth BJ, Durack DT: Infective endocarditis in obstetric and gynecologic practice. *American Journal of Obstetrics and Gynecology* 154:180–188, 1986.
17. Tietze C: The "problem" of repeat abortion. *Family Planning Perspectives* 6:148–150, 1974.
18. Margolis AJ, Davison LA, Hason KH, et al: Therapeutic abortion followup study. *American Journal of Obstetrics and Gynecology* 110:243–249, 1971.
19. Athanasiou R, Oppel W, Michelson L, et al: Psychiatric sequelae to term birth and induced early and late abortion: A longitudinal study. *Family Planning Perspectives* 5:227–231, 1973.

19

❖

Making a Decision About Sterilization

Healthy American men are fertile essentially throughout life, and healthy American women are fertile until about age 51. Most women have completed their childbearing by age 30 to 35, so as a culture, we have many more years of fertility than we need.

Surgical sterilization—tubal sterilization for women or vasectomy for men—is the most popular method of birth control among married couples in the United States. Sterilization offers an extremely high level of effectiveness and the surgical procedures are simple and quick, with few complications and side effects.

The key word with sterilization is permanence. *If there is any chance you might want a pregnancy in the future, you are not ready for a tubal sterilization or a vasectomy. The increasing number of men and women who would like surgery to reverse a previous sterilization shows that the decision about sterilization may be difficult, and needs to be made carefully.*

A couple contemplating sterilization should consider both vasectomy and tubal sterilization. If the two are equally acceptable, the medical recommendation would be vasectomy. Compared to other common kinds of surgery, both vasectomy and tubal ligation are relatively safe, but vasectomy is safer, simpler, and cheaper than tubal sterilization.

Sterilization refers to any procedure that permanently prevents pregnancy, and *surgical* sterilization is the only common method of permanent birth control. (Certain drugs and radiation techniques can result in sterilization, but they are almost never used.)

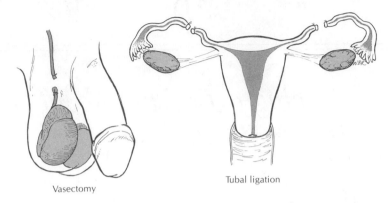

Vasectomy

Tubal ligation

ILLUSTRATION 19-1 Tubal sterilization interrupts the fallopian tubes. Vasectomy interrupts each of the two vas deferens.

Vasectomy is the sterilization operation for men. The vasectomy procedure severs and seals shut each of the two vas deferens, the tubes that transport sperm from the testicles to the penis. The parallel operation for women is called tubal sterilization. Tubal ligation is another term commonly used; it is not a technically accurate term, however, since cautery, clips, or rings are used for tubal closure more often than ligation (tying) with suture thread. Tubal sterilization can be carried out with any one of four common surgical operations; the goal is to block the fallopian tubes, which allow sperm to reach and fertilize an egg from the ovaries. Fertilization almost always occurs in the outer third of the fallopian tube, farthest from the uterus.

None of the sterilization operations involves surgery on the sex glands themselves. The testicles or ovaries continue to produce hormones, and there is no chemical or medical reason to expect a change in sex drive. Male and female sex hormones are carried in the bloodstream, not in the tubes. Sterilization surgery simply blocks transport of egg cells or sperm cells, and when egg and sperm don't meet, pregnancy can't begin (see Illustration 19-1).

Other kinds of surgery can result in sterilization: hysterectomy (removal of the uterus) for women, and in some cases, prostate surgery for men. When sterilization is the primary or sole purpose of surgery, however, these operations will not be recommended, because they involve a higher complication risk than vasectomy or tubal sterilization.

History of Sterilization

Hippocrates described sterilization procedures in ancient Greece. However, wide availability and popularity of surgical sterilization are recent phenomena, partly because of

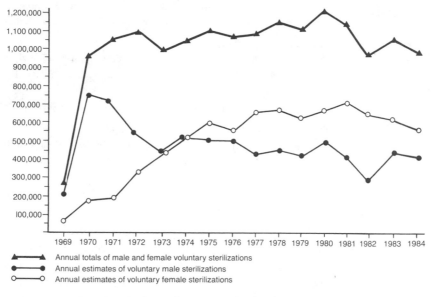

1,200,000
1,100 000
1,000,000
900,000
800,000
700,000
600,000
500,000
400,000
300,000
200,000
100,000

1969 1970 1971 1972 1973 1974 1975 1976 1977 1978 1979 1980 1981 1982 1983 1984

▲——————▲ Annual totals of male and female voluntary sterilizations
●——————● Annual estimates of voluntary male sterilizations
○——————○ Annual estimates of voluntary female sterilizations

ILLUSTRATION 19-2   Surgical sterilization is the leading method of birth
control used by married couples in the United States. These totals,
compiled by the Association for Voluntary Surgical Contraception, do not
include hysterectomies.

the moral and religious restrictions on all forms of birth control that dominated
Western medicine until after World War II, and partly because all surgery was quite
risky until 30 to 40 years ago. Better anesthesia, antibiotics, blood transfusions, and
improved surgical techniques have greatly decreased surgical risks in general. More
than 1 million sterilization procedures have been performed in the United States every
year since 1973 (see Illustration 19-2).

Simple tubal ligation—closing the fallopian tubes with suture thread—was the
earliest sterilization procedure for women, and was described in Western medical
journals in 1880 (1). This technique often failed to prevent pregnancy and has been
replaced with other techniques that add destruction or removal of part of each
fallopian tube to the suturing or ligation approach.

"Band-Aid" surgery, or laparoscopic tubal sterilization, was introduced on a large
scale in the late 1960s. The laparoscope is a tube equipped with light and magnification lenses. It is inserted into your abdomen through a 1-inch incision so that your
surgeon can see your uterus and tubes and seal your tubes with a cauterizing
(burning) instrument, or with rings or clips. Some 200,000 laparoscopic tubal
sterilizations are performed in the United States each year.

Mini-laparotomy is the newest tubal ligation technique. Miniature laparotomy calls
for a 1- to 1 1/2-inch abdominal incision, does not require sophisticated instruments
such as a laparoscope, and can be performed with local or general anesthesia. Your

surgeon simply lifts each fallopian tube out through the small incision, cuts and seals the tubes, and drops the tubes back inside. Mini-laparotomy experience in the United States is limited.

Vasectomy was first described in the late 1890s. It is a simple procedure that is usually done in the physician's office or clinic with local anesthesia. Techniques for ligating (tying) and/or removing a small section of each vas vary slightly, but usually one or two 1/2-inch incisions just through the skin of the scrotum are all that is required. About 5 million vasectomies have been performed in the United States since 1975, and the vast experience with this procedure means that the success rates and immediate complications are well understood. Long-term complications are still under investigation (see Chapter 21).

New sterilization techniques are being developed, and liquid silicone to form a plug that seals the fallopian tubes is already being used in experimental programs. Techniques for closing the tubal openings inside the uterus and for covering the open ends of the tubes are in early stages of investigation. Experimental vasectomy techniques for closing the vas with plugs or valves are under study. The hope is that one or several of these techniques will prove to be more reversible and/or safer than present techniques. Research experience to date is limited, and a real breakthrough in **reversible** sterilization is not likely for some time—probably years.

Effectiveness

Vasectomy and tubal ligation procedures have fewer failures than any of the temporary birth control methods. Overall, the failure rate of commonly used sterilization surgery procedures is about half a percent or less (2).

Many tubal sterilization "failures" actually represent pregnancies that began just before surgery, and many vasectomy "failures" represent pregnancies that began after surgery but before the man's reproductive tract was cleared of sperm. True failures do occur, however, with both vasectomy and tubal ligation, and may be caused by incomplete tubal closure, accidental ligation of a ligament instead of a tube, the presence of an extra tube, an opening or fistula, or regrowth of a tube. Table 19-1 lists typical effectiveness rates for the different sterilization procedures. As you compare rates here with rates for other birth control options, remember that failure rates for temporary birth control methods are for one year of use. Sterilization failure rates are calculated per 1,000 individuals as a one-time risk. A diaphragm failure rate of 2% means that 20 pregnancies occur each year for every 1,000 diaphragm users (two pregnancies for each 100 women); so over a period of five years 100 diaphragm pregnancies would occur. If 1,000 couples rely on vasectomy or tubal sterilization for five years, however, the total number of pregnancies would be 1 to 5.

Reported pregnancy rates after sterilization surgery vary, but it makes sense to select a surgeon who is experienced so your risk for complications or failure will probably be low and your likelihood of pregnancy prevention high.

TABLE 19-1
PREGNANCIES AFTER STERILIZATION SURGERY

STERILIZATION PROCEDURE	PREGNANCIES PER 1,000 PROCEDURES
Vasectomy	2
Laparoscopic tubal sterilization	3
Vaginal or postpartum tubal sterilization	3
Mini-laparotomy tubal sterilization	1–5

SOURCES: Smith GL, Taylor GP, Smith KF: Comparative risks and costs of male and female sterilization. *American Journal of Public Health* 75:370–374, 1985.
Liskin L, Rinehart W: Minilaparotomy and laparoscopy: Safe, effective, and widely used. *Population Reports* Ser C, No 9, May 1985. Baltimore: Johns Hopkins University.

Deciding About Sterilization

Making your own decision about sterilization involves both logical and emotional factors. It is a very personal decision for the man or woman considering surgery, and it is a joint decision for a couple. Feelings deserve full consideration along with facts, and it is important that your decision be made without subtle or overt pressure. **It is a permanent decision**: feelings of regret after sterilization are more likely among people who had misgivings about the surgery beforehand.

If you are uncomfortable about abortion, the effectiveness of sterilization may be its most important advantage for you. Remember that even if 100 couples of average fertility are able to use temporary birth control methods diligently at a 2% failure level, about 10 of the couples will experience at least one unwanted pregnancy every five years.

I had thought about having a tubal ligation after Toni was born, but I wasn't really sure how I would feel if she turned out to have some kind of problem. I didn't worry much about it until I thought I was pregnant *again*. After that scare my mind was made up. I just couldn't see having to worry for the next 20 years.

—WOMAN, 30

Some childless individuals and couples choose sterilization. Concern about serious inherited diseases may be a deciding factor for some. For others, the decision is strictly personal. Some people simply don't want children. Other couples believe that adoption is a more attractive alternative than childbearing. (The number of healthy infants available for adoption is very small compared to the number of couples trying to adopt. The adoption outlook is better for couples who are willing to accept responsibility for older children, children from other ethnic backgrounds or nationalities, or children with known handicaps.)

Most clinicians and sterilization counselors encourage a substantial "thinking-it-over" period if you are very young or have not had children, **because they fear that you may regret your decision later on.** There is no doubt that life situations, feelings, and hopes change over time for most people. Significant changes are a natural part of youth, especially, and clinicians see many patients who request surgery to reconnect the fallopian tubes or vas deferens. **Reversal surgery is not something to count on.** Its success depends on the type of sterilization surgery done initially, and an attempt at reversal may not even be recommended (see the last section in this chapter).

There are no simple formulas for predicting future regret. Regret is not common. Overall at least 90% to 99% of women and men in follow-up studies after sterilization do not regret the decision, and only a small proportion request later reversal (3,4). One study of women seeking tubal reconstruction surgery, however, did find that these women had undergone sterilization at a younger age, with fewer live children than had a comparison group of satisfied sterilization patients (3). In this study the most common reason for reversal was remarriage. In the United States remarriage is also the most common reason given when men seek vasectomy reversal.

Consider your own feelings about the impact of the following major life changes or tragedies before you make a final sterilization decision.

• **Divorce, remarriage, and desire for childbearing with new spouse.** One third to one half of all marriages now end in divorce.
• **Death of a spouse or child.** About 45 out of 100,000 children aged 1 to 15 die in the United States each year (5).
• **A future partner who strongly desires children.** Even if you are fairly sure that you do not want any (or any more) children, would your feelings be altered if a future partner had strong feelings about the issue?

WHICH OF YOU SHOULD BE STERILIZED?

If you have a stable relationship with your partner and each of you feels comfortable about sterilization, vasectomy makes sense as a first choice because it is a less complex procedure than tubal sterilization, has a lower risk of complications, and costs less (2). In many cases, however, one partner (often the woman) will feel more certain about not wanting children in the future than will the other partner, perhaps because pregnancy, childbearing, and parenting can have a different impact on men and women. Often a woman is ready for a sterilization decision several years before her partner.

Hysterectomy can be an appropriate choice if you want to be sterilized and you also have a serious pelvic disease that is likely to require surgery at some future time. For example, if you have severe uterine fibroid tumors that cause pain or heavy bleeding, you might choose hysterectomy rather than tubal ligation now and hysterectomy later. Base your decision on a thorough medical assessment of the likelihood of your future problems and on your own feelings about your alternatives. Your risk of complications with hysterectomy is significantly greater than with tubal ligation, and recovery from surgery will require at least six weeks. Hysterectomy is not a reasonable choice unless there are **good reasons for hysterectomy apart from your desire for sterilization.**

Sometimes the argument is made that hysterectomy for sterilization is justified because hysterectomy eliminates the risk of your developing cancer of the uterus or cervix later on. Detailed analysis of this argument indicates, however, that the overall risk of hysterectomy is too high to justify the operation as a preventive measure.

Legal Aspects of Sterilization

Sterilization surgery historically has been subject to many legal restrictions. Court decisions and laws have struck down many restrictions, and each person has the right to sterilization without having to meet arbitrary qualifications. No state or hospital can impose rigid standards for age, marital status, or previous childbearing. The sterilization decision is up to the person and her/his clinician.

Private hospitals may, if they choose, decline to perform sterilization surgery. Similarly, no surgeon can be compelled to perform sterilization surgery if she/he feels that sterilization is not appropriate in a particular case, or if she/he is opposed to sterilization on religious grounds. Many clinicians are reluctant to consider sterilization for very young or childless patients, but it has become easier to find surgeons willing to respect a patient's sterilization wishes. Your local health department or Planned Parenthood agency may be able to help you with referrals in your community.

You do not have to obtain your spouse's consent if you want to be sterilized. Many hospitals and surgeons, however, **will** ask your spouse to sign a consent form whenever possible. Obviously it is desirable for you and your partner to agree about sterilization, but legally you can make a sterilization decision on your own even if you are married.

Sterilization services for persons under 21 years old are indirectly limited by current federal funding policies, because federal funds cannot be used to pay for sterilization for minors. If you rely on federally subsidized health funds such as welfare or Medicaid, you will not be able to have sterilization surgery through the program until you are 21.

Federally funded health programs also impose special requirements, including a 30-day waiting period, to be sure that each person has given truly informed consent before sterilization surgery. The regulations establish seven steps for consent, and you have a right to all this information before your surgery:

- A full explanation of the procedure
- A description of the possible risks and side effects, including all major life-threatening risks and all common minor risks
- A description of the benefits you can expect
- An explanation of alternative methods of birth control and of the impact of the sterilization procedure, including the fact that you must consider it irreversible
- An offer to answer any questions about the procedure
- A reminder that you are free to withhold or withdraw your consent at any time without prejudicing your future care, and without the loss of other health or welfare benefits to which you might otherwise be entitled
- Written documentation of informed consent, which you yourself must sign

Surgery to Reverse Sterilization

Despite advances in surgical techniques, sterilization reversal still remains an uncertain and costly medical procedure.

For men who have undergone vasectomy, reversal surgery (called vasovasostomy) is a 1 1/2- to 3-hour procedure that often requires general anesthesia. The best results have been reported for surgery done with an operating microscope and very delicate surgical techniques called "microsurgery." The most successful surgeons, using microsurgery, report that 95% of their vasovasostomy patients regain motile sperm, but that pregnancy rates are somewhat lower: 45% to 79% (4). Success with vasovasostomy may depend on how extensive a portion of the vas was removed with the initial sterilization surgery, and whether or not the man has developed antisperm antibodies (see Chapter 21). In some cases the surgeon may even feel that an attempt at reversal is not worthwhile.

Surgery to rejoin the fallopian tubes after female sterilization—called tubal reanastomosis—is also most successful when microsurgery techniques are used. If success seems unlikely, because of the type of tubal ligation procedure originally performed or because of other medical problems, then reanastomosis surgery will not be recommended. As many as 70% of women considering reversal may be advised against it (6). Fallopian tube reanastomosis involves major abdominal surgery, general anesthesia, and hospitalization for five to six days.

Reported rates for successful pregnancy after microsurgery reanastomosis of the fallopian tubes range from about 50% to 80% (6). Reversal success is greatest when a woman has at least 6 cm (2 1/2 inches) of undamaged tube available for repair on each side (7). The type of sterilization procedure performed initially, therefore, influences later reversal success (see Chapter 20).

Ectopic (tubal) pregnancy risks are substantial after tubal reanastomosis surgery. As many as 5% to 25% of pregnancies conceived after reversal surgery are ectopic (7), so early confirmation of pregnancy and early pelvic examination are especially important (see Chapter 8 for information on ectopic pregnancy, including danger signs, and steps in diagnosing pregnancy).

REFERENCES

1. Bordahl PE: Tubal sterilization. A historical review. *Journal of Reproductive Medicine* 30:18–23, 1985.
2. Smith GL, Taylor GP, Smith KF: Comparative risks and costs of male and female sterilization. *American Journal of Public Health* 75:370–374, 1985.
3. Leader A, Galan N, George R, et al: A comparison of definable traits in women requesting reversal of sterilization and women satisfied with sterilization. *American Journal of Obstetrics and Gynecology* 145:198–202, 1983.
4. Liskin L: Male sterilization. *Population Reports*, Ser D, No 4, November–December 1983. Baltimore: Johns Hopkins University.
5. National Center for Health Statistics: Advance report of final mortality statistics, 1982. *Monthly Vital Statistics Report* Vol 33, No 9, Supplement. DHHS Pub No (PHS) 85–1120. Public Health Service. Hyattsville, Md., December 20, 1984.
6. Siegler AM, Hulka J, Peretz A: Reversibility of female sterilization. *Fertility and Sterility* 43:499–510, 1985.
7. Spivak MM, Librach CL, Rosenthal DM: Microsurgical reversal of sterilization: A six-year study. *American Journal of Obstetrics and Gynecology* 154:355–361, 1986.

20

Sterilization Operations for Women

Our son—and second child—was born when I was 31. I went back on Pills for about two years, then switched to a diaphragm, and then I said, "Now wait a minute! I'm 35 and I'll be fertile for 15 more years! Fifteen years of a diaphragm? No! No way!" I couldn't get Joe to have a vasectomy, so I got my tubes tied. Blessed relief.

—WOMAN, 40

There are four different operations that are commonly used to end fertility and interrupt or block a woman's fallopian tubes, and a fifth—tubal closure with silicone plugs—is being used on an experimental basis. Not all of the operations are appropriate for all women, so you will want to discuss the pros and cons of different options with your surgeon beforehand so that together you can choose the best and safest approach for you.

None of the currently available methods for female sterilization should be considered reversible, including the new plug techniques. Success with surgery to reverse a previous tubal sterilization is more likely for some sterilization methods than it is for others, and possible reversibility is one of the main reasons that the tubal plug procedure is being developed. Nonetheless, if you feel there is any chance you may want to have a pregnancy in the future, then you should not have sterilization surgery. There are no research data to show whether women who have had plugs removed do return to normal fertility, and reversal surgery after other tubal sterilization procedures is not something you can count on.

TABLE 20-1
STERILIZATION OPERATIONS FOR WOMEN

MINI-LAP STERILIZATION (MINI-LAPAROTOMY)

Performed: any time
Anesthesia: local or general
Incision: 1- to 2-inch horizontal incision just above the pubic hairline
Tube Closure Techniques: Pomeroy, clip, ring

LAPAROSCOPY STERILIZATION ("BAND-AID" SURGERY)

Performed: any time
Anesthesia: general or local
Incision: 1-inch horizontal incision just below the navel
Tube Closure Techniques: cautery, clip, ring

VAGINAL STERILIZATION

Performed: any time
Anesthesia: general, sometimes local
Incision: 2-inch incision inside the vagina
Tube Closure Techniques: Pomeroy, fimbriectomy, clip, ring

POSTPARTUM STERILIZATION
Performed: within 48 hours after delivery or at the time of cesarean
              section delivery
Anesthesia: general, spinal, or epidural; sometimes local
Incision: 1- to 2-inch horizontal incision just below the navel
Tube Closure Techniques: Pomeroy, fimbriectomy, Irving, clip, ring

---

Sterilization surgery does provide the most effective protection possible against pregnancy except for abstinence, but failures can occur. If an overdue period, breast tenderness, or other symptoms suggest possible pregnancy, then prompt evaluation is essential: ectopic (tubal) pregnancy rates are higher after sterilization than they are among women who conceive using other types of birth control.

The four operations shown in Table 20-1 differ in the type of surgery incision and/or equipment needed to gain access to the fallopian tubes. These are the commonly used surgery options when tubal sterilization is the main reason for surgery.

On occasion sterilization can also be carried out as an extra step when abdominal surgery (laparotomy; see Chapter 48) is needed for some other reason. Also, abdominal surgery is an option if other sterilization methods are inadvisable or impossible because of problems such as extensive pelvic scar tissue from previous infection or surgery. Abdominal tubal ligation requires general anesthesia, a 3- to 5-inch incision, and a

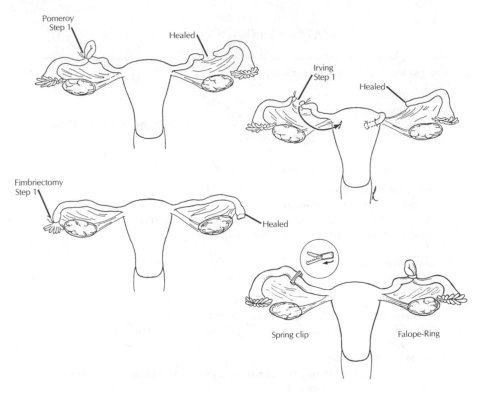

ILLUSTRATION 20-1   Common techniques for closing the fallopian tubes.

longer recovery period, but would otherwise be similar to a mini-lap or the postpartum sterilization described in this chapter.

Techniques for Tubal Closure.   Your surgeon may close your tubes with suture thread and remove a section of each tube, she/he may cauterize your tubes (burn and seal them with an electric cautery instrument), or she/he may apply clips or elastic rings to close each tube.

Common tubal closure techniques are shown in Illustration 20-1. Pomeroy ligation and fimbriectomy can be carried out with any of the tubal ligation operations except laparoscopic tubal ligation. The Irving technique may be used for an abdominal tubal ligation or in conjunction with cesarean section delivery. Cautery, clips, or rings can be used for laparoscopic tubal sterilization.

The closure techniques differ from each other somewhat in failure rates and in the likelihood that reversal surgery would be successful later on. Surgery to reconstruct the fallopian tubes is more successful when tube tissue damage is minimized, so the Pomeroy closure method is more likely to be reversible than laparoscopy with cauterization, for example. As you might suspect, the Pomeroy technique probably has a higher accidental pregnancy rate as well. Since ring sterilization causes tubal damage similar to the Pomeroy method, and clip sterilization damages an even smaller portion of tube, both of these techniques may prove to be relatively favorable for reversal. Fimbriectomy is essentially nonreversible but, as with all tubal ligation methods, can fail to protect against pregnancy in rare cases.

Preparing for Tubal Sterilization

Your surgeon will want to be sure you understand that tubal ligation must be considered permanent and that you are aware of the possible complications. You will probably be asked to sign a consent form; be sure to read about informed consent in Chapter 19. You will also want to **decide in advance what you would like your surgeon to do if the sterilization procedure that you have planned cannot be completed.** In about 7 cases out of 1,000 it is not possible to complete the laparoscopic tubal sterilization, and technical problems are occasionally encountered with the mini-laparotomy and vaginal techniques as well. If problems occur, you have two choices: your surgeon can switch to standard abdominal surgery to perform your tubal ligation while you are still under anesthesia, or she/he can stop. Decide which you prefer, and talk to your surgeon beforehand.

You will also need to decide about anesthesia before your surgery. General anesthesia is the most common choice for sterilization surgery in the United States but local anesthesia with sedation may be an option to consider. The major advantage of general anesthesia is that surgery will be entirely pain-free. Also, general anesthesia may make it easier and quicker for your surgeon to perform the procedure and deal with minor technical difficulties that may arise.

The major advantage of local anesthesia is safety. Serious reactions and even deaths can occur with local anesthesia too, but overall it is safer than general anesthesia. Recovery after surgery is also faster.

Local anesthesia is commonly used for mini-lap sterilization, but this procedure is used much more extensively in other countries than it is in the United States. Local anesthesia is also possible for laparoscopy sterilization, and U.S. statistics show that complication rates are substantially lower for the 15% of women who have laparoscopy with local anesthesia compared to those who have general anesthesia (1). It is possible, however, that the lower rates are influenced in part by factors other than anesthesia. If, for example, patients who have local anesthesia are the most ideal surgery candidates: slender, healthy, and with no history of infection or previous surgery that might make sterilization technically difficult, then lower complication rates would be expected.

Discuss anesthesia options with your surgeon, including your own personal feelings about overall safety versus possible discomfort. Risks are low with either choice.

Finally, be sure you understand any **preoperative instructions** your surgeon has. Laboratory tests such as a blood count for anemia may need to be done in advance, and you will probably be asked not to eat or drink anything during the last 8 to 12 hours before your surgery. If you will be having general anesthesia, this is critical; your surgery will have to be canceled if you have eaten. If you are taking birth control Pills, your surgeon will want you to stop taking them a few weeks before your surgery to avoid any excess risk of blood clotting problems, so you will need to switch to another method such as condoms or a diaphragm. Be sure to continue with effective birth control until your surgery. Tubal sterilization can't protect you in advance!

Surgical Procedures for Sterilization

LAPAROSCOPIC TUBAL STERILIZATION ("BAND-AID" SURGERY)

Laparoscopic tubal sterilization is usually performed in a hospital or surgical center with general anesthesia. Local anesthesia and sedatives or tranquilizers may be an option.

You are positioned on the operating table with your feet in stirrups. Your abdomen and vagina are washed with antiseptic solution, and sterile drapes are placed over your body and legs leaving only a small area on your abdomen and your vaginal area uncovered.

Once anesthesia is complete, your surgeon puts a speculum in your vagina and places a small clamp on your cervix to hold it steady, and then inserts an elevator—a blunt metal rod—into your uterus. These instruments will be used later to move your uterus and tubes into position for clear visualization. If you are having a D&C (see Chapter 47) or an abortion at the same time as your sterilization, it is done at this stage.

Next your surgeon inserts a needle into your abdomen so that carbon dioxide gas can be gently infused through the needle to lift up your abdominal wall and allow your intestines to shift out of the way. When inflation is completed, your surgeon makes a 1-inch incision just below your navel and inserts the laparoscope (see Illustration 20-2) through the incision. Your surgeon is able to see your tubes, uterus, and other abdominal organs through the laparoscope.

Once the laparoscope is in place and your tubes are in view, your surgeon is ready to place clips or rings (sometimes called bands), or carry out cautery to seal each tube. A second instrument for the clip, ring, or cautery may be inserted through a second tiny incision just above your pubic hairline, or the instrument may be inserted through a channel built into the side of the laparoscope. Your surgeon manipulates the elevator

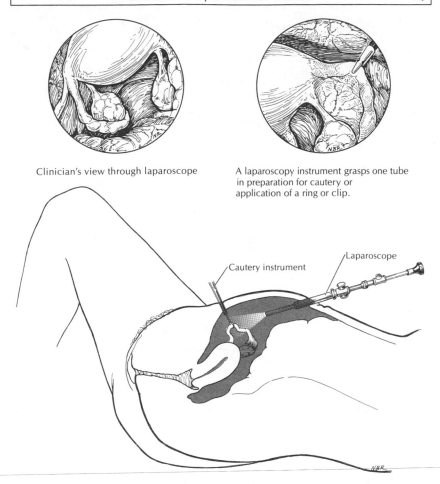

Clinician's view through laparoscope

A laparoscopy instrument grasps one tube in preparation for cautery or application of a ring or clip.

ILLUSTRATION 20-2 The laparoscope light illuminates the abdomen. The tubal sterilization instrument is usually inserted through a second small incision near the pubic hairline. (Reproductive Health Resources, Inc.; used with permission.)

in your uterus to move the uterus and tubes into position so that she/he can grasp one tube and apply the ring or clip or activate cautery to burn and seal 1 to 2 inches of tube. Next, the other tube is located and sealed in the same way. Finally your surgeon inspects both tubes again to be sure that there is no bleeding.

The instruments are removed, and most of the gas escapes from your abdomen. Your incision(s) is closed with one or two stitches (see Illustration 20-3) and covered with one or two Band-Aids.

Open laparoscopy is a term used for a slightly modified laparoscopy technique. With open laparoscopy, the instruments are inserted through a surgical incision slightly larger than the standard laparoscopy incision so that your surgeon can identify each

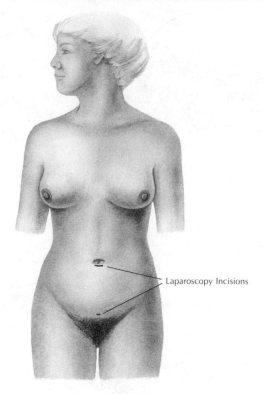

Laparoscopy Incisions

ILLUSTRATION 20-3   Laparoscopic tubal sterilization is performed with one or two small incisions.

layer in the abdominal wall. This technique may help your surgeon avoid puncturing areas where scar tissue may be in the way or bowel may be stuck to the abdominal lining. Open laparoscopy is somewhat more time-consuming, but may be recommended if your surgeon suspects that you have extensive scar tissue.

POSTPARTUM STERILIZATION

In the first 48 hours after full term delivery, surgical sterilization can be carried out very simply. The enlarged uterus remains high in the abdominal cavity (see Illustration 20-4), and the tubes can be reached through a 1- to 2-inch incision just below the navel. If epidural block anesthesia has been used for delivery, it may be possible to perform tubal sterilization immediately after delivery without further anesthesia. Sterilization can also be performed at the same time as cesarean section delivery.

After general, epidural, spinal, or possibly local anesthesia is completed, your abdomen is washed with antiseptic solution, and draped. Your surgeon makes an incision along the curve of your navel and is able to see the top of your uterus and your tubes clearly. The first tube is grasped with a small blunt clamp, lifted out

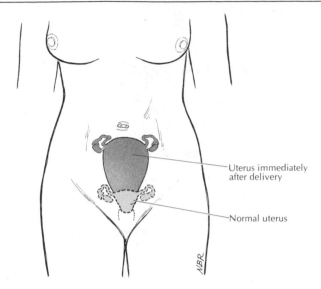

ILLUSTRATION 20-4   Tubal sterilization is easy to perform immediately after delivery, when the uterus and tubes are high in the abdomen.

through the incision, and then a tubal closure procedure is performed. The Pomeroy method (see Illustration 20-5) is the most common because it can easily be performed with the small incision. Alternatively, fimbriectomy or application of rings or clips would be possible.

After the first tube is blocked, it is released and drops back into your abdominal cavity; then the second tube is grasped and the closure procedure repeated. Next your surgeon inspects both tubes to be sure that there is no bleeding, and closes the incision.

The postpartum incision heals quickly and causes minimal discomfort. Most women find that postpartum tubal sterilization does not require any additional recovery time; they are able to leave the hospital two or three days after delivery, just as they normally would.

VAGINAL STERILIZATION

Some women may be able to have tubal sterilization performed through an incision **inside the vagina**. It is most likely to be successful if your uterus, tubes, and ovaries are freely movable, if your pelvic muscles are relatively lax, and if your uterus is not abnormally enlarged.

Because the vagina normally contains many types of bacteria, preoperative cleansing is especially important. Some surgeons recommend antibacterial vaginal suppositories or douches and perhaps antibiotic pills to be taken at home in preparation for surgery, and may also recommend antibiotic pills for the first few days afterward. At the time of surgery, your vagina and vulva are cleansed with antiseptic solution.

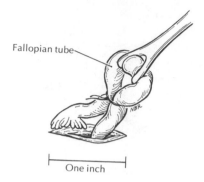

Fallopian tube

One inch

ILLUSTRATION 20-5   A loop of fallopian tube is sutured shut with the Pomeroy technique, and then the top part of the loop is cut away.

Once general anesthesia is complete, your surgeon places a speculum inside your vagina so that she/he can see your cervix and the back of the vagina. If local anesthesia is being used it will be injected after the speculum is in place. A steadying clamp is placed on your cervix, and the surgeon makes a 2-inch incision inside your vagina just below your cervix (see Illustration 20-6). Only a thin layer of connective tissue separates the vagina from the abdominal lining, and when these layers are separated and opened, your surgeon can see the back side of your uterus. She/he manipulates your uterus with the cervical clamp until the first tube is located. Then the tube is grasped and pulled down through the incision into the vagina. Either the Pomeroy or the fimbriectomy technique is usually used (see Illustration 20-1), and the tube is then released back into your abdomen. The second tube is then located and blocked. Your surgeon inspects both tubes to be sure that there is no bleeding and closes the incision.

Your surgeon may permit you to return home the same day, or may recommend overnight hospital observation. Because the incision is small and does not involve an opening in your abdominal muscles, discomfort after surgery is usually minimal and recovery is rapid. Most women are able to resume normal activities (with the exception of intercourse) within one or two weeks. Avoid intercourse until four to six weeks after surgery so that your incision will have plenty of time to heal. The cosmetic results of vaginal surgery are a major advantage for some women because the scar inside the vagina doesn't show.

A disadvantage of vaginal surgery is that infection risk is higher than for the other tubal sterilization techniques because of the large numbers of bacteria normally present in the vagina. Antibiotics may help reduce infection risk, but infection can occur despite antibiotic treatment, and infection rates are still higher than with other sterilization surgery options.

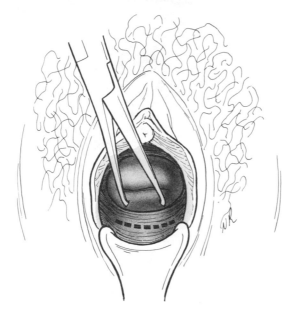

ILLUSTRATION 20-6   Incision for vaginal tubal sterilization.

MINI-LAPAROTOMY

Mini-laparotomy is similar to routine abdominal surgery (laparotomy) except that the incision is only 1 to 1 1/2 inches long instead of 3 to 5 inches long, and the procedure is well suited for local anesthesia. General anesthesia may also be used.

A small patch of hair above your pubic bone may be shaved just before surgery. Your abdomen, inner thighs, and vulva are washed with antiseptic solution and your abdomen is draped. Next, your surgeon inserts a speculum into your vagina, places a clamp on your cervix to hold it steady, and inserts an elevator—a blunt metal instrument—into your uterus. The elevator will be used later to move your uterus and tubes close to the incision opening to bring the tubes into your surgeon's view.

If you are having a local anesthetic, your surgeon injects the drug just under the skin in the area of the incision (see Illustration 20-7). Most women feel an initial stinging sensation with the local anesthetic; the stinging lasts only a few seconds because the anesthetic rapidly blocks the pain nerves to the skin. The anesthetic is then injected into the entire incision area and into the connective tissue and thin peritoneum lining beneath it. During this process you may be aware of a pressure sensation, but you should feel little or no real pain.

Next your surgeon makes the incision about an inch above your pubic bone and uses the elevator to bring your uterus up against the incision (see Illustration 20-8). Your surgeon moves your uterus gently from side to side and locates and grasps the first tube with a blunt clamp. The fallopian tube is brought out through the incision

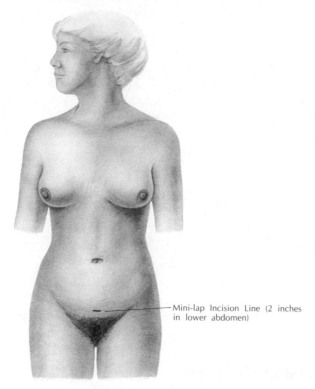

Mini-lap Incision Line (2 inches in lower abdomen)

ILLUSTRATION 20-7   Incision for mini-laparotomy tubal sterilization.

and ligated with the Pomeroy or fimbriectomy technique, or a ring or clip is applied (see Illustration 20-1). The first tube is released into the abdomen; then the second tube is located, grasped, and blocked. The surgeon next checks both tubes to be certain there is no bleeding and closes your incision with stitches.

Recovery after mini-laparotomy is rapid. Most women are able to return home a few hours after surgery and resume normal activities, including intercourse, within one or two days. The incision is very small, and discomfort following surgery is fairly mild.

Mini-laparotomy is suitable only for women who are slender (less than 20% above their ideal weight for height) and have a normal, freely mobile uterus and tubes. It is a relatively uncommon procedure in the United States, and few surgeons have had wide experience with it.

What to Expect After Surgery

After laparoscopic or mini-laparotomy tubal ligation, you can go home once you are able to get up and walk without difficulty and are fully awake. If you have had local

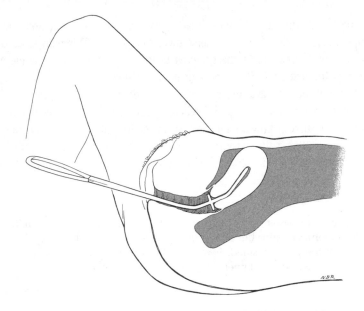

ILLUSTRATION 20-8 A metal elevator raises the uterus so that the uterus and tubes will be closer to the incision.

anesthesia you may be ready to leave as soon as an hour after surgery; after general anesthesia you will stay a little longer, but probably no more than four hours or so. In either case, be sure to arrange for someone to accompany you home from the hospital. After general anesthesia or the sedative used with local anesthesia it will not be safe to drive for at least 24 hours; anesthesia medications slow down your reflexes for some time.

Some women are ready to go home the same day with vaginal tubal ligation, but surgeons sometimes recommend a 24-hour period of hospital observation. Plan on a two- or three-day hospital stay with postpartum sterilization.

I had less discomfort after the operation than I thought I would. My muscles were definitely sore that evening, but I only needed one of the five pain pills my doctor prescribed, and Tylenol was enough after the first night.

—WOMAN, 30

For most women, recovery from tubal sterilization surgery is rapid. If you had general anesthesia, it is common to feel weak, tired, and nauseated during the first 24 hours. You may also notice general muscle soreness from the muscle relaxant drug used with general anesthesia, and a mild sore throat from the windpipe tube. Some women experience shoulder pain after laparoscopic tubal sterilization. This pain is caused by irritation of your diaphragm by the gas used to inflate your abdomen. As the gas is absorbed over the first 24 to 36 hours, your pain will subside.

It is very unusual to have any major problems or delays in recovery. Your pain should not be severe and should be relieved effectively by the prescription pain medication your surgeon provides for the first day or two after surgery. You may find that a nonprescription pain reliever and rest is all you need after the first night. A full bladder can add to your discomfort, so be sure to urinate if pain is bothersome.

I was much drowsier and weaker than I anticipated. By evening I had some abdominal pain, but after I took a pain pill and went to the bathroom the pain subsided. I was able to sleep easily. The next day I was able to go out for dinner. I've been fine ever since.

—WOMAN, 37

It is not uncommon to have some vaginal bleeding or spotting for a few days after surgery. If you had an abortion along with your tubal ligation, bleeding may last several days, and you may have spotting or light bleeding for as long as two or three weeks.

As your incision heals, you may notice thickening or a lump just under the skin. This lump is caused by the regrowth of connective tissue and will gradually diminish in a few months. The scars from laparoscopic tubal sterilization, postpartum tubal sterilization, and mini-laparotomy are usually almost invisible after they have healed.

DANGER SIGNS

Complications after tubal sterilization are uncommon, but it is very important to watch for danger signs of infection, bleeding, or abnormal blood clotting (thrombophlebitis). Get in touch with your surgeon immediately if you develop any of the danger signs listed in Illustration 20-9.

Complications and Risks

Problems serious enough to cause death are very rare. Overall statistics for all methods of tubal sterilization together show that one death occurs for every 25,000 sterilization procedures (2). Researchers from the national Centers for Disease Control analyzed the

20:9   DANGER SIGNS AFTER TUBAL STERILIZATION

Fever (temperature over 100.4 degrees F.)
Pain not relieved by your pain medication or persisting more than
   12 hours
Faintness, chest pain, cough, or shortness of breath
Moderate or heavy bleeding from your incision or from your vagina
Red or tender skin near your incision(s)
Bleeding or oozing from your incision(s)

Possible Ectopic Pregnancy (Long-Term Risk)

Sudden intense pain, or persistent pain, or cramping in the lower
   abdomen, usually localized to one side or the other
Irregular bleeding or spotting with abdominal pain when your
   period is late or after an abnormally light period
Fainting or dizziness that persists more than a few seconds. These
   may be signs of internal bleeding. You will not necessarily have
   any bleeding from your vagina if you have internal bleeding.

Contact your clinician at once or go to a hospital emergency room
if you develop any of these symptoms after surgery.

29 deaths that were reported between 1977 and 1981 and concluded that the following recommendations might help prevent serious complications and deaths (2):

• A windpipe tube should be used during general anesthesia for sterilization (so resuscitation could begin immediately if needed)

• Cautery instruments that use bipolar coagulation are preferable to unipolar instruments for sterilization (to avoid accidental bowel burns)

• A woman using birth control Pills should stop taking them and switch to another method a full month before surgery if possible (to help prevent thrombophlebitis)

Laparoscopy tubal sterilization is one of the most thoroughly studied of all surgical procedures in the United States, and extensive research data on complications of mini-lap are available from other countries. Research reports on complications of vaginal and postpartum tubal sterilization are not as extensive. Because complication rates are so dependent on factors such as the overall health of the group being studied, it is impossible to select one "true" complication rate for each surgery option, and it is difficult to make meaningful comparisons between different research reports.

   For rough comparison, average overall complication rates reported in the 1970s for each of the common sterilization operations are listed in Table 20-2. These rates include both serious and minor complications, and in each case only a small proportion of the total were serious.

TABLE 20-2
TUBAL STERILIZATION COMPLICATION RATES

OPERATION	TOTAL MAJOR AND MINOR COMPLICATIONS PER 100 WOMEN
Laparoscopic tubal sterilization	5.0
Postpartum tubal sterilization	7.8
Vaginal tubal sterilization	11.5
Mini-laparotomy tubal sterilization	7.0

SOURCES: Wortman J, Piotrow PT: Laparoscopic sterilization. II: What are the problems? *Population Reports*, Ser C, No 2, March 1973. Washington, D.C.: George Washington University Medical Center.
Edwards LE, Hakanson EY: Changing status of tubal sterilization. *American Journal of Obstetrics and Gynecology* 115:347–353, 1973.
Wortman J: Female sterilization by mini-laparotomy. *Population Reports*, Ser C, No 5, November 1974. Washington, D.C.: George Washington University Medical Center.

Complication rates are definitely lower for laparoscopy sterilization in the 1980s than the 1970s rate shown in the table, probably less than 2% (1). Complication rates for the other surgery options as well have no doubt decreased with improvements in surgical technique and antibiotics. Comparable recent statistics, however, are not available. The relative safety of the surgery options is probably similar to what it was in the 1970s. Vaginal sterilization in the 1970s had a somewhat higher infection rate that made its overall complication rate slightly higher than the other options. It is likely that infection rates have dropped in the 1980s (as they have with vaginal hysterectomy) because of more effective use of antibiotics and improved surgery. Laparoscopy, mini-lap, and postpartum sterilization have quite similar risks.

Many factors influence complication rates, such as the woman's general health status, specific medical problems, and anatomy. The skill of the surgeon is also an important factor. Laparoscopic tubal complication rates were found to be significantly higher (1 in 20 versus 1 in 200) among women whose surgeons performed fewer than 20 procedures per year compared to women whose surgeons performed 100 or more per year (3). Vaginal surgery complication rates, too, are related to the surgeon's experience (4).

Anesthesia choice also affects risk. Complications directly related to anesthesia are somewhat higher for general anesthesia than for local anesthesia, and rates for other kinds of complications may be affected as well. In a large study of laparoscopy sterilization, 1 woman in 250 had one or more complications (including infection, bleeding, and extra surgery to repair damage) with local anesthesia, compared to 1 in 50 for general anesthesia (1). Both rates are very low compared to other common surgical procedures, and it is possible that the local anesthesia patients were better surgery candidates.

Patient factors also influence risk. Complication rates in the study described above were higher for overweight women (1 in 40), women with diabetes (1 in 12), women with previous pelvic infection or pelvic surgery (1 in 30), and women with lung disease such as asthma (1 in 26) (1).

Remember to put the serious complications of tubal sterilization in perspective with other birth control risks. Surgical sterilization involves a one-time death risk of about 4 in 100,000 procedures. Risks for the temporary methods of birth control are per year. One year of Pill use for a woman over 30 who smokes is a greater death risk than sterilization surgery, and so is two or three years of Pill use for a nonsmoker. Or, from another point of view, sterilization surgery is slightly more dangerous than canoeing but safer than playing football, motorcycling, or driving an automobile as far as chance of death (5).

POSSIBLE COMPLICATIONS
OF STERILIZATION SURGERY

Anesthesia Complications.   As with any surgical procedure, anesthesia complications such as cardiac arrest or death are possible with both general and local anesthesia. This risk is increased if you have asthma or heart disease, are overweight, or if you smoke. Be completely honest in reporting your medical history to your surgeon. The overall risk of anesthesia problems is small. Serious anesthesia complications during laparoscopic tubal sterilization occur in about 1 case in 1,250 to 2,000 (6). General anesthesia complications are probably even rarer with mini-lap, vaginal, and postpartum sterilization.

Damage to Internal Organs.   Injury to the intestines, bladder, cervix, uterus, uterine ligaments, or blood vessels can occur during any tubal sterilization procedure. Injury might occur when instruments are first inserted into the abdomen, or during a cautery, ring, or clip procedure. The carbon dioxide gas used to inflate the abdomen for laparoscopic tubal sterilization can cause injury if gas is released directly into the skin or muscle tissue or if gas pressure in the abdomen interferes with breathing or stimulates changes in the heart rate. These problems are rare.

Further surgery may be required to correct damage or to stop internal bleeding. Your surgeon would perform an immediate laparotomy (see Chapter 48) with a regular 5-inch abdominal incision. Approximately 1 woman in 500 will require further surgery because of laparoscopy complications (1), and further surgery may also be needed if complications occur with mini-lap, vaginal, or postpartum sterilization.

Infection.   The risk of infection in the uterus, tubes, or bladder is increased after any surgery that involves these organs. Infection usually causes pain, fever, and an unusual vaginal discharge. In most cases, infection remains localized in the incision area or in the uterus and tubes and can be effectively treated with antibiotic pills. If the infection spreads to the lining of the abdominal cavity (peritonitis) or if a large collection of pus develops (an abscess), then hospitalization may be necessary so that you can be treated with intravenous antibiotics. In some cases, further surgery may be required to drain an abscess or even to remove the uterus, tubes, and ovaries.

The higher infection risk following vaginal tubal ligation is the primary reason overall complication rates for this procedure are higher than overall rates for the other tubal sterilization methods. Reported rates vary, but typically show that between 1 and 6 patients out of 100 develop infection after vaginal tubal ligation (7). About 1 patient in 1,000 develops an infection that requires further treatment after laparoscopic tubal ligation (1).

Bleeding.   Internal bleeding could occur as a result of damage to a blood vessel or pelvic organ during sterilization surgery. It is likely to be evident during surgery, in which case your surgeon would take any steps necessary to correct it at that time. Later bleeding, though, could occur. With internal blood loss, blood would not come out of your vagina, so your only signs would be abdominal pain, faintness, or weakness, especially when standing up.

Light vaginal bleeding after surgery is common, but significant hemorrhage could occur if instruments used to stabilize your cervix or to position your uterus caused damage or a tear. Heavy bleeding should be reported immediately to your surgeon.

Other Surgical Problems.   As with any type of surgery, your risk for thrombophlebitis (blood clot formation), embolism (clot lodging in the lungs, heart, or brain), and pneumonia is temporarily increased during the immediate postoperative period. These problems are rare in young, healthy women.

CONTRAINDICATIONS

For some women and in some situations, tubal sterilization surgery is not a reasonable idea. If you have active pelvic infection, or are already pregnant and plan to continue your pregnancy, you should not undergo sterilization surgery. Also, surgery should be delayed if you have any significant temporary medical illness. Surgery is safest when you are well, and sterilization surgery is entirely elective. The other conditions listed below may increase your risk of complications, so your decision about sterilization surgery must be weighed especially carefully.

• Pregnancy (except when sterilization is combined with elective abortion)
• Active pelvic infection
• Acute temporary illness
• Previous pelvic infection or abdominal infection
• Previous abdominal surgery

- Abnormal uterine or tubal structure
- Serious medical problems such as heart disease
- Body weight substantially above or below the normal range
- Hernia of the diaphragm (hiatal hernia) or abdominal hernia (laparoscopy risk is increased)

A woman who is pregnant or suspects that she may be pregnant and would plan to continue the pregnancy should not undergo any elective surgery. Many surgeons prefer to schedule tubal ligation during the first week or two after a normal menstrual period to be certain that you are not pregnant at the time of surgery.

Advantages of Tubal Sterilization

No contraceptive method, including tubal sterilization, is 100% effective. The effectiveness rate of tubal sterilization is higher than that of any of the temporary methods of birth control, and tubal sterilization is permanent. The overall risk of minor and major complications and death with tubal surgery is low compared to the risks with long-term use of birth control Pills or an IUD.

Tubal sterilization surgery takes only 15 to 20 minutes. Most women are able to resume normal activity within 24 to 48 hours after laparoscopic, mini-laparotomy, or postpartum tubal sterilization, and within a few days after vaginal surgery.

Tubal sterilization also reduces a woman's future health risks. Risks associated with pregnancy, spontaneous and induced abortion, and ectopic pregnancy are decreased because of her effective protection against pregnancy. Risks for future pelvic infection are also reduced. Infection can occur in the remaining portion of open tube but is less likely than it would be for a woman who has not had sterilization surgery (8).

Long-term Problems
After Sterilization Surgery

Possible long-term effects of tubal sterilization have been a subject of intense controversy, with many research articles analyzing whether a "post-tubal syndrome" (see following section) does or does not exist. Sterilization failure, with unintended pregnancy, must also be considered as a long-term problem, as well as regret after surgery that might lead a woman to seek later reversal surgery. (Tubal sterilization reversal is discussed in Chapter 19, "Making a Decision About Sterilization.")

Tubal sterilization surgery, however, **does not cause any known long-term serious adverse health effects.** Women who have undergone surgical sterilization do not have any greater risks for later serious gynecologic problems or for hysterectomy or pelvic surgery than do comparable women who use other methods of birth control (9).

"POST-TUBAL SYNDROME"

There is no clear-cut definition for post-tubal syndrome. Researchers use this term to encompass a variety of menstrual problems such as irregular menstrual periods, cramps, excessive menstrual flow, bleeding between periods, and premenstrual symptoms such as bloating, irritability, and depression. These issues are very difficult to study because so many women have intermittent problems with menstrual abnormalities throughout the reproductive years **whether or not** they undergo tubal sterilization.

Studies of post-tubal syndrome have produced conflicting results. Several researchers have found identical rates for menstrual cycle irregularities among women with surgical sterilization and comparable women who were not sterilized. Other researchers, however, have been able to document higher rates for abnormal cycle length, and slightly higher rates for moderate to severe cramps and for abnormal bleeding among sterilized women (10). Even in this study, however, many women with cycle problems before surgery actually improved after surgery, and the overall proportion of women with problems was about the same for the tubal sterilization group and the comparison group until four years or more after surgery.

For women who had no previous history of cycle problems, 1 woman in 12 had problems four years after tubal sterilization and 1 woman in 14 in the comparison group had problems. In contrast, 80% of tubal sterilization women with problems **before** surgery also had problems four years later, but only 12% of comparison women did. It is possible that the difference between sterilization patients and the comparison group in this study is actually due to the unexpectedly low rate of problems the comparison group experienced!

The post-tubal syndrome controversy is not yet resolved. It is possible that sterilization surgery might cause subtle damage to the blood supply of a woman's ovaries, and thus cause long-term changes in her menstrual cycle. This is certainly true in the rare cases of severe accidental blood vessel damage during surgery, so the concern about possible long-term effects is plausible. Also, it is possible that newer methods of sterilization with bipolar cautery, clips, or rings may involve less extensive damage and hence have less effect on cycles. This might explain the apparent four-year delay in effects described in the study above. Surgical techniques may have improved during the four-year interval included in this study, so that women sterilized more recently had fewer problems.

STERILIZATION FAILURE

Sterilization failure, with conception and pregnancy after surgery, is quite rare. Reported rates range from 1 pregnancy for every 1,000 procedures to 1 for every 80 procedures, with rates of 1 failure in 200 to 300 procedures most typical, and very similar for all the commonly used techniques (9). Failure rates for the clip method are perhaps slightly higher than for the ring, cautery, or surgical techniques.

Apparent failure can occur if a woman has already conceived immediately before surgery. This type of "failure" is quite common, and probably reflects the human propensity to believe that next week's surgery will protect us tonight. Pregnancy can also occur if the surgery is not properly done so that one or both tubes are not correctly identified or completely blocked. Pregnancy can occur if a tube spontaneously rejoins during the healing process or if a hole or fistula forms in the tube that is large enough to allow for passage of sperm and/or an egg (11).

Failures most often occur within the first two years after surgery (12), but rare pregnancies are possible years or even decades later.

Ectopic Pregnancy.   Because tubal sterilization protects so effectively against all pregnancy, a woman's risk for ectopic pregnancy is much lower after tubal sterilization than it would be if she used no birth control or a temporary method of birth control.

If tubal sterilization fails, however, and the woman does become pregnant, then ectopic pregnancy is a serious concern (13). At least 16% and as many as 50% of sterilization failure pregnancies are ectopic (12,13), so prompt confirmation of pregnancy and evaluation for possible ectopic pregnancy are absolutely essential. Unsuspected ectopic pregnancy is a grave health threat. As the pregnancy grows, rupture of the tube is possible with sudden, massive internal hemorrhage. Ectopic pregnancy is a leading cause of death associated with pregnancy.

Any woman who has had surgical sterilization should remember the danger signs of possible ectopic pregnancy shown in Illustration 20-9. Also, keeping track of menstrual cycles will still be necessary so you can recognize that your period is overdue. A sensitive pregnancy test (see Chapter 8) will be needed as soon as possible if you have any suspicion of possible pregnancy.

Experimental Methods
of Female Sterilization

Researchers hope to find new sterilization techniques that may be readily reversible and/or simpler, safer, and less expensive than existing surgical options. Many different kinds of experimental methods are being developed, and may be options already for a woman who is interested in enrolling in a research study program.

TUBAL PLUG

Silicone plugs are being tested in the United States (9). To place the plugs (called Ovabloc) the clinician uses a hysteroscope. The slender lighted tube, inserted through the cervical canal, allows the clinician to see the inside of the uterus and locate the two fallopian tube openings at the top of the uterine cavity (see Chapter 46 for further information on hysteroscopy). Liquid silicone is then squirted into each tube. The silicone hardens rapidly to form a plug.

From the patient's point of view this procedure is fairly similar to insertion of an IUD. General anesthesia is not required, and it can be carried out in an office setting. Recovery is rapid.

Success with forming plugs has been good (80% or more) and subsequent pregnancy rates fairly low (about 1%) (9). Researchers hope that this method will also have good reversibility. Hysteroscopy could be used again later to remove the plugs if the woman wished to become pregnant. No research data, however, are yet available to show what proportion of women might return to normal fertility after removal.

CHEMICAL TUBE CLOSURE

MCA (methyl-cyanoacrylate) is a chemical that adheres to tissue and also hardens after placement. It is used with an insertion tube and balloon that expands inside the uterus to push the MCA to the upper part of the uterus where the fallopian tube openings are. This method is already approved for use in Canada and for research use in the United States. The MCA and insertion device, called Femcept, is successful in blocking both tubes for 87% to 98% of patients after two applications, one month apart.

A Femcept procedure would be similar to IUD insertion. Special instruments such as a hysteroscope are not required, and it does not require general anesthesia or an operating room facility.

Quinacrine is a drug commonly used in the past to prevent malaria. In high concentration it also causes local tissue fibrosis. Sterilization with quinacrine involves placing tablets of the drug inside the uterine cavity to induce fibrosis and scarring near the tube openings. The tablets can be placed with a slender plastic inserter similar to an IUD inserter. Several insertions, spaced one month apart, may be necessary. Research on this method is fairly extensive in other countries, but very limited in the United States (14).

For further information about sterilization research studies, or programs in your area, you can contact the Association for Voluntary Surgical Contraception, 122 East 42nd Street, New York, N.Y. 10168, 212-351-2500.

REFERENCES

1. DeStefano F, Greenspan JR, Dicker RC, et al: Complications of interval laparoscopic tubal sterilization. *Obstetrics and Gynecology* 61:153–158, 1983.
2. Peterson HB, DeStefano F, Rubin GL, et al: Deaths attributable to tubal sterilization in the United States, 1977 to 1981. *American Journal of Obstetrics and Gynecology* 146:131–136, 1983.

3. Phillips AJ, Keith D, Hulka J, et al: Gynecologic laparoscopy in 1975. *Journal of Reproductive Medicine* 16:105–117, 1976.

4. Akhter MS: Vaginal versus abdominal tubal ligation. *American Journal of Obstetrics and Gynecology* 115:491–496, 1973.

5. Hatcher RA, Guest FJ, Stewart FH, et al: *Contraceptive Technology 1986–1987* (ed 13). New York: Irvington Publishers, 1986.

6. Phillips JM (ed): *Endoscopic Female Sterilization. A Comparison of Methods*. Downey, Ca: American Association of Gynecologic Laparoscopists, 1983.

7. Wortman J, Piotro P: Colpotomy: The vaginal approach. *Population Reports,* Ser C, No 3, June 1973. Washington, DC: George Washington University Medical Center.

8. Phillips AJ, d'Ablaing G III: Acute salpingitis subsequent to tubal ligation. *Obstetrics and Gynecology* 67:55S–58S, 1986.

9. Liskin L, Rinehart W: Minilaparotomy and laparoscopy: Safe, effective, and widely used. *Population Reports* Ser C, No 9, May 1985. Baltimore: Johns Hopkins University.

10. DeStefano F, Perlman JA, Peterson HB, et al: Long-term risk of menstrual disturbances after tubal sterilization. *American Journal of Obstetrics and Gynecology* 152:835–841, 1985.

11. Soderstrom RM: Sterilization failures and their causes. *American Journal of Obstetrics and Gynecology* 152:395–403, 1985.

12. DeStefano F, Peterson HB, Layde PM, et al: Risk of ectopic pregnancy following tubal sterilization. *Obstetrics and Gynecology* 60:326–330, 1982.

13. McCausland A: High rate of ectopic pregnancy following laparoscopic tubal coagulation failures. *American Journal of Obstetrics and Gynecology* 136:97–101, 1980.

14. Kessel E, Zipper J, Mumford SD: Quinacrine nonsurgical female sterilization: A reassessment of safety and efficacy. *Fertility and Sterility* 44:293–298, 1985.

21

❖

Vasectomy:
The Sterilization Procedure
for Men

*Vasectomy is a simple 20-minute office procedure. Its purpose is to provide permanent birth control, and **permanent is the key word**. Vasectomy reversal surgery may be possible if you later regret sterilization, but reversal does not assure that fertility will return (see Chapter 19).*

Risks and complications with vasectomy are minimal. Your surgeon will want to be sure, however, that you don't have any medical problems that would increase your risk with surgery.

*Special precautions may be needed if your **blood clotting is not normal** because of anticoagulant (blood-thinning) medication or a bleeding disease such as hemophilia. **Infection** of the skin or reproductive tract should be treated and cured before your surgery. Infection can interfere with the healing process and increases your risk of postoperative complications.*

*Vasectomy may be more difficult to perform if you have a **hernia**, previous hernia repair, an **undescended testicle**, or other abnormalities. Your clinician will evaluate these problems before your surgery, and in some cases will recommend general anesthesia and surgery in a hospital setting.*

PREPARING FOR SURGERY

Your clinician will review your medical history and perform a general physical exam, and may order a blood test for anemia or abnormal bleeding tendencies. She/he will want to be sure that you understand that the surgery is permanent and that you understand the possible complications of the procedure. You may be asked to sign a consent form.

Your surgeon will probably recommend a thorough shower or bath just before your surgery appointment, and may ask you to trim the hairs from your scrotum yourself. (You will not have to shave the pubic hair above your penis.)

Arrange for someone to accompany you and drive you home after your surgery. Bring snug jockey shorts or an athletic supporter with you. Make plans so that you can stay at home and be quiet for the first 48 hours after surgery. Some surgeons also recommend that you have an ice pack ready for use after your procedure.

THE VASECTOMY PROCEDURE

First, your scrotum area will be cleaned, shaved, and draped with a sterile cloth. Your surgeon may give you a mild sedative or tranquilizer such as Valium.

Your surgeon first locates each vas deferens where it passes just under the skin along the middle of your scrotum above your testicles (see Illustration 21-1). Next, she/he injects a local anesthetic similar to Novocain to make a small area of your skin numb. The anesthetic takes effect within a few minutes—much more quickly than dental anesthetic—and most men find that the anesthetic procedure is not particularly painful.

After the anesthetic has taken effect, your surgeon makes a 1/2-inch incision through the skin and thin muscle layer of the scrotum. Next, she/he identifies the first vas and lifts it through the incision with scissors or a small clamp. A 1/2- to 1-inch section of the vas is removed, and then the two cut ends are tied and/or cauterized to seal them shut. Some surgeons then fold each cut end back on itself or cover each end with connective tissue to insure that they will remain separated. Next, the other vas is located and sealed. Your surgeon may use just one incision in the midline or two incisions, one on each side. Once both tubes are tied, your surgeon closes your incision(s) with one or two stitches. (Some surgeons use absorbable thread that does not need to be removed, and others use standard silk thread, in which case your stitches will need to be removed in about four days.)

Your surgeon places a small gauze bandage over the incision, which is held in place by an athletic supporter or scrotal suspensory.

WHAT TO EXPECT AFTER SURGERY

You will be advised to rest for the first 24 to 48 hours after surgery, because rest decreases the likelihood of swelling and of blood collecting (hematoma) in the scrotal area. An ice pack may also help prevent swelling and will relieve discomfort. You may have a dull ache or dragging sensation in your scrotum for the first few days, and wearing an athletic supporter or jockey shorts often helps relieve this sensation. Use a supporter as long as you are more comfortable with it than without it. Pain is usually mild and will probably be relieved by nonprescription pain medication such as aspirin.

Most men feel able to return to work and normal activities the day after surgery, but strenuous activities, straining, and lifting should be avoided for the first week or so.

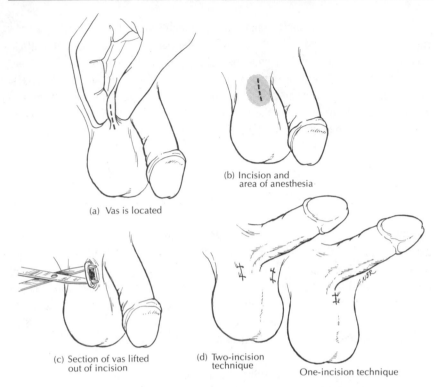

(a) Vas is located

(b) Incision and area of anesthesia

(c) Section of vas lifted out of incision

(d) Two-incision technique

One-incision technique

ILLUSTRATION 21-1   **Vasectomy is usually performed using local anesthesia in an office or clinic setting.**

Keep your incision area dry for the first 24 to 48 hours. You can bathe or shower after that time. Tub soaks in plain warm water several times a day (beginning after 48 hours) may speed the healing process.

Recommendations regarding intercourse vary, but in most cases surgeons say that you can resume intercourse as soon as you think it would be comfortable. **Remember that the vasectomy does not provide immediate contraceptive protection.** You must rely upon another birth control method until your postoperative sperm counts show zero sperm.

POSTOPERATIVE SPERM COUNTS

Live sperm are present in your semen for some time after vasectomy because mature sperm are stored in the part of your vas deferens above the vasectomy site. Most men have to ejaculate 10 to 20 times to clear sperm completely from the reproductive tract. For most men, live sperm are absent after about two weeks, but the time interval could be as long as ten weeks or more (1).

The only way to be certain that your semen is free of sperm is to have a sperm count, a microscopic examination of a semen sample. Arrange for your sperm counts when you see your surgeon for a postoperative checkup. You will simply take a fresh semen sample to your surgeon's office or to a lab, and it will be examined for sperm. Use another form of birth control until you have had two consecutive sperm counts that show no sperm at all.

Some clinicians recommend that you see your regular clinician for a sperm count once a year to detect possible regrowth of the vas. The likelihood of regrowth is very small, but a sperm count is a simple, cheap, and harmless test that could help you prevent unwanted pregnancy.

PROBLEMS AND RISKS

About three men out of 100 will experience some problem after vasectomy (1). Problems are almost always minor, and require simple treatment only. No vasectomy-related deaths have been reported in the United States, but deaths have occurred in other countries due to tetanus infection.

One or 2 men out of 100 will develop a blood clot (hematoma) under the skin in the incision area. In most cases, the surgeon must reopen the incision to remove the clot and prevent further bleeding.

Infection can develop in the incision itself or in the vas, testes, or other parts of your scrotum, and 1 or 2 out of 100 men develop infection following vasectomy. In some cases, infection is severe enough to cause fever, pain, and swelling of the scrotum. Treatment with antibiotics usually results in prompt healing, but if a pus pocket (abscess) develops, surgery to drain the infection may be necessary.

Painful swelling of the sperm-carrying tubules on top of each testicle (epididymitis) or the testicles themselves as a consequence of sperm engorgement occurs in less than 1% of men. Swelling usually subsides within a week and is treated by rest, cold packs, and wearing a support.

Formation of a granuloma—a lump of inflammatory tissue—occurs in a small percentage of men. A granuloma can be caused by leakage of sperm from the cut end of the vas, but usually does not cause symptoms or require treatment. A granuloma can become infected and may increase your risk of tube regrowth and lead to vasectomy failure.

Danger Signs.   For the first week or so after surgery you will need to watch for signs of possible vasectomy problems. Call your surgeon immediately if you have any of the symptoms shown in Illustration 21-2.

LONG-TERM EFFECTS OF VASECTOMY

There are no known harmful, long-term effects associated with vasectomy. Several reports appeared between 1968 and 1971 concerning men who developed antibodies to sperm following vasectomy, and there was active debate about the possibility that such

---

21:2 DANGER SIGNS AFTER VASECTOMY

Fever (temperature over 100.4 degrees F.)
Bleeding that is prolonged or heavy. A small amount of bleeding and black-and-blue skin near the incision are normal.
Excessive pain or swelling that is not relieved by aspirin and an ice pack

Contact your clinician at once or go to a hospital emergency room if you develop any of these symptoms after surgery.

---

antibodies could cause arthritis and other problems. Sperm antibodies are special proteins that would attach to any sperm they encounter, just as polio antibodies coat polio viruses once you've been immunized. Considerable research in recent years has confirmed the antibody finding.

About one half to two thirds of men develop antibodies to sperm after vasectomy (1). Similar antibodies are also found in some men who have not had vasectomy and also in some women, and possible effects of antisperm antibodies have been the subject of extensive research over the last two decades. Antisperm antibodies do appear to be a factor in fertility problems. When antibodies are present in the male or the female, a couple's chance for conception is reduced. In relation to vasectomy, this effect of antisperm antibodies is significant only if the man later seeks vasectomy reversal in hopes of restoring fertility.

Possible medical effects of antisperm antibodies have also been explored extensively. Researchers were concerned that antibody formation to other body tissues might occur, or that antibodies circulating in the bloodstream might affect other organs such as the kidneys, or that the body's antibody response pattern in general might be altered. So far, however, no adverse medical effects of antisperm antibodies have been found (1). Further reassurance comes from statistical follow-up studies of men who have had vasectomy compared to men who have not. Vasectomy men do not have higher rates for disease of the immune system (1).

Vasectomy impact on heart disease risk has also been studied extensively. A study published in 1978 triggered extensive debate (2). This study involved five vasectomized monkeys and five nonvasectomized monkeys fed high cholesterol diets and then examined for evidence of blood vessel damage. The vasectomized monkeys had more severe damage and the researcher speculated that this might be a risk for heart disease. Subsequent studies have not confirmed this finding in monkeys (3), and statistical data on humans have been carefully analyzed for any link between vasectomy and heart disease. So far there is no evidence that vasectomy has any effect on heart disease rates (4,5).

ADVANTAGES OF VASECTOMY

Vasectomy is extremely effective: about 1 failure is reported for every 1,000 procedures (1). Vasectomy is more effective than any temporary method of birth control. Vasectomy failure is calculated as a one-time (remaining lifetime) rate; failure rates for temporary methods of birth control are calculated for each year of use. The overall risk of problems or complications is lower for vasectomy than for tubal ligation surgery (6). The risk is very low compared to the risks associated with temporary birth control for women. Vasectomy is permanent. Surgery requires only 20 minutes, and recovery is rapid. Most men feel able to resume normal activities within 24 to 48 hours. Vasectomy does not cause any change in hormone levels or in the appearance or volume of semen. There is no medical reason to expect vasectomy to cause a change in sex drive.

REFERENCES

1. Liskin L: Vasectomy—safe and simple. *Population Reports* Ser D, No 4, November–December 1983. Baltimore: The Johns Hopkins University.
2. Alexander NJ, Clarkson TB: Vasectomy increases the severity of diet-induced atherosclerosis in *Macaca fascicularis. Science* 201:538–541, 1978.
3. Lauersen NH, Muchmore E, Shulman S, et al: Vasectomy and atherosclerosis in *Macaca fascicularis.* New findings in a controversial issue. *Journal of Reproductive Medicine* 28:750–758, 1983.
4. Perrin EB, Woods JS, Namekata T, et al: Long-term effect of vasectomy on coronary heart disease. *American Journal of Public Health* 74:128–132, 1984.
5. Massey FJ, Bernstein GS, O'Fallon WM, et al: Vasectomy and health: Results from a large cohort study. *Journal of the American Medical Association* 252:1023–1029, 1984.
6. Smith GL, Taylor GP, Smith KF: Comparative risks and costs of male and female sterilization. *American Journal of Public Health* 75:370–374, 1985.

22

❖

Basic Facts About Reproductive Tract Infection

*It is a rare woman indeed who lives her entire life without ever once having a reproductive tract infection. Not even celibacy is an absolute guarantee: yeast infections (candidiasis) can arise quite spontaneously. **However, most infections are transmitted through sexual intimacy.** Even cancer of the cervix now appears to be a sexually transmitted disease.*

"Sexually transmitted disease" (STD) has replaced "venereal disease" (VD) as the official and popular generic term clinicians, journalists, and others use for this group of illnesses. STD is a clearer term, and doesn't carry the moral stigma VD does; the images of brothels, syphilis, and disfigured bodies don't immediately come to mind. Today the term STD calls up more accurate images for the 80s: chlamydia, worrisome changes in Pap smears, and possible fertility problems.

STDs are epidemic in Americans aged 15 to 34. Mild ailments such as yeast and trichomonas can make life miserable, but they aren't serious health threats. Chlamydia, gonorrhea, herpes, syphilis, hepatitis, AIDS, and genital warts are. STDs can be major threats to fertility, health, relationships—even life.

STDs are biologically sexist infections, generally causing more havoc in the reproductive tracts of women than of men. *Pelvic inflammatory disease (PID), a serious complication of chlamydia, gonorrhea, and other bacterial infections, may involuntarily sterilize up to 100,000 U.S. women each year (1), and is a leading cause of ectopic pregnancy as well. PID is also directly responsible for 300,000 hospitalizations each year for women, countless major surgical procedures necessary to treat infection and its sequelae, and about 3 deaths each year for every 1 million women age 15 to 44 (2). STDs are directly linked to a risk of death for women (and men) when:*

- *A woman develops overwhelming PID infection*
- *Major surgery is necessary to control PID or to repair PID damage that is causing pain or infertility*
- *Ectopic pregnancy occurs later as a result of scarring from PID*
- *A woman or a man is infected with the wart virus strains (human papillomavirus) that are reponsible for cervical cancer and are also associated with penile cancer*
- *A woman or a man acquires hepatitis B through sexual exposure*
- *A woman or a man acquires AIDS virus through sexual exposure*
- *An infant suffers birth defects or serious illness because it is infected by its parent's STD during pregnancy or at the time of birth*

STD risks are serious risks, and becoming more so every day. Not just inconvenient, or embarrassing, or uncomfortable: STDs are significant killers, especially for women. And nice people do get STDs. If you are having intercourse, you need a working knowledge of your STD risk, symptoms to watch for in yourself and your sexual partner, and prevention strategies. Read on.

Protecting Yourself from Infection

I've been on the road seven years for my company, spending at least one night a week in a hotel with a bunch of other businessmen. There was the usual playing around, picking up local girls in the hotel bar. I never did that, but I saw a lot of it. Saw a lot of tired-looking guys in the coffee shop the next morning too!

It's been different in the last couple of years. The playboy types are being more careful. Nobody wants to get—or give—some godawful disease, and from what you read, godawful diseases are everywhere.

—MAN, 32

Herpes lasts forever. Chlamydia or gonorrhea could take away fertility without any clear warning of trouble. Some strains of the virus that causes genital warts can lead to cervical cancer. *Clearly, it is best to avoid STDs altogether.*

My husband had an affair after we'd been married four years. He wasn't willing to stop seeing her so we separated. After a few weeks of moping around I started going out with Jeff, and three months after the separation Jeff and I decided to move in together.

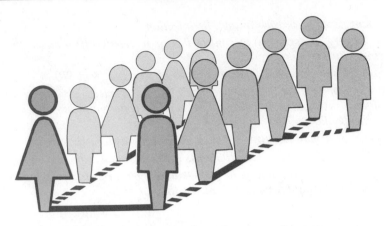

ILLUSTRATION 22-1   In the United States in the 80s, a perfectly "ordinary" man or woman can have an extraordinarily high risk for STD.

> Soon after that I found out I had chlamydia. My first assumption was that I got it from Jeff, but after talking to my doctor I realized that I had in essence been exposed to *five* people's germs in the last few months! My ex-husband, his girlfriend, the guy she used to date, Jeff, and Jeff's former girlfriend!
>
> —WOMAN, 29

Reducing your risk of infection requires your best efforts to be clearheaded, direct, honest, and brave. At least it is comforting to know that measures to protect yourself from one infection will protect you from all of them! Some guidelines for preventing sexually transmitted infection follow:

1. **Your infection risk is highest when you have more than one sex partner or when your partner has more than one sex partner.** Think about STDs any time you are not celibate or living in a long-term, strictly monogamous relationship. See Illustration 22-1 to understand the effects of multiple partners on your risk of infection. If you have more than one partner, then it is quite likely that your partners also have more than one partner each, and all these human beings must be counted in tallying STD exposure risk. Recent but definitely ended relationships count, and so do relationships that weren't significant . . . they count especially!

Reproductive tract infections are transmitted by sexual intimacy: skin to skin, or mucous membrane to mucous membrane. Intercourse, oral sex, and anal sex can all transmit infection. Infections are prevalent among heterosexual men, heterosexual women, homosexual men, and bisexual men and women. STDs are less common among lesbian women. **Infection rates are highest for people between the ages of 15 and 34,** but you can acquire a sexual infection at any age.

2. **Use condoms or a diaphragm with spermicide to help prevent infection.** These products also provide good birth control protection, but it is entirely reasonable to use them even if you are also taking birth control Pills or have already had sterilization surgery. Condoms or a diaphragm with spermicide can reduce your risk of acquiring an STD by half, or even more (3). Research has documented lower rates for gonorrhea and PID among barrier users, and there is some evidence that condoms and spermicides may also help prevent transmission of the viruses that cause herpes, genital warts, and AIDS as well. In the absence of a dual commitment to monogamy, barriers are essential; you can reduce your infection risk if you will use them every time you have intercourse.

Remember, though, that protection is not 100%, and barrier birth control methods will not protect you against warts or herpes infection on the skin of your partner's scrotum, nor could they protect him from similar ailments on your vulva or anus. So, clearheaded and honest risk assessment are important even if you are using barrier products.

3. **Have a frank conversation about infections before you become sexually intimate with a new partner.** It is hard to have a serious conversation about contagious diseases when you are in love (or even when you are not). However, playing fair means you tell him about any past or present infections you've had, and he does the same for you. (If it is just unimaginable to you to have such a conversation, you might want to reevaluate why you are contemplating sexual intimacy with him when intimacy with words isn't there yet.) Try something like this:

> I know this is hard for me and probably for you too, but can we talk
> about sex and infections for a minute? I want you to know that I don't
> have any symptoms of anything at all right now, and I had a good checkup
> two months ago. I did have trich two years ago, but I got a prescription
> that cleared it up. I had a boyfriend in college who had warts on his pe-
> nis, but I didn't get them. So I think I'm fine.
> What about you? Have you ever had anything?

It can be done. It's a great way to begin a grown-up, honest relationship.

4. **Avoid all sexual intimacy if either of you has even mild symptoms of infection.** In the white heat phase of romance when your lover seems absolutely perfect, it may never even occur to you to think of physical flaws. Try to marshal all your clearheadedness and *look*. And *ask*. It is hard, too, to notice your own symptoms in the early phases of love, but if you feel sore and tender or have an unusual discharge, it is best to postpone lovemaking and see your clinician.

5. **Avoid all sexual intimacy if you have any reason at all to suspect either of you has an infection.** If a previous lover calls and says he has gonorrhea, see your clinician first even though you feel entirely well. If your partner says he had a

discharge from his penis for a while but it seems to be cleared up, have him see his clinician first.

Some clinicians think it is prudent to avoid intercourse with a man if a previous partner of his developed cervical cancer, just as a man would be wise to avoid intercourse with a woman who has cervical cancer. Both cervical and penile cancer are linked to wart virus infection, and the wart virus may be present with no obvious symptoms.

6. **Consider pelvic infection risk when you choose a method of birth control.** Women who use birth control Pills have lower rates for PID than do women who are not using contraception. Oral contraceptives may protect users from having sexual infections **ascend** from the vagina into the uterus and tubes. Birth control Pills decrease menstrual bleeding so bacteria have less blood to thrive on; and they help maintain a thick, sticky plug of mucus in the cervical canal for much of the cycle, which may act as a physical barrier to the ascent of pathogens (infection-causing organisms). On the other hand, women who use Pills tend to have a more extensive area of delicate cervical canal lining tissue extending from the cervical opening out across the external surface of the cervix. This tissue may be less resistant to infection than the hardy tissue that normally covers the surface of the cervix. So it may be that Pills **simultaneously increase cervical infection risk** and **decrease the risk of infection in your uterus and tubes.** Further research is needed to clarify Pill/infection relationship more precisely. Many women who are not in long-term monogamous relationships choose to use Pills *and* a diaphragm, Pills *and* a sponge, or Pills *and* condoms for excellent contraception and protection from infection as well.

IUDs increase the likelihood that bacteria in the vagina and cervix will ascend into the uterus and tubes. IUDs increase menstrual blood loss and cramping and the IUD string may provide a pathway through the cervical canal for easier passage of bacteria.

7. **Worry about sex partners—not hot tubs and toilet seats.** Although it appears that pathogens can survive for a brief time on toilet seats, towels, and perhaps even in hot tubs, there is no evidence that anyone has ever acquired an infection from these sites. These pathogens need warm, moist mucous membrane environments for survival.

I had gonorrhea when I was 18, warts when I was 22, and trich four times. I have to get Pap smears every six months. Who knows whether I can get pregnant or not. I want to settle down with one guy—who wants to settle down with me—and stop worrying about who's going to give who what. Why can't people be more like snow geese and mate for life?

—WOMAN, 25

Manifestations of Reproductive Tract Infection

There are close to 25 bacteria, viruses, parasites, and other pathogens that cause illness when they are transmitted via sexual intimacy. Only the ten or so common American pathogens will be discussed in detail in this chapter. If you recently had a date in Jakarta, Malawi, or another exotic tropical location and now have symptoms of infection, you may have made the acquaintance of one of the rarer STDs, so see your clinician and be sure you inform her/him about your travels, and read Chapter 29 for some details on the more uncommon STDs.

It is important to understand in the beginning just how a bout of infection causes temporary or permanent harm to your body. Infections can attack one structure only, your cervix alone or your labia alone, for example. Some types of infection tend to **ascend**; that is, pathogens are deposited in the vagina and on the surface of the cervix during intercourse, then move upward through the cervical canal—perhaps carried by swimming sperm cells—to the uterus. (See the illustrations in Chapter 2 for a review of a woman's reproductive tract structures.) Uterine muscle contractions may push pathogens into the tubes to invade the ovaries and the entire pelvis, and bacteria or viruses may even enter the bloodstream to travel throughout the body.

THE BACTERIAL INFECTION PROCESS

Three very common infections—chlamydia, gonorrhea, and bacterial vaginosis—are caused by one-celled bacteria organisms. Each illness has its own specific bacterial pathogen, so each is diagnosed and treated in a different way. (See Illustration 22-2 to learn what *Chlamydia trachomatis* looks like under an electron microscope.)

Some bacteria attach to the surface of normal body tissue cells, and some live within host cells, such as gonorrhea and chlamydia. Some types thrive on oxygen (aerobic bacteria), while others are very intolerant of oxygen (anaerobic). Gonorrhea bacteria cannot survive in an oxygen-rich environment and chlamydia is exquisitely fussy about its environment and only thrives when conditions are absolutely perfect. This fastidiousness is the reason that until quite recently it has been very difficult and expensive to test for chlamydia: technicians simply couldn't keep the organism alive long enough to diagnose the disease.

In the 1940s the first drugs capable of killing harmful bacteria became widely available—the antibiotics. Antibiotic chemicals work by invading bacterial cells and deactivating them. The "broad spectrum" antibiotics destroy many different types of bacteria. Other types of antibiotic drugs are effective for only a few bacterial pathogens.

Many kinds of bacteria normally live in the intestine (where they are essential for digestion) and on the outer surfaces of the body, including the vaginal cavity. The uterus and other internal pelvic organs, however, are normally free of bacteria. The

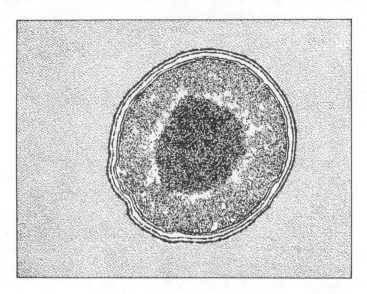

ILLUSTRATION 22-2   *Chlamydia's* elementary body is magnified 118,000 times
in this illustration. The tiny bacteria can survive only inside other cells.

uterine cavity and cervix are protected by mucus that has a mild germ-killing
(antibacterial) effect and constantly coats and cleanses the lining of the uterus and
cervix. The occasional bacterium that enters the uterus usually is destroyed by white
cells from the bloodstream.

No matter what kind of bacteria is present or where in your body infection occurs,
the infection process is fairly predictable. Bacteria are nourished by the fluid or tissue
that they attack, and then produce waste products that they release into the invaded
tissues. Body defenses sense the presence of bacteria and send white blood cells into the
area to attack them. The infected area becomes warm, red, and swollen because of the
increased blood flow and the accumulation of pus, which is composed of dead bacteria,
dead white blood cells, and fluid. Bacterial waste products can be poisonous and can
cause fever, chills, and malaise (feeling tired and achy) when they enter your
circulation and travel to the rest of your body. Toxic shock syndrome is an example of
an illness caused by the poisonous (toxic) chemicals released by certain types of
Staphylococcus aureus bacteria.

Your cells can be destroyed by bacteria directly, or indirectly by the excessive
swelling and poisonous bacterial wastes. Even when all bacteria are eradicated, tissues
may heal slowly and may never completely return to normal.

**Your body's normal infection defenses can be overwhelmed if a large number of
bacteria or an unusually aggressive kind of bacteria invades your body.** A large number
of bacteria can enter your uterus on medical instruments during a D&C (see Chapter
47), an endometrial biopsy (see Chapter 4), or insertion of an IUD; contamination is
more likely if your cervix is infected or you have vaginitis at the time.

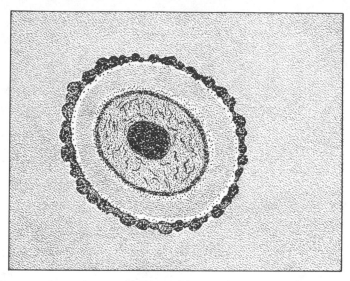

ILLUSTRATION 22-3   The herpes virus particles can lie dormant in nerve pathways for months or years.

Your normal infection defenses may prove inadequate if your uterus contains blood or unexpelled fetal or placental tissue after a miscarriage or abortion. These substances are ideal sites for bacterial growth, and your infection-fighting white blood cells have difficulty reaching them inside the uterus. The presence of an IUD may also interfere with your infection defenses. Diabetes and some medications, such as cortisone, can reduce your body defenses against all kinds of infection.

Reproductive tract infection is rare during a normal pregnancy, but after delivery your cervical opening does not shrink to normal size for several weeks, and the lining of your uterus does not have its normal mucus protection. Infection risk is high during the first few weeks after delivery, miscarriage, or abortion.

The risk that STD infection might spread upward to your uterus and fallopian tubes is higher during your menstrual period than at other times in your cycle. Bleeding seems to facilitate bacterial spread and blood enhances bacterial growth. Women with reproductive tract infection often say that they first noticed symptoms two or three days after the beginning of a menstrual period.

Your defense against infection is impaired if you have scarring or damage from infection in the past; and you may have repeated attacks months or years after your initial infection.

THE VIRAL INFECTION PROCESS

Viruses are tiny organisms made of the nucleic acids DNA or RNA. They are much smaller than bacteria. (See Illustration 22-3 to learn what the genital herpes virus

COMMON SITES FOR STD SYMPTOMS

	Trichomonas	Candida	Bacterial Vaginosis	Chlamydia	Gonorrhea	Herpes	Genital Warts	Aids	Viral Hepatitis	Syphilis
Vulva	■	■	■	■	■	■	■			■
Bartholin's glands				■	■					
Vagina	■	■	■	■	■					■
Rectum*		■		■	■	■				■
Cervix	■		■	■	■	■				■
Uterus				■	■					
Tubes				■	■					
Ovaries				■	■					
Pelvis				■	■	■				
Systemic						■		■	■	■
Urethra, bladder**	■			■	■					

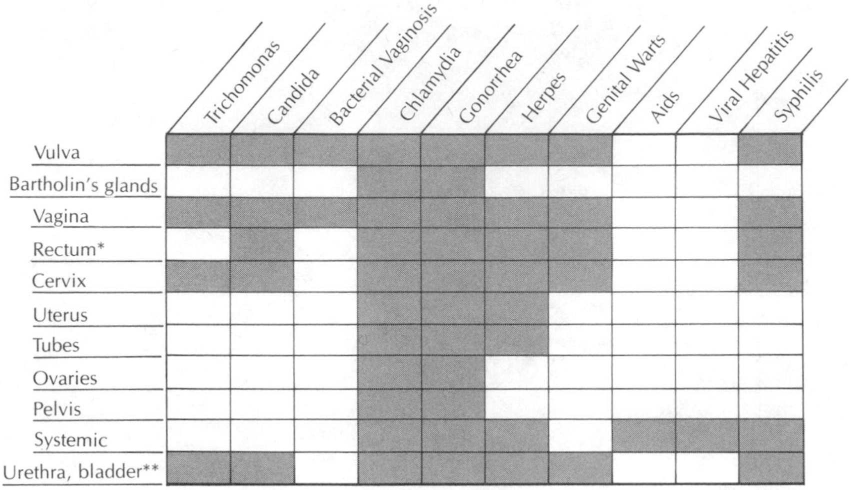

*Vulnerable to infection with anal intercourse and oral/anal contact

**SEE Chapter 23 for details on urinary tract infections.

ILLUSTRATION 22-4 Common sites for STD symptoms.

looks like under an electron microscope.) Viruses invade normal cells, take over the cell's metabolic functions, and feed themselves with the cell's own fuel.

Herpes, viral hepatitis, and genital warts are common infections that are caused by viruses.

Antibiotics are ineffective against viral illness. The body's own immune system controls viral infections by recognizing the invader (the antigen) and mobilizing an antibody response. Antibodies coat and kill the foreign virus particles and mark them so macrophages—giant cells that do "mop-up" duty for the infection-fighting system—can destroy what's left of the virus. A clinician may help you through a viral illness by providing medication to relieve symptoms and possibly by giving you antibiotics to control any bacterial infection that attacks susceptible, virus-weakened tissues.

We do understand how to **prevent** some viral illness. Childhood vaccinations for measles, mumps, smallpox, rubella, and polio are all examples of effective **immunization** against virus disease. Vaccination triggers an initial antibody response, which remains ready for immediate activation if the same virus antigen enters the body again.

So far there are very few drugs that are effective in treating a virus infection once it has begun. Acyclovir, a drug to help control herpes, is one example, and research is under way to find more antiviral drugs that are not too toxic to use.

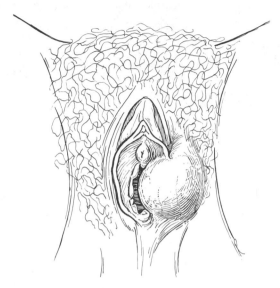

ILLUSTRATION 22-5   An infected Bartholin's gland.

SITES OF INFECTION

Symptoms of bacterial or viral infection can appear in any or all parts of a woman's reproductive tract, and some infections cause symptoms in other parts of the body completely removed from the reproductive tract. Pain, discharge, itching, and skin lesions (blisters, warts, or sores) can be mild, moderate, or severe. You could have only fever and malaise and not suspect a reproductive tract infection at all. You could be entirely symptom-free. If you are having intercourse—and particularly if you or your sex partner has **another** partner—consider the possibility of STD any time you suspect you are ill. Illustration 22-4 shows common sites for symptoms with the ten STDs discussed in this chapter.

Vulvar Symptoms.   When you have a cervical or vaginal infection, you will be likely to notice symptoms of itching, redness, or discharge **only on your vulva, if at all,** because the vulva is rich in nerve receptors and the cervix and vagina aren't. Although the vagina is actually the main site of infection, discharge coming fom the vagina reaches the vulva, where its irritating effects are much more likely to be evident.

Genital warts, herpes blisters, and the chancre of primary syphilis all appear very commonly on the labia and other vulvar structures, including the area around the anus.

Bartholin's Gland Infection.   Bartholin's glands are normally inconspicuous (see Chapter 2). If a gland is invaded by infection, however, it becomes very conspicuous: an exquisitely tender, hot lump that can become as large as a lime (see Illustration 22-5). Infection is often caused by chlamydia or gonorrhea, but can also be caused by other kinds of bacteria.

An initial episode of infection can cause scarring of the gland duct and impair or block drainage of normal gland secretions. If this occurs, then subsequent, repeated attacks of infection are likely. Also, scarring can lead to gradual accumulation of gland secretions trapped within the gland, forming a large cyst.

Vaginal Symptoms.   Vaginal infections are some of the most common maladies any clinician ever sees. Herpes blisters, genital warts, and the chancre of primary syphilis can all appear in the vagina. With these culprits, however, you may not notice any symptoms at all because there are few nerve receptors for pain and discomfort in the vagina. The discharges of yeast infection (candidiasis), bacterial vaginosis, trichomonas, and many types of cervicitis may be abundantly evident when they cause large amounts of leaky vaginal discharge. In some cases the amount of discharge is truly copious. In other cases, though, the amount of discharge may be so modest that it is not apparent externally, although you might notice discharge adhering to the vaginal wall during your own speculum exam or even with a finger inside your vagina. You are, however, quite likely to notice irritation of your vulva caused by exposure to discharge coming from a vaginal infection. Vaginitis is discussed in detail in Chapter 23.

Rectal Symptoms.   Herpes blisters, genital warts, and the chancre of primary syphilis can all appear in the area around the rectum. Women who have anal intercourse or anal/oral sexual contact can experience rectal pain and discharge from rectal gonorrhea, chlamydia, herpes, and warts, and from a number of intestinal infections such as amebiasis, giardiasis, or shigellosis.

Cervical Symptoms.   Herpes blisters, genital warts, and the chancre of primary syphilis can all appear on the surface of the cervix. When infection actually invades the cervix, the condition is called cervicitis. **Cervicitis** is inflammation of the cervix (the ending "itis" means inflammation). Inflammation can also be caused by chemicals or foreign bodies. If you have mild cervicitis, you may not notice any symptoms at all. A more severe case of cervicitis can cause profuse, pus-like discharge with an objectionable odor that persists throughout your cycle. Discharge is often thin or of a mucous consistency, and gray-white or yellow in color. Cervicitis may cause pain during intercourse or when you touch your cervix, spotting or bleeding after intercourse, or even abdominal pain and back pain.

Chlamydia, gonorrhea, trichomonas, herpes, and candida organisms can cause cervicitis. If you have a chlamydial infection your clinician may call the condition mucopurulent cervicitis. Common bacteria that are normally present in the vagina can also cause cervicitis if they invade the mucus glands in the cervical canal and begin to multiply. Chemicals in vaginal hygiene products can also cause inflammation.

Your clinician may suspect cervicitis on the basis of your symptoms, the appearance of your cervix, a microscopic examination of cervical discharge, or an abnormal Pap smear that shows inflammatory cells (see Chapter 35). If cervicitis is severe, your clinician will find that your cervix is swollen, reddened, and possibly tender to the touch. **You may have a pus discharge from your cervix,** and the surface of your cervix may look abnormal. Your clinician may use terms like eroded (raw) or friable (crumbly) to describe the appearance of your cervix.

Tests for chlamydia and gonorrhea are essential if you have cervicitis, because both of these pathogens thrive in the endocervical (cervical canal) environment. Your clinician may prepare a wet smear (see Chapter 4) to look for trichomonas or yeast organisms, or excessive vaginal bacteria.

If the surface of your cervix appears abnormal or if you have an area of erosion, your clinician may use a colposcope (see Chapter 4) to distinguish between simple inflammation and precancerous ulceration. Biopsy (also described in Chapter 4) of abnormal areas is sometimes helpful in making a precise diagnosis. If you have genital warts on your cervix, your clinician will want to remove them because of the possible increased risk of cervical cancer. (Read Chapter 35 for more details.) If your clinician finds that you have chlamydia, gonorrhea, yeast, or trichomonas infection, she/he will treat it. If a chemical irritant is causing cervicitis, your clinician will advise you to avoid it.

Prolonged or repeated problems with cervicitis may lead you to consider cryosurgery, which is described in Chapter 4. Prolonged cervicitis may make it difficult or impossible for you to become pregnant; abnormal mucus production interferes with sperm's ability to penetrate your cervical canal.

Treatment for your partner is crucial if your cervicitis is caused by chlamydia, gonorrhea, or trichomonas infection, and you must avoid intercourse until your cervicitis is cured. You also may be advised to avoid intercourse or have your partner use condoms while you are being treated for other types of cervicitis.

Symptoms in the Uterus, Tubes, Ovaries, and Pelvis.   Chlamydia and gonorrhea are the two infections most likely to ascend from the vagina through the cervix to invade the internal reproductive organs and cause pain, vaginal discharge or bleeding, chills, and fever. Some terms your clinician may use in describing these conditions are endometritis (uterine lining is infected), myometritis (uterine lining and uterine muscle wall are infected), salpingitis (fallopian tubes are infected), oophoritis (ovary is infected), and pelvic peritonitis (membrane lining of the abdomen is infected).

Pelvic inflammatory disease is an extremely serious complication of chlamydia, gonorrhea, and other bacterial infections because it can impair fertility and health, and may even be life-threatening. PID is discussed in detail in Chapter 25.

Systemic Symptoms.   Acquired immunodeficiency syndrome (AIDS), viral hepatitis, and syphilis are infections that may be transmitted through sexual intimacy but have few manifestations in the reproductive tract per se, with the exception of the usually painless and often unnoticed ulcer, called a chancre, of primary syphilis. The manifestations of these illnesses are discussed in detail in Chapter 28. Pelvic inflammatory disease can cause fever and generalized malaise (feeling tired, achy, and ill). An initial outbreak of herpes can cause fever, malaise, and swollen lymph glands. The rash of secondary syphilis can appear over large areas of skin.

Urinary Tract Symptoms.   Because the distance from the vagina to the urethra is only about 1/2 inch, and because the urethra itself is only an inch long, it isn't surprising that chlamydia, gonorrhea, herpes, and trichomonas organisms can colonize the urethra, bladder, and even the kidneys. These infections are discussed in detail in Chapter 38, "Bladder and Kidney Problems."

Coping with Infection

If you are having symptoms, or are worried about a possible STD, contact your clinician. She/he should be able to schedule the exam and tests you need without delay, or refer you promptly to an appropriate resource. If you don't have a clinician, you can call your local health department or Planned Parenthood clinic. Both are almost certain to provide STD evaluation and treatment themselves, as well as referral suggestions for private care if that is what you prefer.

The diseases covered in this chapter have different symptoms and require different treatments. They even have lots of different names. See Table 22-1 for a list of infections and their aliases. Each disease is discussed in more detail in the following chapters. Certain basic facts about transmission and cure, however, apply to all of them.

1. **Don't wait for symptoms to go away.** Infections are very unlikely to vanish without treatment. Symptoms may come and go, but you will need treatment to get a genuine cure.

2. **If you think you need to be tested for infection, be sure to ask for testing.** Your clinician may not automatically test you for any sexual infections when you have a checkup unless you let her/him know you are concerned. If you have oral sex or anal sex be sure to tell your clinician so you can be examined thoroughly for an accurate diagnosis. Also, antibiotic treatment may be different for a throat infection than for a reproductive tract infection.

3. **Know the warning signs of infection.** Although it is not uncommon for both men and women to have a contagious reproductive tract infection with no symptoms

22:6   STD (Sexually Transmitted Disease) DANGER SIGNS

Abnormal vaginal discharge
Pain or burning with urination or bowel movements
Itching around your vulva, rectum, or pubic hair
Blisters, warts, bumps, or sores of any kind around your vulva
    or rectum
Abnormal bleeding, or bleeding after intercourse
Pain with intercourse, either near the opening of your vagina or
    deep inside
Pain in your pelvis or back
Menstrual cramps that are unusually severe
Tenderness in your pelvis with pressure or jarring, such as when
    you cough or run
Chills
Fever (temperature over 100.4 degrees F.)
General tired, achy feeling (malaise)

See your clinician immediately or go to a hospital emergency room
if you develop any of these signs.

whatsoever, see your clinician right away if you develop any of the symptoms shown in Illustration 22-6.

4. **Don't ignore even mild symptoms in yourself or your partner.** The most commonly reported STD is chlamydia, and chlamydia may not cause any dramatic symptoms for you or your partner.

5. **An examination and lab tests are the only way to learn what kind of infection—or infections—you have.** Remember that chlamydia, gonorrhea, and other illnesses can coexist. You must be tested if you suspect that you have been exposed to an infection. Be sure you ask your clinician to give you the specific name(s) of your infection(s).

Leftover medicines from your seventh yeast infection may be just what you need to cure your eighth one! In general, however, you'll need an exam, lab tests, and a new prescription for any infection. Don't take any leftover antibiotics before you see your clinician and do not douche before your exam; if you do, your tests may not be accurate. Your clinician cannot diagnose a discharge that isn't there.

None of the common infections responds to exactly the same kind of treatment; chlamydia medicine will not help a trichomonas infection, for example. You may have more than one infection at the same time, and you will need two separate and distinct courses of treatment. If you are itching and miserable and have to wait three days for your appointment, frequent soaks in a bathtub full of plain warm water (sitz bath) may relieve your symptoms. Betadine douche used according to the directions on the package is often an effective interim treatment for mild vaginitis, and does not require a prescription. Two dangers with self-treatment for vaginitis are the possibility that you

TABLE 22-1
INFECTIONS AND THEIR ALIASES[a]

TRICHOMONAS

Trich
Trichomoniasis
Trichomonas vaginalis

BACTERIAL VAGINOSIS

Nonspecific vaginitis
Gardnerella vaginalis
Bacterial vaginitis
Hemophilus vaginalis
Corynebacterium vaginalis
Anaerobic vaginosis

GONORRHEA

Neisseria gonorrhoeae
G.C.
Clap
Gonococcus
Drip

GENITAL WARTS

Venereal warts
Condylomata acuminata
Flat condylomata
HPV warts
Human papillomavirus (HPV) warts
Papovavirus warts

HERPES

Genital herpes
Herpes simplex type 2
Herpes genitalis
HSV

**ACQUIRED IMMUNODEFICIENCY
  SYNDROME**

AIDS
Acquired Immune Deficiency
  Syndrome
HIV infection
HTLV-III/LAV infection

YEAST

Candida albicans
Fungus infection
Monilia
Candidiasis

TOXIC SHOCK SYNDROME

TSS

CHLAMYDIA

Chlamydia trachomatis
Mucopurulent cervicitis
Nongonococcal urethritis (in men)

PELVIC INFLAMMATORY DISEASE

PID
Pelvic infection
Polymicrobial pelvic infection

CERVICAL INTRAEPITHELIAL NEOPLASIA

CIN
Abnormal Pap smear
Class III or IV Pap
Precancerous cell changes
Dysplasia

VIRAL HEPATITIS

Hepatitis B
Venereal hepatitis

SYPHILIS

Syph
Treponema pallidum
Lues

LYMPHOGRANULOMA VENEREUM

LGV
Chlamydia trachomatis
Tropical bubo

PUBIC LICE

Crabs
Papillon d'amour
Phthirus pubis
Pediculosis pubis

MOLLUSCUM CONTAGIOSUM

Poxvirus
Molluscum

SCABIES

Sarcoptes scabiei
Mites

---

[a]For some reason neither the medical world nor the general public has been able to settle on one name for sexual infections. Here is a list of terms the authors use, along with some medical and lay aliases.

might have chlamydia or gonorrhea and remain untreated and unaware because no test was done, and that your treatment might interfere with tests your clinician performs later to diagnose the cause of infection.

6. **If you have an STD, your partner needs to be treated at the same time you are.** It may be awkward or embarrassing, but fair play really does mandate full disclosure to any sex partners you've had, particularly in the past 30 days. (If syphilis is the issue, you'll need to tell partners going back six months.) Being honest and complete about partner exposure is important as a public health responsibility—and it is also important for your own health. You are likely to get reinfected immediately unless your partner(s) is treated along with you. Many clinicians are willing to give you medicine to take to your partner yourself, but in some cases your partner must be seen himself for treatment. Ask your clinician to tell you where your partner should go for treatment. Sometimes men have clear symptoms of infection, but often they do not. Burning, pain, discharge, or skin irritation may be present with many of the common infections, but it is also possible for a man to have no outward signs of infection. You cannot assume that he is infection-free just because he has no symptoms.

7. **Use all the medicines you are given, and use medicines correctly.** Infections tend to feel better before they are completely cured (thank goodness). But be diligent about your medication schedule, and use the full course recommended so that you will be sure of a cure.

Tell your clinician if you are using any other prescription or nonprescription medications.

If you have ever had any kind of allergic reaction to penicillin, you must not use penicillin, ampicillin, or any drug with a "cillin" ending. Be sure to tell your clinician about your history of allergy. She/he is likely to prescribe tetracycline or another substitute antibiotic.

Do not take tetracycline if you are pregnant or suspect that you could be pregnant and intend to continue the pregnancy. Tetracycline may cause dark stains on the permanent teeth of a fetus that is exposed to the pregnant woman's tetracycline. Avoid milk, all milk products, antacids, and iron, vitamin, and mineral supplements one hour before and two hours after each tetracycline pill. The calcium in these products decreases your body's ability to absorb and use tetracycline, with the result that the drug may not be fully effective. Avoid sunbathing and prolonged sun exposure of any kind while you are taking tetracycline, because you may develop a skin rash. Never use tetracycline after the expiration date on the package; serious side effects have been reported with outdated or degraded pills.

If you are pregnant or suspect you are pregnant, **do not use sulfa drugs, acyclovir (Zovirax), or lindane** (the active ingredient in many treatments for pubic lice and scabies). **Avoid metronidazole (Flagyl)** in the first trimester of pregnancy.

Make sure you know the exact name and danger signs for the particular drug your clinician prescribes. Diarrhea, for example, is a common and fairly harmless side effect with ampicillin; diarrhea with some other less common antibiotics may be a sign of serious trouble.

8. **Find out from your clinician whether you will need a follow-up exam.** A repeat test for you and your partner is crucial if you have chlamydia or gonorrhea, but you may be able to tell for yourself whether your yeast, trichomonas, or bacterial vaginosis is under control. Even these infections can be stubborn, so see your clinician for repeat tests if you suspect that you still have a problem. It may be especially important to have follow-up tests when you have been treated with antibiotics such as ampicillin or tetracycline, because these drugs may **promote** the growth of yeast while they cure the other infection. Some clinicians routinely provide a prescription for yeast medication along with such antibiotics so that you can have the prescription filled later if you develop symptoms.

9. **Avoid intercourse or have your partner use condoms until you are certain both you and your partner have been cured.** Intercourse is likely to be painful as long as you have symptoms anyway.

10. **Infections can cause abnormal Pap smears.** Bacterial vaginosis, yeast, trichomonas, herpes, chlamydia, and gonorrhea can cause significant inflammation of the cervix; and inflammation can cause abnormal but noncancerous cell changes. It is common to have abnormal Pap smears during an infection. Have your Pap test repeated when your infection is cleared up, in 6 to 12 weeks. When you are free from inflammation, your Pap test is more likely to give an accurate report on the presence or absence of premalignant or malignant cervical cells.

REFERENCES

1. Cates W Jr: Sexually transmitted diseases: The national view. *Cutis* 33:69–80, 1984.
2. Grimes DA: Deaths due to sexually transmitted diseases: The forgotten component of reproductive mortality. *Journal of the American Medical Association* 255:1727–1729, 1986.
3. Stone KM, Grimes DA, Magder LS: Personal protection against sexually transmitted diseases. *American Journal of Obstetrics and Gynecology* 155:180–188, 1986.

Vaginitis: Trichomonas, Yeast, and Bacterial Vaginosis

Trichomonas, yeast, and bacterial vaginosis are exceedingly common maladies that cause physical and emotional distress, but are not likely to cause serious health problems among basically healthy people. These are the infections that cause maddening itchiness and drippiness, fear of smelling bad, and a sense that your sexual attractiveness has probably plummeted to zero. No small problems these, especially when you are on your third round of treatment for the same infection in a year's time. If your clinician seems to minimize the significance of these infections, it is because your health is not likely to be threatened. It is entirely normal for you to feel as though your infection is quite a big deal indeed.

Trichomonas Vaginitis
("Trich," Trichomoniasis, Trichomonas vaginalis; Pronounced "Trick")

Trichomonas is caused by a one-celled protozoan called a trichomonad (see Illustration 23-1). Infection is usually transmitted by sexual intimacy. The trichomonad is not quite as delicate as the chlamydia or gonorrhea bacterium, so it may be possible for trichomonads to survive for up to 24 hours on wet towels or bathing suits. This finding may explain why trichomonas outbreaks occasionally occur among institutionalized women (1).

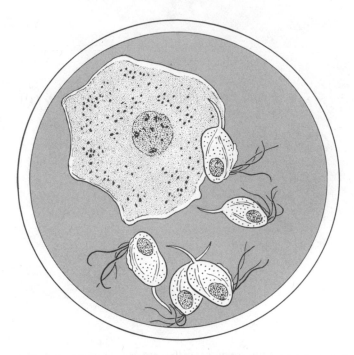

ILLUSTRATION 23-1   The one-celled protozoan that causes trichomonas. A whip-like tail allows the trichomonad to move rapidly.

Symptoms.   Trichomonas is apt to produce a frothy, thin, greenish white or grayish vaginal discharge, intense itching, redness, an objectionable odor, pain, and/or frequency of urination. It may produce no symptoms at all in women, and usually produces no symptoms in men. When men do have symptoms, they are likely to have discharge, burning with urination, or irritation.

I've had vaginitis before, but trich was something else! I had gallons of discharge, and it really burned. One day I was fine, and the next day I couldn't even go to work. It was the first time in my life I demanded an immediate appointment with my doctor.

—WOMAN, 31

Diagnosis.   Your clinician will prepare a wet smear by mixing a sample of your discharge with a drop of salt solution (normal saline) and examining it under a microscope. Trichomonas organisms often can be easily identified because they swim quite rapidly with their whip-like tails. Trichomonads are sometimes identified on a

Pap smear or in the sediment of a urine specimen. Trichomonas can also cause small, dark red spots (petechiae) on your cervix. Your vaginal secretions are likely to be more alkaline than normal, and your clinician may use a strip of pH paper to check acidity. The pH is likely to exceed 5.0.

Treatment.   The most effective drug for treatment of trichomonas is metronidazole. Some brand names for metronidazole are Flagyl, Metryl, Protostat, and Satric. For simplicity's sake the name Flagyl is used in this discussion. Flagyl is an antibiotic that is given in pill form. Your clinician may recommend either (2):

• A single 2,000-mg dose, or
• Three 250-mg doses every day for seven days

One-day treatment is certainly less of a bother. There is some evidence that the seven-day regimen may be slightly more effective, however (1).
   Your partner(s) must be treated at the same time you are.
   Side effects of Flagyl may include an allergic reaction; nausea and/or diarrhea; dryness of the mouth; a tinny, metallic taste; a depression in the white blood cell count (leukopenia); and intolerance to alcohol—many (not all) people who drink alcohol within 24 hours after Flagyl therapy experience nausea, vomiting, headache, and/or flushing.
   The FDA-approved information leaflet for physicians that accompanies each package of Flagyl begins with the following statement (3):

WARNING

Metronidazole *[generic name for Flagyl]* has been shown to be carcino-genic *[cancer-producing]* in mice and rats. Unnecessary use of the drug should be avoided. Its use should be reserved for the conditions described in the Indications and Usage section below.

The "Indications and Usage" section says that Flagyl (for both you and your partner) should be used only when your clinician has done lab tests to be sure trichomonads are present and when you have definite symptoms of inflammation caused by these organisms. There is no evidence that the drug causes cancer in human beings.
   The FDA-approved instructions also recommend that you have a white blood cell count performed both before and after treatment, because Flagyl may temporarily decrease your body's ability to produce white blood cells (leukocytes). **A white cell**

count is especially important before taking a second course of Flagyl. Diminished white blood cell production could impair your body's ability to fight infection of any kind.

If you have a severe, stubborn infection and choose to take a second course of Flagyl, observe the following precautions: (1) Have another exam and a microscopic examination of your discharge to be certain trichomonads are still present. (2) Have a white blood cell count. (3) Be certain that you are not pregnant. (4) Make sure that your partner(s) and anyone he may have had intercourse with are treated. (5) Wait at least four to six weeks after your first course of treatment.

Do not use Flagyl at all if you are in the first trimester of pregnancy, and avoid the one-day treatment in later stages of pregnancy. It may be best to stay away from Flagyl completely when you are pregnant and to use clotrimazole suppositories, hypertonic saline douches, and other topical medications to relieve your symptoms. Do not nurse while you are using Flagyl because the drug appears in breast milk. You can take the single-dose treatment if you interrupt your breastfeeding for 24 hours afterward. Medications such as antibiotic vaginal suppositories are not as effective as Flagyl and do not kill trichomonads in your urinary system (or in your partner), so reinfection is quite likely.

Prognosis. Trichomonas can occasionally be cured with antibiotic vaginal suppositories such as clotrimazole or antibiotic douches, and can almost always be cured with Flagyl. Reinfection is quite common and recurrence in some cases may occur because the trichomonas strain is resistant to Flagyl, or medications such as phenobarbital taken simultaneously have reduced Flagyl's effectiveness. Yeast infections often flare up after a trichomonas infection. Trichomonas does not attack or harm your uterus or tubes, and your fertility should not be affected once the infection is cured.

You should avoid intercourse during treatment and your partner should use condoms for the first four to six weeks after that to avoid reexposure until you can be sure that your treatment has been successful, and that your partner(s) has completed treatment.

A small percentage of female infants born to women with an active trichomonas infection will acquire the disease. Infection in infants often vanishes in a few weeks, once the mother's estrogen hormone leaves the baby's circulation.

Yeast Infection
(Monilia, Candida, Fungus Infection)

Yeast is a very common fungus *(Candida albicans)* that normally exists in harmony with other organisms in your body (see Illustration 23-2). When it overgrows, you are likely to have symptoms. Yeast is usually not sexually transmitted.

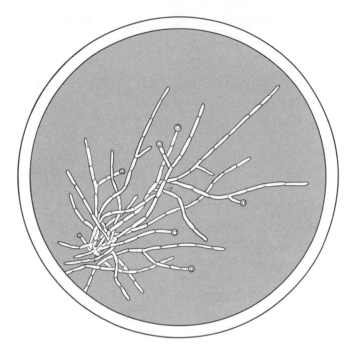

ILLUSTRATION 23-2   Yeast infection is caused by an overgrowth of *Candida albicans,* a ubiquitous fungus.

Symptoms.   Yeast infection causes a thick, white, cottage-cheese-like discharge, itching, redness, or swelling around the labia, and sometimes itching and redness on the upper thighs. Burning and/or itching may be most obvious after intercourse, and itching is frequently severe. Some women notice a faint, sweet, "yeasty" smell. Some women have no symptoms at all. Men may be symptom-free, or may develop urethritis, sores on the penis, or inflammation of the tip of the penis.

Diagnosis.   Your clinician will mix a sample of your discharge with a drop of potassium hydroxide solution and examine it under a microscope. Long, branching yeast colonies are easy to see and may also appear on your Pap smear. Vaginal acidity is likely to be normal (pH of 4.5 or less). Your clinician may also examine a sample of your discharge by staining, or may send a sample to a lab for culture.

Treatment.   Yeast infections are usually treated with antibiotic vaginal cream or suppositories such as Monistat (miconazole), Gyne-Lotrimin or Mycelex (clotrimazole), or Femstat (butoconazole). For an initial yeast infection attack, three different medication schedules provide similar cure rates with either **miconazole or clotrimazole** (2):

- One 100-mg dose each day for seven days
- One 200-mg dose each day for three days
- A single 500-mg dose (clotrimazole only)

Butoconazole cream, one 100-mg dose each day for three days, is the newest yeast treatment alternative, and small studies show cure rates similar to those for miconazole and clotrimazole (4). Nystatin cream or suppositories (brand names such as Mycostatin, Nilstat, and others) are probably somewhat less effective, and require 7 to 14 days of treatment.

The safety of these products has not been established during the first trimester of pregnancy and when breastfeeding. Treatment of partners probably isn't necessary, but healing will be quicker if you avoid intercourse during treatment.

Store suppositories in the refrigerator to prevent melting. You can use tampons or pads to reduce vaginal discharge caused by melting suppositories. Cream containing a yeast-killing agent or a combination of yeast-killer and cortisone, such as Mycolog Cream, can be applied to the skin around the entrance to your vagina and on your thighs to reduce swelling and itching and make you more comfortable until the vaginal yeast treatment has a chance to overcome your infection. Another alternative for skin treatment is lotion containing miconazole; and the lotion may be preferable because it is less likely to leave a persistent moist residue that may aggravate skin problems.

Gentian violet suppositories (Hyva) or tampons (Genapax) once or twice a day for 12 to 14 days may be used to cure yeast. These cause purple stains on clothing, so use pads or panty shields. Boric acid powder (600 mg once a day) dissolved in a douche or inserted in the vagina in gelatin capsules is another alternative. This substance, however, is classified as a poison and possible toxicity issues have not been studied sufficiently to allow firm conclusions about its safety.

There is some evidence that potassium sorbate is effective against yeast infections. This chemical is used as a preservative in food and by vintners to control yeast in wine production, and can be used in douche or suppository form. One commercial vaginal suppository—Summer's Eve—contains 3% potassium sorbate.

Plain yogurt made with live culture is very popular as a yeast remedy. Some women who have tried it recommend eating yogurt, and others insert yogurt into the vagina. There is no research to indicate what, if any, therapeutic effect yogurt has. Similarly, some women use lactobacillus in a capsule or douche to control yeast infections. Lactobacilli are harmless bacteria that normally inhabit the vagina; advocates of this treatment feel that it may help restore the balance of the vaginal ecosystem. There are no scientific studies to determine whether or not lactobacillus therapy is effective.

Prognosis.   Medication will almost always cure yeast infections, but reinfection is extremely common. Your symptoms should improve within a day or two and be completely gone within two weeks. Yeast does not attack or harm your uterus or tubes and should not affect your fertility once you are cured. Babies born to women with active yeast infections are more likely to develop thrush, an oral yeast infection.

Problems with Recurring Yeast.   Repeated yeast attacks are miserable for the unfortunate woman who has them, and effective treatment is not clear-cut. Spontaneous yeast attacks can occur months, weeks, or even just a few days after treatment. Exactly what prompts repeated attacks is not known, but probably depends mainly on the woman's current susceptibility. Yeast is ubiquitous: yeast organisms are present almost everywhere in our environment. At least 20% of normal women, and 40% of pregnant women, carry yeast in their vaginas with no symptoms at all. Yeast is also a "normal" inhabitant of the intestinal tract. So no specific exposure or source of yeast is necessary to start a yeast vaginal infection attack.

The fact that yeast is ubiquitous also means that efforts to rid the body of all yeast organisms "once and for all" are unrealistic. Yeast is almost sure to return as soon as medication is stopped. A more reasonable goal is to reduce temporary yeast overgrowth (in the vagina) in hopes that the normal state of affairs, a few yeast organisms living in harmony with normal vaginal bacteria, can be reestablished.

Persistent yeast problems are especially likely during pregnancy. Women who take birth control Pills also have higher yeast colonization rates than women using other birth control methods. Research is not clear, however, on whether Pill users have more symptomatic yeast attacks. Women with diabetes are often plagued by yeast, possibly because of their higher blood sugar (and therefore vaginal sugar) level. It is very unlikely, however, that vaginal yeast would be a first sign of diabetes. Some clinicians recommend diabetes testing for women who have repeated yeast attacks, but many do not. Other, more significant, signs of diabetes would almost surely be obvious. Yeast is also a common problem for women who are significantly overweight.

If you are suffering with recurring yeast attacks, the following suggestions may help you regain control of your vaginal environment.

First, be sure the problem really is yeast. A yeast infection in May does not guarantee that vaginal discharge in October is also yeast. If you have been exposed to a new partner (or your partner has possible exposure), another exam is essential to be sure that you don't have a sexually transmitted culprit like trichomonas or bacterial vaginosis that is causing symptoms similar to your previous yeast attack.

Consider prolonged and/or intermittent treatment. If this is your second or third yeast attack within a few months, choose the seven-day treatment plan and ask your clinician about refills for your medication. You may want to try a 7- to 14-day initial treatment followed by 1- or 2-day treatment each month to prevent flare-ups.

Yeast medication taken by mouth such as nystatin or ketoconazole can temporarily eradicate yeast in the mouth and intestinal tract. Research so far has not shown any persuasive improvement in initial cure rates for yeast vaginitis by this treatment as compared to vaginal medication, but long-term treatment can reduce the number of recurring infection attacks (5). Be sure to discuss possible adverse effects of oral medication with your clinician. Side effects are not common, but ketoconazole can cause liver toxicity in rare cases.

Use yeast treatment whenever you take other antibiotics. Refill your yeast medication and use it during treatment for other vaginal infections or whenever you take antibiotics for unrelated problems like ear infection or strep throat.

Consider evaluation and/or treatment for your sexual partner. Sexual transmission is not usually a primary source of yeast problems, but for some women it can be. One researcher found that unsuspected yeast infection in a partner's mouth or semen was the source of yeast for women with recurring yeast infection problems. Yeast medication taken by mouth is likely to cure your partner's infection (6).

Maintain a good level of basic genital health. When you keep your vulva clean, dry, and healthy, you are less likely to get infections.

Bathe carefully every day with water and a mild soap, and ask your partner to do the same. Wipe front to back, to avoid bringing bowel bacteria into your vaginal area. Wear cotton underpants. Avoid nylon underpants and pantyhose, and very tight jeans and other pants, because they tend to hold moisture in the vulvar area.

Avoid bath oils, bubble baths, and hygiene sprays if you are frequently bothered by tender, irritated skin around your vulva. Avoid douching, which can irritate your vaginal lining and make you more vulnerable to infection. Avoid deodorant tampons and pads. Lose weight if you are overweight. Extra pounds mean less exposure of the vulva to air, so the vulvar environment can become too moist.

If you use extra lubrication for intercourse, try contraceptive foam, cream, or gel. All these products offer good lubrication and can help destroy infectious organisms to some degree. A good second choice for lubrication, without germ-killing capability, is a water-soluble lubricant such as K-Y Jelly, which is available in drugstores without a prescription. **Avoid petroleum jelly lubricants** such as Vaseline, because they tend to stay in the vagina, are hard to wash away, and may even promote infection.

Maintain a good level of general health. Infections seem to crop up most frequently when times are hard: after an illness, during exam week, during a long battle siege with your partner. That is why you might have six infections in one year, and then no infections for eight years. Try to maintain a healthy physical and emotional equilibrium, and you may prevent infections (and have a happier life).

Your partner should wash his penis carefully with soap and water daily and use condoms for intercourse until your infection is cleared.

I used to get yeast as regular as clockwork right after each period. I would see my doctor, get suppositories, and use them faithfully for two weeks; then maybe the next cycle I wouldn't have problems. But in the cycle after that yeast always came back. Now my doctor gives me suppositories to have on hand all the time. I store them in the refrigerator. Every month I use them for three days after my period stops. I haven't had any itching or discharge in a year.

—WOMAN, 36

Bacterial Vaginosis
(Nonspecific Vaginitis, Corynebacterium vaginalis, Gardnerella vaginalis, Bacterial Vaginitis)

There is no clear, commonly accepted definition of this condition. There isn't even real agreement on its name! Bacterial vaginitis is the most common term. **Bacterial vaginosis** may be a better term, however, and will be used in this discussion. Vaginitis implies irritation of the vagina, and generally the vagina is not irritated or inflamed with this condition. Vaginosis simply implies the presence of an abnormal process (not inflammation) in the vagina. (Changing the name of this infection from vaginitis to vaginosis is a bit like getting promoted from corporal to sergeant: a little more status, but still a little ignored and misunderstood.)

It is generally felt that bacterial vaginosis is caused by an overgrowth of normal vaginal organisms, a mixture of the *Gardnerella vaginalis* bacterium and other oxygen-intolerant bacteria. The infection may be transmitted via sexual intimacy or may arise spontaneously, and is more likely to occur among women with more than one sex partner, IUD users, and women who have cervicitis (1).

True vaginal inflammation caused by bacteria, literal bacterial *vaginitis,* also does exist. For example, young girls who have not yet begun to menstruate may have gonorrheal vaginitis rather than the more typical adult gonorrheal cervicitis. Also, other rarer types of vaginal bacterial infection undoubtedly do exist. Inflammation caused by a small, comma-shaped bacterium is one example. The identity of this culprit is not yet known, but several researchers have reported on cases they have found. It can be eradicated with antibiotics such as penicillin, ampicillin, and amoxicillin.

Symptoms.   Bacterial vaginosis discharge is white or gray and adherent. It may be thick or watery, and it may have an objectionable odor. Pain on urination, and/or pain or burning in the vagina or vulva during intercourse, may also be symptoms. Itching and redness are likely to be absent or mild. It is unclear what symptoms, if any, men have.

Diagnosis.   Your clinician will take a sample of your discharge and look at it immediately under a microscope. She/he looks for stippled cells coated with bacteria on your slide. These cells are called "clue cells" and are shown in Illustration 23-3. Gardnerella bacteria may also be detected on your Pap smear. The diagnosis is often made by eliminating the possibility of trichomonas or yeast infections on the microscopic examination and eliminating the possibility of chlamydia or gonorrhea with culture tests. She/he may mix a couple of drops of potassium hydroxide with your discharge. If the mixture gives off a fishy odor, it helps confirm the presence of bacterial vaginosis.

Vaginal pH is likely to be slightly alkaline (4.7 or higher).

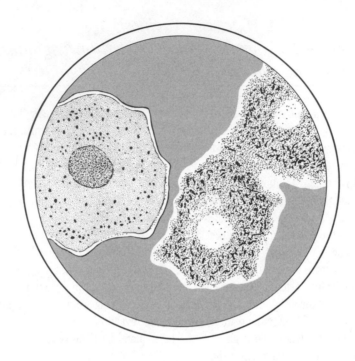

ILLUSTRATION 23-3   Clue cells, normal vaginal lining cells coated with clumps of bacteria, are visible under the microscope when bacterial vaginosis discharge is examined.

Treatment.   Oral antibiotics such as metronidazole (500 mg twice daily), or ampicillin or amoxicillin (500 mg four times daily) for seven days are the initial treatment recommended by the Centers for Disease Control (2). It is possible to treat you and your partner simultaneously. Routine partner treatment, however, is not recommended by national STD authorities (2), and research so far does not show a definite benefit in the cure rate for women whose partner has been treated. Partner treatment may be reasonable, however, if your infection recurs after treatment or you suspect sexual transmission as its cause. If your partner will not seek treatment, you may be given ampicillin to take to him. **Be sure to tell him not to take it if he is allergic to penicillin.** If he is, he needs another type of antibiotic.

Sulfa-based creams and suppositories (Furacin, Sultrin Triple Sulfa, Vagitrol, AVC) relieve symptoms for many women, but are unlikely to cure infection, and vaginal treatment has the disadvantage that your partner is not treated at the same time you are. An over-the-counter antibacterial douche such as Betadine (povidone-iodine) is often prescribed along with the oral antibiotics. You may find douches less messy than vaginal suppositories or cream.

Bacterial vaginosis can coexist with other STDs such as trichomonas and chlamydial mucopurulent cervicitis, so your clinician will check you carefully for these infections as well.

Prognosis.   Bacterial vaginosis usually improves promptly with treatment, but reinfection is common. Some researchers believe bacterial vaginosis may lead to uterine and fallopian tube infection with the same organisms that cause the vaginal infections (7), and may also cause infections during and after pregnancy (1). Clearly it is important to take this infection seriously and be certain you are cured.

REFERENCES

1. Holmes KK, Mardh P-A, Sparling PF, et al: *Sexually Transmitted Diseases.* New York: McGraw-Hill, 1984.
2. Centers for Disease Control: 1985 STD treatment guidelines. *Morbidity and Mortality Weekly Report, Supplement* Vol 34, No 4S, October 18, 1985.
3. *Physicians' Desk Reference* (ed 40). Oradell, N.J.: Medical Economics Company, 1986.
4. Butoconazole for vulvovaginal candidiasis. *Medical Letter on Drugs and Therapeutics* 28:68, 1986.
5. Sobel JD: Recurrent vulvovaginal candidiasis. A prospective study of the efficacy of maintenance ketoconazole therapy. *New England Journal of Medicine* 314:1455–1458, 1986.
6. Horowitz BJ, Edelstein SW, Lippman L: Sexual transmission of *Candida. Obstetrics and Gynecology* 69:882–886, 1987.
7. Paavonen J, Lehtinen M, Teisala K, et al: *Haemophilus influenzae* causes purulent salpingitis. *American Journal of Obstetrics and Gynecology* 151:338–339, 1985.

Toxic Shock Syndrome (TSS)

Until 1979, toxic shock syndrome (TSS) was a little known and very rare disease of interest only to a handful of medical specialists. In 1980, researchers confirmed a link between tampon use and the occurrence of TSS. Suddenly, the choice of menstrual protection was a very serious medical issue, and warnings appeared on tampon boxes (see Danger Signs in Illustration 24-1). Today 20 to 30 cases of TSS are reported in the United States each month (1), and 2,815 cases later we know quite a bit more about prevention and treatment.

Researchers believe that toxic shock syndrome is caused by TSST-1, a specific protein toxin (poison) released by some strains of *Staphylococcus aureus* bacteria (2). (This bacterial family produces many different toxins—including the "poison" responsible for common food poisoning.) *Staphylococcus* is not likely to be sexually transmitted.

Although TSS can occur in men and in children, **most of the cases reported have occurred in women during their menstrual period** or, less commonly, in the first few weeks after childbirth. The majority of TSS cases are associated with the use of tampons. Even with tampon use the risk of TSS is low. Researchers estimate that TSS during menstrual days occurs in about 5 women out of 100,000 each year. TSS risk at other times during the cycle is even lower, probably less than 1 out of 100,000 women annually.

TSS cases have also been reported for women using vaginal contraceptive sponges (3) and for diaphragm users (4). Whether or not these products increase a woman's risk for TSS, however, is not clear. Researchers in one study estimated that 8 sponge users out of 100,000 developed TSS each year, and concluded that sponge use multiplied TSS risk at least eightfold compared to "normal" risk (3). Other researchers, however, believe that an accurate estimate of "normal" risk is not possible with existing data (5), so the sponge risk comparison may not be meaningful.

The possible risks of pregnancy, and some of the risks associated with other birth control options, are higher, so sponge use may be entirely reasonable despite TSS risk. TSS rates for diaphragm users are very low. Only a handful of cases of TSS in this group have been reported, and so far there is no statistical evidence that using a diaphragm increases the risk above the level that all women face (6). So far TSS has not been linked to use of the cervical cap. Nevertheless, women using any of these methods need to be aware of TSS and its signs. Women who use birth control Pills have about half the risk for TSS that noncontraceptors have (6).

The precise role that tampons play is not known. Stagnant blood in or behind a tampon would make an ideal site for bacterial growth. Tampons have been used for many years while TSS is a new problem. What has changed? Some researchers believe that genetic mutation in *Staphylococcus* has allowed a new, hardier, or more toxic strain of this bacterium to evolve.

Other researchers point to recent changes in tampons themselves. Several tampon manufacturers introduced synthetic "superabsorbent" fibers in their products in the late 1970s. Rely tampon, withdrawn from sale by Procter & Gamble in 1980, was one of the most popular of the many superabsorbent brands on the market. How new tampon technology might be linked to TSS is not known. Perhaps superabsorbent tampons simply hold more blood longer inside the vagina to promote bacterial growth. In mid 1985 all remaining superabsorbent brands of tampons were removed from the market by their manufacturers. Nevertheless, TSS cases have been reported among users of all the major tampon brands, old and new, and even among women who use natural sponges for menstrual hygiene.

An intriguing laboratory study (7) has demonstrated a link between low magnesium levels and production of toxin by *Staphylococcus*. Researchers found that tampons made of polyacrylate rayon, or polyester foam containing carboxymethyl cellulose, absorbed and bound magnesium from a culture medium. Production of TSS toxin was accelerated in culture, and this effect was reversed when additional magnesium was added to the fluid. This preliminary finding will no doubt lead to further research. According to a Centers for Disease Control spokesperson (1), there is no evidence from this in vitro study to warrant daily magnesium supplementation in an attempt to prevent TSS.

SYMPTOMS, DIAGNOSIS, AND TREATMENT

TSS could occur after *Staphylococcus* infection anywhere in the body (with serious injury, for example). For most women TSS victims, however, silent infection in the vagina has been the source of the problem. Typically, the disease begins with sudden high fever, diarrhea, vomiting, muscle ache, inflamed eyes, and after a day or two, widespread rash that looks like sunburn. In severe cases there may be kidney, heart, liver, and blood-clotting problems, and severe low blood pressure (shock). The disease can be fatal—about 2% to 3% of TSS victims die of its complications (1)—but more commonly, it occurs in a mild or moderate form that resolves completely when toxin exposure is ended.

Your clinician will diagnose TSS based on your symptoms. A vaginal culture to look for *Staphylococcus aureus* organisms may help to confirm the diagnosis.

Mild cases of TSS can be treated on an outpatient basis, but you will need to be hospitalized if your case is severe. Therapy consists of antibiotics known to be effective against *Staphylococcus aureus*, supportive intravenous fluids if there is a risk of shock, and possibly corticosteroids to control fever and blood pressure.

Prognosis.   TSS sometimes recurs. A recent study indicates that appropriate antibiotic therapy and eliminating the use of tampons may decrease the risk of recurrence to less than 5% (8).

MINIMIZING TSS RISKS

You yourself can decrease your risk of having an initial or recurrent attack of TSS. Some suggestions:

• Your risk for TSS is almost entirely eliminated if you use sanitary pads instead of tampons. Even if you choose to use tampons, your risk for TSS is quite low.
• Be careful that you don't leave your diaphragm or contraceptive sponge in your vagina any longer than the recommended time period. Don't use a diaphragm or sponge during a menstrual period or the first 12 weeks after giving birth. TSS risk is increased whenever you are bleeding and after pregnancy.
• If you think you may have had mild TSS symptoms in the past (one or more of the danger signs below), discuss these with your clinician. A culture to find out whether you have *Staphylococcus* in your vagina may be reasonable.
• Women who choose to use tampons can take steps to reduce their TSS risks: avoid all tampons with superabsorbent fibers. Don't use leftover "super plus" tampons that have been taken off the market. "Super plus" tampons until recently contained a fiber called polyacrylate, so read labels carefully. Although the precise role of the fiber content isn't understood, it may be prudent to use cotton and rayon fiber tampons.
• Don't leave a tampon in place more than eight hours
• Wash your hands before inserting a tampon, and insert the tampon carefully to avoid carrying bacteria from your skin or rectum into your vagina
• Allow a tampon-free interval every day; for example, use pads at night
• If you have had TSS, it is safest to stop using tampons entirely. Also, it may be advisable to avoid using a diaphragm or contraceptive sponge.
• Watch the newspaper for new recommendations from the Centers for Disease Control and the Food and Drug Administration as the TSS story continues to unfold

Watch for TSS danger signs during your period (Illustration 24-1). If one or more danger signs occur, **stop using tampons (or sponges or diaphragm) and see your clinician immediately.** Be sure your case is reported to the Centers for Disease Control,

24:1   TOXIC SHOCK SYNDROME DANGER SIGNS

Fever (temperature of 101 degrees F. or more)
Diarrhea
Vomiting
Muscle aches
Rash (like sunburn)

Contact your clinician immediately or go to a hospital emergency room if these symptoms occur during a menstrual period, or while you are wearing a diaphragm or sponge for birth control.

Meningitis and Special Pathogens Branch, 1600 Clifton Road, N.E., Atlanta, Georgia 30333.

REFERENCES

1. Oxtoby, Margaret J., Epidemiologist, Meningitis and Special Pathogens Branch, Division of Bacterial Disease, Centers for Disease Control. Personal communication, February, 1986.
2. Editor: Prevention and treatment of toxic shock syndrome: A retrospective look. *Journal of the American Medical Association* 252:3411–3412, 1984.
3. Faich G, Pearson K, Fleming D, et al: Toxic shock syndrome and the vaginal contraceptive sponge. *Journal of the American Medical Association* 255:216–218, 1985.
4. Baehler EA, Dillon WP, Dryja DM, et al: The effects of prolonged retention of diaphragms on colonization by *Staphylococcus aureus* of the lower genital tract. *Fertility and Sterility* 39:162–166, 1983.
5. Petitti D, D'Agostino RB, Oldman MJ. Nonmenstrual toxic shock syndrome: Methodological problems in estimating incidence and delineating risk factors. *Journal of Reproductive Medicine* 32:10–16 1987.
6. Lanes SF, Poole C, Dreyer NA, et al: Toxic shock syndrome, contraceptive methods, and vaginitis. *American Journal of Obstetrics and Gynecology* 15:989–991, 1986.
7. Mills JT, Parsonnet J, Tsai Y-C, et al: Control of production of toxic-shock-syndrome toxin-1 (TSST-1) by magnesium ion. *Journal of Infectious Diseases* 151:1158–1161, 1985.
8. Helgerson SD, Mallery BL, Foster LR: Toxic shock syndrome in Oregon: Risk of recurrence. *Journal of the American Medical Association* 252:3402–3404, 1984.

Chlamydia, Gonorrhea, and Pelvic Inflammatory Disease (PID)

Chlamydia and gonorrhea are among the most common STDs. If you've never even heard of chlamydia you are not alone; until just a few years ago this organism was so hard to identify that laboratories were rarely able to prove its existence. So even though chlamydia has been around forever, we are only now able to understand its extraordinary role in reproductive tract infection. Gonorrhea has been well understood for decades.

A review of the bacterial infection process described in Chapter 22 would probably be helpful before you read on.

Chlamydia and gonorrhea are alike in many ways. Both are bacteria. Both are transmitted in adults only by sexual intimacy. Both establish their first beachhead in the endocervix, the inch-long canal that leads from the vagina to the uterus. Both are likely to be symptom-free in both women and men in the early stages. Both can cause pelvic inflammatory disease (PID); that is, they infect the uterus, tubes, and other internal pelvic structures if the bacteria aren't eradicated promptly. Both can cause widespread damage to pelvic structures resulting in chronic pain, infertility, and a high risk of ectopic pregnancy. An infant born to a mother infected with either gonorrhea or chlamydia can acquire infection at the time of birth. And to complicate matters further, the two infections often coexist.

The fallopian tubes are delicate structures with quite narrow passageways, and won't tolerate much inflammation without becoming obstructed or permanently scarred. Once the tubes are blocked, sperm and egg can no longer reach each other. Chlamydia probably accounts for about 25% of all cases of PID in the United States each year;

about 50% of cases are caused by gonorrhea, and the remainder by mycoplasma and other less common bacteria, or combinations of one or more bacteria.

Chlamydia
(Chlamydia trachomatis, Mucopurulent Cervicitis, Male Nongonococcal Urethritis)

Chlamydial infections are caused by the *Chlamydia trachomatis* bacterium, which is an obligate intracellular organism; that is, it cannot survive except inside another cell. Between 3 million and 10 million cases occur each year in the United States. (Chlamydia is not an official reportable disease, so we can only guess at the true number of cases.) For adults chlamydia is transmitted by sexual intimacy.

Symptoms.   It is quite common for women and men to have absolutely no symptoms for weeks or months with chlamydia. When symptoms do occur, you are likely to notice an unusual yellowish vaginal discharge that actually originates from your cervix. Chlamydia can invade the uterus and tubes and cause pelvic pain and tenderness, painful urination, painful intercourse, abnormal vaginal bleeding, bleeding after intercourse, and/or fever. Chlamydia infection in the uterus or tubes does not always cause dramatic symptoms. Damage occurs in some cases so quietly that the woman has no symptoms that would alert her to the need for treatment. Researchers believe that swimming sperm cells can carry chlamydia organisms upward into the uterus and tubes (1). Chlamydia most often attacks the reproductive tract, but can attack the urethra and bladder as well, and cause frequent, burning urination.

Symptoms in men can include urinary frequency, burning with urination, and a clear or white penile discharge. In men the disease may be called nongonococcal urethritis (NGU).

Diagnosis.   Your clinician will suspect chlamydia if you have a typical chlamydial cervical discharge and if your cervix has red, swollen areas and seems friable (crumbly). Pap test results may also raise the suspicion of chlamydia. A Pap test, however, is not an accurate way to determine your diagnosis (2). Your clinician can confirm the diagnosis with laboratory tests such as culture, monoclonal antibody test, immunofluorescence, or enzyme immunoassay. (If these sound like expensive, sophisticated tests, they are. Because chlamydia is such a fastidious organism, fairly high technology is required to diagnose it successfully outside its normal environment.) Your clinician may also look for white blood cells in a sample of your discharge. Because gonorrhea often coexists with chlamydia your clinician will also collect a cervical discharge sample for a gonorrhea culture. If you also have gonorrhea, you will be treated for both infections at the same time (see the section on gonorrhea for treatment).

Treatment.   Many clinicians, and national STD experts at the Centers for Disease Control, advocate presumptive treatment for chlamydia; that is, treatment based on your symptoms and physical exam and begun before test results are available, or given without testing if necessary.

For chlamydial cervicitis, with no evidence of infection spread to the uterus or tubes, treatment options recommended by the Centers for Disease Control are (3):

- **(Preferred)** Doxycycline, 100-mg capsules taken two times a day for seven days,
- or Tetracycline, 500-mg capsules taken four times a day for seven days
- or (allergic to tetracycline or during pregnancy) Erythromycin, 500-mg capsules taken four times a day for seven days, or 250-mg capsules taken four times a day for 14 days

Although doxycycline (Doryx, Vibramycin) is a bit more expensive than tetracycline, it may be a better choice. Doxycycline is taken twice a day compared to four times a day with tetracycline, is less likely to cause intestinal upset, and maintains higher blood levels of antibiotic than tetracycline (see Chapter 22 for instructions about using tetracycline). Also, doxycycline absorption is not blocked by milk and food so it can be taken with meals whereas good tetracycline absorption requires careful dose timing to avoid mixing it with milk in the stomach.

If chlamydia has invaded your uterus and tubes and you have pelvic inflammatory disease, your clinician may feel you need to be hospitalized so your infection can be treated with intravenous (IV) antibiotics. Read the section entitled "Pelvic Inflammatory Disease (PID)" in this chapter to learn more about treatment approaches.

Your partner(s) must be treated at the same time you are. Also, you and your partner(s) will need follow-up exams four to seven days after treatment is completed to be sure you are cured. You should avoid intercourse until your follow-up test shows you are free of chlamydia, and your partner should use condoms if there is any doubt that he has been thoroughly treated and cured.

Prognosis.   Overall rates and time lapse for the spread of chlamydial infection from the cervix upward to the uterine cavity and tubes are not known. In one study, however, 40% of women with chlamydial cervicitis also had evidence of uterine infection in biopsies taken as part of the study. Some, but not all, of these patients had abdominal pain, uterine tenderness, or abnormal bleeding suggesting mild PID at the time they were tested (4). These results indicate that aggressive treatment for chlamydia is essential, and full PID treatment should be considered if there is any evidence whatsoever of uterine spread.

Once infection has reached the fallopian tubes, you are at risk for scarring, tubal obstruction, infertility, and ectopic pregnancy. The longer your infection remains untreated, the greater the likelihood of permanent damage. Repeated episodes of infection also increase the risk of permanent damage.

Infected pregnant women may be at increased risk for spontaneous abortion, stillbirth, and postpartum fever. Babies born to infected women are at risk for eye infections and pneumonia.

Gonorrhea
(Neisseria gonorrhoeae, GC, Clap)

Gonorrhea is caused by the *Neisseria gonorrhoeae* bacterium. About 2 million cases occur each year in the United States. Among adults, it is transmitted via sexual intimacy.

Symptoms.   It is quite common for women and men to have absolutely no symptoms with gonorrhea, especially in the early stages. A woman's first clue may very well be her partner's penile discharge, burning, or frequency of urination.

At first I was shocked that my doctor wanted to do a gonorrhea test as part of my regular checkup. Why spend the extra money when I didn't feel sick and neither did Charlie? Still, it was reassuring to find out I don't have gonorrhea smoldering inside.

—WOMAN, 23

Many cases of gonorrhea among women are first detected by a routine gonorrhea culture. When symptoms do occur, they can include unusual discharge, painful urination, painful intercourse, pelvic pain or tenderness, unusual vaginal bleeding, bleeding after intercourse, and/or fever. Gonorrhea most often attacks the reproductive tract, but can attack the throat, eyes, and rectum as well.

Diagnosis.   Your clinician cannot diagnose gonorrhea on the basis of an examination alone. Immediate microscopic examination of discharge or a stained slide from the discharge may suggest gonorrhea, but accurate diagnosis for a woman is based on a culture test, which takes about 48 hours to complete. If you do have gonorrhea, a blood sample should be taken to check for syphilis as well (syphilis is much less common than gonorrhea, however).

Treatment.   Because one in four men and two in five women who have gonorrhea also have chlamydia (3), your treatment should be designed to cure both infections. Your partner(s) must be treated at the same time you are.

Gonorrhea is quickly eradicated in about 95% of cases by a single (large) dose of ampicillin, amoxicillin, or penicillin. Probenecid is used along with these drugs to increase their effectiveness. Probenecid temporarily slows down kidney excretion of penicillin-type antibiotics so that a high bloodstream antibiotic level can be quickly achieved and sustained. **After an initial single-dose treatment for gonorrhea you should take tetracycline or doxycycline faithfully for seven days to cure chlamydia as well.** Erythromycin will be substituted if you are pregnant. Tetracycline and doxycycline are also effective against gonorrhea, but are not preferred treatments because cure depends on precise and faithful doses over the entire seven days. **Anyone (woman or man) exposed to a partner with gonorrhea should be treated.** An exam and cultures should also be done, but treatment should be started immediately even if no symptoms are present.

Treatment options recommended by the Centers for Disease Control for uncomplicated gonorrhea infection, with no evidence of infection spread to the uterus or tubes, are (5):

An initial antibiotic single dose of:

- Amoxicillin, 3 grams (six capsules) taken all at once, **plus** Probenecid, 1 gram (two capsules) taken at the same time
- or Ampicillin, 3.5 grams (seven capsules) taken all at once, **plus** Probenecid, 1 gram (two capsules) taken at the same time
- or Penicillin injection (procaine penicillin, 4.8 million units total given by injection into muscle in two different sites), **plus** Probenecid, 1 gram (two capsules) taken at the same time

Followed by:

- Tetracycline, 500-mg capsules taken four times a day for seven days
- or Doxycycline, 100-mg capsules taken two times a day for seven days
- or (if you are allergic to tetracycline or pregnant) Erythromycin base or stearate, 500-mg capsules taken four times a day for seven days, or Erythromycin ethylsuccinate, 800-mg capsules taken four times a day for seven days

If you are allergic to penicillin, you can be treated with tetracycline or doxycycline, or with an injection of spectinomycin (2 grams) or ceftriaxone (250 mg). Tell your clinician if you have ever had any unusual reaction to penicillin, ampicillin, or tetracycline in the past. Also tell your clinician if you think you could be pregnant. Be sure to read Chapter 22 for instructions on taking antibiotic drugs.

If you have abdominal pain and tenderness or other signs that gonorrhea has spread to your uterus and tubes and caused pelvic inflammatory disease, you will need longer, more intensive treatment with antibiotics. Your clinician may recommend that you be admitted to the hospital for intravenous antibiotic therapy. **Gonorrhea infection in your uterus and tubes is a serious threat to your health and to your fertility.**

Gonorrhea throat infection requires treatment with ceftriaxone or doxycycline; penicillin-type antibiotics are not effective. Rectal infection is best treated with penicillin or spectinomycin injection.

You and your partner will need to be cultured again four to seven days after treatment to be sure you are cured. Follow-up tests are essential because some strains of gonorrhea are resistant to penicillin, and further treatment is necessary to eradicate the disease.

Avoid intercourse until cultures for both you and your partner (including rectal cultures) prove that you are both cured. Reinfection is quite common, especially if your partner isn't treated at the same time you are. Remember that condoms or the sperm-killing chemicals in diaphragm creams and gels, foam, sponges, and spermicidal condoms may help cut your risk of acquiring gonorrhea again in the future.

Penicillin-Resistant Gonorrhea.   Some strains of gonorrhea bacteria produce a chemical (penicillinase) that inactivates penicillin antibodies. These organisms, called **PPNG** (penicillinase-producing *Neisseria gonorrhoeae*) are not eradicated by penicillin treatment. Treatment with ceftriaxone or spectinomycin is necessary. PPNG strains are becoming an increasing problem. The number of cases is increasing (abut 17,000 in the United States in 1986, compared to 9,000 in 1985), and cases are no longer localized to Florida, New York City, and Los Angeles, where almost all cases have occurred in the past (6). **PPNG means that follow-up tests to confirm your cure are absolutely essential after gonorrhea treatment.** PPNG is particularly serious for women because ineffective gonorrhea treatment involves a high risk for pelvic infection.

Prognosis.   Once untreated gonorrhea infection has reached the fallopian tubes, you have up to a 40% risk of scarring, tubal obstruction, and infertility (7). The longer gonorrhea remains untreated, the greater the likelihood of permanent damage. Each time you have a repeat episode of gonorrhea, your risk of irreversible damage increases. Read the section entitled "Pelvic Inflammatory Disease" in this chapter for more details.

Untreated people are also at risk for a syndrome caused by disseminated gonococcal infection, which can include septicemia (blood poisoning), arthritis, skin problems, and heart and brain infections.

Babies born to infected women are at risk for eye infections, pneumonia, anorectal infections, and scalp abscesses at the site of fetal monitors (7).

Pelvic Inflammatory Disease (PID)

Pelvic infection and pelvic inflammatory disease (PID) are general terms for infection anywhere in a woman's pelvic organs. Your clinician may also use more precise terms to indicate which specific areas are infected:

• Endometritis: infection of the endometrium or lining of the uterus
• Myometritis: infection of the muscular layers of the uterus
• Salpingitis: infection of the fallopian tubes
• Oophoritis: infection of the ovaries

25:1   PELVIC INFECTION (PID) DANGER SIGNS

Cramping or persistent abdominal pain or back pain
Abdominal tenderness with pressure or jarring, such as walking,
    coughing, jumping, or intercourse
Abdominal pain with bowel movements or urination
Abnormal vaginal discharge, bleeding, or spotting
Fever (temperature over 100.4 degrees F.)
Chills or malaise (fatigue, aching)

Contact your clinician immediately or go to a hospital emergency
room if you develop any of these signs.

- Unilateral: affects one side of paired structures such as the tubes or ovaries
- Bilateral: affects both sides of paired structures such as the tubes or ovaries
- Pelvic abscess: walled-off pocket of infection in the pelvic cavity
- Peritonitis: infection of the peritoneum, a thin, strong membrane that lines the abdominal cavity
- Pelvic inflammatory disease (PID): generic term for infections in the uterus, tubes, ovaries, and/or pelvis

PID attacks more than 1 million women a year in the United States, and some 300,000 of them are hospitalized for treatment (7). Most cases of PID are thought to be polymicrobial in nature; that is, two or more types of pathogens are present at the same time. Chlamydia or gonorrhea is a culprit in over half of all PID.

Symptoms.   Symptoms of pelvic infection can be very dramatic, with sudden, severe pelvic pain, a temperature of 102 to 104 degrees (Fahrenheit), shaking chills, unusual vaginal discharge, and vaginal bleeding. But infection symptoms can also be very subtle: annoying, persistent, mild abdominal pain or backache, or pain that you notice only during intercourse, or slightly increased vaginal discharge. Your symptoms depend on the location of your infection, the type of bacteria causing it, and how quickly the bacteria multiply and spread. Gonorrheal PID is likely to have a dramatic onset, while chlamydial PID may be quite insidious.

If your symptoms are severe, your need for treatment will be obvious. Subtle symptoms are a real problem, however, because it is easy to ignore them and put off calling your clinician. Indolent, smoldering infection is a leading cause of infertility; it can permanently scar and obstruct your fallopian tubes just as a dramatic infection can. Infection danger signs are shown in Illustration 25-1.

You are unlikely to have all these danger signs. Fever, for example, only occurs in about one third of cases. If you suspect infection, have an examination immediately to be certain. Suspect infection especially if you have an IUD, if you think you may have been exposed to chlamydia or gonorrhea, or if you have recently had a baby, a miscarriage, an abortion, or pelvic surgery.

Diagnosis.   Your clinician will need to examine you to decide whether or not you have a pelvic infection. One of the most important clues is **tenderness** in your uterus, tubes, or ovaries during pelvic examination. If your uterus is tender or if moving your cervix back and forth (which jars the uterus, tubes, and ovaries) causes pain, your clinician will suspect infection. Sometimes infection is obvious, but sometimes it is difficult for your clinician to be certain. Even if there is some doubt, it is probably better to go ahead with treatment anyway. There is nothing to be gained by waiting until the infection becomes severe.

A bacterial culture from your cervix may help to identify the specific bacteria causing your infection and determine which antibiotic would be most effective. **Chlamydia and gonorrhea tests are essential,** and your clinician may recommend other tests to help determine the cause, extent, and severity of your infection. Culture results are not always clear-cut, however. Since bacteria are normally present in the vagina, your culture is likely to show growth of several of these bacteria. It may be difficult to determine which type(s) of bacteria is responsible for your pelvic infection and which types just happen to live harmlessly in your vagina.

A blood count can determine whether your body defense cells have been stimulated. When you have an active infection, the number of white cells in your bloodstream is elevated and your blood proteins are altered so that your blood cell sedimentation rate is speeded up.

If your clinician suspects that you may have an abscess, she/he may recommend a sonogram (see Chapter 4). An abscess is a localized pocket of fluid containing pus and bacteria. Abscess formation in a fallopian tube or in the pelvic cavity impairs the effectiveness of antibiotics and normal body defenses against infection. Sonography uses sound waves to identify localized swelling or fluid collection and can provide your clinician with information about abscess size and location. This helps your clinician decide whether surgical treatment to drain the abscess is necessary, and your progress can be followed by sonography once antibiotic treatment has begun.

In some cases, surgery will be necessary for diagnosing pelvic infection. If your symptoms are so severe that your clinician suspects you could have appendicitis or an abscess, she/he will consider surgery. Either exploratory laparoscopy, viewing the inside of your abdomen through a lighted tube inserted through a 1-inch incision just below your navel (see Chapter 48), or laparotomy, a 5-inch surgical opening in your lower abdomen, might be recommended.

Treatment.   Your treatment will depend on how severe your infection is. You will be hospitalized if any of these conditions are present (5):

• You are gravely ill
• Surgical emergencies such as appendicitis or ectopic pregnancy are suspected
• Your clinician isn't sure of your diagnosis
• Your clinician suspects you have a pelvic abscess
• You are pregnant
• You have not responded to previous antibiotic treatment, or clinical follow-up after 48 to 72 hours of outpatient treatment cannot be arranged

• For any reason you cannot be treated on an outpatient basis (living in a remote area, significant intellectual impairment, or mental illness)

In the hospital your antibiotics can be administered directly into a vein in higher, more effective doses than you could absorb through your stomach. Some experts recommend that all women with PID be hospitalized for treatment (7).

Hospital treatment for suspected chlamydia and/or gonorrhea is likely to be intravenous doxycycline and cefoxitin for at least four days and at least two days after you are free of fever, followed by doxycycline pills after you go home to total 10 to 14 days of therapy (5). If your clinician suspects other bacteria are causing your infection, if you have an IUD-related infection, or if you have an abscess, she/he may prescribe other drugs.

Oral antibiotics, pain medication, and rest at home will cure pelvic infection in some cases. Your clinician also might be able to arrange for intravenous antibiotic treatment for you at home or at an outpatient facility. While you are being treated at home, pretend that you are in the hospital. **The importance of complete rest cannot be overemphasized.** Rest enables your body defenses to function at their best. Antibiotics do part of the job, but your own internal defenses are crucial in your cure. Your clinician will also recommend **pelvic rest**; by that she/he means no intercourse, no active sports, and no other activity that jars or bounces your pelvis.

Antibiotics recommended by the Centers for Disease Control for outpatient treatment of PID are (5):

• Cefoxitin injection, 2 grams injected into muscle, **plus** Probenecid, 1 gram (two capsules) taken at the same time, **plus** Doxycycline, 100-mg taken two times a day for 10 to 14 days
• or Amoxicillin, 3 grams (six capsules) taken all at once, **plus** Probenecid and Doxycycline as above
• or Ampicillin, 3.5 grams (seven capsules) taken all at once, **plus** Probenecid **and** Doxycycline as above
• or Penicillin injection (Aqueous Procaine Penicillin G), 4.8 million units total given by injection into muscle at two sites, **plus** Probenecid **and** Doxycycline as above
• or Ceftriaxone injection (250 mg into muscle at 1 site) **plus** Doxycycline as above

Your sexual partner(s) must be treated at the same time you are with one dose of ampicillin or amoxicillin and seven days' treatment with doxycycline or tetracycline. Partner treatment is essential whether or not your partner has any symptoms, and whether or not he is tested for STD infection. Treatment is reasonable even if he is tested and the results for gonorrhea and chlamydia are negative. Tests are not 100% reliable and if your partner does continue to carry gonorrhea or chlamydia, you are likely to become reinfected when you resume intercourse. With PID your stakes are high. Another PID attack would be a serious threat to your health and fertility, and far more hazardous than the minor risk your partner assumes by completing an effective course of antibiotics. Read the sections on chlamydia and gonorrhea in this chapter, and Chapter 22, for more specific information on taking antibiotics.

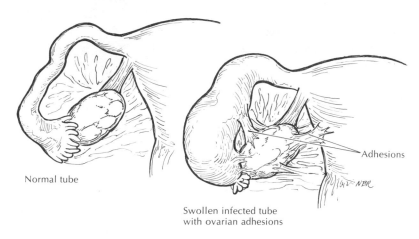

Normal tube

Adhesions

Swollen infected tube
with ovarian adhesions

ILLUSTRATION 25-2   Pelvic infection can cause the fallopian tubes to become grossly swollen and distended.

Your clinician will want you to return for a checkup after 48 to 72 hours and again after one or two weeks. At that time, she/he will evaluate your improvement to decide whether you are ready to resume your normal activities.

If your infection does not improve with antibiotic treatment, whether you are in the hospital or at home, your clinician will probably recommend a sonogram or other tests and will consider surgery to drain an abscess or remove infected tissue. When infection is truly severe and antibiotic treatment is not working well, it may be necessary to remove the infected organs. Severe infection might mean removing one or both tubes, the uterus, and possibly even your ovaries. Hysterectomy is discussed in Chapter 49.

Permanent damage is especially likely if infection involves your fallopian tubes. The inner lining of the tubes is delicate and easily damaged by infection. The tube walls are thin and pliable, so fluid or pus accumulation can cause massive swelling. A fluid-filled tube that looks like a fat sausage or balloon is called a pus tube (pyosalpinx) or a fluid tube (hydrosalpinx) and is fairly common with pelvic infection. Infection can cause such severe scarring that the open end (near the ovary) of one or both tubes is literally sealed shut. Even if the tubes are not blocked, irreversible infection damage to the lining may still cause infertility. Tube lining cells provide an essential environment for sperm and for a newly fertilized egg. Infection can also trigger growth of scar tissue bands (adhesions) that can distort the shape of the tubes. Infected fallopian tubes are shown in Illustration 25-2.

Pelvic abscess is another serious complication that can occur with infection. Pus and live bacteria leaking from the open end of a fallopian tube can enter the abdominal cavity itself and cause peritonitis, widespread infection throughout the lining of the abdomen (peritoneum). In many cases, pus collects in a puddle, and your body's normal defenses attempt to prevent its spread by producing a scar tissue wall to separate it from the rest of your abdomen. A walled-off collection of pus and active bacteria is called an abscess.

Antibiotic medications are often ineffective in treating an abscess, for antibiotics and infection-fighting white blood cells carried in your bloodstream cannot penetrate an abscess very effectively. When you have an abscess, the symptoms are likely to persist despite antibiotic treatment. Surgery may be necessary to drain the pus and bacteria so that healing can begin.

Infection that occurs after pregnancy, abortion, or miscarriage is a special situation. Your clinician will carefully evaluate the size of your uterus and may recommend a sonogram to assess whether there is evidence of any retained fetal or placental tissue. If there is, she/he will recommend uterine scraping (D&C or vacuum curettage, Chapters 47 and 18). A D&C may also be considered if you do not respond promptly to antibiotic treatment. Your clinician will probably prescribe a drug such as Methergine (methylergonovine) (Chapter 18) to stimulate uterine contraction and help prevent accumulation of blood inside your uterus.

If your infection is associated with an IUD, then your clinician will probably recommend that the IUD be removed; this is essential if future fertility is an issue for you. In some cases, when infection is mild and limited to your uterus, infection can be treated effectively with your IUD in place. If infection is severe or if it does not respond promptly to treatment, then your IUD should definitely be removed.

Prognosis. If pelvic infection is limited to the uterus itself, antibiotic treatment usually resolves the problem rapidly and completely with little likelihood of permanent damage or future complications. If infection has involved your fallopian tubes, ovaries, or abdominal cavity, however, long-term consequences are of significant concern. Irreversible fallopian tube damage may lead to four serious long-term problems:

First of all, **infertility** is possible because of infection damage. Second, the incidence of **tubal (ectopic) pregnancy**—pregnancy that implants and grows in the fallopian tube or elsewhere rather than the uterus—is increased after pelvic infection, for partial obstruction of a tube can delay or obstruct passage of the fertilized egg to the uterus. Third, there is a significant risk that **repeated episodes of infection** will occur in the future. Finally, scar tissue (adhesions) formed during infection can be a source of **continuing pelvic pain,** sometimes severe enough to require later surgery.

It is important to remember that chlamydia, gonorrhea, and other types of pelvic infection do not always cause infertility. Your clinician will stress the possibility of permanent damage and infertility when you have an infection, but **you cannot assume that you are infertile**. Many women have unwanted pregnancies because they assumed, quite naturally, that they would not need birth control after a warning from their clinician. If you do not want to be pregnant, you will need to continue using birth control. Your clinician can tell from examination that there may be tubal scarring that could impair your fertility, but she/he cannot tell for sure whether you are able to conceive or not. Hysterosalpingography (see Chapter 10) to determine

TABLE 25-1
REPEATED PID AND INFERTILITY RISK

NUMBER OF PID EPISODES	% OF WOMEN WHO BECOME INFERTILE
1	11
2	23
3	54

SOURCE: Westrom L: Incidence, prevalence, and trends of acute pelvic inflammatory disease and its consequences in industrial countries. *American Journal of Obstetrics and Gynecology* 138:880–892, 1980.

whether or not your tubes are blocked would probably answer the question, but is medically unwise. Hysterosalpingography might trigger another bout of infection.

If you have had a pelvic infection, it is absolutely essential to protect yourself from any further exposure to chlamydia and gonorrhea. Your health and your fertility are at stake. **Your partner(s) must be treated,** and so must any other woman or man with whom either of you has had intercourse, **whether or not they have symptoms and whether or not they have been tested.** Both men and women can carry early infection with no symptoms at all. **Your body does not build effective immunity to chlamydia and gonorrhea.** If you are exposed to chlamydia or gonorrhea a second time, your risk of developing a second serious pelvic infection may be even higher than it was the first time, and your risk for infertility increases (see Table 25-1).

I had PID twice, when I was 18 and 20. I didn't feel too bad either time, so I didn't get worked up about it. Then I got married and couldn't get pregnant in two years of trying. My tubes were blocked, I finally found out. I went to an infertility specialist. Now my husband and I have to decide if we want to adopt, or spend five thousand dollars a month for however many months it takes to have in vitro fertilization. The success rate is only 25%. If I'd seen a doctor sooner about PID, would things be different today? What if I'd only had PID once instead of twice? I go nuts thinking about this stuff.

—WOMAN, 24

PID involuntarily sterilizes 100,000 U.S. women a year (8), and can also be associated with chronic pain and depression.

25:3   ECTOPIC PREGNANCY DANGER SIGNS

Sudden intense pain, or persistent pain, or cramping in the lower abdomen, usually localized to one side or the other

Irregular bleeding or spotting with abdominal pain when your period is late or after an abnormally light period

Fainting or dizziness that persists more than a few seconds. These may be signs of internal bleeding. You will not necessarily have any bleeding from your vagina if you have internal bleeding.

Contact your clinician immediately or go to a hospital emergency room if you develop any of these signs.

Ectopic pregnancy can be a life-threatening consequence of PID. Common ectopic pregnancy sites and symptoms are described in Chapter 8. Ruptured ectopic pregnancy is a **leading cause of death during pregnancy**. Internal bleeding occurs most often between four and eight weeks after conception, when the growing pregnancy stretches and tears the fallopian tube. Internal hemorrhage can be massive and silent—with no vaginal blood loss at all. Bleeding may cause pain in the abdomen or in the shoulder when it irritates the lining of the abdominal cavity under the diaphragm.

If you have ever had PID, always be alert to the ectopic pregnancy danger signs shown in Illustration 25-3.

REFERENCES

1. Wiesmeier E, Rosenthal DL, Weideman S: Detection of chlamydial cervicitis with Papanicolaou-stained smears and cultures in a university student population. *Journal of Reproductive Medicine* 32:251–253, 1987.

2. Friberg J, Confino E, Suarez M, et al: *Chlamydia trachomatis* attached to spermatozoa recovered from the peritoneal cavity of patients with salpingitis. *Journal of Reproductive Medicine* 32:120–122, 1987.

3. Centers for Disease Control: Chlamydia trachomatis infections: Policy guidelines for prevention and control. *Morbidity and Mortality Weekly Report, Supplement* Vol 34, No 3S, 1985.

4. Paavonen J, Kiviat N, Brunham RC, et al: Prevalence and manifestations of endometritis among women with cervicitis. *American Journal of Obstetrics and Gynecology* 152:280–286, 1985.

5. Centers for Disease Control: Sexually transmitted diseases treatment guidelines, 1985. *Morbidity and Mortality Weekly Report, Supplement* Vol 31, No 4S, 1985.

6. Centers for Disease Control: Penicillinase-producing *Neisseria gonorrhea*—United States, 1986. *Morbidity and Mortality Weekly Report* 36:107–108, 1987.

7. Hatcher RA, Guest FJ, Stewart FH, et al: *Contraceptive Technology 1988–1989* (ed 14). New York: Irvington Publishers, in press.

8. Cates W Jr: Sexually transmitted diseases: The national view. *Cutis* 33:69–80, 1984.

26

❖

Herpes Infection (Herpes Simplex Type 2, Genital Herpes)

Herpes genital infection is caused by Herpes simplex type 2 *virus, a tiny DNA particle. Its close relative,* Herpes simplex type 1, *causes infections of the mouth, lips, and skin commonly called cold sores, canker sores, and fever blisters. Type 1 usually does not attack below the waist, and type 2 usually stays below the waist. Spread outside normal territory is possible with either type 1 or 2, so oral sex is unwise if either partner has active herpes infection of either type. (Read Chapter 22 for a review of the basic principles of viral infection and treatment, and an illustration of the herpes virus.)*

Herpes genital infection is a recurrent, incurable, sexually transmitted illness. The initial infection—the first outbreak of symptoms—may be fairly severe and can cause blisters, fever, swollen nodes, and malaise. Recurrent attacks are usually milder. In the United States about 200,000 people experience a symptomatic new infection each year, and perhaps 20 million harbor the virus (1). Herpes is an increasingly common STD, as is evident in Illustration 26-1. Initial outbreaks usually last about 12 days, and recurrences about 5 days. During latent periods the virus retreats to the dorsal nerve root ganglia (see Illustration 26-2), where it remains alive but dormant.

Symptoms. Single or multiple small, extremely painful blisters (similar to cold sores on the lips or nose) appear on the vulva or buttocks. Occasionally they appear on the cervix, where they may be completely unnoticed. After about two days, the blisters open and small painful ulcers remain. You may also have vulvar swelling, fever, and enlarged, tender lymph nodes in your abdomen, especially the first time you are infected. An outbreak may be preceded by a tingling or itching sensation in the area where sores later appear. Initial symptoms usually appear about one

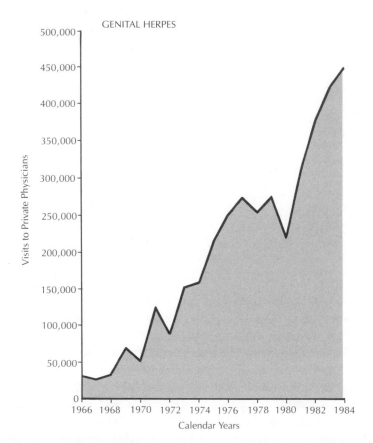

ILLUSTRATION 26-1 Genital herpes has increased about tenfold in the last two decades.

week after you are exposed, but may occur as soon as 1 day or as late as 26 days after exposure (2). In men, blisters usually are located on the penis and appear somewhat drier.

There is a wide variation in how herpes is expressed. Some people have 1 blister during an outbreak and others more than 20. Some heal in a week while others need up to three weeks to feel well. Some people have recurrences once every few months while others have one or more a month. Approximately 10% of those who have a symptomatic initial attack never have a recurrence.

Some people have no symptoms whatsoever. Research on the prevalence of blood antibody against herpes shows that many (perhaps even most) people who have acquired herpes are not aware of it. Their symptoms must have been entirely absent, or too minimal to be noticed (2). Transmission of herpes by an asymptomatic sexual partner is discussed later in this chapter.

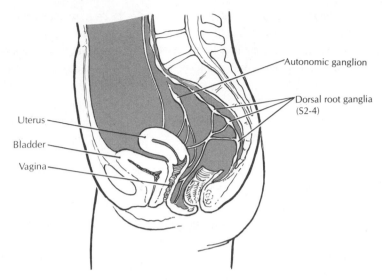

ILLUSTRATION 26-2   **The genital herpes virus retreats to the dorsal nerve root ganglia during dormant periods.**

Special Precautions.   Herpes virus is quite contagious. Both herpes type 1 and herpes type 2 can be accidentally spread from an initial site to the eye, where serious infection damage is possible. Infants and children also can acquire herpes infection of the mouth or lips through accidental contact.

If you have herpes blisters or ulcers, be very careful to wash your hands thoroughly and dry them if you touch your herpes sores. Do not kiss your infant or children if you have active herpes in or near your mouth. Also, it makes sense to avoid sharing towels, washcloths, and toothbrushes while you have active herpes. Transmission of the virus has not been proven for indirect exposure such as through towels, but the virus can remain alive for several hours in a moist environment.

Special precautions are also necessary during pregnancy. Read the last part of this section for specific pregnancy recommendations.

Diagnosis.   Your clinician will suspect herpes if you have typical blisters or ulcers present at the time you are examined and/or describe a typical recurrent pattern of illness. A Pap smear or stained microscopic slide may reveal multinucleated giant cells with inclusions inside the nucleus. A culture or immunologic test smear for herpes, taken with a cotton swab from an active herpes blister or ulcer, can confirm the diagnosis. If you suspect you have herpes, try to see your clinician during an outbreak if possible.

Treatment.   There is no known cure for herpes. Your clinician will provide you with pain-relieving pills and/or antibacterial ointment to prevent bacterial invasion in the virus ulcers, and will probably recommend cool sitz baths using baking soda or

Domeboro solution, and cold, wet medicated compresses to decrease your discomfort. Sores will heal spontaneously in one to four weeks with little or no scarring.

If you are experiencing your first herpes attack and your symptoms have been present for six days or less, your clinician may recommend acyclovir. Acyclovir does not cure herpes, but does help relieve symptoms and shorten the time for healing. Acyclovir inhibits the virus's ability to use proteins, so its ability to multiply is retarded. It is marketed under the trade name Zovirax and is available in ointment and pill form. (An intravenous form is also available for severely ill people with impaired immune systems.)

The ointment was previously used for treatment of initial herpes attacks, but is not as effective as the newer pill form. Oral acyclovir taken on a continuous basis also reduces the frequency of recurrent attacks (1). It will not necessarily prevent the transmission of herpes to your sex partner(s), however. The Food and Drug Administration (FDA) has approved three oral acyclovir regimens.

For an initial outbreak, recommended treatment is one 200-mg capsule every four hours while awake, totaling five a day, for ten days.

For short-term recurrence therapy, the schedule is one 200-mg capsule every four hours while you are awake, totaling five capsules daily for five days, beginning with your very earliest symptoms of a herpes attack. This regimen is recommended to shorten recurrent attacks.

For long-term recurrence therapy, take one 200-mg capsule three times a day for no more than six months. If this regimen fails to improve your symptoms, your clinician may step up your dosage to five capsules a day. The safety and effectiveness of acyclovir used longer than six months has not been established.

Oral acyclovir reduces the duration of symptoms, speeds healing in initial outbreaks, and relieves pain for some initial attack sufferers. In studies of people with frequent recurrences, daily acyclovir suppressed outbreaks in two out of every three patients and reduced the frequency and severity in the others (3,4). However, some study subjects have noted that a first recurrence after oral acyclovir therapy is ended is likely to be fairly severe (5).

No studies have been done to evaluate the effect of oral acyclovir on the fetus or nursing infant, so avoid the drug if you are pregnant or breastfeeding, unless you and your clinician strongly believe that benefits outweigh unknown potential risks. There is some evidence that high concentrations of acyclovir in animals can cause chromosome damage, and the manufacturer suggests that this finding be taken into consideration as you decide whether or not to use the drug during pregnancy or breastfeeding.

Headache, diarrhea, nausea and/or vomiting, and dizziness are fairly common side effects of oral acyclovir therapy, but generally are not severe enough to stop therapy. Two theoretical concerns must await more experience with oral acyclovir: whether the virus can become resistant to the drug and whether there are side effects associated with extended use (6).

Remember that acyclovir is more likely to help if you begin treatment with your earliest possible signs of attack, including any tingling or itching you can identify before blisters actually appear.

Deciding about long-term suppression treatment is not always easy. Treatment is quite expensive ($2 to $4 per day), and long-term risks are not known. If your herpes is frequent and severe, treatment may be a godsend for your life. If attacks are mild and infrequent, treatment may not be worthwhile. Ask your clinician for a copy of "Important Information Concerning Genital Herpes and Its Treatment with Zovirax (Acyclovir) Capsules," a pamphlet produced by the manufacturer of Zovirax.

Many other techniques for curing or ameliorating herpes have been tried in the past, all without any success. These include photoinactivation with neutral red dye and fluorescent light, ether, nitrous oxide, lysine, and smallpox vaccination. None of these approaches has been shown to cure herpes. It is especially important to avoid photoinactivation treatment, because it can cause viral mutations that might predispose you to develop skin cancer; whether this actually occurs is not known.

Living with Herpes

On good days I think of herpes as nature's own braking system—a way to slow me down and help me be more circumspect sexually. On bad days I think of it as a permanent curse I don't deserve, driving away men who won't risk being my lover.

—WOMAN, 22

Many people who have herpes experience recurrences at least occasionally, and some sufferers have recurrences more than once a month. What determines your likelihood and frequency of recurrence is not known. Triggers such as stress, inadequate nutrition, lack of rest, illness, or exposure to extreme heat or cold seem to prompt a recurrence for some people. Others don't notice any particular trigger. Some women notice that recurrences happen at a particular time in the menstrual cycle.

You are highly contagious when you have active sores during your initial attack and also during recurrences. Viral shedding—the clearest indication of the possibility of transmission—occurs for two to ten days in the initial episode and two to five days in recurrent episodes. **Viral shedding also occurs intermittently during latent periods.** Viral shedding means that a culture of genital secretions shows definite evidence of the herpes virus, and this can occur even when the person has no apparent sores at the time. One study of pregnant women known to have herpes found that about 1% to 2% of cultures taken during an asymptomatic time were positive for herpes (7).

No one knows how likely transmission is when viral shedding occurs without any symptoms. Sexual transmission of the virus by an asymptomatic person can definitely occur, however, and is an important issue (8). Studies of people experiencing an initial herpes attack have found that **most cases of genital herpes were transmitted by partners who had no symptoms or had atypical or undiagnosed symptoms**. In one study, 35% of partners had no previous history of herpes symptoms, and 9% were themselves experiencing a primary attack, acquired from another recent sexual partner (9).

Cultures from active sores show 100 to 1,000 times more herpes virus than cultures of genital secretions during asymptomatic shedding episodes (2), so the risk of transmission is likely to be much greater when active sores are present.

Deciding on appropriate precautions may not be easy if you have herpes, or your partner does. In some cases it may be difficult to tell for sure whether early signs of a recurrence are beginning, and you need to decide how you feel about possible exposure risk from asymptomatic shedding.

At a minimum, **you must avoid intercourse and oral sex when sores** are present. Wait until the sores are completely healed and the skin looks entirely normal. Condoms may protect against herpes sores on the penis that are completely covered by the condom, but they cannot protect against sores on other parts of his skin (or yours). So it may be better not to rely on condoms and **avoid all contact with herpes sores**. Herpes can even attack the skin on your hands if a tiny scratch on your hand comes into contact with an active herpes sore on genital skin or mucous membrane.

You should also **avoid intercourse and oral sex when you suspect**, or your partner suspects, that **the first subtle signs of a herpes recurrence** may be starting. Watch for tingling or slight redness in usual attack areas. If you have even the slightest doubt, you should avoid intercourse or, at the very least, your partner should use condoms.

If you want to be a little more cautious your partner could use condoms several weeks after each attack; and using condoms as a routine practice is an entirely reasonable idea. **Condoms are especially important during pregnancy** if the man has herpes and the woman does not. A first attack of herpes during pregnancy is a serious risk for the baby. Pregnancy precautions are discussed in the next section of this chapter.

If you have herpes, you will have to think about how you will manage your sexual life, given the risk that you can transmit herpes to a partner. You will probably want to find your own way to tell potential lovers that you have herpes, and you will have to decide **when** to talk about herpes.

> The only wrong time to tell somebody is after sex. That's what happened to me. And people who say it's no big deal? I read once that it is "simply a benign chronic dermatologic condition." No it isn't. It is a threat to relationships, old ones and new ones.
>
> —WOMAN, 26

Despite the difficulties involved in maintaining prevention and despite the uncertainties about viral shedding, transmission of herpes to your partner can be avoided successfully. In one small study, more than half of the herpes victims reported that their present partner did not have herpes and that they had not transmitted herpes to a partner. An effective herpes vaccine would be of great help for herpes sufferers and their uninfected partners, and a new generation of herpes-free people in the future. Researchers report that vaccine development is feasible, but financially unlikely because of the low profit and possible liability risk a manufacturer would face (10). These are serious problems with all vaccines today. Write to your legislators!

Herpes support groups exist in many cities. You may find that a support group is a good source of practical advice about living with herpes, and a source of solace as well. See the "Resources" section at the end of this chapter for details.

If you have herpes **you also need to be especially faithful about routine pelvic exams and Pap smears once a year.** Having herpes means that your risk for precancerous abnormalities and cervical cancer is higher than average, and so is your risk for skin cancer on the vulva. Risk statistics are probably higher for women with herpes because women who have herpes are also more likely than average to have HPV, human papillomavirus, as well. HPV causes genital warts (see Chapter 27) and is an important culprit in cervical and vulvar cancer. HPV infection can occur with no outward signs that might alert you to the problem, so Pap smears are essential. Also, it is possible that herpes itself may play a role in cervical cancer risk.

Pregnancy Precautions.   Most women who have herpes have successful pregnancies and normal deliveries despite this problem. It is essential, however, to begin prenatal care early and be sure that your clinician is aware of your herpes history. Women who have herpes have a higher than average miscarriage rate. Most important, an infant exposed to active herpes infection at the time of vaginal delivery may acquire herpes, which can cause severe illness or even death for a newborn. Your goal is to be sure that your baby is not exposed. If you have active herpes at the end of pregnancy, you will need a cesarean section delivery.

• Have your first prenatal exam within the first six to eight weeks of pregnancy; this helps insure that your pregnancy dates will be accurately assessed in case cesarean section is needed

• Be faithful about your prenatal visit schedule. This helps insure that your dates are accurately assessed.

• Tell your clinician if **either you or your partner has ever had herpes.** In either case you should have herpes testing during the last few weeks of pregnancy **even if neither of you has had an attack in years.**

• **Do whatever you can to avoid having a first attack of herpes while you are pregnant.** If your partner has herpes and you do not, be especially careful about precautions to avoid all contact with active sores. Using condoms routinely throughout pregnancy to protect against possible exposure through asymptomatic viral shedding should be seriously considered.

• If you notice signs of a recurrence close to your expected delivery date (due date), contact your clinician immediately

• Be sure you have a careful exam to look for any signs of herpes as soon as you start labor or your water breaks

If you have signs of herpes or your recent cultures have been positive for herpes, you will need a cesarean section.

SUGGESTED READING

The Helper. A newsletter published quarterly by the Herpes Resource Center, Box 100, Palo Alto, California 94302. Up-to-date and detailed information on herpes treatment and research in clear and understandable language. A must for herpes sufferers. Subscription fee is $20 per year.

Sacks, Stephen L.: *The Truth About Herpes.* Vancouver: Verdant Press, 1986. Clear, easy-to-read, and detailed information about herpes written in question-and-answer format.

RESOURCES

The Herpes Resource Center. An information service for herpes sufferers, co-sponsored by the American Social Health Association and the Herpes Resource Center. Ask about HRC's newsletter, *The Helper,* and other publications available. Write to Herpes Resource Center, 260 Sheridan Avenue, Palo Alto, California 94306, or telephone 415-328-7710. (*Not* a toll-free call. Long distance rates apply.)

HELP. Local herpes support groups are active in many communities. Check your telephone directory for a HELP listing or contact the Herpes Resource Center for a listing of HELP chapters.

REFERENCES

1. Hatcher RA, Guest FJ, Stewart FH, et al: *Contraceptive Technology 1986–1987* (ed 13). New York: Irvington Publishers, 1986.
2. Corey L, Spear PG: Infections with herpes simplex virus. *New England Journal of Medicine* 314:686–690, 1986.
3. Douglas JM, Critchlow C, Benedetti J, et al: A double-blind study of oral acyclovir for suppression of recurrences of genital herpes simplex infection. *New England Journal of Medicine* 310:1551–1556, 1984.
4. Straus SE, Takiff HE, Seidlin M, et al: Suppression of frequently recurring genital herpes. A placebo-controlled double-blind trial of oral acyclovir. *New England Journal of Medicine* 310:1545–1550, 1984.
5. FDA-approved product labeling for oral acyclovir, January 1985. Manufacturer's information for physicians can be found in *Physicians' Desk Reference* (ed 40). Oradell, N.J.: Medical Economics Co., 1986.
6. Whittington WL, Cates W Jr: Acyclovir therapy for genital herpes: enthusiasm and caution in equal doses. *Journal of the American Medical Association* 251:2116–2117, 1984.
7. Harger JH, Meyer MP, Amortegui AJ: Changes in the frequency of genital herpes recurrences as a function of time. *Obstetrics and Gynecology* 67:637–641, 1986.
8. Rooney JF, Felser JM, Ostrove JM, et al: Acquisition of genital herpes from an asymptomatic sexual partner. *New England Journal of Medicine* 314:1561–1564, 1986.
9. Mertz GJ, Schmidt O, Jourden JL, et al: Frequency of acquisition of first-episode genital infection with herpes simplex virus from symptomatic and asymptomatic source contacts. *Sexually Transmitted Diseases* 12:33–39, 1985.
10. American Social Health Association: Vaccines, Part 1. *Helper* 9:1–6, 1987.

27

❖

Genital Warts
(Human Papillomavirus)

*Clinicians and their patients used to believe that warts on genital skin were just like warts on any other skin: a nuisance, none too alluring, but not dangerous. Recent research teaches us that **genital warts can be quite dangerous**, indeed, because they can be associated with precancerous and cancerous cell changes on the cervix and other genital areas. Prompt, aggressive treatment for genital warts has become essential.*

Genital warts may also be called venereal warts, Condylomata acuminata, flat condylomata, human papillomavirus (HPV) warts, or papovavirus warts. They look like garden variety warts on other parts of the body and, like other warts, are caused by a virus. Genital warts are caused by human papillomavirus (HPV), a slowly growing DNA virus. They are the most common *viral* sexually transmitted disease in the United States, accounting for some 3 million cases a year, more new cases than for the much more infamous viral STD, herpes. And the incidence of warts is increasing to epidemic proportions in this country (see Illustration 27-1).

More than 40 distinct strains of HPV have been identified. Some are responsible for common but quite benign annoyances like plantar warts (on the feet) or common warts on the hands. These types are not precancerous. Several strains of genital HPV, though, are now believed to be essential culprits in triggering the development of cervical cancer, vaginal cancer, vulvar cancer, and penile cancer. These strains tend to cause flat smooth warts that may be quite inconspicuous to the naked eye, or even completely inapparent. Unfortunately, there is no simple test yet available to identify which specific strain a victim of genital warts has, so all genital warts must be considered potentially precancerous.

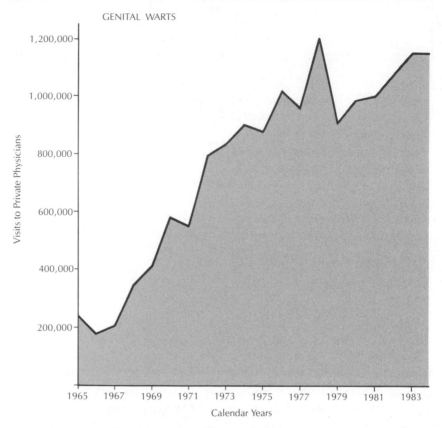

GENITAL WARTS

ILLUSTRATION 27-1   Genital warts is the leading STD (sexually transmitted disease) in the United States.

SYMPTOMS

Dry, painless warts appear on the vulva, cervix, inside the vagina, and/or around the anus. (Afflicted men usually have warts on the penis and sometimes on the anus or scrotum.) Warts may be small or large, single or multiple, raised or flat. If left untreated, they may go away spontaneously, but are more likely to grow in size and number, merge, and take on a cauliflower-like appearance. Warts are usually firm and rough, and are flesh colored or grayish-white. Symptoms are likely to become apparent one to three months after exposure. Time from exposure to wart growth, however, is variable and may be many months or even years. Also, warts may be very inconspicuous—a small, very flat penile wart or flat cervical wart may be difficult even for a physician to detect (see Illustration 27-2). For these reasons some wart victims are unable to identify the original contact source of their infection.

Wart virus infection involving the cervix is unlikely to cause symptoms you would notice. An abnormal Pap smear result showing warty cell changes called atypia, koilocytosis, or dyskeratosis may be your first sign of a wart problem.

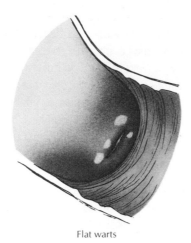

Flat warts

ILLUSTRATION 27-2   Flat warts on a woman's cervix mean she is at risk for cervical cancer.

DIAGNOSIS

Your clinician can usually diagnose warts by appearance alone. They can sometimes be confused with condylomata lata, the moist, flat sores sometimes associated with secondary syphilis. If there is any question, your clinician will draw a blood sample to test for syphilis. **Skin cancer on the vulva may also be mistaken for genital warts,** and your clinician may recommend biopsy to determine which disease is present in your case. This is essential if you have "warts" that persist despite repeated treatment. Your clinician is likely to recommend tests for other STDs as part of the diagnostic process.

Thorough evaluation is essential. Wart virus infection is quite likely to involve several areas. About half the women with vulvar warts in one study also had wart virus infection involving the cervix (1). A woman with cervical infection may also have unsuspected, inconspicuous vulvar warts. Colposcopy—to examine your vulvar skin, vagina, and cervix through a magnifying lens with a powerful light source—will be recommended. Your clinician can use a dilute vinegar solution swabbed on your skin along with colposcopy to identify areas of dense cell growth that appear white through the colposcope. These areas of wart virus infection may be invisible to the naked eye. Your partner also will need a colposcopy exam to identify any areas of wart virus infection he may have.

TREATMENT

Seek treatment promptly. Genital wart virus is contagious, and your warts are likely to grow and spread. Extensive warts are harder to treat (and more miserable). Your partner(s) must be treated at the same time you are.

If the warts are on your vulva or anus there are several treatment options. Your clinician may recommend freezing the warts with liquid nitrogen or a cryosurgery instrument (see Chapter 4), or she/he may use cautery to burn off the warts. Depending on where your warts are located and how extensive they are, you may need local anesthesia or even general anesthesia for wart treatment using these techniques. Your clinician may even recommend laser treatment to eradicate warts, especially if your warts are persisting or recurring despite other treatment.

In some cases a simpler approach using a caustic chemical such as trichloroacetic acid or podophyllin painted directly on your warts may be reasonable. Treatment failure rates with this method are fairly high, however. Chemical treatment will involve visits once or twice a week to your clinician's office. Your clinician may first put a lubricant jelly on surrounding normal skin to prevent burns, although treatments usually are not painful. You will be asked to wash off the podophyllin one to four hours after each treatment; trichloroacetic acid should be washed off after 12 hours. Warts may go away after three to four applications, or you may need quite a few treatments.

Warts inside the vagina or on the cervix cannot be treated with podophyllin. Your clinician will use cautery, freezing, or laser instead, or may recommend fluorouracil (Efudex) cream.

I guess I got warts from the guy I dated last summer while I was working at Yellowstone. I went to the health clinic a couple of times in the fall quarter and they put medicine on them, but it didn't help much.

By Christmas vacation they were driving me crazy. The clinic doctor said I would *have* to come in once a week till they were entirely gone. I did, and they were gone by spring break.

—WOMAN, 19

You should not be treated with podophyllin if you are pregnant, because it is not known whether podophyllin causes fetal abnormalities. If you are planning a pregnancy in the near future and have genital warts, be sure your warts are treated first. Warts may grow very rapidly during pregnancy, and could even constrict your vaginal opening so much that you would need a Cesarean delivery. Your baby may have an increased risk of developing wart-like growths on the larynx (voice box) if exposed to genital wart virus during delivery.

Podophyllin treatment is not effective in some cases, and the drug can cause toxic reactions if it is applied too liberally or the individual is sensitive to it. Researchers also question whether repeated application of podophyllin may itself have a carcinogenic effect. Alternative treatments are therefore receiving increasing attention.

Warts are often associated with bacterial or trichomonas vaginal infections. Wart treatment is more likely to be effective if any other infection present is treated effectively, and your clinician may ask you to use antibacterial vaginal cream faithfully until your warts have responded to treatment.

Condoms may protect against penile warts that are entirely covered by the condom, but they cannot protect against warts located elsewhere on your partner's genital skin, or on your skin. You should avoid intercourse while you are being treated for **warts on your skin,** while you are healing, and until both of you are free of warts. If you are being treated for **warts on the cervix,** your partner should use condoms routinely at least until your cervix has healed and your Pap smears have returned to normal. Thereafter, using condoms as a routine practice is an entirely reasonable idea as well.

PROGNOSIS

Warts can be treated effectively, and your risk of permanent scarring is greatly decreased if you seek treatment promptly. Warts sometimes become giant condylomata, a condition that is benign but very destructive and quite difficult to treat without extensive tissue damage. Reinfection can occur, particularly if your partner isn't treated at the same time you are. Recurrence of warts in some cases may occur even without new exposure. Dormant virus may remain in the skin cells for weeks or months and flare up later.

Warts do not attack or harm your uterus or tubes. Your fertility should not be directly affected. If treatment for warts requires cervical cryosurgery or laser, however, damage to cervical mucus glands is possible, and might impair fertility (see Chapter 4). And cervical cancer resulting from wart virus infection is likely to require hysterectomy.

The greatest concern is the relationship between genital warts, particularly flat warts on the cervix, and cervical cancer. Research suggests that these warts may be precursors or possibly cocarcinogens that work with other factors to lead to cancer (2,3,4,5,6). Some strains of the wart virus, types 16, 18, and 33 specifically, are strongly implicated in cervical cancer development. A routine pelvic exam could miss these flat warts, so if you have been exposed to warts or have vulvar warts, your clinician will recommend a colposcopic exam (see Chapter 4) for a closer look at your cervix, vagina, and vulva. Women who have evidence of wart virus infection involving the cervix are quite likely to have precancerous cervix abnormalities as well. About 11% of such women in one study already had cervical intraepithelial neoplasia (CIN) at the time of their initial evaluation, and 33% developed CIN within the next 12 months (7). (Precancerous and cancerous diseases of the cervix are described in detail in Chapter 35.)

The most important risk factors statistically linked to cervical cancer are attributes that relate directly to overall STD risk. These include intercourse before age 20, exposure to more than one male partner or a partner who is not monogamous, and previous infection with other STDs such as herpes. It may be that statistics document these risk factors because they also correlate with a higher risk of acquiring HPV infection.

Smoking and the use of birth control Pills are also cervical cancer risk factors, and they too appear to be statistically linked to HPV risk. Smokers in one study were four times as likely as nonsmokers to develop genital warts, and women who used birth control Pills five years or more were ten times as likely to develop warts (8). This study does not prove that Pills or smoking made women more susceptible to warts. It may be that Pill users and smokers had more warts because their lives were different from those of the control women in ways that the research project did not measure. Its findings are significant, however, because it shows that **all the cervical cancer risk factors may be linked to wart virus**. Also, it means that **women who smoke or are long-term birth control Pill users need to pay close attention to wart virus risk, and be very faithful about Pap smears.**

It is absolutely essential that genital warts—especially cervical ones—be aggressively treated and eradicated. Colposcopic examination and biopsy of suspicious areas are crucial. Be diligent about follow-up care, annual Pap smears, and pelvic exams if you have had warts, because recurrence is common. Also, you are at higher than average risk for cervical cancer, vaginal cancer, and vulvar cancer thereafter. A man who has had genital warts needs special surveillance for penile cancer. Using condoms routinely would be prudent.

REFERENCES

1. Reid R, Greenberg M, Jenson AB, et al: Sexually transmitted papillomavirus infections. *American Journal of Obstetrics and Gynecology* 156:212–222, 1987.
2. Crum CP, Ikenberg H, Richart RM, et al: Human papillomavirus type 16 and early cervical neoplasia. *New England Journal of Medicine* 310:880–883, 1984.
3. Guijon FB, Paraskevas M, Brunham R: The association of sexually transmitted diseases with cervical intraepithelial neoplasia: A case-control study. *American Journal of Obstetrics and Gynecology* 151:185–190, 1985.
4. Smotkin D, Berek JS, Fu YS, et al: Human papillomavirus deoxyribonucleic acid in adenocarcinoma and adenosquamous carcinoma of the uterine cervix. *Obstetrics and Gynecology* 68:241–244, 1986.
5. Schneider A, Sawada E, Gissmann L, et al: Human papillomavirus in women with a history of abnormal Papanicolaou smears and in their male partners. *Obstetrics and Gynecology* 69:554–562, 1987.
6. Winkler B, Richart RM: Human papillomavirus and gynecologic neoplasia. *Current Problems in Obstetrics, Gynecology and Fertility* 10:55–90, 1987.
7. Nash JD, Burke TW, Hoskins WJ: Biologic course of cervical human papillomavirus infection. *Obstetrics and Gynecology* 69:160–162, 1987.
8. Daling JR, Sherman KJ, Weiss NS: Risk factors for condyloma acuminatum in women. *Sexually Transmitted Diseases* 13:16–18, 1986.

28

AIDS

(Acquired Immunodeficiency Syndrome), Viral Hepatitis, and Syphilis

Between the mid 1950s and early 1980s, industrialized societies experienced a brief reprieve from the fear of fatal sexually transmitted illness. Prior to that time and since, the dark side of sexual freedom has been the risk of acquiring an infection that might progress to severe illness and death, with little or no hope of cure.

Before the 1950s, syphilis was the fearsome menace; men and women lived under its shadow for 400 years at least, possibly for 1,000 years or more (1). (During the fear reprieve, cervical and penile cancer caused by genital warts actually were a threat to life but their menace was not known, and the role of sexual transmission in viral hepatitis was not widely recognized.) In 1983 the cause of AIDS was definitely shown to be a virus that could be transmitted through sexual intimacy (and some other routes), and the brief reprieve from fear ended. AIDS, so inexorable and deadly, may even surpass syphilis in its terrible devastation.

These are the diseases that cannot be ignored. Calculated romantic risks with trichomonas infection or even with herpes or gonorrhea may seem reasonable, but when the possible consequence is incurable illness, suffering, and death, the concept of rational risk taking just doesn't apply.

Both quality and quantity count. Intercourse with just one partner from an AIDS high-risk group is very dangerous; more dangerous than intercourse with several low-risk partners. Exposure to multiple partners, however, means you also have indirect exposure to many other unknown partners, past and present. You are at risk for all sexually transmitted diseases, including AIDS, hepatitis, and syphilis.

You may already have a friend or family member who has been touched by the AIDS epidemic, but most likely that friend or relative is male. Nevertheless, there are aspects of this illness that are extremely important for women to understand, such as which women are at risk for AIDS, steps to prevent infection, and what risks are associated with pregnancy and delivery. **Women have no special protection against AIDS.** There is even some evidence that women are at greater risk than men when exposed to AIDS through heterosexual intercourse. A woman is quite likely to become infected with just one exposure to infected semen. Protect your own life by respecting the AIDS risk factors.

If there is any chance at all that you may have been exposed to the AIDS virus, you will need careful evaluation and testing before you consider pregnancy. Until you can be sure you do not have the virus, you should take every possible precaution to avoid pregnancy. If you are infected with AIDS virus, pregnancy may be dangerous for you, and your baby is very likely to develop severe AIDS problems as well.

AIDS (Acquired Immunodeficiency Syndrome)

Researchers who write about AIDS use very precise terminology, and so to understand their findings you will need to know a few of the terms they use. Here are four to get you started. Each will be described in greater detail later in the chapter:

- **HIV** (human immunodeficiency virus) is the name of the virus that causes AIDS and related illnesses. Until 1986 it was called HTLV-III in the United States, which stands for human T-lymphotropic virus type III, or HTLV-III/LAV. The additional letters stand for lymphadenopathy-associated virus. LAV is the term used by the French scientists who first identified this virus. These two independently discovered viruses are either virtually or absolutely identical.
- **ARC** describes an illness associated with mild, intermittent symptoms such as swollen lymph glands, fatigue, and fever. The abbreviation stands for AIDS-related complex.
- **PGL** means an illness associated with persistent swollen lymph glands in many parts of the body. The abbreviation stands for persistent generalized lymphadenopathy. PGL is often associated with ARC.
- **AIDS** describes a serious illness that includes laboratory evidence of impaired immunity and one or more opportunistic infections. The abbreviation stands for acquired immunodeficiency syndrome.

AIDS was discovered in 1981 when a cluster of four cases occurred in Los Angeles. Four young and otherwise healthy men were afflicted with a rare and peculiar type of pneumonia, *Pneumocystis carinii* pneumonia, that previously was a problem only among frail cancer or transplant patients or severely malnourished children. Like all people with AIDS, these men had profound, irreversible loss of immune defenses, and were unable to combat infection of any kind. The cause of AIDS was elusive until 1983, when scientists in France and the United States isolated HIV virus. This virus invades T cells, members of the white blood cell's infection-fighting team. T cells infected with AIDS virus are unable to perform their normal defense functions. Instead, they become AIDS virus factories, producing new virus particles in prodigious numbers and releasing them to attack other T cells.

Scientists were soon able to develop a sensitive blood test to detect the presence of antibodies to HIV, indirect evidence that the virus is present. A person infected with AIDS virus may have disease symptoms such as AIDS-related complex, persistent generalized lymphadenopathy, or advanced AIDS disease, or the person may have no noticeable symptoms at all. Even if no symptoms are present, however, active virus is present in the blood of an infected person and also in semen; virus also may be present in saliva, tears, breast milk, and vaginal and cervical secretions (2,3,4,5). Much like hepatitis B, AIDS is transmitted through sexual intimacy (particularly intercourse with ejaculation of semen), exposure to blood from an infected person, or transmission during or soon after pregnancy from an infected woman to her fetus or newborn. Most AIDS cases in the United States so far have been among members of one or more of the following high-risk groups (2):

• Homosexual or bisexual men
• People who use illicit intravenous drugs
• People with hemophilia treated prior to 1985 with clotting factors derived from pooled, donated blood
• Sex partners of people with AIDS or of people carrying the AIDS virus
• Children of women infected with the virus

Infection acquired through blood transfusion accounted for 1% to 2% of AIDS cases until 1985, when effective tests were introduced to screen donated blood for AIDS prior to its use.

Spread between homosexual men has accounted for more than 65% of cases in the United States. Initial public information on AIDS stressed the role of extraordinary sexual promiscuity in AIDS transmission. Perhaps for this reason, most of the HIV-positive homosexual and bisexual men actually identified through screening did not believe that they were at high risk. AIDS is not simply a homosexual disease, however. Studies in central Africa have found equal infection rates for men and women, and heterosexual transmission of the virus has been definitely documented. Based on U.S. statistics, the risks for acquiring AIDS virus through heterosexual intercourse are higher for a woman exposed to an infected man than they are for a man exposed to an infected woman, as is true with other sexual infections. For homosexual men, rectal intercourse may be of particular importance, with receptive anal intercourse carrying the greatest risk. Researchers suspect that small tears in the rectum caused by intercourse may facilitate entry into the bloodstream of virus from infected semen. Vaginal intercourse and oral/genital sex can also transmit the virus.

Exposure to the virus in infected blood explains transmission through blood transfusion (prior to 1985), through hemophilia treatment with blood products, and through needle sharing among illegal intravenous drug users. Shared needles and

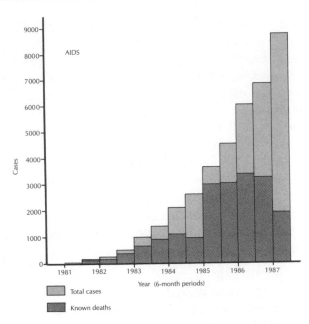

ILLUSTRATION 28-1   If the AIDS epidemic curve continues its steep rise, this disease may become a leading cause of death in the United States within just a few years. Both women and men are at risk. It can be spread through heterosexual intercourse as well as homosexual exposure.

SOURCES: Centers for Disease Control:Update:Acquired Immunodeficiency Syndrome—United States. *Morbidity and Mortality Weekly Report* 34:245–248, 1985; and Personal Communication, Robert H. Byers, Ph.D., Statistician, AIDS Program, U.S. Centers for Disease Control, Atlanta, Georgia, July, 1987.

injection equipment can carry the virus from an infected person to the next user. Accidental puncture injury by a needle or a medical or dental instrument contaminated with AIDS virus is a potential danger for health workers. Transmission of hepatitis virus is known to occur in this way, but the risk for HIV transmission so far appears to be much lower than hepatitis transmission following such accidental exposure.

There is no evidence that AIDS is transmitted through immune globulin or hepatitis B vaccine, or through food, mosquitoes or other insects, or casual contact (2).

There can be no doubt that AIDS is a very serious epidemic now, and has a potentially catastrophic future. The number of new AIDS cases reported in the United States has approximately doubled every 6 to 12 months since 1981. Illustration 28-1 shows AIDS cases already reported, and new cases predicted through 1986. This steeply rising curve is almost certain to continue for at least several years because the reservoir of people already infected with the virus but not yet ill is huge. Researchers estimate that as many as 1 to 2 million Americans have already been infected. Many of the people already infected know that they are in high-risk groups already, and some are no doubt taking precautions so that they don't infect other people. Others may be unknowingly spreading the virus. Unless sexual practices change drastically in our population or a cure for the disease is found, the epidemic is likely to continue.

It is not surprising that the AIDS epidemic first became apparent in the homosexual community and among intravenous drug users. The rates for all sexually transmitted diseases are high in these groups. **There is no reason to believe, however, that AIDS will remain confined to high-risk groups.** Heterosexual transmission does occur and the disease already has a foothold among women drug users, prostitutes (particularly those who use drugs), and sexual partners of infected bisexual men. Researchers have found that 10% of heterosexual intravenous drug users in San Francisco have blood test evidence of AIDS virus infection. In New York City, needle sharing between homosexual and heterosexual addicts appears to be more common, and 50% of intravenous drug users test positive for AIDS antibody (6). Unsuspected AIDS virus infection has also been detected in screening of heterosexual members of a social/sexual club (popularly known as a "swing club") in Minnesota (7). No one can be certain how slowly or quickly the virus will spread among heterosexual people in the future. Infection rate curves may be even more severe than curves for other viral infections such as herpes, warts, or hepatitis. Two unique characteristics may contribute to epidemic spread for AIDS:

• **HIV contagiousness is continuous and may persist permanently**
• **Symptoms of AIDS may not be apparent until five years or more after exposure.** HIV has an exceptionally long incubation period. During this time the man or woman is **contagious to others**, but may not be aware that the virus is present, and there are no external signs that might alert a sexual partner to his or her risk of exposure.

If sexual practices and drug use with hypodermic needles in the United States remain unchanged, and if effective prevention and treatment for AIDS are not found, AIDS could conceivably become a leading cause of death in the nation within one or two decades. It is already the leading cause of death among young men in New York City, San Francisco, and Los Angeles, and among women between the ages of 25 and 29 in New York City.

SYMPTOMS

The official medical definition of AIDS is specific and quite restrictive. A definite (reportable) diagnosis of AIDS is made only if the man or woman has one of the AIDS-associated cancers such as Kaposi's sarcoma, or a rare type of persistent pneumonia (chronic lymphoid interstitial pneumonitis), or a severe opportunistic infection. Cancers and infections associated with AIDS are shown in Table 28-1. An opportunistic infection is one caused by microorganisms that are not able to invade a human host who has normal infection defenses. Researchers believe, however, that the AIDS virus is actually responsible for a whole range of additional problems.

With AIDS or AIDS-related complex (ARC) a man or woman is likely to experience severe fatigue, recurrent fever, weight loss, diarrhea, and malaise, with additional

TABLE 28-1
CANCERS AND OPPORTUNISTIC INFECTIONS IN AIDS

CANCERS

Kaposi's sarcoma
Non-Hodgkin's lymphoma
Brain lymphoma

INFECTIONS

Pneumocystis carinii	Cryptococcus	Cytomegalovirus
Toxoplasma	Candida (yeast)	Herpes simplex virus
Cryptosporidia	Aspergillus	Varicella-zoster virus
Isospora	Histoplasma	JC virus
Strongyloides	Coccidioides	Nocardia
Mycobacteria	Salmonella	Legionella
(including tuberculosis)		

SOURCE: Adapted from Holmes KK, Mardh P-A, Sparling PF, et al: *Sexually Transmitted Diseases.* New York: McGraw-Hill, 1984.

symptoms depending on the specific type of opportunistic infection or cancer involved. Kaposi's sarcoma usually begins as one or more purple patches on the skin, similar in appearance to a bruise. Patches can arise anywhere on the body and may progress to a lump or plaque. Kaposi's sarcoma may also involve the lymph nodes, the lining of the intestinal tract, or the lungs, where it can cause lethal damage to lung function. In most cases, however, the cancer itself is not the direct cause of death.

Complications of severe infection are responsible for most AIDS deaths. Although treatment for most of the infections is known, treatment success for a person who has AIDS is severely compromised because normal infection defenses are absent.

In addition to infection and Kaposi's sarcoma, AIDS virus probably also increases susceptibility to other kinds of cancer including some forms of lymphoma and squamous cell rectal, oral, and vaginal cancer. AIDS virus can also infect brain tissue and cause neurologic problems and progressive brain disease in some cases.

Mild or early forms of HIV infection also exist. Some people may experience an initial illness similar to mononucleosis soon after exposure to the virus. Symptoms such as fever, malaise, intestinal upset, sore throat, and diarrhea are similar to symptoms with other mild viral infections such as flu, and are not likely to be identified as HIV infection. After these symptoms subside, the man or woman may have no further symptoms whatsoever for months or even years.

For some people, the HIV virus causes a pattern of milder, intermittent symptoms, AIDS-Related Complex (ARC), such as fatigue, swollen lymph glands, fever, drenching night sweats, profound diarrhea, and weight loss associated with laboratory evidence of impaired immune defenses. Lymph node swelling may be extensive and persistent, and is called PGL (persistent generalized lymphadenopathy). People who have ARC or PGL are statistically more likely to develop AIDS itself within subsequent months than are people who have evidence of HIV antibody but no symptoms.

Researchers do not know why some people infected with the virus are well, others have mild symptoms, and still others have devastating disease. They suspect there may be "cofactors" that can accelerate illness. Suspected cofactors include recreational drug use and other sexually transmitted infections.

DIAGNOSIS

AIDS is diagnosed when opportunistic infections and/or malignancies occur in a person with evidence of compromised immunity.

Sensitive blood tests to detect antibody to the HIV virus are widely available, and are used to test those who may have AIDS, persons at high risk for AIDS, and donated blood prior to its use. If the initial screening is positive, it is repeated and additional tests such as the Western Blot are performed to be certain that the positive test result is correct, and that HIV virus is in fact present.

Anyone who has a confirmed, positive blood test result for AIDS virus antibody must be presumed to have active virus present, and must be presumed to be contagious through unprotected sexual contact and shared drug needles or syringes. This is true even if the person has no symptoms whatsoever and appears to be completely healthy.

TREATMENT

No cure for AIDS is known. Treatment is available, however, for many of the infections and cancers that afflict AIDS patients.

Numerous antiviral medications are being tested in experimental treatment programs, but researchers are cautious in predicting future success. Most drugs that can kill viruses are also quite toxic, and finding ways to combat viral illnesses generally has been a slow and frustrating effort. Drugs that are safe yet effective in eradicating viruses have not yet been found for many of the common viral illnesses that humans experience.

PROGNOSIS

Once AIDS is diagnosed, the prognosis is bleak. Approximately half of all known AIDS patients have already died, including 80% of patients diagnosed before 1985.

No one knows what the future holds for people who have blood test evidence of AIDS virus but do not have the disease. Experts estimate that at least 25% to 50% will develop AIDS, but acknowledge that the rate may prove to be even higher (8). Accurate prediction may not be possible for another five years or more because the incubation period for AIDS can be so long.

PREVENTION

With AIDS, prevention is the only weapon now available. AIDS prevention requires the same steps as prevention of any other sexually transmitted disease (see Chapter 22), but some specific high-risk situations bear special mention. AIDS is a risk for women as well as men. High-risk situations include:

- Intercourse with anyone who has AIDS or has blood test evidence of HIV virus
- Intercourse with any member of a high-risk group, including homosexual or bisexual men; men or women intravenous drug users; prostitutes; and men treated for hemophilia
- Sharing needles or injection equipment in illicit drug use

If you have one or more of these risk factors, **testing for evidence of AIDS exposure is essential before you consider pregnancy.** Testing before pregnancy is also recommended for women and men who were born in parts of the world where heterosexual spread of the virus is more significant, such as Haiti and central Africa, and for women who have been (or are) prostitutes. You also need careful evaluation to help you determine when pregnancy might be safe. If you were exposed to AIDS risk in the past, but the exposure ended, blood tests that remain negative for six months after your last possible exposure to AIDS can give you assurance that you did not become infected with the virus. An AIDS expert in your area can help you determine how long you need to wait for your follow-up tests.

Pregnancy is not safe if you have continuing exposure to AIDS risk. The normal immune system changes that occur in pregnancy may accelerate severe AIDS problems for a woman who has the virus, and the infection is very likely to be transmitted to the baby.

A selective attitude in making decisions about sexual intimacy, and being certain that you know your partner well enough to be aware of possible risk factors in his or her history, are essential. Exposure to large numbers of sexual partners is also an important common denominator in AIDS risk for some high-risk groups. **The use of condoms is a reasonable precaution,** but condoms cannot provide 100% protection and their effectiveness in reducing virus transmission and perhaps AIDS risk is not definitely documented in research. One laboratory study has shown that latex condoms do prevent transmission of HIV from one tissue culture to another when the virus is present in a concentration similar to that found in semen (8). Lower rates for HIV antibodies have also been found for prostitutes in Zaire who reported routine condom use with partners (9). Nevertheless, **saying no to intercourse when you have any question about possible high-risk factors may be a life-preserving decision.**

If your are using condoms to minimize STD (sexually transmitted disease) risk, it makes sense to choose a latex condom brand that has a spermicidal lubricant. Latex condoms are less permeable than natural skin condoms, and the spermicide may help kill STD organisms. Some sexual practices are safe, and some are definitely dangerous

TABLE 28-2
SAFE SEX PRACTICES

SAFE	RISKY	DANGEROUS
Dry kissing	Wet kissing	Oral sex without a condom
Masturbation on healthy skin	Masturbation on open/broken skin	Vaginal intercourse without a condom
External watersports (urination)	Oral sex on a woman	Anal intercourse without a condom
Touching	Amphetamines (speed)	Internal watersports (urination)
Fantasy	Amyl nitrite (poppers)	Intravenous drugs
	Alcohol	Sharing a needle
	Marijuana	Fisting (anal penetration with a hand or fist)
		Rimming (oral-anal stimulation)

POSSIBLY SAFE
Vaginal intercourse with a condom
Anal intercourse with a condom
Oral sex with a condom

Adapted from Charlottesville AIDS Resource Network brochure, entitled "Safe Sex," developed for the American College Health Association, 1986.

(see Table 28-2). The goal in safe sex is to avoid sharing body fluids. Semen, blood, menstrual blood, urine, feces, and saliva may harbor the AIDS virus as well as hepatitis-B, chlamydia, gonorrhea, and syphilis. Contact between these body fluids and any mucous membrane (mouth, vagina, penis, rectum) can transmit disease, and so can contact with an open cut or sore on skin. Anal intercourse and anal penetration with a hand or fist (fisting) can be especially dangerous because the rectal lining is delicate and if it is bruised or torn, virus or bacteria may enter the bloodstream easily. Illicit drugs and alcohol are on the risky list because of the effect they may have on judgment and also because they may adversely affect normal immune responses.

Remember, too, that you may be exposed through decisions your partner makes now, or made in the past. You are at risk if you are a woman whose male sex partner was or is exposed to intravenous drugs, intercourse with prostitutes, or to homosexual intimacy. In some cities, as many as 57% of female prostitutes tested show antibody evidence of HIV infection (10). A man is at risk if his female partner was or is an intravenous drug user, a prostitute, or is a present or former sex partner of an infected person.

When sex is at stake people just seem to have more difficulty being honest. One of my friends had to have an abortion because her boyfriend told her he had a vasectomy. It was just a lie; he wanted sex with her so badly that he simply made it up. Really, he is a basically honest person.

It makes me wonder just how honest people will be about the sexual parts of their past lives. Can you really trust someone who knows that sex will be out if you find out about a heavy drug summer three years ago, or a brief gay affair? I'm not even sure I could be honest.

—WOMAN, 28

If you work in the health care field, or dentistry, you should also be aware of potential exposure at your job. AIDS transmission is not likely to be a serious threat for health workers, but precautions to avoid accidental exposure are certainly reasonable. Handle used needles or medical equipment carefully, don't recap needles, and wear gloves and eye goggles whenever exposure to blood or other body fluids from patients is possible, especially if you have any cuts or scratches on your hands. Read and follow the recommendations of the Public Health Service. The recommendations are detailed, and are updated periodically; to obtain them contact your local health department or the Public Health Service, Centers for Disease Control, 1600 Clifton Road, NE, Atlanta, Georgia 30333.

Transmission of the AIDS virus is also possible through artificial insemination with donor semen. If you have insemination treatment, be sure that the donor has been tested for the AIDS virus antibody. This is a routine practice at reputable fertility treatment programs. Some experts recommend that donor semen be frozen and stored for at least three months before use. A blood test may not show evidence of AIDS virus until six weeks after exposure. The three-month storage interval allows time for the donor to be retested to detect recent infection before his semen is released. Only a handful of AIDS cases have occurred through artificial insemination, however, and this approach has the disadvantage that frozen semen is significantly less effective in achieving pregnancy than is fresh semen.

Viral Hepatitis

Hepatitis, inflammation of the liver, is a potentially life-threatening illness caused in most cases by virus infection. **The common types of hepatitis, named A, B, and non-A non-B, can be transmitted through sexual intimacy.** In other respects, each type is quite distinct.

Hepatitis A, formerly called infectious hepatitis, primarily affects children and young adults, and is spread through close contact (in institutions and day care centers, for example) that exposes victims to oral secretions or feces of an infected person. It can also be spread through contaminated food or water, or very rarely through blood transfusion. Uncooked shellfish harvested from contaminated water is a common infection source. Sexual intimacy is a potential means of spread, particularly if sexual intimacy exposes you to your partner's feces.

Hepatitis A is usually a mild illness that resolves completely within 6 to 12 weeks. Symptoms are likely to begin about three weeks after exposure, but may be so mild that the victim is not aware of the illness. Severe illness is very rare and fewer than 5 in 1,000 hepatitis A victims die of the disease.

Hepatitis B was formerly called serum hepatitis. Sexual contact (homosexual and/or heterosexual) is probably the most important route for its spread in the United States (1). It is also transmitted through shared needles and other injection equipment among drug users. Health workers exposed to accidental injury from contaminated needles or dental or surgical instruments are vulnerable to infection. Hepatitis B can be spread between family members. The route for such spread is not known, but active virus may be present in the tears, sweat, saliva, vaginal secretions, or semen of an infected person as well as in her/his blood. An infected woman is likely to transmit hepatitis B to her infant, especially if she is a carrier or if her illness occurs during the last three months of pregnancy. Transfusion with contaminated blood was formerly an important means of hepatitis B transmission, but sensitive laboratory tests are now used to detect it in donated blood, so this route of spread is rare.

Hepatitis B may be a mild or even inapparent illness, or may cause severe symptoms. Symptoms usually appear 2 to 3 months after exposure, but could begin as early as 1 month or as late as 18 months later. Among hepatitis B victims who do have symptoms, approximately 1% develop severe liver failure, which is fatal in 75% of cases (1). Another serious problem is persistent infection, which can occur with no apparent symptoms (a carrier state) or can lead to chronic liver disease. Persistent infection can cause permanent liver scarring and liver failure, and is linked to later development of liver cancer.

In the United States, approximately 200,000 people develop hepatitis B infection each year (11); approximately 25% of them develop significant symptoms and 5% require hospital care. Hepatitis B is extremely common in some parts of the world such as Southeast Asia, parts of Africa, and the Pacific Islands, where most people acquire

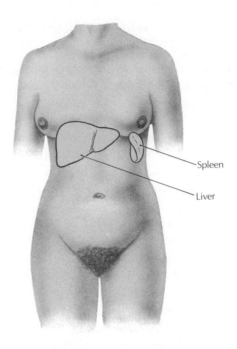

Spleen

Liver

ILLUSTRATION 28-2   Hepatitis can be a sexually transmitted disease. It causes
tenderness and enlargement of the liver and spleen in some cases.

the infection at birth or during childhood and as many as 5% to 15% are virus
carriers.

Non-A non-B hepatitis is an illness similar in most respects to hepatitis B, but
patients with this virus show no evidence of either the hepatitis B virus or the A virus.
Researchers believe it is caused by one or more viruses as yet not identified. Non-A
non-B hepatitis accounts for less than 15% of all hepatitis cases, but is responsible for
most cases of transfusion hepatitis that now occur. The **delta virus**, also known as
hepatitis D, is a virus that piggybacks with hepatitis B. Both may be acquired at the
same time, or a carrier of hepatitis B may later acquire the delta virus, and experience
a second episode of hepatitis symptoms. Delta virus is likely to be associated with
needle drug abuse.

SYMPTOMS

Symptoms, when they occur, are similar for all types of hepatitis. Low-grade fever,
fatigue, headache, and generalized muscle aches may precede symptoms of disrupted
liver function. Loss of appetite, nausea, vomiting, indigestion, and abdominal pain are

common. Yellow pigments called bilirubin accumulate in the bloodstream when liver cells fail to convert them for excretion or liver swelling blocks bile passages. High bilirubin results in jaundice, a yellow cast to the skin and eyes, and also in dark urine and clay-colored or white stools, signals of liver disease. In some cases hepatitis is accompanied by skin rash, joint pain, and arthritis symptoms.

DIAGNOSIS

Your clinician is likely to suspect hepatitis if you have some or all of the symptoms described above. She/he will review your medical history for possible recent exposure, and to determine whether you are in a high-risk category for hepatitis (see the section entitled "Prevention"). Jaundice may be evident, and in some cases, tenderness high in the abdomen on the right side and enlargement of the liver and/or spleen can be detected during physical examination (see Illustration 28-2).

You will need blood tests to confirm the diagnosis, to determine which type of hepatitis you have, and to assess the extent of liver impairment.

TREATMENT

No effective drug to cure hepatitis is available, so the goal in your treatment is to assure an optimal chance for your own body defenses to overcome the illness. If you are severely ill, hospitalization may be necessary. In most cases, though, rest and supportive care at home are sufficient. A nutritious diet and complete avoidance of alcohol will be recommended until blood tests show that normal liver function has been restored. Medications containing estrogen such as birth control Pills and postmenopausal hormone treatment must also be stopped until your liver returns to normal, because the liver helps excrete estrogen. If liver function is disrupted by hepatitis, high estrogen levels may accumulate.

PROGNOSIS

For most hepatitis patients the virus is eliminated and liver function returns to normal within 6 to 12 weeks. New liver cells regenerate to replace damaged tissue so successfully that no evidence of previous hepatitis is likely to remain after healing is complete. Antibodies against the specific type of hepatitis involved remain and confer lifetime immunity against another attack by the same virus.

For some people, however, virus infection persists. Approximately 5% to 10% of hepatitis B victims and as many as 30% of non-A non-B victims have evidence of continuing virus infection. Some have no symptoms of liver disease while others show persistent symptoms, a disease called chronic active hepatitis. Chronic hepatitis can lead to permanent, irreversible liver damage (cirrhosis) and is also linked to a high risk for later development of liver cancer.

PREVENTION

Hepatitis risks are another good reason to think carefully about consequences when you are considering sexual intimacy. It is one of the sexually transmitted ailments that can cause permanent disability or even death. Read Chapter 22 for ways to minimize your risks for all sexually transmitted disease.

Hepatitis A and hepatitis B can be prevented effectively by treatment with immune globulin immediately after exposure. A vaccine is available to prevent hepatitis B. Staying away from shared needles and from intimacy with infected people will prevent transmission in many cases.

An immune globulin injection provides temporary, passive, immune protection. It is prepared from pooled blood from blood donations and contains antibodies against hepatitis that were produced by the donors, so protection lasts only while those antibodies are still circulating in your body. Fortunately, manufacturing steps used in preparation of immune globulin appear to eliminate viruses such as AIDS that would otherwise be a risk for recipients of pooled blood, and there is no evidence that AIDS virus has been transmitted by this route (2). Immune globulin injections effective against both hepatitis A and B are available; its effectiveness against non-A non-B hepatitis is not known. You must get your A injection within two weeks of exposure and your B injection within eight days of exposure. When given promptly, globulin can prevent at least 80% of hepatitis A and about 75% of hepatitis B cases that would otherwise be expected.

Vaccination to induce long-term immunity is available for hepatitis B. Vaccination involves a series of three injections given over six months. The vaccine contains chemicals similar enough to the B virus that your body's immune defenses triggered by the vaccine are also effective against the real virus if exposure occurs later on. Immunity lasts four years or more, and prevents at least 80% or 90% of hepatitis B cases that would otherwise occur. In some cases a vaccine booster dose may be recommended after five years. Temporary soreness in the arm after vaccination is common. Other adverse reactions are rare. Testing for previous hepatitis exposure is not necessary for vaccination.

Vaccination against hepatitis B is quite expensive ($150 or more for the series), but is recommended (11) for people at high risk of hepatitis B exposure:

- Health care workers exposed to possible needle-stick or instrument injury, including students in nursing, medicine, dentistry, laboratory technology, and allied health professions, and health personnel who work in a laboratory, operating room, cancer or dialysis unit, blood drawing or intravenous therapy service, emergency room, blood bank, or dental service. This category also includes mortuary workers.
- Household contacts of a person infected with hepatitis B
- Sexual partner(s) of a person infected with hepatitis B
- Heterosexual people with multiple partners; risk increases with increasing number of partners and is extremely high among prostitutes

- Homosexual men with multiple partners (homosexual women are not at high risk)
- People planning travel or an extended visit to areas where hepatitis B rates are high, such as Southeast Asia, parts of Africa, and the Pacific Islands. Vaccination should begin six months before travel.
- Clients and staff of institutions for the developmentally disabled
- People receiving hemodialysis or treatment with blood products for clotting disorders such as hemophilia
- Prison inmates
- People who use illicit injectable drugs

If exposure to hepatitis B has already occurred, then immediate treatment within eight days with immune globulin to provide temporary protection is recommended for:

- Sexual partner(s) of a person who has hepatitis B virus
- An infant born to a woman who has evidence of hepatitis B
- Anyone exposed to blood from an infected person by needle stick, puncture wound, or blood contact with the eye or mouth

Immune globulin treatment should be started as soon as possible after exposure, and vaccination to provide long-term immunity will be recommended at the same time in most cases.

No vaccine is yet available for hepatitis A. Treatment with immune globulin can provide temporary protection if it is administered within two weeks after exposure. Immune globulin shots are recommended (11) after hepatitis A exposure for:

- Sexual partner(s) of a person with hepatitis A
- Household contacts of an infected person
- Staff and fellow clients if the infected person is a member of a day care center or lives in an institution

Globulin treatment is also recommended prior to travel (and every four months while away) for anyone visiting an area where hepatitis A rates are high.

Little is known about **prevention of non-A non-B hepatitis.** There is some evidence that immune globulin may protect against non-A non-B, and treatment is recommended for anyone exposed to blood from an infected person by accidental needle stick or injury.

Syphilis
(Lues, Treponema pallidum Infection)

Treponema pallidum, the microorganism that causes syphilis, was responsible for untold human suffering and death prior to the 1940s, when penicillin first became available for clinical use. Its modern name was acquired in 1530 from a poem about an afflicted shepherd written at the height of a severe syphilis epidemic in Europe. It was also called the Great Pox, in contrast to smallpox, another serious health threat at the time.

In the United States, syphilis declined from an all-time high of nearly 400 cases per 100,000 people in 1943 to a low of less than 10 in 1977 (1). Rates increased slightly between 1977 and 1982 and then steadily declined until 1987 when a marked increase in reported cases occurred. Nearly doubled syphilis rates were reported for some areas (California, Florida, New York) during the first three months of 1987, and the overall U.S. annual rate rose 23%, from 10.9 to 13 cases annually for every 100,000 people. The increase occurred mainly among heterosexual people. Experts are worried (12). Because syphilis is still with us, routine premarital blood testing is widespread. In most Health Department STD clinics, people with gonorrhea or another sexually transmitted infection are routinely tested for syphilis.

T. pallidum is a very small, spiral-shaped, motile bacterium. It is not visible on a routine microscope slide, but can be seen with a special dark-field microscope. *Treponema* cannot be grown in bacterial culture, so dark-field microscopy and blood tests to measure antibody evidence of infection are the only means for detecting syphilis.

Syphilis is a highly contagious, fickle disease. The risk of acquiring syphilis is about 30% if you have intercourse with an infected person. Exposure to only a few organisms, perhaps as few as 50, may be sufficient to transmit the disease.

Once acquired, the disease has a long and variable course. The initial symptoms are often overlooked, and the highly contagious victim is often unaware of infection. Later or secondary symptoms may be mild or severe, and may mimic other diseases. Syphilis is also contagious during the secondary phase. If untreated, secondary syphilis may subside during a latency period only to return months or even years later. The most serious consequences of late syphilis—meningitis, brain damage, heart disease, and aneurysm (weakening and ballooning in the walls of large blood vessels leading from the heart)—can occur among untreated women or men decades after the initial infection.

SYMPTOMS

Primary Syphilis.   The primary or first disease stage occurs about three weeks after sexual exposure. The range of time from exposure to the onset of symptoms may be anywhere from 9 to 90 days. Usually the first symptom is at the site of sexual contact: a sore called a chancre (pronounced "shanker"). The chancre is usually painless; there may be a hardened, red-rimmed sore or pimple-like area on the edge of your vagina, cervix, vulva, or mouth, or on your partner's penis. These are the most common locations, but the chancre may also appear on the fingertip, lip, breast, anus, or almost anywhere there is intimate contact between you and your infected partner. During this primary stage, syphilis is extremely infectious. **Only a small percentage of women who develop a chancre will notice it,** because it is painless and may be deep inside the vagina. In two to six weeks the chancre will disappear, even without treatment.

Secondary Syphilis. The second stage occurs as soon as one week or as long as six months after the chancre heals. Symptoms tend to last three to six months but may come and go for several years. They include rash, especially on the palms of the hands and soles of the feet, fever, a sore throat, headache, a sore mouth, loss of appetite, nausea, and inflamed eyes. Scalp hair may fall out in patches. (Syphilis is sometimes called "haircut.") Sores called condylomata lata may appear around the genitals and anus; these sores are moist, broad-based, and about ¼ inch across. Other possible symptoms include pain in the joints, generalized lymph node swelling, and enlarged liver and spleen. In severe cases, the kidneys or brain may be involved as well. **You are highly infectious** in the secondary phase of syphilis, and the infection can be spread from any affected site.

Tertiary Syphilis. After 10 to 20 years, signs of tertiary syphilis such as heart disease, brain damage, spinal cord damage, and blindness may develop. Fortunately, these serious consequences do not occur if syphilis is treated. If untreated, 15% to 40% of syphilis victims will eventually suffer incapacity or death from the disease.

Congenital Syphilis. Syphilis can spread to infect a developing fetus if a pregnant woman has syphilis at the time she conceives or if she acquires syphilis during pregnancy. Infection during pregnancy commonly causes miscarriage, stillbirth, and many different kinds of severe birth defects.

DIAGNOSIS

A man I had dated a few times called me and said he had syphilis, and I nearly died! I went to the health department, and their tests showed I had gonorrhea, not syphilis. I never thought I'd be *relieved* to find out I had gonorrhea!

—WOMAN, 22

Your clinician will look first for a chancre, rash, or flat, moist genital sore, the outward signs of primary and secondary syphilis. If you have a chancre or secondary syphilis sores, it may be possible to identify the syphilis organism in a drop of secretions examined by dark-field microscopy. Syphilis is usually confirmed by testing your blood to determine whether you have syphilis antibodies, which appear about six to seven weeks after the disease begins. If you suspect you may have been exposed to syphilis and your first blood test is normal, have the test repeated about six weeks later.

It is not uncommon for a syphilis blood test to be positive even though the person does **not** have syphilis. False-positive test results occur most commonly during pregnancy, during a temporary illness with fever caused by some other problem, or after a recent immunization. People suffering from lupus erythematosus or thyroid disease and narcotic addicts may also have falsely positive syphilis blood test results. An initial positive blood test result, therefore, should be followed up with additional, more specific tests to be certain that syphilis is really present.

TREATMENT

The high-dose penicillin or ampicillin treatment given for gonorrhea will destroy early incubating syphilis within ten days of exposure but will not destroy syphilis that has progressed to the chancre stage or beyond. Longer-acting penicillin or tetracycline preparations are used for the treatment of primary, secondary, or tertiary syphilis.

Treatment recommended by the Centers for Disease Control for early syphilis (less than one year duration) is benzathine penicillin G, 2.4 million units in one injection (13). For a person allergic to penicillin, tetracycline, 500 mg taken four times a day **very faithfully** for 15 days, is recommended. The effectiveness of tetracycline and other alternative treatments such as erythromycin is not entirely established, so follow-up tests ordered by your clinician to be sure of a cure are especially important.

If syphilis has been present for one year or more, if its duration is uncertain, or if signs of brain infection or late syphilis are present, then more prolonged, intensive treatment will be needed. A spinal tap to check for syphilis in the brain and spinal fluid is also recommended to be sure that a brain infection is not overlooked.

For all stages of syphilis, **you and your partner(s) must be treated at the same time**. Avoid intercourse and all sexual intimacy for at least a month and until repeat tests prove that you and your partner are cured. In some cases syphilis blood tests may remain positive for one to three years or longer even when you have been completely cured, but conscientious follow-up is essential. You need to be absolutely certain that the syphilis is gone and you are no longer infectious.

PROGNOSIS

Syphilis can be cured with antibiotics. Reinfection is possible if your partner is not treated at the same time you are. If you are cured in the primary or secondary stage, permanent damage will be prevented.

A blood test for syphilis is essential during the first four months of pregnancy whether you think you have been exposed or not. Syphilis can seriously harm or even kill a developing fetus, but can be treated and cured during pregnancy. Read Chapter 22, "Basic Facts About Reproductive Tract Infection," for tips on preventing infection in the future.

PREVENTION

Syphilis is one of the very good reasons to take sexually transmitted disease risks seriously. Its prevention requires the same precautions as any other sexually transmitted infection. Detailed recommendations for reducing your own personal STD risk are discussed in Chapter 22.

SUGGESTED READING

DeVita, Vincent T.; Hellman, S.; and Rosenberg, S.A. (editors): *AIDS: Etiology, Diagnosis, Treatment, and Prevention.* This 1985 book (384 pages, illustrated) is quite technical but includes recent research findings and current references. It can be ordered ($38 plus tax) from J.B. Lippincott Co., P.O. Box 1630, Hagerstown, Maryland 21741.

Gong, Victor (editor): *Understanding AIDS: A Comprehensive Guide.* New Brunswick, New Jersey: Rutgers University Press, 1985. 228 pages. A clear, understandable and reasonably priced ($9.95 in paperback) introduction to AIDS issues.

Mandel, Bea, and Mandel, Byron: *Play Safe: How to Avoid Getting Sexually Transmitted Diseases.* This book explains, in easy-to-understand terminology, what STDs are, how they are and are not transmitted, how to prevent them, and what to do if you get one. To order a copy ($4.95) write to: Center for Health Information, P.O. Box 4636, Foster City, California 94404. 415-345-6669.

Mayer, Ken, and Pizer, Hank: *The AIDS Fact Book.* New York: Bantam Books, 1983. This 135-page book is written primarily for the gay community, but is broad enough for the general public.

Ulene, Art: *Safe Sex in a Dangerous World: Understanding and Coping with the Threat of AIDS.* New York: Random House, 1987. The essential, clear, inexpensive ($3.95) guide for all sexually active people in the AIDS era.

RESOURCES

For further information about AIDS, hepatitis, and syphilis, and the location of local sites for AIDS testing, call your city, county, or state health department.

Specialized medical services as well as support groups for AIDS patients and their friends and families are organized in many cities. Your local health department, county medical society, or local AIDS foundation may be able to put you in touch with local services.

The U.S. Public Health Service has established a toll-free AIDS hotline for telephone information: 1-800-342-AIDS (in Atlanta call 329-1290). This number gives you a four-minute taped message of up-to-date AIDS information, followed by another toll-free number to call for more information from a nontaped human being.

Written materials developed by the Public Health Service are also available, free of charge, from AIDS, Suite 700, 1555 Wilson Boulevard, Rosslyn, Virginia 22209, and AIDS, P.O. Box 14252, Washington, D.C. 20044, and Office of Public Inquires, Centers for Disease Control, Building 1, Room B-63, 1600 Clifton Road, Atlanta, Georgia 30333.

REFERENCES

1. Holmes KK, Mardh P-A, Sparling PF, et al: *Sexually Transmitted Diseases.* New York: McGraw-Hill, 1984.
2. Curran JW, Morgan WM, Hardy AM, et al: The epidemiology of AIDS: Current status and future prospects. *Science* 229:1352–1357, 1985.
3. Vogt MW, Craven DE, Crawford DF, et al: Isolation of HTLV-III/LAV from cervical secretions of women at risk for AIDS. *Lancet* 1:525–527, 1986.
4. Wofsy CB, Hauer LB, Michaelis BA, et al: Isolation of AIDS-associated retrovirus from genital secretions of women with antibodies to the virus. *Lancet* 1:527–529, 1986.
5. Food and Drug Administration: Progress on AIDS. *FDA Drug Bulletin* 15:27–32, 1985.
6. Chaisson RE, Moss AR, Onishi R, et al: Human immunodeficiency virus infection in heterosexual intravenous drug users in San Francisco. *American Journal of Public Health* 77:169–172, 1987.
7. Positive HTLV-III/LAV antibody results for sexually active female members of social/sexual clubs—Minnesota. *Morbidity and Mortality Weekly Report* 35:697–699, 1986.
8. Francis DP, Chin J: The prevention of acquired immunodeficiency syndrome in the United States. *Journal of the American Medical Association* 257:1357–1366, 1987.
9. Mann J, Quinn TC, Piot P, et al: Condom use and HIV infection among prostitutes in Zaire. *New England Journal of Medicine* 316:345, 1987.
10. Centers for Disease Control: Antibody to human immunodeficiency virus in female prostitutes. *Morbidity and Mortality Weekly Report* 36:157–161, 1987.
11. Centers for Disease Control: Update on Hepatitis B prevention. *Morbidity and Mortality Weekly Report* 36:353–360, 1987.
12. Centers for Disease Control: Increases in primary and secondary syphilis—United States. *Morbidity and Mortality Weekly Report* 36:393–396, 1987.
13. Centers for Disease Control: 1985 STD treatment guidelines. *Morbidity and Mortality Weekly Report, Supplement* Vol 34, No 4S, 1985.

Pubic Lice, Molluscum Contagiosum, Mycoplasma, and Others

This chapter describes some character actors, mystery walk-ons, and bit players in the STD story. Some, like pubic lice, we have understood for centuries and some, like mycoplasma, we don't understand today. You'll develop an appreciation for the great breadth and scope of sexual infection.

Pubic Lice
(Crabs, Phthirus pubis, Pediculosis Pubis)

Pubic lice are parasites, small bloodsucking insects much like head lice, except that they tend to inhabit the pubic area rather than the scalp. (Very hairy people may find that pubic lice spread to chest hair, underarms, and the scalp on occasion.) They are commonly transmitted by sexual intimacy, but you may also be infested by sharing clothing or a bed with an infested person. Pubic lice are slightly more common among women than men.

SYMPTOMS

Lice cause mild to intense itching in pubic hair areas. You may be able to see tiny lice (see Illustration 29-1) moving about, or feel egg cases as small bumps along the length of a pubic hair. Scratching can cause irritation of the external urinary opening (urethritis) or even lead to bladder infection (see Chapter 38).

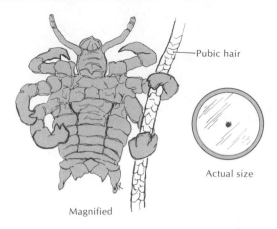

Pubic hair

Actual size

Magnified

ILLUSTRATION 29-1   The crab louse, or *"papillon d'amour"* (butterfly of love), as the French say.

DIAGNOSIS

Your clinician will inspect your pubic hair carefully for lice and/or egg cases called nits. (Now you know what nit-picking really means!) If you have found and removed lice yourself, you might put them in an envelope and show them to your clinician to confirm the diagnosis.

TREATMENT

A prescription cream, lotion, or shampoo called Kwell kills pubic lice. Kwell is a 1% solution of the potent pesticide lindane, and it **should not be used by pregnant women or children less than 10 years old.** Several nonprescription products (such as Rid, A-200 Pyrinate, or Triple X) are also available and are often effective treatments for pubic lice. **Your sexual partner(s) must be treated when you are.**

Kwell Cream or Lotion.   Bathe or shower thoroughly, dry yourself completely, and apply cream or lotion to all affected areas. Wash the cream or lotion off thoroughly after eight hours and put on freshly laundered clothes. Repeat in seven days if living lice are still visible.

Kwell Shampoo.   Shampoo all affected areas thoroughly for four minutes, then rinse completely. Comb your pubic hair with a fine-toothed comb to remove egg cases. Repeat in seven days if living lice are still visible.

All Treatments.   Change clothes and bedding at the time you treat yourself and wash them in hot water. Wash combs and brushes in Kwell shampoo. Pubic lice can live about 24 hours once they leave the body, and egg cases can survive six days. All articles are safe to use after that time.

Don't exceed the amount and duration of medication indicated in your instructions because pesticide overdose can be quite toxic. Also, do not use lice medication on your eyelashes (1). Your clinician can provide ophthalmic ointment if treatment is needed.

PROGNOSIS

Pubic lice are easy to cure although itching may persist for a while even after all lice are killed. Reinfestation is unlikely if all infested people are treated at the same time. Lice are not a serious health risk except in certain countries where lice carry disease. Pubic lice do not carry disease in the United States.

Scabies (Sarcoptes scabiei, Mites)

Scabies are tiny mites that burrow under the skin, where the female lays her eggs. They are usually transmitted by sexual intimacy, but you may also be infested by body contact or sharing clothing or a bed with an infested person. It is not uncommon for scabies to affect an entire household.

SYMPTOMS

Small bumps on your wrists or fingers (or on your partner's penis) and itching that seems worse at night are the major symptoms. Scratching can cause raw skin and bacterial infections. People who are especially sensitive to scabies may develop reddish brown nodules a month or more after infestation begins.

DIAGNOSIS

Your clinician will probably diagnose scabies simply by examining you for characteristic sores and itching, especially if you know you have had intimate contact with someone who has scabies. She/he may scrape a sore and look at a specimen under a microscope for eggs or mites.

TREATMENT

A prescription cream or lotion called Kwell kills scabies (1). Kwell is a 1% solution of the potent pesticide lindane, and it **should not be used by pregnant women or children less than 10 years old. Your sexual partner(s) must be treated at the same time you are, as must all others, adults and children, with whom you have close body contact.**

Bathe and dry yourself thoroughly, then apply a thin coat of cream or lotion all over your body from the neck down. Wash it off completely after eight hours. One treatment usually eradicates scabies. Repeat treatment in seven days if you are *certain* you still have living mites. Itching may persist for a while even after all mites are killed.

Alternate treatments include crotamiton (10%) applied each night for two nights, then washed off 24 hours after the second application, or sulfur (6%) in petrolatum applied each night for three nights. You can bathe just before each nightly application.

Change your clothes and bedding at the time you treat yourself and wash them in hot water or dry-clean them.

PROGNOSIS

Scabies are fairly easy to cure, and reinfestation is unlikely if all affected people are treated at the same time.

Molluscum Contagiosum

This illness sounds a lot worse than it is! It is a viral infection caused by *Molluscum contagiosum,* a member of the poxvirus group. In sexually active men and women the illness is usually spread by sexual contact, and in children transmission is usually by simple skin contact (2).

SYMPTOMS

The classic molluscum presentation is a cluster of round, 1/4-inch, smooth, shiny, flesh-colored or white bumps with a little dimple in the middle (see Illustration 29-2). The bumps are usually painless but occasionally feel itchy or tender. Adults usually have bumps on their genital skin, thighs, and abdomen, while children are usually affected on their arms, legs, and trunk.

DIAGNOSIS

Examination alone is usually adequate to diagnose molluscum. Your clinician may want to examine a specimen of tissue or fluid from a bump under a microscope and look for typical "molluscum bodies" inside cells. Your diagnosis will include testing for other STDs.

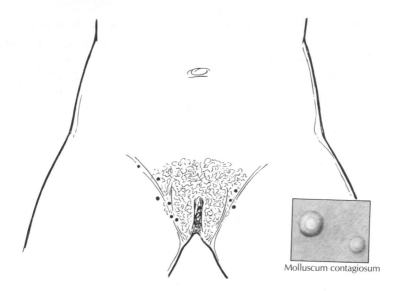

Molluscum contagiosum

ILLUSTRATION 29-2   Molluscum contagiosum causes small painless bumps that are likely to be mistaken for pimples when they first appear. Each bump contains a small white kernel. The bumps appear dark in this illustration for clarity; on real human skin the bumps are the same color as skin or even a little lighter.

TREATMENT

You are more likely to want treatment because of the way molluscum looks than because of any bothersome symptoms. Your sexual partner(s) needs to be treated when you are to avoid reinfection. Scraping with local anesthesia, freezing with liquid nitrogen, or application of caustics such as silver nitrate or podophyllin will eradicate the bumps. They will go away on their own, usually without scarring, in 6 to 36 months, but treatment will help prevent spread on your own body or to another person.

PROGNOSIS

Molluscum is a benign, if bothersome, infection that poses no serious health risks and resolves completely with or without treatment. Reinfection is possible if all infected people are not treated at the same time.

Mycoplasma

The mycoplasmas are the smallest free-living organisms, somewhere between viruses and bacteria in size. They are ubiquitous and associated with a wide variety of mild to severe illnesses. Quite often mycoplasmas can be found in people who have no signs of illness whatever. In adults, most cases of illness are thought to be sexually transmitted. Women may be more vulnerable to infection than men.

Genital mycoplasmas, particularly *Mycoplasma hominis* and *Ureaplasma urealyticum*, are poorly understood at present, and are the focus of active current research. These organisms can be found in the reproductive tracts of roughly half all sexually active men and women (3).

SYMPTOMS

Mycoplasmas are implicated in a wide range of illnesses, but in no case is their role clear. They may be involved in nongonococcal urethritis and prostatitis in men. In women they have been associated with:

• Vaginitis
• Pelvic inflammatory disease
• Fever following abortion
• Fever following delivery
• Spontaneous abortion
• Low birth weight infants
• Infertility
• Kidney infection
• Ectopic pregnancy

DIAGNOSIS

Mycoplasma infection is diagnosed on the basis of a laboratory culture of samples of fluid from the vagina or other sites. *Ureaplasma urealyticum* results are available in one to two days and *Mycoplasma hominis* in about seven days (3). Your diagnosis will include tests for other sexually transmitted infections.

TREATMENT

Mycoplasmas respond to oral antibiotics such as tetracycline and doxycycline. (See Chapter 22 for advice on using these drugs safely and effectively.) Your sexual partner(s) should probably be treated when you are.

PROGNOSIS

An understanding of your risks in the face of mycoplasma infection may have to await the results of more research. It is difficult to clarify the role of an organism that is everywhere and that sometimes causes illness and sometimes doesn't. Certainly the issues of infertility, abortion, and fetal and infant illness are crucial. For now, your clinician will suspect mycoplasma when reproductive tract infection presents itself, and will eradicate mycoplasma when she/he finds it.

Other Infections

This book covers only the reproductive tract infections that commonly occur in the United States. There are a number of other sexually transmitted diseases that are rarely seen here but are fairly common in other parts of the world. You might suspect these infections if you have a sexual partner who has recently returned from another country, or if you have been traveling—and romancing—yourself. Be sure to mention this to your clinician; otherwise she/he may have trouble diagnosing your illness.

Just so you will have an idea of the range of other illnesses that can be transmitted through varying forms of sexual contact, and in varying latitudes, consider this (exotic) list.

- Cytomegalovirus infection
- Group B streptococcus infection
- Shigellosis
- Salmonellosis
- Amebiasis
- Giardiasis
- Donovanosis (granuloma inguinale)
- Chancroid
- Lymphogranuloma venereum

This would probably be a good time to go back to Chapter 22 and read the section on how to prevent STDs.

REFERENCES

1. Centers for Disease Control: Sexually transmitted diseases treatment guidelines, 1985. *Morbidity and Mortality Weekly Report, Supplement* Vol 34, No 4S, October 18, 1985.
2. Margolis S: Genital warts and molluscum contagiosum. *Urologic Clinics of North America* 11:163–170, 1984.
3. Holmes KK, Mardh P-A, Sparling PF, et al: *Sexually Transmitted Diseases.* New York: McGraw-Hill, 1984.

30

❖

Premenstrual Syndrome (PMS)

"It's a prostaglandin problem."
"It's a mental illness."
"It's a progesterone deficiency."
"It's the feminist issue of the 80s."
"It's a vitamin deficiency."
"It's just part of being a woman."
"It's an endorphin deficiency."

There are passionate advocates for each of these positions. Perhaps none of these statements is true. Perhaps they all are, in one way or another.

Rigorous scientific study of premenstrual syndrome (PMS) is in its infancy, and it will be several years before the results of large-scale, careful clinical studies are reported. Today we have only partial answers about what causes PMS, and what makes it better. For many thoughtful women and their clinicians, PMS is a clear reminder that our bodies and souls are great mysteries to this day.

PMS: A Provisional Description

There is good consensus that premenstrual syndrome is a real phenomenon. Women with PMS experience recurring physical and/or emotional problems in the luteal (postovulatory) phase of their menstrual cycles. Symptoms are most likely to recur in the seven to ten days just before the menstrual period begins. This definition implies

TABLE 30-1
SYMPTOMS OF PREMENSTRUAL SYNDROME

EMOTIONAL SYMPTOMS

Anxiety	Feeling withdrawn
Depression	Irritability
Tension	Mood swings
Crying spells	Difficulty concentrating

PHYSICAL SYMPTOMS

Acne	Backache
Constipation	Menstrual-like cramps
Food cravings	Upset stomach
Headache	Fatigue and lethargy
Weight gain	Muscle spasms
Clumsiness	Insomnia
Itching	Cyclic asthma
Abdominal bloating and heaviness	Breast swelling and tenderness
Fluid retention; swollen ankles or fingers	Increased or decreased appetite or thirst

two corollaries: One, a woman can have PMS **only if she ovulates,** so technically the syndrome cannot occur among birth control Pill users, prepubescent women, pregnant women, postmenopausal women, and others who don't ovulate. Two, there must be at least some days, perhaps 7 to 12 or so in each cycle, when symptoms are absent or only minimally noticeable. Birth control Pill users and other women who do not ovulate do sometimes experience symptoms similar to PMS that merit evaluation and treatment, but most clinicians would not term these problems PMS.

It is not the nature of the symptoms but their **cyclicity** that determines the diagnosis of PMS.

SYMPTOMS OF PMS

Psychic and somatic manifestations of PMS are legion. Emotional symptoms are somewhat more common than physical symptoms. Commonly reported problems are listed in Table 30-1.

Without question, other types of cyclic problems could be added to these lists. Some researchers believe PMS symptoms can be grouped into clusters of problems that tend to appear together, but others feel this theory is not logical because many women experience problems in several of the clusters.

Symptoms can be mild, moderate, or severe enough to be truly incapacitating. Studies have shown that women's suicide attempts, psychiatric hospital admissions, and violent criminal acts are most likely to occur in the premenstrual days.

It is next to impossible to determine how many women have PMS. Perhaps 20% to 40% of women feel that PMS significantly interferes with daily living. In one 1985 study 20% of women reported that they had sought help from a physician for PMS problems (1).

Severe Symptoms.   If PMS symptoms are so bad that you feel you are losing control—in danger of hurting yourself or your children, destroying your job, or thinking of suicide—**don't get stuck on the PMS part. Get help.** These are serious warning signs and you need urgent treatment. Although your symptoms may indeed be cyclic, it is important to face the underlying problems.

Severe PMS can be a warning that you need to spend time, energy, and effort on restoring emotional well-being, and you will probably need more help than the vitamins, minerals, or other medications discussed in this chapter. Symptoms originating from serious psychiatric problems such as depression or panic attacks are often most severe during the premenstrual phase each month. Treating just the PMS part, however, is not enough (2). It makes sense to begin with a psychotherapist you can trust.

Causes of PMS

I get kind of silent and withdrawn; not really sad, but it's hard for me to be around people. I feel bloated, like somebody slipped in and cinched up all my waistbands, and my breasts get sore. I'd kill for chocolate, and I cry watching television. Sometimes I have clean-up attacks and work for hours alphabetizing the spice rack and cleaning out closets. It's hard to imagine that all that strangeness could have one cause!

—WOMAN, 40

The cause—or causes—of premenstrual syndrome are not clearly understood. There are investigators who are convinced PMS has one cause, and there are investigators just as convinced that PMS is a collection of ailments, each with its own cause and its own therapy. At least four different PMS theories merit mention because each has its stalwart advocates.

PROGESTERONE DEFICIENCY

Dalton has long held that in her own clinical experience supplementing natural progesterone in vaginal or rectal suppository form during the luteal phase dramatically helps PMS sufferers (3). Progesterone has a calming effect on the central nervous system and also helps the kidneys excrete salt, which may help with fluid retention symptoms. Other researchers have found contradictory results. Six placebo-controlled studies of natural progesterone treatment have been reported, and five out of six found no difference between progesterone and placebo (4,5).

VITAMIN DEFICIENCY

Abraham, developer of Optivite brand vitamin/mineral supplements, hypothesizes that low levels of vitamin B_6 (pyridoxine) and magnesium contribute to premenstrual problems. This researcher noted improvement in women who took 200 to 800 mg of B_6 daily (6). Vitamin B_6 plays a crucial role in the synthesis of dopamine, a key chemical in both physical and emotional well-being. Other researchers have reported disappointing results with B_6 (6). **Do not overdose on B_6.** Toxicity has been reported at a level of 500 mg per day.

PROSTAGLANDIN EXCESS

Budoff has studied the effect of antiprostaglandin drugs on PMS (7), and there is some research evidence that prostaglandin hormones may play a role in causing PMS symptoms (8). Prostaglandins stimulate muscle contraction in the uterus and elsewhere, and antiprostaglandin drugs inhibit this effect. A wide range of problems including cramps, headache, and backache improved. Although antiprostaglandins are primarily used for relief of menstrual cramps, there may be a role for them in PMS treatment, at least for some women. Antiprostaglandin drugs such as ibuprofen (Advil, Nuprin, Motrin) are discussed in detail in Chapter 31.

ENDORPHIN DEFICIENCY

Some researchers and PMS activists describe PMS as a neuroendocrine disorder originating in the brain and pituitary gland. The theory is that levels of endorphins, opium-like chemicals manufactured by the brain, fluctuate during the luteal phase of the cycle in response to ovarian hormone activity. Sudden decreases in endorphin levels may cause tension, anxiety, and irritability. Changing levels of endorphins may also stimulate the release of prolactin from the pituitary gland and cause breast pain or tenderness, and endorphins may also alter the body's ability to excrete fluids (9). If there is one theory with any promise of accounting for most or all of the symptoms associated with PMS, it may be hormone-mediated changes in endorphin levels, and low endorphin levels have been documented for PMS patients compared to women without PMS symptoms in one 1985 study (10). Future research will provide a clearer answer.

OTHER THEORIES

Other hypotheses for the cause of PMS have been investigated, including allergy to progesterone or other hormones, fluid retention, psychological factors, sleep disorder, and hypoglycemia. No doubt other causes will be postulated and studied in the future.

CONCLUSION

There are overwhelming difficulties in interpreting the data we have so far on PMS. We know, for example, that human beings are often inaccurate when they are asked to recall problems they experienced in the past, and many PMS studies have relied on such retrospective reporting of symptoms. We know also that women in this culture have been conditioned—subtly or overtly—to experience premenstrual and menstrual problems.

Another complicating factor is that researchers themselves can bias their study outcomes unless very strict scientific protocols are followed; much PMS work in the past has lacked rigorous attention to such protocols. Also, many PMS studies have focused on atypical groups of women such as prison inmates or patients in special gynecologic clinics. Results of studies in such populations may not have any particular relevance for women in general.

Finally there is the placebo effect to consider. A placebo is an inert pill (or ointment or injection) used in scientific studies for comparison with a real drug under investigation. In many medical studies the comparison of outcomes between real drugs and placebos is the basis for the conclusions of the research.

Norman Cousins has called the placebo "the doctor who resides within." **Many people do get better on placebos.** Perhaps they feel better simply because by taking the "drug" they are making a concrete effort to get better: perhaps because they truly believe the "drug" will make them get better, and perhaps because they respond positively to the kind and caring intervention of the person providing the therapy. The positive response to placebos is a **real** response and not one to be devalued, so it is often difficult to evaluate how much good the "real" drug under study is doing. Researchers try to override the confounding nature of the placebo response by having placebo subjects and drug subjects "cross over" in the middle of the study: that is, placebo subjects begin taking the drug, and drug subjects begin taking the placebo. Many PMS studies in the past have failed to include placebo and cross over protocols, so study results are hard to interpret. Fortunately, good, rigorous PMS studies are now under way.

CYCLE DAY	DATE	BASAL BODY TEMPERATURE (Measure in morning first thing before you get out of bed. Circle daily temperature. Connect the daily circles.)	DAILY WEIGHT	Bleed (X)	No Discharge (X)	Discharge (X)	Describe discharge when present	INTERCOURSE (X)	breasts sore	depressed	salty food	bloated	Additional Comments
1	9/10		117	X									Advil for cramps
2	9/11		117	X									
3	9/12		116	X									
4	9/13		117	X									
5	9/14		116		X			X					3 drinks at party
6	9/15		117		X			X					
7	9/16		117		X								
8	9/17		118		X								
9	9/18		117			X	thick						
10	9/19		117			X	thick	XX					
11	9/20		117			X	clear						
12	9/21		118			X	clear, lots						
13	9/22		117			X	clear	X					
14	9/23		117		X								
15	9/24		117		X								
16	9/25		118		X								
17	9/26		118		X								
18	9/27		119		X			X	X		X		pretzels!
19	9/28		119		X			X	X				
20	9/29		120		X			X					
21	9/30		120						X	X			withdrawn
22	10/1		118						X	X	X		
23	10/2		118							X			
24	10/3		117										
25	10/4		118										
26	10/5		117					X					
27	10/6		117			X	thick						
28	/												
29	/												
30	/												
31	/												
32	/												
33	/												
34	/												
35	/												

Calendar Calculations

Shortest cycle in last 8: _____ days. First fertile day in this cycle is cycle day _____.
Longest cycle in last 8: _____ days. Last fertile day in this cycle is cycle day _____.
Cycle length for this cycle _____ days. (Complete at end of cycle.)

Name _____

Month _____

Year _____

ILLUSTRATION 30-1   Weight gain, breast tenderness, and depression show clear cyclic patterns. The patterns of craving for salty food and a bloated feeling are less clear, but still possibly cyclic.

For the present, the authors of this book must conclude that we don't know what causes PMS. In the absence of a demonstrable unifying theory we can only assume that PMS is a **group of problems**; some we know how to treat, and some we do not. If there is a magic bullet, nobody has found it yet.

Do-It-Yourself PMS Care

If you are genuinely, miserably suffering and you think you have PMS, see your clinician without delay. However, if you feel basically well, you may first want to try some steps on your own for relief.

CHARTING

The first step is to begin immediately to **record your symptoms**. You will need at least two or three months of day-to-day charting to learn whether your symptoms, whatever their nature, are indeed cyclic. You will need a chart similar to the sample in Illustration 30-1 so that you can record your cycle day, date, basal body temperature, vaginal discharge patterns, weight, and your PMS symptoms each and every day. Look for cyclic patterns: Do you have symptoms that recur in most cycles? Do symptoms appear after ovulation? Do you have a week or more of symptom-free days early in your cycle? (See Chapter 6 for instructions on recording your cyclic body changes.)

You might consider keeping a daily chart record of what you eat and drink as well, at least for one or two cycles. You'll be able to watch for **cyclic** changes in appetite or thirst, and for fluctuations in your patterns of eating sweets, salty food, and the like. A food log will be a better diagnostic tool for you if you can avoid "being extra good" about what you eat and drink, and simply eat and drink as you normally would.

VITAMINS AND NONPRESCRIPTION DRUGS

Vitamin B_6 (pyridoxine) helps the body synthesize catecholamines (chemicals that regulate the transmission of nerve impulses), and may be helpful if you have postovulatory anxiety or depression. A dose of 25 to 50 mg twice a day may be beneficial but be careful to avoid excessive doses. A 1983 U.S. Food and Drug Administration panel on over-the-counter drugs concluded that B_6 was safe in normal doses but that data were insufficient to determine its effectiveness in treating PMS (11). Many clinicians, however, feel that B_6 does help some women. Even though B_6 is a water-soluble vitamin, excessive doses may be toxic. Serious neurologic (nerve) problems have been reported. Most problems reported occurred after use of 2,000 mg per day or more, but in one case the dose was only 500 mg (12).

Vitamin E (alpha-tocopherol), 400 IU (International Units) twice a day, has been helpful for some women who have premenstrual breast tenderness. Vitamin E may alter certain hormones and lipids, but the mechanism by which it helps breast tenderness is not understood.

There are special premenstrual vitamin and mineral supplements available in drugstores. You may want to compare prices and determine whether special PMS preparations or individual vitamins and minerals will be your best buy.

While you are shopping (or watching TV for that matter), you will no doubt notice that many over-the-counter medications are available for relief of menstrual symptoms. The Food and Drug Administration advisory panel reviewed all nonprescription premenstrual and menstrual medications in 1983 (11), and ranked active ingredients for effectiveness and safety. Table 30-2 lists the active ingredients the panel approved. You will find that most over-the-counter products have two or three ingredients. The FDA panel found these combinations safe and effective:

TABLE 30-2
OVER-THE-COUNTER
PREMENSTRUAL AND MENSTRUAL MEDICATIONS:
ACTIVE INGREDIENTS APPROVED FOR
SAFETY AND EFFECTIVENESS

PAIN (CRAMPS, HEADACHE)

Aspirin and other salicylates (analgesic)
Acetaminophen (analgesic)
Caffeine (analgesic properties when used in combination with another
  pain reliever)

FLUID RETENTION AND BLOATING

Ammonium chloride[a] (diuretic)
Caffeine (diuretic properties)
Pamabrom (diuretic)
Pyrilamine maleate (antihistamine—effective diuretic when used in
  combination)

FATIGUE

Caffeine (stimulant)

MOOD CHANGES

Pyrilamine maleate (antihistamine—effective when used in combination)

---

[a]Avoid ammonium chloride if you have impaired liver or kidney function; also, effectiveness
diminishes after four to five days.

SOURCE: Adapted from Willis J: Doing something about menstrual discomforts. *FDA Consumer,*
June 1983.

• Analgesic and diuretic
• Analgesic, antihistamine, and diuretic
• Antihistamine and diuretic
• Any two diuretics with varying actions, such as ammonium chloride and caffeine

These products are designed to counteract specific symptoms, not PMS as a whole, and
the FDA effectiveness judgment applies only to the specific symptom(s) listed by the
drug company in its application to the FDA. Analgesics such as aspirin or acetaminophen (Tylenol and others) are likely to be helpful in relieving pain of any kind,
including pain of headache, backache, menstrual cramps, or breast tenderness associ-

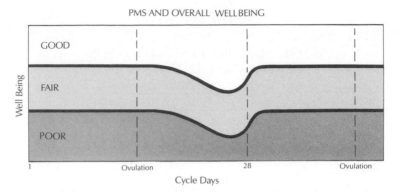

PMS AND OVERALL WELLBEING

ILLUSTRATION 30-2   A dip in well-being is less debilitating if overall well-being is high to begin with.

ated with PMS. If menstrual-like cramps are a significant factor in your PMS symptoms, you may also want to consider newer over-the-counter or prescription drugs such as ibuprofen (Advil, Nuprin, Motrin). Ibuprofen provides a good analgesic effect and is particularly helpful for uterine cramping. These options are discussed in detail in Chapter 31.

Diuretics contained in over-the-counter products are less potent than the prescription diuretics discussed later in this chapter. For this reason they are probably safer than prescription alternatives, but also less effective. Safer still, and probably more effective, is careful attention to diet. Mild nonprescription diuretics cannot compensate for excessive salt intake, and getting control of salt is likely to solve the problem without drugs.

You should avoid caffeine-containing drugs if you are having PMS problems. Caffeine does have a mild diuretic effect, and is approved as an antidote to fatigue, but it also has other central nervous system effects that may aggravate PMS symptoms (see the section titled "Eliminating Toxins" later in this chapter).

Antihistamines are commonly used for treating allergies, but they also have some effects on mood as well (a calm or even drowsy reaction). They do not specifically counteract PMS mood problems, so you may not find them helpful.

OVERALL WELL-BEING

If you are feeling physically and emotionally well to begin with, a premenstrual dip in your well-being will be less troublesome (see Illustration 30-2). Most people would agree with this simple principle, but putting it into action takes some real effort.

Why is it so hard to take good care of yourself? I know what I do: I talk about it a lot more than I do it! I treat my body like it's invincible!

TABLE 30-3
DAILY INTAKE RECOMMENDATIONS

PROTEIN

Fish, poultry
Whole grains
Legumes
Limit dairy products to two servings daily
Limit red meat to less than 3 ounces daily

FATS

Limit to polyunsaturated vegetable oils

VITAMINS

Increase green leafy vegetables

CARBOHYDRATES

Whole grains
Legumes
Seeds and nuts
Limit refined sugar to 5 tsp daily
Eliminate chocolate, candy, cake, pastry, ice cream

I spent three weeks in Houston recently at a training course for work, and by the end of the course I felt fantastic! When I stopped to figure out why, it was simple. I ate well, exercised every day, slept enough, didn't drink much, and cut way back on smoking since we didn't smoke in class all day. I was learning job skills I would use, and the trainers were fun and thoughtful. I was away from home, so I didn't have all those maddening little chores that eat up leisure time. I felt just wonderful.

The question is, can I keep it up at home? Will I even be able to remember how good I felt?

—WOMAN, 34

It is hard to take good care of yourself. Most people find it takes weeks or even months of constant vigilance before new, healthier patterns become second nature. Feeling strong and peaceful is the extraordinary payoff.

Diet. A daily diet oriented to well-being and PMS control is low in salt, refined sugar, and fat, high in complex carbohydrates (about 65% of your total intake), and moderate in protein (no more than 20% of your total intake). See Table 30-3 for more detailed dietary recommendations.

Many women find that eating five or six small meals a day helps them stay on a more even metabolic keel. **Keeping your blood sugar level fairly steady throughout the day is an important PMS goal.** Low blood sugar (hypoglycemia) can cause many symptoms familiar to PMS sufferers: irritability, fatigue, and depression especially. You might not even be aware that what you really need is something to eat. Fasting can cause hypoglycemia, so skipping meals is a very poor idea if you have PMS. **The most important low blood sugar trigger, though, is eating refined sugar.**

When you eat sugar (a chocolate chip cookie, for example), it is rapidly absorbed and enters your bloodstream within just a few minutes. So initially you will experience a sudden rise in blood sugar. Within a few more minutes, however, your body responds to the sugar rise by releasing insulin; insulin's job is to reduce the level of sugar in your blood by sending the sugar into body cells (especially fat cells). As a consequence, your blood sugar level drops rapidly, and quite profoundly, about 20 minutes or so after the cookie. Your final blood sugar level is likely to be lower than the level you started with, and you may experience hypoglycemia symptoms. This insulin response explains why it is so hard to eat just one chocolate chip cookie. When blood sugar starts to fall, it is normal to want another cookie.

Cookies are not a good way to counteract hypoglycemia symptoms, however. Prevention is key. Being sure to eat healthy meals at regular intervals throughout the day is an important first step. The complex carbohydrates and protein in your healthy foods are digested and absorbed more slowly than refined sugar, so you insure that a steady, gradual supply of nutrients (including sugar) is entering your bloodstream. The second step in preventing hypoglycemia is to avoid dosing yourself with refined sugar. You know the culprits: cookies, ice cream, candy, and their relatives. Remember to count soft drinks too, and fruit juices, especially if they are artificially sweetened.

Decreasing salt (sodium) intake will help control premenstrual fluid retention. As a rule, watching your salt means keeping your sodium intake to less than 2,000 mg a day. Sodium that occurs naturally in meat, dairy products, vegetables, and fruit provides all you will normally need.

If you are like most Americans, your sodium intake is about 4,000 to 6,000 mg a day, so it may take some real effort to bring your consumption down to a healthier level. (Just one teaspoon of salt contains 2,000 mg!) Give yourself a few weeks to make a gradual adjustment to low-salt living. The basic principles of low-salt nutrition are:

- Eliminate table salt
- Don't add salt in cooking
- Drink plenty of water (to help your kidneys excrete salt)
- Eat fresh rather than processed food

TABLE 30-4
HIDDEN SOURCES OF SODIUM

FRESH FOODS COMPARED TO PROCESSED FOOD ALTERNATIVES

	Milligrams of Sodium	
	Fresh	*Processed*
Corn, 1 cup	1	390 (canned)
Flounder, broiled with butter, 4 1/2 oz	285	810 (frozen)
Oatmeal, 3/4 cup	1	280 (instant)
Rice, 1/2 cup	1	570 (minute variety)
Beef stew, 1 cup	290	1,220 (canned)

COMMON PRODUCTS THAT ARE HIGH IN SODIUM

Baking powder	Garlic salt
Baking soda	Onion salt
Soy sauce	Celery salt
Tamari sauce	MSG (monosodium glutamate)
Worcestershire sauce	Many nonprescription antacids
Catsup	Saccharin
Pickles	Quick baking mix
Olives	Instant pudding
Cocoa mix	Meats, canned or salted
Cottage cheese	[b]Smoked herring
Feta cheese	[a]Canned shrimp
Blue cheese	[a]Chipped, dried beef
Parmesan cheese	[a]Ham
Roquefort cheese	Wieners
American pasteurized processed cheese	[a]Canned chili
[a]Sauerkraut, canned	[a]Frozen meat loaf dinner
Pancake mix	[a]Frozen turkey dinner
Stuffing mix	[b]Fast food chicken dinner
[a]Soups, canned or dehydrated	[a]Bacon
[a]Tomato sauce	Meat tenderizer

[a] = more than 1,000 mg sodium/serving
[b] = more than 2,000 mg sodium/serving

SOURCES: U.S. Department of Agriculture: *The Sodium Content of Your Food.* Washington, D.C.: U.S. Government Printing Office, 1980.
The Intelligent Person's Guide to Calories and Sodium. New York: The Jeffrey Weiss Group, not dated.
Jacobson M, Liebman BF, Moyer G: *Salt: The Brand Name Guide to Sodium.* New York: Workman Publishing, 1983.

• Become a label reader
• Change your ordering patterns in restaurants

Read food product labels for salt or sodium content. If salt content is given rather than sodium, simply multiply the salt milligram figure by 0.4 to get a sodium equivalent. Generally, if one serving of a product contains more than 150 mg or so of sodium, consider trying something else to eat. Not all food products quantify sodium content. Remember that processed food ingredients are listed in order of quantity, so if salt or sodium appears in the first half dozen ingredients, the product is probably too salty for you. Many preservatives and food additives used in processed foods also contain sodium, so watch for sodium in any form.

Canned, frozen, dehydrated, and other processed foods are likely to be astoundingly high in hidden sodium. The convenience of processed foods is more than offset by the hidden sodium for those who are trying to limit sodium intake. Table 30-4 lists a sampling of products high in hidden sodium. You may also want to check your bookstore or the Government Printing Office for an inexpensive guide to sodium content in foods.

You can control your sodium intake in restaurants by ordering pasta and meat without sauces, and by dressing salads with lemon or oil and vinegar, and by staying away from soups. If you do choose to order a dressing or meat sauce, have it served on the side and use it sparingly.

I've been off salt for three years, and now the taste of it is unbearable! Salt really overwhelms food flavor. I'm never even tempted to use it.

—WOMAN, 42

Even *The New York Times* food critic Craig Claiborne came to the conclusion that salt robs food of subtle flavor, and that other more healthful seasonings add more gustatory pleasure. As an alternative, try lemon juice or vinegar. Their sour flavor stimulates your tastebuds and decreases the need for salt.

Exercise.   Exercise stimulates the production of endorphins, the brain's own opium-like chemicals. Endorphins are a major reason you feel so good after a workout, swim, or run. Start with a program of brisk walking if you are out of shape, then choose an aerobic exercise you enjoy enough to do regularly. You want to increase your heart rate by 50% for 30 minutes, three to five times a week. Benefits include cardiovascular fitness, muscle tone, weight control or reduction, decrease in fluid retention, and increase in self-esteem. A regular exercise program may be the most reliable do-it-yourself way to control PMS symptoms.

Eliminating Toxins.   Alcohol, nicotine, caffeine, and recreational drugs are toxins. Try to eliminate all of them. A strong association between caffeine consumption and the presence and severity of PMS symptoms has been documented in one study of 295 college women. Women who drank four or more caffeine-containing beverages daily were seven times more likely to experience moderate or severe PMS symptoms compared to women who consumed no caffeine. The primary caffeine source for these women was cola beverages (13).

Alcohol tolerance may be decreased premenstrually so be especially careful to control your intake at that time. Remember that caffeine-like chemicals are in tea, soft drinks, and some kinds of chocolate as well as in coffee.

Rest.   Most people feel best with about seven hours of sleep each night, but you could need more or less. Let your body be your guide. Some women find that an earlier bedtime helps them cope more effectively during the premenstrual week.

Stress Reduction.   Meditation and yoga are excellent stress reduction techniques to incorporate into daily living. Stress reduction workshops can help you tailor a program to your individual needs. First learn to be attentive to what parts of life are stressful for you, and try to eliminate as much stress as you can, especially on premenstrual days. These are the days for a babysitter, for delegating the dishes to someone else, a massage, an evening out, starting the novel you've been eager to read, or for seeing a friend you've been missing. Be good to yourself, and ask for a little extra tenderness from the people who love you as well.

Coping with Emotions.   If you are like many women, the most troublesome aspect of PMS is the intensity of your own emotional responses during premenstrual days. You may find your own feelings of anger and frustration quite foreign and definitely uncomfortable. For most women anger is a frightening emotion even when there are sound, logical reasons for it, and when 99 out of 100 independent observers would say the anger is justified.

Another way of thinking about the PMS emotional patterns my patients describe is that women tend to be abnormally pleasant and nice three weeks out of four. They fail to experience or express normal annoyance and anger a great deal of the time, and are dismayed when these emotions surface during premenstrual days. Who wouldn't be angry about an alcoholic husband, or a dead-end job?

—GYNECOLOGIST, 40

For some women, PMS days may be an important window to a part of themselves that is rarely seen. Try to listen to your feelings and identify the aspects of your life that are causing conflict and anger. Anger itself is unpleasant and often unhelpful; it can, however, help you to find priorities for change and the strength that will be necessary to accomplish it.

If your premenstrual symptoms are more emotional than physical and if your own efforts at improving your well-being aren't making a significant difference in how you feel, perhaps a psychotherapist can help. A psychiatrist, psychologist, psychiatric social worker, or other mental health professional can often help clarify complex emotional issues when they are hard to understand and cope with on your own. Most of us have not been trained in the skills for true self-knowledge; we lack even a vocabulary for describing our deepest feelings.

Therapeutic approaches range from short-term work to change a specific behavior, to long-term insight therapy to help you uncover the very nature of your personality. Ask your friends and your clinician for names of therapists. When you are selecting a therapist, it is entirely appropriate to ask about her/his therapeutic approach, fees, insurance coverage, and other policies. Probably the best way to choose a therapist is to make an appointment for an initial visit, talk together for 45 to 50 minutes, and then decide if the therapist is someone with whom you will be able to talk freely. If the answer is no, keep looking. Psychotherapy can be helpful only when you trust your therapist and when you tell all the truth you can possibly tell.

There is no clear evidence to show which kind of psychotherapy will help with emotional PMS problems, so therapy will likely be individualized to your own specific needs. Your therapist may or may not recommend drugs to control mood, anxiety, or depression. In general, such medications are used only on a short-term basis when daily living is a true struggle. Many people in therapy begin to feel better right away because it is a relief to have a skilled advocate to talk to. However, don't be discouraged if it takes a few weeks or even months to notice improvement. It often does. If after a few months of therapy you aren't feeling better, reevaluate your feelings about therapy and talk them over with your therapist.

If you live in a good-sized town you might also check to see if there is a PMS support group in existence for women who want to learn more about PMS and compare their insights.

Seeing Your Clinician for Help with PMS

When your own PMS management efforts aren't working, your clinician may be able to help. When you go for your appointment, be sure to take along your cycle charts and food logs if you have them, and the names and dosages of any medications, over-the-counter drugs, or vitamin/mineral supplements you take.

Your clinician can help you assess whether PMS is a plausible cause for your symptoms. Illnesses such as diabetes can cause PMS-like symptoms, so your clinician will want to know about any other symptoms you may have noticed, and your family medical history, to determine whether you should be tested for diabetes. Your clinician will also try to assess whether PMS is the central problem or whether a more serious psychiatric problem is involved, with cyclic patterns of crisis. Problems like depression are very common (and serious), and are often worst for women during premenstrual days. If you are having depression, you need and deserve professional help to overcome it. PMS treatment should be a secondary concern.

There are no specific physical examination steps or laboratory tests that can confirm a diagnosis of PMS, and extensive hormone tests are not likely to be helpful in its evaluation or treatment (14). If your cycle charts show normal ovulatory cycle patterns, however, it is very likely that your hormones are functioning fine. Your clinician may be able to help you identify chart patterns if you are uncertain.

If you aren't already charting your cyclic symptoms, she/he will want you to begin charting at once. Your clinician's initial recommendations about diet, rest, exercise, and vitamin supplementation are likely to be quite similar to those in the previous section, "Do-It-Yourself PMS Care."

If these recommendations don't bring relief, or if you are already following these recommendations on your own, it may be time for other measures.

DIURETICS FOR FLUID RETENTION

If demonstrable cyclic weight gain and fluid retention are not relieved by limiting your salt intake, it may make sense to try a prescription diuretic every other day in the premenstrual weeks. Diuretics work by increasing your kidney's ability to excrete sodium and water in urine, so the amount of fluid surrounding body tissue cells will be diminished. (Your kidneys do an amazing amount of work. They filter 180 liters of fluid a day, return 99% of it to your body, and excrete 1%.)

Prescription diuretics are powerful drugs with a very real potential for causing side effects, so never use them without a clinician's supervision. Diuretics do not obviate the need for limiting salt intake; in fact, using a lot of salt while taking a prescription diuretic can lead to markedly decreased potassium levels, weakness, and lethargy.

If you are considering a course of prescription diuretics to control cyclic fluid retention, read Table 30-5 carefully. It contains specific comments about diuretics frequently used for control of PMS symptoms. Also, be aware of the following general precautions for diuretic use:

• Inform your clinician promptly if you develop any of these warning signs: thirst, dry mouth, weakness, lethargy, drowsiness, restlessness, muscle cramps or pain, muscle fatigue, racing or irregular heartbeat, very low urine volume, dizziness, nausea, or vomiting

TABLE 30-5
COMMONLY PRESCRIBED DIURETICS

TYPE	BRAND NAME(S)	COMMENTS
Thiazides	Diuril HydroDiuril	Probably the safest diuretics.
		May cause serious drop in blood cell production and also inflammation of the pancreas.
		Jaundice from liver problems and disturbance in blood sugar regulation may occur.
		Allergy reactions are possible, including rash, fever, and asthma-like symptoms.
Potassium-sparing	Spironolactone	May cause breast enlargement, menstrual disturbance.
		Breast cancer has been reported, but cause and effect not established.
		Has caused liver and endocrine tumors in lab animals.
		Avoid potassium supplements, including potassium-based salt substitutes.
	Dyrenium	Have blood monitored regularly.
		Do not use in combination with another potassium-sparing diuretic.
Combinations	Aldactazide	Spironolactone plus a thiazide. Read spironolactone above.
	Dyazide Maxzide	Dyrenium plus a thiazide. Read dyrenium above.
Loop (furosemide)	Lasix	Do not exceed prescribed dose (as with all prescription drugs).
		Inform your clinician if you are on phenytoin (Dilantin) therapy.
		Have serum calcium monitored regularly.
		Inform your clinician if you are on indomethacin (Indocin) therapy.

SOURCES: AMA Department of Drugs: *AMA Drug Evaluations* (ed 4). Chicago: American Medical Association, 1980.
The Obstetrician's & Gynecologist's Compendium of Drug Therapy 1981–82. New York: Biomedical Information, 1982.

• If you take diuretics more than four or five days in a month, have your electrolytes (potassium, sodium, chloride, bicarbonate) tested regularly
• Fasting (not eating) is unwise while you are taking diuretics, and you should contact your clinician if you have significant diarrhea or vomiting because your electrolytes may be altered
• Inform your clinician promptly if you suspect you are pregnant
• Do not use diuretics while breastfeeding
• Do not use diuretics if you have liver or kidney disease
• Inform your clinician if you are receiving lithium therapy
• Avoid high salt intake, which can cause a serious decrease in potassium levels
• Latent diabetes may become apparent. Insulin requirements for diabetics may change.

HORMONE TREATMENT

One small study showed that effectively shutting down the ovaries with a GnRH agonist, a drug that blocks the action of hormones on the ovaries, relieved PMS for six of eight women (15). This approach, equivalent to temporary menopause, is too drastic to be a reasonable treatment for PMS; the study does, however, provide evidence for the role of hormones in PMS.

Some clinicians are willing to try a course of hormone therapy when other treatment approaches have not provided relief. Hormones will not be recommended for all women, however, just as birth control Pills would not be recommended for all women, because of possible increased risk of heart attack, stroke, or other health problem (see Chapter 13 for more details on guidelines for safe Pill use). Your clinician may ask you to have a lipid panel blood test before treatment to check your levels of cholesterol and triglycerides. Hormone treatment may not be advisable for a woman whose lipids are elevated.

A high-progestational-activity birth control Pill such as Lo/Ovral, Nordette, or Triphasil, or a progestin-only Minipill such as Micronor, Nor-Q.D., or Ovrette, are possible choices for hormone therapy. Birth control Pills stop ovulation completely, so at least theoretically PMS should not exist. And some women find that they do not have PMS symptoms when they take birth control Pills. Others, though, continue with symptoms unchanged and some even find that PMS symptoms are more severe. Progestin-only Minipills do not consistently block ovulation, and provide a significantly lower dose of progestin than do birth control Pills. Because they do not contain estrogen, Minipills may be an option for women 35 to 40 who are likely to be advised not to use regular birth control Pills. A woman using Minipills may find that PMS symptoms improve, are unchanged, or are more severe.

Natural progesterone (one to four 100- to 400-mg rectal or vaginal suppositories daily) is the PMS treatment advocated by Dalton. Unlike the synthetic hormones used in birth control Pills, natural progesterone cannot withstand stomach acid. Consequently, it must be administered in suppository form so it can be absorbed directly into the bloodstream through the vaginal lining or rectum. No commercial progesterone products for PMS use are available (suppositories are compounded by a pharmacist) and there is very little research information available regarding possible side effects or hazards of suppository treatment. Natural progesterone suppositories may cause spotting, bleeding, and weight change. Rectal suppositories can cause soreness, diarrhea, and flatulence.

OTHER MEDICATIONS

If you have very severe breast tenderness that persists despite your best self-help measures and prescription analgesics, then **bromocriptine treatment** may be an option to consider. Bromocriptine was originally developed for treatment of abnormal milk production or hormone suppression caused by excessive prolactin hormone levels. (Treatment with bromocriptine is discussed in more detail in Chapter 10.) Several studies of bromocriptine (Parlodel) have reported success in alleviating **premenstrual breast tenderness and pain** (16), apparently by decreasing the release of prolactin hormone from the pituitary gland; in other words, bromocriptine slows down hormonal stimulation of breast tissue. Bromocriptine **does not alleviate other symptoms** of PMS.

Serious adverse side effects with the drug are rare, but bothersome side effects are common (see Chapter 10). The drug is not recommended for women who have high blood pressure or who are taking phenothiazine (Thorazine, Stelazine), and should be used with care in women using other medications that may affect blood pressure. Some success in treating more generalized PMS symptoms has been reported with low dose danazol treatment. This drug blunts cyclic hormone patterns, but used in low doses (200 mg daily) does not stop ovulation or menstrual periods (17). Side effects and complications of danazol treatment are discussed in Chapter 10.

Xanax (alprazolam), a tranquilizer in the Valium family, also has been investigated for treatment of severe PMS. Researchers in one study reported that intermittent, low dose Xanax (0.25 mg three times daily for the last week of each cycle) was significantly better than placebo in relieveing PMS symptoms (18). A decision to use tranquilizers, however, deserves careful thought. Drug dependence (addiction) is a possible risk, and can be a much more difficult problem than PMS.

The people who are *certain* they know how to cure PMS can't prove it. The people who read all the medical journals say they *don't know* what it is or how to cure it. And here I am, really struggling for a week out of every month. It's disheartening. I will try anything that makes sense to me and won't hurt me. Maybe we'll figure PMS out some day.

—WOMAN, 33

REFERENCES

1. Friedman D, Jaffe A: Influence of life-style on the premenstrual syndrome: Analysis of a questionnaire survey. *Journal of Reproductive Medicine* 30:715–719, 1985.
2. Harrison WM, Rabkin JG, Endicott J: Psychiatric evaluation of premenstrual changes. *Psychosomatics* 26:789–799, 1985.
3. Dalton K: *The Premenstrual Syndrome and Progesterone Therapy* (ed 2). London: William Heinemann Medical Books, 1984.
4. Maxson WS: The use of progesterone in the treatment of PMS. *Clinical Obsetrics and Gynecology* 30:465–477, 1987.
5. Dennerstein L, Spencer-Gardner C, Gotts G: Progesterone and the premenstrual syndrome: A double blind crossover trial. *British Medical Journal* 290:1617–1621, 1985.
6. Abraham GE: Nutritional factors in the etiology of the premenstrual syndrome. *Journal of Reproductive Medicine* 28:446–464, 1983.
7. Budoff PW: Zomepirac sodium in the treatment of primary dysmenorrhea syndrome. *New England Journal of Medicine* 307:714–719, 1982.
8. Puolakka J, Makarainen L, Viinikka L, et al: Biochemical and clinical effects of treating the premenstrual syndrome with prostaglandin synthesis precursors. *Journal of Reproductive Medicine* 30:149–153, 1985.
9. Reid RL: Endogenous opiate peptides and premenstrual syndrome. *Seminars in Reproductive Endocrinology* 5:191–197, 1987.
10. Chuong CJ, Coulam CB, Kao PC, et al: Neuropeptide levels in premenstrual syndrome. *Fertility and Sterility* 44:760–765, 1985.
11. Willis J: Doing something about menstrual discomforts. *FDA Consumer,* June 1983.
12. Berger A, Schaumburg HH: More on neuropathy from pyridoxine abuse. *New England Journal of Medicine* 311:986–987, 1984.
13. Rossignol AM: Caffeine-containing beverages and premenstrual syndrome in young women. *American Journal of Public Health* 75:1335–1337, 1985.
14. Sondheimer SJ, Freeman EW, Scharlop B, et al: Hormonal changes in premenstrual syndrome. *Psychosomatics* 26:803–816, 1985.
15. Muse KN, Cetel NS, Futterman LA, et al: The premenstrual syndrome: Effects of "medical ovariectomy." *New England Journal of Medicine* 311:1345–1349, 1984.
16. Ylostalo P: Cyclical or continuous treatment of the premenstrual syndrome (PMS) with bromocriptine. *European Journal of Obstetrics, Gynecology, and Reproductive Biology* 17:337–343, 1984.
17. Sarno AP, Miller EJ, Lundblad EG: Premenstrual syndrome: Beneficial effects of periodic, low-dose danazol. *Obsetrics and Gynecology* 70:33–36, 1987.
18. Smith S, Rinehart VS, Ruddock VE, et al: Treatment of premenstrual syndrome with alprazolam: Results of a double-blind, placebo-controlled, randomized crossover clinical trial. *Obstetrics and Gynecology* 70:37–43, 1987.

31

❖

*Painful Periods
(Dysmenorrhea)*

Women in the future will look back on 1975 to 1985 as the landmark decade when the cause of "normal" menstrual cramps was finally discovered and reasonably effective treatment for cramps became widely available. These break-throughs are important because cramps are so common and painful, and because cramps interfere with life very significantly for many women. Cramps are responsible for 600 million lost working hours each year in this country (1). Our understanding of the cause and treatment of menstrual pain puts to rest all the terrible old theories about psychological causes for cramps.

The specific chemical culprit—excessive levels of prostaglandin hormone—has been identified, and medications that reduce prostaglandin production with few side effects are here. Assuming that you don't have an underlying gynecologic problem causing your menstrual cramps, you can now expect to find relief.

Primary and Secondary Dysmenorrhea

Menstrual cramps (dysmenorrhea) can be caused by specific medical problems such as endometriosis, pelvic infection, fibroid tumors (benign leiomyoma of the uterus), or ovarian cysts. Cramps associated with these conditions typically appear for the first time when a woman is in her 20s or 30s. Your clinician will call this condition **secondary dysmenorrhea,** for the cramps are secondary to (caused by) another medical problem. An IUD (intrauterine device) can also cause secondary dysmenorrhea.

Most women who have menstrual cramps don't have any underlying illness, however. Severe, disabling cramps without underlying illness is called **primary dysmenorrhea**. In addition to cramps, primary dysmenorrhea can cause backache, leg pain, nausea, vomiting, diarrhea, headache, and dizziness. As many as 70% of women experience at least some cramping pain during menstrual flow (2), and 15% of women have cramps severe enough to be disabling. Typically, a young woman may begin menstrual periods with somewhat irregular cycles and little pain during the first year or two, and then begin to have serious cramps when ovulation patterns and her regular cycle become established. Young women with severe cramps may be unable to manage normal daily activities for the first 24 to 36 hours of each menstrual period. Primary dysmenorrhea symptoms rarely last more than two days with each cycle, and severe cramps often subside somewhat on their own when a woman reaches her later 20s or has a full term pregnancy.

MENSTRUAL CRAMPS—THE CAUSE

Prostaglandin hormone is the cause of cramps in primary dysmenorrhea. Prostaglandins are actually a family of closely related hormones with names such as prostaglandin F_2 and prostaglandin E_2; they are present in many body tissues. Uterine lining cells (endometrial cells) normally manufacture prostaglandin, and the prostaglandin concentration is higher during the luteal phase of the menstrual cycle—the two weeks or so after ovulation occurs—than it is during the early part of the cycle. When menstrual bleeding begins, prostaglandin is released by the endometrial cells as they are shed from the uterine lining. Women who have severe cramps have significantly higher levels of prostaglandin in their menstrual fluid than women who do not have cramps.

Prostaglandin hormone stimulates contraction of uterine smooth muscle cells. If excessive prostaglandin is present, the normal contraction response can become a strong, painful spasm. Blood flow to the uterine muscle may be reduced because spasm constricts the uterine blood vessels. Reduced blood flow means inadequate oxygen—and that means pain. Excessive prostaglandin release is also responsible for contraction of smooth muscle in the intestinal tract; hence the diarrhea, nausea, and vomiting that often accompany severe dysmenorrhea. Headache and dizziness, too, may be the result of high prostaglandin levels.

The role of progesterone hormone in cramps is paradoxical. The direct effect of natural progesterone on uterine muscle is to reduce contractility, or cramping, and progestin medications may also have this result. On the other hand, cramps are unlikely to be severe unless ovulation has occurred, and progesterone is released from the ovary only when ovulation has occurred. Steady progestin exposure with birth control Pills or a progestin IUD tends to reduce or eliminate cramps, and treatment with progestin, particularly medroxyprogesterone acetate (Provera, 10 mg each day) for the last ten days of each cycle, was one alternative in combating cramps before antiprostaglandin drugs were developed. Progestin added to postmenopausal hormone treatment may increase cramping, and some women using birth control Pills find that cramps are a problem with some progestins but not others.

Conquering Menstrual Cramps

Dysmenorrhea pain can begin a day or two before menstrual bleeding. Typically, it is worst during your first one or two days of bleeding, and then subsides. If the pain you are having is not at the right time for a normal period, is severe, lasts longer than two or three days, and you aren't sure that it is plain old cramps, you should think about other possible causes for lower abdominal or uterine pain.

Remember that women who have endometriosis and uterine fibroids often have problems with dysmenorrhea as well. In some cases, treatment specifically for dysmenorrhea is helpful, but often the underlying problem must be tackled directly to control pain. If pelvic infection or an IUD seems to be the pain source, then careful management of the underlying problem is essential. **Pain can be a warning sign of pelvic infection, early pregnancy problems, or unsuspected IUD infection.**

In any event, your first step should be a thorough examination to be certain you don't have a medical problem that is causing your cramps.

Your medical history and pelvic exam alone may provide enough information for your clinician to determine whether your cramps are caused by primary dysmenorrhea or by another medical problem. If there is any doubt, further evaluation will be needed. Blood tests may show evidence of an infection response, and uterine fibroids may be confirmed by an ultrasound exam (test procedures are described in Chapter 4). If the pain is severe and its cause is uncertain despite an exam and initial tests, laparoscopy may be recommended. This procedure permits your clinician to look at your uterus, tubes, and ovaries through a narrow, illuminated tube inserted just below your navel. (See Chapter 48 for a description of laparoscopy.)

For mild, normal cramps of primary dysmenorrhea, your best home therapy may be all you need. Aspirin or acetaminophen may provide good relief, and low-dose antiprostaglandin pain relievers are available without a prescription. Table 31-1 lists commonly used prescription and nonprescription antiprostaglandin preparations.

Also, avoid prolonged standing or walking on hard pavement, and try back massage, a heating pad, tub soaks, exercise to put endorphins—your brain's natural pain relievers—to work, and rest. One stiff drink may help, because alcohol relaxes the uterine muscle. Orgasm also helps relax the uterine muscle, and will decrease congestion in your pelvis. Warning: Pennyroyal, an herbal "remedy," can cause serious and even fatal poisoning (see Chapter 18).

If cramps are bothersome despite your own efforts, then by all means talk to your clinician about a prescription for antiprostaglandin medication.

TABLE 31-1
COMMONLY USED ANTIPROSTAGLANDIN DRUGS

DRUG NAME: BRAND NAME[a]	COMMONLY PRESCRIBED DOSE	STRENGTH OF TABLET	MAXIMUM DOSE IN 24 HOURS ( ) = NUMBER OF TABLETS
IBUPROFEN			
Advil	1–2 tablets every 4–6	200 mg	(6) 1,200 mg
Nuprin	hours. No Rx needed.	200 mg	(6) 1,200 mg
Motrin, Rufen	1 tablet every 4 hours	400 mg	(6) 2,400 mg
Motrin, Rufen		600 mg	(4) 2,400 mg
Motrin		800 mg	(3) 2,400 mg
FENOPROFEN CALCIUM			
Nalfon	1 tablet every 4–6 hours	200 mg	(16) 3,200 mg
		300 mg	(10) 3,200 mg
		600 mg	(5) 3,200 mg
MEFENAMIC ACID			
Ponstel	2 tablets initially, then 1 every 6 hours	250 mg	(5) 1,250 mg to start (4) 1,000 mg other days
NAPROXEN SODIUM			
Anaprox	2 tablets initially, then 1 every 6–8 hours	275 mg	(5) 1,375 mg
NAPROXEN			
Naprosyn	2 tablets initially, then 1 every 6–8 hours	250 mg 375 mg 500 mg	(5) 1,250 mg

[a]Other drugs, such as indomethacin (Indocin), phenylbutazone (Butazolidin), sulindac (Clinoril), piroxicam (Feldene), tolmetin (Tolectin), and meclofenamate (Meclomen), are also effective antiprostaglandin drugs, but are not usually used for treatment of dysmenorrhea. Their side effects tend to be more severe. Zomepirac (Zomax), another member of this drug family, was withdrawn from sale by the manufacturer in 1983, and suprofen (Suprol) was withdrawn in 1987, because of serious adverse reactions.

I had cramps that made me stay in bed doubled up for about a day. I'd feel weak, sweaty, and sick at my stomach. I'd live on ginger ale. Sometimes I could make it to work and sometimes not. Just your usual agony. Now I don't miss a beat, even on the first day of my period. I keep the pills in my purse all the time in case I start my period away from home. Great drug!

—WOMAN, 26

Overall, at least 80% of women treated for cramps with antiprostaglandin medication can expect good relief. There are several closely related drugs called prostaglandin synthetase inhibitors that have similar effects. All of them decrease production of prostaglandin within normal body cells, including uterine lining cells. For most women any of the commonly used antiprostaglandin drugs is likely to be effective. They are not identical, however, so if one is not effective or side effects are a problem, then trying an alternative is reasonable. Many studies of antiprostaglandin drugs used for cramps have been published (3), and reported success rates for relieving pain range from about 60% to more than 90% for various products in various studies. Unfortunately, results are not comparable from one study to another because of differences in study design, so the relative effectiveness of different products is not yet clear.

These drugs belong to a large drug family called nonsteroidal anti-inflammatory drugs (NSAIDs). Aspirin is a member of the NSAID family, and many of the NSAIDs were originally developed for treatment of arthritis as alternatives to aspirin. Arthritis treatment often requires prolonged use of medications at quite high daily doses, so research evidence on possible risks and complications for NSAIDs is fairly extensive; generally they have side effects and adverse effects similar to those for aspirin.

SIDE EFFECTS

Side effects are not usually a problem for women using antiprostaglandin medications to combat menstrual cramps. Most common are nausea and heartburn, and taking the medication with food or milk may alleviate these problems.

Serious complications are very rare. **Women who have had a severe allergic reaction to aspirin such as asthma, hives, runny nose, itching or rash, swelling or shock, however, should not take antiprostaglandin drugs.** They do not contain aspirin, but are chemically similar enough that an allergic reaction is quite likely. If you have ulcer disease or kidney disease you should also avoid antiprostaglandin drugs (4). Like aspirin, they can cause stomach irritation that could be a significant hazard for a woman with bleeding ulcers. With serious kidney disease a drop in the prostaglandin level may be harmful because blood flow to the kidney may be decreased as a result. Other possible side effects are listed in Table 31-2.

TABLE 31-2
POSSIBLE SIDE EFFECTS
OF ANTIPROSTAGLANDIN DRUGS[a]

SEVERE (SEE DANGER SIGNS IN ILLUSTRATION 31-1)

Allergic reaction. Do not use these drugs if you have had an allergic reaction to aspirin such as asthma, hives, runny nose, itching or rash, swelling or shock. Although these drugs do not contain aspirin, people who are allergic to aspirin are likely to be allergic to them as well.

Meningitis. Severe persistent headaches, fever, muscle aches, and lab tests confirming aseptic meningitis (inflammation of the covering of the brain with no detectable infectious agent) have been reported. This is extremely rare. Patients recovered after stopping the drug.

UNCOMMON (EXPERIENCED BY AT LEAST 1% OF USERS)

Nausea and vomiting	Indigestion
Headache	Bloating and flatulence
Heartburn	Itching
Dizziness	Skin eruptions
Nervousness	Ringing ears
Abdominal or stomach pain	Loss of appetite
Constipation	Fluid retention and
Diarrhea	swelling

RARE (EXPERIENCED BY LESS THAN 1% OF USERS)

Irritability	Palpitations
Depression	Visual disturbances
Kidney damage	Liver function changes
Jaundice	Hepatitis
Dry eyes and mouth	Heart failure
Bronchial spasm	Hair loss
Hearing loss	Dream abnormality, insomnia
Malaise	Elevated blood pressure
Abdominal pain with fever,	Change in anticoagulant drug effect
chills, nausea, and vomiting	Prolonged blood clotting time
Allergic reaction	and other blood disorders
(see "Severe" above)	Ulcer, stomach, or intestinal
	bleeding

---

[a]Reported for patients using medication continuously for arthritis.

SOURCES: *Physicians' Desk Reference* (ed 41). Oradell, N.J.: Medical Economics Co., 1987.
Lawson JM, Grady MJ: Ibuprofen-induced aseptic meningitis in a previously healthy patient. *Western Journal of Medicine* 143:386–387, 1985.

31:1   ANTIPROSTAGLANDIN DRUG DANGER SIGNS
Blurred vision, spots in your vision, or a change in color vision Jaundice Abdominal or stomach pain Signs of intestinal bleeding (black stools or vomiting blood) Weight gain or swelling Bloody urine An allergic reaction or skin rash Fever, headache, muscle aches Stop taking the medication and contact your clinician at once if you develop any of these problems.

Although serious complications with these drugs are rare, you should watch for **danger signs of serious trouble**. Stop taking medication and contact your clinician if you develop any of the problems listed in Illustration 31-1.

Also, you should not take antiprostaglandin medication if you are pregnant or think you might be pregnant, because during the last three months of pregnancy these drugs may cause heart problems for the fetus or problems during labor and delivery for the pregnant woman. There are no reports of fetal damage from the drugs taken early in pregnancy, but there is also no research to prove that they are safe, so if you are trying to become pregnant it is especially important to wait until regular menstrual bleeding has begun before taking your first dose each month.

DOSAGE SCHEDULE

Since antiprostaglandin drugs work by preventing uterine spasm, it is best to take your first dose **before** your cramps have become severe. You may want to begin medication at the very first sign of menstrual bleeding. Then take additional tablets as directed in your prescription, or as you feel cramps just beginning to reappear. Although you should not exceed the recommended maximum 24-hour dose, you are likely to find that taking additional doses early in the day provides better relief throughout the day than trying to bear the pain while you space out your doses.

Do not worry if you notice a decrease in menstrual flow while you are taking antiprostaglandin medication. Your bleeding may even stop temporarily. Overall menstrual blood loss is decreased for medication users—a beneficial side effect.

WHAT TO EXPECT

Finding the medication and dose schedule that is best for you may require some experimenting. Also, you may find that cramps are worse some months than others, and will need to adjust your doses accordingly. You may not be able to eliminate cramps entirely, but it is reasonable to expect your treatment to control them well enough that you are able to continue your normal daily activities without difficulty.

If your initial cycle is not successful, plan to begin your medication sooner next time and be sure you are taking the full, recommended amount. You may want to carry your medication with you to avoid a delay when your period or symptoms begin. Even an hour can make a difference, and once cramps are severe your treatment will not be effective as quickly.

OTHER TREATMENT OPTIONS

After two or three months, talk to your clinician again if you still don't have good pain control. Changing to a different antiprostaglandin drug may be of help. "Stronger" pain medication is actually less likely to be effective in treating cramps than the antiprostaglandin drugs, and side effects are a bigger problem. Other options, though, such as birth control Pills to stop ovulation or progestin pills for the last ten days of each month, may be possibilities.

If your cramps persist despite treatment, you may need further evaluation to be sure that an unsuspected gynecologic problem is not your real problem.

Treatment with acupuncture may be another possibility to consider. Weekly acupuncture sessions continued through three menstrual cycles resulted in significant improvement for 10 out of 11 patients in a small but carefully designed 1987 study (5).

Surgery to sever nerves to the uterus is another option. Before antiprostaglandin drugs and birth control Pills, this drastic approach was one of the few options for women with disabling symptoms. In the past, abdominal surgery requiring hospitalization, a five-inch abdominal incision, and four to six weeks' convalescence was necessary. Laparoscopy surgery to sever uterine nerves may now be a possibility (6). Laparoscopy can be performed at an outpatient surgical facility without hospitalization, and little convalescence is involved. Laparoscopy instruments are inserted into the abdominal cavity through a one-inch incision below the navel. Laparoscopy surgery is described in Chapter 48.

Birth Control and Menstrual Cramps

Your menstrual cramps can be increased or decreased to some extent by your contraceptive method. Birth control Pill users rarely have cramps; they do not ovulate so they don't experience the normal increase in prostaglandin synthesis that occurs in the postovulatory cyclic phase. The Pill user's uterine lining is also thinner, so prostaglandin production may be lower.

IUDs tend to increase menstrual cramping for many users. The Progestasert IUD is an exception. This IUD releases a steady low level of progestin, which reduces the amount of cyclic endometrial growth, so cramps are likely to be decreased. For much the same reason, progestin-only Minipills may decrease the likelihood and severity of cramps.

Some diaphragm users find that cramps are more severe when the diaphragm is in place, perhaps because of rim pressure on pelvic nerves and muscles. Condoms, vaginal spermicides, sponges, and fertility awareness methods should not alter menstrual cramping.

REFERENCES

1. Dawood MY: Dysmenorrhea. *Journal of Reproductive Medicine* 30:154–167, 1985.
2. Andersch B, Milson I: An epidemiologic study of young women with dysmenorrhea. *American Journal of Obstetrics and Gynecology* 144:655–660, 1982.
3. Owen PR: Prostaglandin synthetase inhibitors in the treatment of primary dysmenorrhea. *American Journal of Obstetrics and Gynecology* 148:96–103, 1984.
4. Drugs for rheumatoid arthritis. *Medical Letter on Drugs and Therapeutics* 27:25–28, 1985.
5. Helms JM: Acupuncture for the management of primary dysmenorrhea. *Obstetrics and Gynecology* 69:51–56, 1987.
6. Lichten EM, Bombard J: Surgical treatment of primary dysmenorrhea with laparoscopic uterine nerve ablation. *Journal of Reproductive Medicine* 32:37–41, 1987.

32

❖

Abnormal Bleeding

Regular menstrual periods are not as regular as you might think. Some women have a consistent, predictable interval between periods, but most women have cycles that vary in length, and many women have variations of a week or more.

It is almost universal that women don't like unpredictable periods. They are annoying at best, and at worst they cause profound anxiety. Nuisance or ominous early warning? Most women want help from their clinicians to learn the answer. Sometimes the answer is clear and sometimes not. If you are over 30, it is best not to delay evaluation of abnormal bleeding, even if it isn't bothering you very much.

The average cycle is somewhere between 24 and 32 days long, counting from the first day of one menstrual period to the first day of the next period. Menstrual bleeding usually lasts three to seven days and totals 4 or 5 tablespoons of fluid, one third of which is blood. If your bleeding differs substantially from these averages, your clinician may use terms like:

• Oligomenorrhea: Infrequent flow, often irregular intervals
• Hypomenorrhea: Scant flow but regular intervals
• Hypermenorrhea: Excessive flow but regular intervals
• Menorrhagia: Prolonged flow
• Metrorrhagia: Irregular flow, short intervals
• Menometrorrhagia: Prolonged and irregular flow
• Spotting: Light, irregular flow, often prolonged; the term metrorrhagia could also be used

Any vaginal bleeding that does not correspond to an average normal pattern should be reported to your clinician. If you are over 30, you must see your clinician promptly even if your unusual bleeding is not heavy or troublesome. Your clinician will want to evaluate you carefully for cancer of the uterus or cervix. If you are under 30, the likelihood of cancer is remote; you may not need extensive evaluation unless the problem is persistent, bleeding is very heavy, you have cramps or other signs of infection, or you are trying to become pregnant. Women who are taking combined estrogen and progestin treatment after menopause often have light flow following each monthly cycle of medication. **Any other bleeding at all, even the tiniest pink or red or brown trace, that occurs after menopause must be evaluated promptly.**

Abnormal bleeding is an extremely common problem, and is most likely to occur early and late in the reproductive years. Between ages 14 and 25, when menstrual patterns are just being established, irregular menstrual cycles are likely to mean that ovulation is not yet occurring on a completely regular monthly basis. The chance of cancer is extremely low, but the possibility of problems such as infection and complications of unsuspected pregnancy demands careful evaluation. Disruptions in ovulation are also common late in the reproductive years. Women 35 to 50 also are more likely to have other kinds of problems such as polyps or uterine fibroids.

There are numerous possible causes for abnormal bleeding, most of them not too frightening. Among the rare causes, however, are several kinds of gynecologic cancer, so your faithful persistence in following through with the necessary tests and procedures is crucial. You need to be sure you and your clinician arrive at a good understanding of the cause of the abnormality. In most cases, your problems with bleeding will also be solved, or at least corrected, at the same time.

Two specific types of bleeding merit special mention here, midcycle spotting and bleeding after intercourse.

Midcycle Spotting.   About 10% of women have spotting or light bleeding for one or two days at the time of ovulation. This bleeding is probably triggered by the temporary drop in estrogen production that occurs with ovulation. If this is the cause of your spotting, your next period should begin almost exactly 14 days later.

Bleeding After Intercourse.   Even if your abnormal bleeding occurs only after intercourse, you will still need evaluation. Your cervix is likely to be the source of bleeding. There may be no serious problem at all, or your bleeding could be the first warning of a more serious problem such as infection or cervical or uterine cancer.

BLEEDING EMERGENCY

One morning, out of the blue, I woke up in a pool of blood. I thought
I was going to faint from fear, or blood loss, or both! Bill rushed me
to the emergency room with a beach towel between my legs. It turned
out to be just my IUD, and I was fine, but it was an utterly terrifying
experience.

—WOMAN, 33

In rare cases bleeding may be heavy enough to constitute a real emergency. Persistent
bleeding that is moderate or heavy can lead to anemia. In most cases this is a gradual
process and your clinician will be able to detect anemia with a simple office blood test.
Treatment to control your bleeding and iron supplements will enable your body to
replace the red blood cells you have lost, and your blood count will gradually return to
normal over a period of several weeks. Be sure that you continue taking iron for at
least three months; you need to replace the iron stores in your body.

Sudden heavy blood loss can be severe enough to lead to hemorrhagic shock. Early
signs of shock include severe fatigue, feeling faint or weak, or feeling dizzy when
sitting or standing up. If you have heavy bleeding and develop any of these symptoms,
call your clinician immediately or go to the emergency room at a nearby hospital.

Sudden bleeding that totals more than 1 or 2 cups should also be reported to your
clinician; if bleeding this heavy persists more than a few hours, emergency evaluation
will be needed.

Clots are quite common when bleeding is heavy. Clots mean that the pace of your
bleeding is rapid enough that anticlotting factors normally present in uterine secretions
are not sufficient to keep up with the amount of bleeding present. Clots can form
inside the uterus, and expelling them often causes severe but temporary crampy pain.

Clots can also form in the vagina if blood pools there while you are quiet or lying
down. The pool of clots and blood from the vagina is likely to gush out the next time
you stand up, do something active, or sit on the toilet. This can be very disconcerting,
since it appears as if you have had sudden massive bleeding, The total amount of
bleeding over several hours, rather than the amount in one gush, is a more accurate
measure of your overall blood loss. If you have more than four or five soaked pads
within two hours, you should call your clinician.

PREGNANCY CAUSES
OF ABNORMAL BLEEDING

• Spontaneous bleeding in early pregnancy (no apparent harm)
• Miscarriage (spontaneous abortion)

• Ectopic (tubal) pregnancy
• Abnormal pregnancy (molar pregnancy)

If **pregnancy** is even a remote possibility, your clinician is likely to think first about pregnancy problems as a cause for abnormal bleeding. Pregnancy complications are described in detail in Chapter 8. A review of your history, a physical exam, and a sensitive pregnancy test should settle the issue.

VAGINAL CAUSES
OF ABNORMAL BLEEDING

• Vaginal infection (vaginitis; see Chapter 23)
• Vaginal warts (see Chapter 27)
• Vaginal atrophy (see Chapter 34)
• Vaginal injury (see Chapter 39)
• Foreign body
• Vaginal cancer (see Chapter 41)

Bleeding because of **vaginal problems** is rare. Vaginal infection can occasionally be severe enough to cause bloody discharge and vaginal warts may bleed with even minimal trauma. Also, a forgotten tampon, diaphragm, or other foreign body can cause bloody discharge. Injury caused by intercourse, a tampon inserter, or the edge of a cervical cap or diaphragm rim is possible, but very rare.

Vaginal injury sufficient to cause bleeding is somewhat more common after menopause. When estrogen hormone levels are low, the vaginal lining is thin (atrophic) and loses some of its elasticity. Even minimal trauma during intercourse or douching may be enough to tear the delicate lining and cause bleeding.

Vaginal cancer is very, very rare, even among DES daughters, but bleeding may be its first sign. Special evaluation needs for DES daughters are discussed in Chapter 42.

CERVICAL CAUSES
OF ABNORMAL BLEEDING

• Cervical infection (see Chapters 22 and 40)
• Warts (see Chapter 27)
• Herpes (see Chapter 26)
• Syphilis (see Chapter 28)
• Ectropion (see Chapter 40)
• Cervical polyps (see Chapter 40)
• Cervical cancer (see Chapter 41)

Bleeding originating from the **cervix** is most likely to occur after intercourse. Intercourse, or inserting a diaphragm or spermicide, may bump the cervix and start bleeding if the surface of the cervix is damaged or especially fragile.

The normal, adult covering of the cervix is a smooth, tough layer of cells called squamous epithelium. Part of the cervical surface near the opening of the canal may be covered by delicate, mucus-secreting epithelium that lines the canal and extends out into the surface in young women, a normal variation called ectropion. Cervical damage during childbirth may also bring canal lining tissue onto the outer surface. When ectropion is present, trauma is more likely to cause bleeding.

Infection on the surface of the cervix or in the outer part of the canal is a more serious problem that can cause bleeding. Cervical warts, herpes ulcers, syphilis ulcers, and bacterial infections such as chlamydia and gonorrhea all can cause bloody discharge. A cervical polyp, a benign tongue of extra cervical tissue protruding from the canal, is likely to bleed whenever it is touched. For a woman who has missed her routine Pap smears, cervical bleeding can be the first symptom of cervical cancer.

UTERINE CAUSES
OF ABNORMAL BLEEDING

• Uterine polyps (see Chapter 40)
• Benign fibroid tumors (see Chapter 40)
• Uterine infection (see Chapter 25)
• Endometriosis (see Chapter 36)
• IUD (see Chapter 14)
• Hyperplasia (see Chapter 40)
• Uterine cancer (see Chapter 41)

The **uterus** is the actual origin of abnormal bleeding whenever hormone disruption is the underlying cause. Hormone problems are discussed later in this chapter. Diseases of the uterus itself also can lead to bleeding. Polyps in the uterine lining are common. These are almost always benign, and tend to form and grow when estrogen levels are high. Polyps typically cause intermittent, painless spotting or bleeding in between normal periods.

Benign tumors of the uterine wall commonly cause excessively heavy flow during periods, but can also cause spotting or bleeding between periods. These tumors, called fibroids, or leiomyoma, or fibroadenoma, are often multiple and can cause crampy pain as well as bleeding.

The combination of abnormal bleeding and pain also can signal either infection in the uterus or endometriosis. An IUD could also be the cause of pain and bleeding, and the possibility of infection associated with IUD use should be carefully considered.

Abnormal bleeding without pain can be the first symptom of uterine cancer, and of uterine hyperplasia, abnormal thickening of the uterine lining, a precancerous alteration in some cases.

The **fallopian tubes** very rarely cause abnormal bleeding. Infection in the tubes (salpingitis) is almost always accompanied by infection in the uterus as well. Bleeding or bloody discharge is likely to accompany this problem. When recurrent or long-term infection in the tube spreads to involve the nearby ovaries, hormone production by the ovaries may be affected and may lead to bleeding. Cancer originating in the fallopian tube is exceedingly rare, but could cause watery, bloody discharge as well as pain.

OVARIAN CAUSES OF ABNORMAL BLEEDING

• Follicular cyst (see Chapter 40)
• Corpus luteum cyst (see Chapter 40)
• Polycystic ovary disease (see Chapter 40)
• Ovarian cancer (see Chapter 41)

The **ovaries** are directly involved in abnormal bleeding whenever disrupted hormone patterns are its cause. In some cases, abnormalities within the ovary cause the problem. In other cases, the ovaries are bystanders—responding as they should respond, but to improper signs from the pituitary gland.

Benign cysts of the ovary are so common that every woman is likely to encounter this problem at some time in her life. A small cyst (fluid-filled sac) normally forms in the ovary at the site of ovulation each month. Prior to ovulation this would be called a follicular cyst—corresponding to the follicle in which the ripening egg is developing. After the egg is extruded, this same group of cells shifts its hormone apparatus to the manufacture of progesterone and is called the corpus luteum cyst. A completely normal follicle or corpus luteum cyst may be 3 to 20 mm in diameter. The occasional formation of a much larger yet still normal cyst, perhaps as large as 50 mm (2 inches), is not unusual. A large cyst may be painful, and your clinician is likely to be able to feel it because its presence makes that ovary larger than normal. Formation of a large cyst is often accompanied by a delay in the normal sequence of hormone patterns. If the preovulatory phase is prolonged by a large follicle cyst, or ovulation fails to occur as it should, then your menstrual period is likely to be delayed. When bleeding does finally occur, it may be heavier than it normally would be. Also it may follow an atypical bleeding pattern—intermittent or prolonged, for example.

If your clinician suggests that your symptoms are caused by a benign cyst, then waiting a month or so for it to resolve may be all the treatment you need. Once your functional cyst (clinicians use this term for both follicular and corpus luteum cysts) is resolved, your normal cyclic hormone patterns will probably resume quite promptly.

Ultrasound examination, using sound waves and a sonar receiver to construct a picture of your pelvic organs, may be helpful. The actual size of the cyst can be measured accurately with ultrasound, and the picture can also confirm that it is an entirely fluid-filled cyst and not a tumor (solid mass of cells).

If the cyst is very large, if you are having severe pain, or if your age (over 30) or medical history raises a question of ovarian tumor, then your clinician may feel that surgery is indicated to determine your diagnosis for certain. In some cases laparoscopy may be appropriate. With this procedure, your pelvic organs are visualized through a lighted tube inserted into the abdomen through a small incision below your navel (see Chapter 48). In other cases, laparotomy allows your surgeon to see, biopsy, and, if necessary, remove all or part of the abnormal ovary. Laparotomy is major abdominal surgery and will require hospitalization for several days and four to six weeks for recovery (also described in Chapter 48).

Ovarian tumors are not common, especially before the age of 40. Some do produce hormones and cause abnormal bleeding. Also, the possibility of a tumor must be considered whenever one or both ovaries are larger than normal. Your faithfulness in follow-up, to be sure that your cyst completely disappears and your ovary returns to normal size, is essential.

Polycystic ovary disease is probably not truly a disease of the ovaries. Rather, the ovaries are innocent victims of hormone disturbances that originate elsewhere. Persistent ovulation failure, with fairly steady low to moderate levels of pituitary hormone release, leads to this disease. The ovaries are stimulated, but not enough to prompt full maturity of the follicle and egg. Ovulation does not occur. Continuous growth of early follicles eventually results in enlarged, thickened ovaries with many small early follicles in various stages of growth and regression. Estrogen is produced by these early follicles. Amenorrhea, lack of menstrual bleeding, can result or bleeding may be irregular. Infrequent light bleeding, prolonged intermittent bleeding, or unpredictable episodes of heavier bleeding may all occur. These are examples of **dysfunctional uterine bleeding**, the name given to abnormal bleeding patterns that occur when ovulation fails. Management of this problem is described in the section titled "Dysfunctional Uterine Bleeding."

OTHER CAUSES
OF ABNORMAL BLEEDING

• Hormone treatment: tablets, shots, or creams
• Thorazine and other drugs used for psychiatric problems
• Aspirin, antiprostaglandin drugs
• Anticoagulant drugs
• Blood clotting or platelet disorders
• Leukemia
• Liver disease

- High blood pressure
- Low levels of thyroid hormone
- Adrenal gland tumor

Diseases that slow blood clotting are examples of the rare **causes outside the reproductive system of abnormal vaginal bleeding**. Hereditary bleeding disorders and platelet diseases as well as leukemia are in this group. Anticoagulant drugs, aspirin, and antiprostaglandin medications can also interfere with clotting. These problems should be considered especially if a woman suddenly develops a very heavy flow but retains her normal cyclic timing.

Serious medical disorders such as very low thyroid hormone levels, adrenal gland tumor, high blood pressure, and liver disease can also cause abnormal bleeding patterns. Medications used for treatment of psychiatric problems, epilepsy, and many other serious disorders also may alter hormone balance and lead to abnormal bleeding.

And, of course, hormone medications, whether administered orally in tablet form, by injection, or in cream, all can alter hormone balance and potentially can cause abnormal bleeding patterns. Birth control Pills are in this category (see Chapter 13). Estrogen-containing medications are the most common culprits, but treatment with synthetic or natural progestin can also lead to bleeding problems.

DIAGNOSIS AND TREATMENT OF IRREGULAR BLEEDING

A review of your symptoms, medical history, pelvic examination, and simple lab tests are likely to pinpoint your diagnosis if the underlying problem is pregnancy, a vaginal or cervical problem, or pelvic infection. If you are over age 30, or there is any question about the cause of your bleeding, your clinician will probably recommend endometrial biopsy (see Chapter 4) or a D&C (dilation and curettage; see Chapter 47) to be sure you don't have uterine cancer. The D&C may also serve as a treatment in some cases: heavy bleeding from almost any cause can usually be stopped, at least temporarily, with D&C, and endometrial polyps can be detected and removed during the procedure.

If the cause of your abnormal periods is a specific problem such as infection or fibroids, your treatment will be directed to that particular problem. If your clinician does find evidence of a serious medical problem or severely abnormal hormone levels, she/he will probably recommend further tests and may refer you to a specialist in that particular medical area or to an endocrinologist, a hormone specialist, for full evaluation.

If your clinician tells you that your irregular bleeding is caused by **hormone imbalance**, she/he probably means that you have a temporary alteration in your estrogen and progesterone production that either delayed your period or caused it to start early. Stress or illness may have suppressed ovulation for one or two cycles; if this is the cause, your irregular bleeding is likely to resolve itself without treatment. Your hormones, also, will return to normal.

Sometimes hormone problems are not temporary. Persistent ovulation failure is quite a common problem. When irregular bleeding is occurring, the likely cause of ovulation failure is a disruption in the normal pattern of hormone signals between the pituitary gland and the ovary. Even slight alterations in the hormone levels, or the timing of their release, can be enough to block ovulation. Once started, an abnormal pattern may become self-reinforcing, and may lead to polycystic ovary disease. This problem is discussed in detail in Chapter 40.

DYSFUNCTIONAL UTERINE BLEEDING

Dysfunctional uterine bleeding (DUB) is a descriptive term used for abnormal bleeding patterns that are caused by the absence of ovulation. DUB occurs because steady exposure to estrogen, without orderly episodes of progesterone, disturbs the normal sequence and timing of growth in the uterine lining. Progesterone, which is produced by the ovary only after ovulation has occurred, is responsible for the final maturation of the lining and its underlying blood vessels. This prepares the lining for menstruation by assuring that all of the surface layer is ready to fall off neatly, and all at once, or within a few days. Steady estrogen exposure results in growth of the lining, but some areas may be thicker than others, or out of synchrony, so bleeding can begin from one area, only to be followed a few days later by bleeding from another area. In some cases, bleeding is light, although unpredictable and possibly prolonged. Moderate to heavy bleeding persistent enough to cause anemia is not uncommon. And in some cases, hemorrhage can be severe enough to require hospitalization and even blood transfusion.

The initial goal in treatment of dysfunctional bleeding is to control the bleeding. If bleeding is very heavy or has been very prolonged, then your clinician will probably begin with high doses of estrogen. Estrogen is almost always effective in stopping bleeding temporarily.

If bleeding is light or moderate, or estrogen has temporarily stopped it, then cyclic treatment with synthetic progestin or with combined estrogen and progestin is a reasonable plan. For a young woman who has heavy bleeding or needs birth control protection, birth control Pills may be a logical choice. Your clinician may recommend as many as four tablets daily used for an initial five- to seven-day treatment to gain control of bleeding. After the first treatment week, Pills are stopped and a fairly heavy (and crampy) period should start within two or three days. The next 21-day cycle of Pills is started on the fifth day after bleeding, at the normal dose of one tablet daily. The amount of bleeding during periods will decrease after the first Pill cycle or two are completed.

Treatment with progestin alone can be used for a young woman who does not need birth control or for an older woman who should not take birth control Pills. Typical progestin treatment would be Provera (medroxyprogesterone acetate), 10 mg daily for ten days every four to eight weeks. Bleeding after the initial ten-day treatment may be quite heavy as the uterus expels whatever lining has built up in the weeks or months preceding. Subsequent progestin-induced periods, however, should be more reasonable.

If cyclic hormone treatment with birth control Pills or with progestin fails to induce bleeding two to seven days later, or if abnormal bleeding persists despite treatment, then reevaluation is necessary. If treatment is successful, then it should be continued until spontaneous ovulation cycles return or pregnancy is desired.

Pregnancy is quite unlikely unless regular ovulation is occurring. If you want to be pregnant, let your clinician know. Treatment to induce ovulation can be started whenever you wish, and will be successful in at least four out of five women (1). Ovulation induction will probably require medication and monthly visits to your clinician. See Chapter 10 for more information on fertility treatment. Treatment to induce ovulation requires fairly intensive medical supervision and side effects are more common during ovulation induction than with progestin or birth control Pill management of anovulation (the absence of ovulation). For these reasons, ovulation induction is not recommended unless you are actually trying to achieve pregnancy.

Excess hair growth, or **hirsutism**, is another rather common concern. In most cases, a hereditary pattern rather than a disease is responsible. Genetic factors govern the number of hair follicles present in the skin as well as their sensitivity and response to hormones. So hormone levels that are entirely normal can, in some women, stimulate growth of more facial and body hair than average. Persistent anovulation, however, is often accompanied by slightly elevated production of male hormones. Approximately 70% of women with persistent anovulation also have problems with hirsutism (1). Read the section on polycystic ovary disease (a cause of persistent anovulation) in Chapter 40 for more information on evaluation and treatment of hirsutism.

REFERENCE

1. Speroff L, Glass RH, Kase NG: *Clinical Gynecologic Endocrinology and Infertility* (ed 3). Baltimore: Williams & Wilkins, 1983.

33

❖

Absence of
Menstrual Periods
(Amenorrhea)

If your menstrual periods fail to start, or disappear once begun, it is absolutely natural to be anxious. Unintended pregnancy may be your leading fear, or a serious internal disorder that might impair your health or future fertility. Once medical evaluation provides assurance about these issues, however, you may be tempted to ignore the problem. Menstrual bleeding is something that you may be just as happy to do without. Don't do it.

Prolonged absence of periods can mean your normal hormone patterns are seriously disrupted. You will need to have regular exams and tests to monitor your hormones, and possibly hormone treatment as well. Persistently abnormal hormone levels, if untreated, can put you at risk for serious consequences later. If your lack of periods is being caused by hormone levels that are consistently low, with little or no estrogen production in your ovaries, then you may lose bone density and face serious illness and deformity from the fragile bones of osteoporosis within just a few years. If your estrogen production is consistently high, this too can block cyclic patterns, and in the future you will face excess risk for uterine cancer, and possibly breast cancer as well.

If you are between 15 and 45 and are not having menstrual periods, the first cause you and your clinician will think about is pregnancy; an examination and pregnancy test will be the first step in your evaluation. Almost every woman can expect to miss a few periods in her lifetime for reasons other than pregnancy, however. If unusual stress or illness has temporarily interrupted your hormone cycles, your periods should return spontaneously within a month or two. Short episodes of amenorrhea ("a" means without; "menorrhea" means menstrual flow) are so common that your clinician will probably not recommend any diagnostic tests unless:

• You have missed three or more periods in a row
• You have other symptoms such as breast milk production, headache, vision changes, difficulty with coordination, or growth of body hair
• You are 16 years old and have never had a menstrual period
• You are 14 years old, have never had a menstrual period, and have not had any breast development or pubic hair growth

Long lapses between periods, lasting six months or even more, are quite common with persistent physical stress. Women who have problems with anorexia nervosa, or some other serious medical problem, may find that periods vanish when symptoms of their other problem are severe. This is particularly likely if weight loss is part of the picture. Women athletes, too, may find that a serious competitive training schedule causes periods to stop. Even though these causes are common and quite predictable, **the same rules for evaluation and treatment of amenorrhea still apply.** Risks for later consequences are involved no matter what is causing your hormone abnormality.

Amenorrhea means total absence of menstrual bleeding, not one drop. The evaluation steps described in this chapter are specifically for amenorrhea. Hormone abnormalities, and causes similar to the ones that can stop periods completely, may also lead to irregular menstrual patterns or a marked change in the amount of bleeding you have—less or more. These problems are discussed in Chapter 32. Evaluation steps for amenorrhea are described in the last section of this chapter.

Causes and
Treatment of Amenorrhea

Menstrual bleeding may be absent because of problems in the uterus, cervix, vaginal opening, ovaries, pituitary gland (located in the center of the brain), or the brain itself (hypothalamus). (You may want to review the hormone cycle that governs menstrual periods. See Chapter 2.)

When abnormal hormone patterns are the cause of amenorrhea, other signs of hormone disruption may also occur. Breast milk secretions (galactorrhea), problems with acne, a marked change in hair growth, and—more rare—a change in voice or sex drive or enlargement of the clitoris are symptoms your clinician will want to know about.

ABSENCE OF OVULATION

The most common cause of amenorrhea is absence of ovulation. When ovulation does not occur, your ovary does not produce progesterone; and without progesterone, menstrual bleeding may cease or become irregular. Absence of ovulation is not directly harmful and is quite common. Some women ovulate only occasionally throughout their entire menstrual years.

Lack of ovulation is an immediate problem if you are trying to become pregnant. In this situation, your clinician can prescribe drugs to induce ovulation (see Chapter 10).

Even if you are not trying to conceive, however, you will need ongoing treatment. Without ovulation, your ovaries produce only estrogen, which exposes your body to a steady continuous level of estrogen. If your estrogen level is moderate or high, then you are risking excessive stimulation of the uterine lining (adenomatous hyperplasia) or uterine cancer. Researchers also believe that high estrogen levels increase your breast cancer risk. For this reason, your clinician may recommend monthly treatment with synthetic progestin pills such as medroxyprogesterone acetate (Provera) to interrupt the steady estrogen level. A common treatment pattern is Provera, 10 mg daily for 10 to 14 days of each month.

If your estrogen level is moderate or high, then you will have menstrual bleeding beginning two to seven days after each batch of progestin pills. **If you have bleeding at any other time, your clinician will want to know about it.** Unexpected bleeding could mean that you already have uterine hyperplasia, or it could mean that your body has restarted its own cycle and that ovulation has occurred. If you have had problems with abnormal bleeding, or your clinician suspects that you have already had prolonged estrogen exposure, then endometrial biopsy to check for hyperplasia may be recommended before you begin treatment. (See Chapter 4 for more on endometrial biopsy.)

You do need to continue with birth control if you do not want to be pregnant. Ovulation can occur at any time and you will have no way to predict its return in advance.

If you fail to have bleeding after taking your progestin pills, your clinician will want to know. Lack of bleeding probably means that your estrogen level has dropped—and is now too low. This hormone pattern most often is caused by problems in the brain (hypothalamus).

PROBLEMS IN THE BRAIN

Absent periods are often caused by a problem in the brain itself (hypothalamic amenorrhea). When the amount of hormone released from your hypothalamus is too low, the pituitary gland is not stimulated, and your ovaries in turn are not stimulated to produce normal estrogen and progesterone. There is no direct test for hypothalamic amenorrhea. Your clinician can confirm this diagnosis only by testing you for other causes of amenorrhea and determining that none of the others is present.

Illness, physical or mental stress, travel, a new job, rapid or extreme weight loss, beginning college, entering prison, and other stressful events can suppress hypothalamic hormones.

Amenorrhea that occurs after you stop using birth control Pills is usually caused by hypothalamic hormone suppression. If your menstrual periods do not return spontaneously within three to six months after you stop taking Pills, see your clinician for a full evaluation. The connection between your Pills and your missed periods could be only a coincidence. Also, you will need to consider treatment if the problem lasts six months or more.

Suddenly I stopped having periods when I was the healthiest I've ever been! I was doing training runs every day, running races lots of weekends, and swimming when the weather was bad. Was my body telling me something? Was I pushing too hard?

—WOMAN RUNNER, 28

Hypothalamic amenorrhea is a fairly common problem for women athletes. Competitive sports or physically demanding disciplines such as ballet are stressors and are also associated with a low body fat level. When the amount of body fat drops below approximately 20% of body weight, the likelihood of amenorrhea is substantial. A woman in this situation may find that her menstrual cycles cease whenever she drops below a specific critical weight.

Critical weight depends on overall body size, and there is no precise formula to predict it. For one woman, dropping below 112 pounds might be the limit; for another it might be 98 pounds.

Anorexia nervosa is another increasingly common cause of hypothalamic amenorrhea. Rapid weight loss, low body fat percentage, and sustained body weight below a critical level lead to low hypothalamic hormone production.

Sometimes, disappearance of menstrual periods is the first clear evidence for the woman or her family that disciplined attention to controlling weight is slipping toward the serious pattern of anorexia. Women age 10 to 30 are at greatest risk. Other signs that should be a warning include:

- Weight loss of 25%, or weight 15% below normal range
- Preoccupation with food and/or eating, such as hoarding, or markedly peculiar eating habits
- Inability to recognize or admit that weight and/or eating patterns are not ideal
- Conviction that strict weight control is necessary because of serious fatness problems, despite a normal or slender body structure
- Episodes of binging (often in secret) and/or vomiting
- Use of laxatives
- Excessive physical activity (hyperactivity)
- Excessive water drinking
- Appearance of fine, pale hair in areas previously free of hair

Anorexia is a severe illness, and early treatment is the best hope. It most often affects young women with high aspirations and every social and economic reason to expect success, and so is especially tragic. Evaluation of the amenorrhea itself should be completed even when anorexia is suspected or already evident. Treatment may be needed for the hormone deficit as well as psychotherapy to work on the anorexia problem.

No matter what the cause, hypothalamic amenorrhea means that hormone levels are low. Pituitary hormone production is depressed, and estrogen production by the ovary is depressed. If low estrogen persists, then symptoms and problems typical of menopause, such as vaginal dryness, are likely to occur. Particularly important is the possibility of significant loss in bone density and strength (osteoporosis).

A young woman athlete who begins losing bone density in her twenties is likely to encounter very serious medical problems as a result. Despite excellent exercise and diet, significant bone loss among athletes with amenorrhea has been demonstrated (1). Bone density below normal has also been documented for anorexia patients (2).

If hypothalamic amenorrhea persists more than a few months, estrogen replacement therapy is essential. Cyclic treatment similar to that sometimes prescribed for menopausal women is the most common approach. Young women need a slightly higher estrogen dose, however. Conjugated estrogen (Premarin), 1.25 mg daily for the first 25 days of each month, with medroxyprogesterone acetate (Provera), 10 mg daily added for the last 14 estrogen days, is a typical regimen. Menstrual bleeding should occur sometime during the five or six no-drug days at the end of each month. If bleeding occurs at any other time, the cyclic hormones should be stopped to see if spontaneous menstrual cycling has resumed. This cyclic therapy does not provide effective birth control protection. If contraception is a goal, then birth control Pills are a reasonable choice. Regular low-dose birth control Pills provide sufficient estrogen to protect bone density.

LOW PRODUCTION OF THYROID HORMONE

Insufficient hormone production by the thyroid gland (hypothyroidism) can cause amenorrhea. If production of thyroid hormone is low, the pituitary gland increases its production of thyroid-stimulating hormone (TSH) in an attempt to compensate. High levels of TSH, in turn, are often accompanied by high levels of prolactin hormone. This overproduction can cause amenorrhea and sometimes breast milk secretion as well. Prolactin stimulates breast milk production. Testing for thyroid hormone alone may not be sufficient since high TSH, compensating for thyroid insufficiency, may be maintaining normal output levels from the thyroid gland despite its impairment. This is a rare cause of amenorrhea, but worth attention because a simple blood test for TSH can detect it, and treatment with thyroid hormone easily and promptly cures the whole problem.

STRUCTURAL ABNORMALITIES

If you have never had any periods, your clinician will look for structural abnormalities during your exam, such as a hymen that completely closes the entrance to your vagina (imperforate hymen) or an obstruction in your cervical canal. These problems are easily corrected by minor surgery or by dilating your cervical opening. Other structural abnormalities, such as a missing uterus or missing vagina, are extremely rare, and would probably be evident at the time of your first pelvic examination.

PROBLEMS WITH THE UTERINE LINING

If treatment with estrogen and progestin fails to trigger bleeding, your clinician will know that you have an **unresponsive uterus**. This condition usually means that your uterine lining tissue has been scarred or damaged by infection and/or scraping, such as with a D&C (see Chapter 47). Your clinician may call this Asherman's syndrome. Regrowth of uterine lining can sometimes be stimulated by hormone treatment. Your clinician may also consider hysteroscopy, to look inside your uterus through a narrow lighted instrument. With hysteroscopy it may be possible to locate and remove tiny strands of scar tissue present in the uterine lining (hysteroscopy is described in Chapter 46). In some cases a soft inflatable bag may be inserted temporarily to hold your uterine walls apart so that lining tissue has an opportunity to cover the inner walls more completely.

PITUITARY GLAND TUMOR

A tumor in your pituitary gland can interfere with normal hormone production and stop your periods. Very small tumors are quite common, and usually cause no problems whatsoever. Often they are discovered, or suspected, when amenorrhea or breast milk production (galactorrhea) occurs because of higher than normal levels of prolactin hormone produced by the tumor cells. Even if prolactin is high, the tumor may be so small that it cannot be identified. A larger tumor, however, may also cause symptoms such as headache or vision problems. Pituitary tumors are almost always benign (not cancerous) and grow quite slowly.

One of the main purposes of medical evaluation for your amenorrhea is to be certain that you do not have a pituitary tumor large enough to risk damage to nearby structures in the brain. If your prolactin level is elevated, therefore, you will need to be faithful about follow-up. You will also need an x-ray of the pituitary area ("coned down view of the sella turcica") initially and then at least once a year until your problem is resolved. If the x-ray is not normal, your clinician will recommend a CAT scan (computerized axial tomography) to pinpoint the tumor and determine its size.

If the tumor is large, your clinician will probably refer you to a specialist in endocrinology, neurology, or neurosurgery. Your treatment, though, is likely to begin with an oral medication called bromocriptine (Parlodel). This drug effectively blocks prolactin production and also causes the tumor to shrink. In most cases, milk production and breast pain rapidly resolve and normal menstrual cycles, with ovulation, return promptly. Treatment with bromocriptine, including side effects and risks, is discussed in Chapter 10. In some cases, drug treatment is all that is needed. Surgery to remove the tumor, however, may also be an option.

If the tumor is small, then you may not need treatment for the tumor unless you are having problems with breast pain or are trying to become pregnant. You will need to have prolactin tests and an x-ray every year, and you may also need to have estrogen and progestin hormone replacement to protect your bones.

MENOPAUSE OR PREMATURE MENOPAUSE

At menopause your ovaries stop responding to hormones from the pituitary gland. If ovary response stops before age 45, you may have premature menopause, and there is no known treatment. In rare cases, ovary failure can be caused by diseases such as diabetes, rheumatoid arthritis, and thyroiditis. If this is the situation, then resumption of normal ovary function and even pregnancy is possible in some instances. If you are younger than 30 or would like to be pregnant, your clinician may recommend further evaluation. Also, you will need hormone replacement therapy. Premature menopause is very rare.

DELAYED PUBERTY

Delayed puberty means that your ovaries fail to become responsive to pituitary stimulation at a normal age, and this condition is a possibility if you have not yet begun to have menstrual periods by age 16. Normal age ranges for puberty events are shown in Chapter 2. Late puberty may be simply a family pattern, but evaluation will be needed to be sure that rare problems like chromosome abnormalities (see the following section), birth defects involving the ovaries or uterus, or abnormalities in the brain centers that control cyclic hormones are not responsible for the delay.

Evaluation is likely to start with a review of your medical and family history and a physical exam. Initial laboratory tests will also be needed, including a blood test for the pituitary hormones FSH and LH, which are responsible for stimulating normal ovary function at puberty, as well as x-rays to document bone age, and skull x-rays to detect malformation or tumor in the brain. Further evaluation depends on the initial findings, and referral to a specialist in endocrinology may be needed.

ABNORMAL CHROMOSOME (GENE) STRUCTURE

Abnormal chromosome (gene) structure can result in ovaries that fail to produce estrogen and progesterone despite normal pituitary hormone stimulation. Your clinician will be particularly concerned about this possibility if you have not yet started periods by age 16, or if you do not have breast and pubic hair development by age 14. Chromosome abnormalities are rare and require individualized evaluation and treatment.

Steps in Evaluation and Follow-up

Your clinician will probably follow a fairly standard step-by-step procedure to determine the cause of your amenorrhea (see Illustration 33-1).

Your evaluation will start with a review of your history and symptoms, and a physical exam. Serious medical problems such as kidney failure, cystic fibrosis, and colitis can cause irregular menstrual cycles or amenorrhea, and so can illicit drugs, especially heroin (3). Your clinician will need to know about any drugs or medications you are taking. Some prescription drugs used for psychiatric problems (including Compazine, Stelazine, and Thorazine), Temaril, used for skin problems, and the blood pressure medication reserpine can cause elevated prolactin levels. High prolactin also occurs normally as a result of intense nipple stimulation; prolactin is high during pregnancy, and breastfeeding triggers a surge in prolactin with each feeding.

Your clinician will also need to know about your recent dietary habits. Weight loss, malnutrition, and excessive dietary carotene may be significant. A vegetarian diet with restricted calories is especially likely to cause abnormal cyclic hormone patterns (4). High carotene levels, from a daily intake of about 1 pound of carrots, was found to be the cause of amenorrhea for nine women in a recent study, and periods resumed when carotene intake was reduced (5).

Assuming your exam is normal, and you are not pregnant, then your first evaluation steps will be simple blood tests for thyroid-stimulating hormone (TSH) and prolactin, along with progestin pills or an injection to see whether bleeding can be triggered easily. If you are having breast milk production, your clinician will also order x-rays early in the evaluation process to check for pituitary tumor.

Progestin pills or an injection, called a progestin challenge test, is quite likely to induce bleeding within two to seven days. If you happen to be ovulating spontaneously just at the time you take progestin, then bleeding will begin after 14 days. Anything more than a few drops is a positive result, and means that your problem is absence of ovulation. If you have no bleeding at all, then further tests will be necessary to pinpoint the problem.

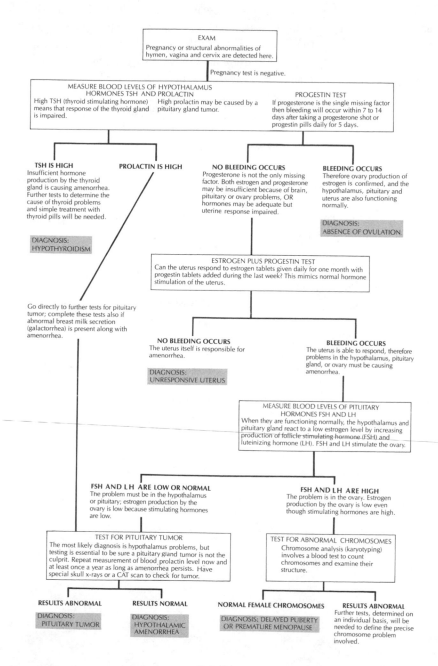

EXAM
Pregnancy or structural abnormalities of hymen, vagina and cervix are detected here.

Pregnancy test is negative.

MEASURE BLOOD LEVELS OF HYPOTHALAMUS HORMONES TSH AND PROLACTIN
High TSH (thyroid stimulating hormone) means that response of the thyroid gland is impaired.   High prolactin may be caused by a pituitary gland tumor.

PROGESTIN TEST
If progesterone is the single missing factor then bleeding will occur within 7 to 14 days after taking a progesterone shot or progestin pills daily for 5 days.

TSH IS HIGH
Insufficient hormone production by the thyroid gland is causing amenorrhea. Further tests to determine the cause of thyroid problems and simple treatment with thyroid pills will be needed.

DIAGNOSIS:
HYPOTHYROIDISM

PROLACTIN IS HIGH

NO BLEEDING OCCURS
Progesterone is not the only missing factor. Both estrogen and progesterone may be insufficient because of brain, pituitary or ovary problems, OR hormones may be adequate but uterine response impaired.

BLEEDING OCCURS
Therefore ovary production of estrogen is confirmed, and the hypothalamus, pituitary and uterus are also functioning normally.

DIAGNOSIS:
ABSENCE OF OVULATION

ESTROGEN PLUS PROGESTIN TEST
Can the uterus respond to estrogen tablets given daily for one month with progestin tablets added during the last week? This mimics normal hormone stimulation of the uterus.

Go directly to further tests for pituitary tumor; complete these tests also if abnormal breast milk secretion (galactorrhea) is present along with amenorrhea.

NO BLEEDING OCCURS
The uterus itself is responsible for amenorrhea.

DIAGNOSIS:
UNRESPONSIVE UTERUS

BLEEDING OCCURS
The uterus is able to respond, therefore problems in the hypothalamus, pituitary gland, or ovary must be causing amenorrhea.

MEASURE BLOOD LEVELS OF PITUITARY HORMONES FSH AND LH
When they are functioning normally, the hypothalamus and pituitary gland react to a low estrogen level by increasing production of follicle stimulating hormone (FSH) and luteinizing hormone (LH). FSH and LH stimulate the ovary.

FSH AND LH ARE LOW OR NORMAL
The problem must be in the hypothalamus or pituitary; estrogen production by the ovary is low because stimulating hormones are low.

FSH AND LH ARE HIGH
The problem is in the ovary. Estrogen production by the ovary is low even though stimulating hormones are high.

TEST FOR PITUITARY TUMOR
The most likely diagnosis is hypothalamus problems, but testing is essential to be sure a pituitary gland tumor is not the culprit. Repeat measurement of blood prolactin level now and at least once a year as long as amenorrhea persists. Have special skull x-rays or a CAT scan to check for tumor.

TEST FOR ABNORMAL CHROMOSOMES
Chromosome analysis (karyotyping) involves a blood test to count chromosomes and examine their structure.

RESULTS ABNORMAL
DIAGNOSIS:
PITUITARY TUMOR

RESULTS NORMAL
DIAGNOSIS:
HYPOTHALAMIC
AMENORRHEA

NORMAL FEMALE CHROMOSOMES
DIAGNOSIS: DELAYED PUBERTY OR PREMATURE MENOPAUSE

RESULTS ABNORMAL
Further tests, determined on an individual basis, will be needed to define the precise chromosome problem involved.

ILLUSTRATION 33-1   Your clinician will follow a step-by-step procedure for evaluating amenorrhea.

Thorough evaluation of amenorrhea is absolutely essential. It is a fairly complicated problem, and you may need to be patient and persistent. Be sure that you have all the necessary tests and that you understand your test results and recommended treatment. The main goal of evaluation is to be sure that you don't have a pituitary tumor, and to determine whether hormone treatment is needed to protect your bones. If you want to be pregnant now, then further treatment to induce ovulation will be needed (see Chapter 10), otherwise ovulation and regular cycles are not essential as long as you are faithful about follow-up and replacement hormones.

Remember that you will need reevaluation at least once every 12 months as long as amenorrhea persists. A pituitary tumor can be very tiny and can grow so slowly that it is detected only after several repeated examinations. And remember to **think about pregnancy**. Without normal cycles you are not likely to conceive, but **in some cases ovulation returns with no advance warning**. If you do not want to be pregnant, then good birth control protection makes sense.

REFERENCES

1. Drinkwater BL, Nilson K, Chesnut CH III, et al: Bone mineral content of amenorrheic and eumenorrheic athletes. *New England Journal of Medicine* 311:277–281, 1984.
2. Rigotti NA, Nussbaum SR, Herzog DB, et al: Osteoporosis in women with anorexia nervosa. *New England Journal of Medicine* 311:1601–1606, 1984.
3. Neinstein LS: Menstrual dysfunction in pathophysiologic states. *Western Journal of Medicine* 143:476–484, 1985.
4. Pirke KM, Schweiger U, Laessle R, et al: Dieting influences the menstrual cycle: Vegetarian versus nonvegetarian diet. *Fertility and Sterility* 46:1083–1088, 1986.
5. Kemmann E, Pasquale SA, Skaf R: Amenorrhea associated with carotenemia. *Journal of the American Medical Association* 249:926–929, 1983.

34

Menopause

If you grew up in India, China, or Africa, you would probably believe that the good life begins at menopause. In many cultures, women past the childbearing years are respected and revered for their wisdom; younger women take over child care (at last), and relatives look to older women for advice on all important family matters. Older American women aren't always so fortunate. In our youth-worshiping culture, some women even dread menopause.

Many female mammals bear young until they die, and reproduction is often the cause of death. Ours is an unusual species in that female reproductive function ceases well before the end of life. If indeed evolutionary changes happen for a reason, then we can assume that nature intends for postmenopausal women to have a significant role in our culture; we Americans may have some important lessons to learn from other cultures.

Menopause is a normal process, not a medical problem or disease, but many women do have at least some troublesome symptoms associated with it. Common symptoms and their relationship to hormone changes that your body undergoes are discussed in the first section of this chapter. Menopause also brings new health priorities. Some of the new and essential health tasks after menopause are:

Protecting Health Against Serious Disease. The overall risk of serious illnesses like heart disease and cancer increases substantially after age 40 or 50. Your own preventive health efforts take on more importance, and new routine health screening tests will be needed. Read Chapter 7 for specific recommendations.

Protecting Bone Health.   Good calcium balance to insure bone strength is a lifelong necessity. For many women, however, the lower hormone levels of menopause mean serious jeopardy to their bones. Active steps will be needed. Read the section "Maintaining Strong Bones" for preventive recommendations.

Weighing the Personal Pros and Cons of Hormone Treatment.   Hormone treatment is discussed at length in this chapter because it is both complex and controversial. Many women, however, find that they can manage their own menopausal problems, and others may need to consider alternatives to estrogen.

Finding Postmenopausal Zest.   PMZ, postmenopausal zest, is a wonderful health concept developed by Sadja Greenwood, M.D., in her book on menopause (see "Suggested Reading"). It belongs on the list of essential health tasks because PMZ building blocks—nutrition, exercise, and personal stress management—are essential defenses against inevitable adversities during the second half of life. When friends or family members are seriously ill, or major changes occur in your life, your own health risks are high too. Knowing your personal route to PMZ will help protect your health. Also, you are almost certain to feel better, and to accomplish more of whatever you want to do.

The most creative force in the world is the menopausal woman with zest.

—MARGARET MEAD

Physical and Hormone Changes of Menopause

The transition from the reproductive phase of a woman's life cycle into the postreproductive phase is called the **climacteric**. Menopause, the cessation of menstrual periods, is the most obvious event, but many other changes occur as well.

Approximately 50% of women undergo menopause at or before age 51, although the normal age range is fairly wide, 45 to 55. The timing of menopause is not predictable. You may follow the same pattern that your mother and sisters experience(d), or your menopause may be earlier or later. Factors like age at the onset of periods or pregnancy history do not correlate with menopause age, although smoking is linked to earlier menopause. Smoking speeds up the body's breakdown of estrogen so that women who smoke have lower overall estrogen levels than do nonsmokers both before and after menopause (1). **Climacteric changes begin considerably before** menopause. A significant decline in fertility occurs in the mid 40s. The reason for this decline is not known, but a decrease in the number of maturing ovary follicles and a gradual decrease in ovarian estrogen production also occur at about this time.

Menstrual changes heralding menopause vary from individual to individual. Some women experience several years of irregular menstrual cycles or prolonged intervals between periods. For other women, the changes in menstrual patterns are more abrupt: previously normal and predictable monthly cycles are followed by complete cessation of bleeding. Women who undergo premature menopause because of surgical removal of the ovaries have extremely precipitous hormone changes, and symptoms related to menopause are often quite severe.

As the climacteric nears completion, ovarian estrogen production declines to low levels. The ovary is no longer responsive to follicle-stimulating hormone (FSH) produced by the pituitary gland in the brain. Release of pituitary FSH, therefore, rises to high levels because its output is triggered by low levels of estrogen. Pituitary release of FSH's companion, luteinizing hormone (LH), rises after menstrual periods cease, and both FSH and LH levels remain elevated throughout the postmenopausal years.

Before menopause, developing egg follicles in the ovary are the source of most of a woman's estrogen. Production of this type of estrogen, called estradiol, falls to about one tenth of its previous level during the climacteric transition. Estrone, another form of estrogen, assumes greater importance. Estrone is manufactured by many body tissues, including body fat cells. The raw material required for estrone production is a precursor called androstenedione, which is produced throughout life by the ovaries and by the adrenal glands. Even after menopause, therefore, the ovaries continue to contribute to estrogen production (2). Overall, the level of estrogen is high enough so that approximately 15% of women continue to have evidence of an estrogen effect on the vaginal lining, and remain quite free of the low estrogen symptoms described in the next section.

COMMON SYMPTOMS AND PROBLEMS

In the past, low estrogen levels and "menopause syndrome" were accepted as the causes of a host of problems, ranging from hot flashes to irrationality and decrepitude. Research, however, has shown that estrogen lack can be unequivocally blamed for only certain specific problems. **Problems that are clearly improved by estrogen replacement therapy include hot flashes, thinning (atrophy) and dryness of vaginal and urinary tract lining tissue, and loss of bone strength caused by osteoporosis.** Women, of course, are quite likely to notice many other changes during the climacteric years. Aging is responsible for some of these changes, and some may originate in personal, social, and economic stresses also common during this phase of life. And some no doubt will be linked by future researchers to as yet unappreciated hormone effects.

Hot Flashes. The occurrence of hot flashes (flushes) is an almost universal symptom of the climacteric. A flush usually begins as a sudden wave of heat in the trunk or chest that radiates to the head, arms, and legs. Perspiration and reddening of neck and facial skin may accompany the heat wave. For some women, flushes are brief and infrequent. For others, they can be severe enough and frequent enough to be disabling, interrupting sleep at night or interfering with work and normal daytime activities.

Skin temperature and heart rate both rise during a hot flash, and although episodes often seem random and unprovoked, many women find that environmental heat, from heavy clothing or a stuffy room, for example, can trigger attacks. Certain medical problems including excessive thyroid activity, night fevers, and rare tumors can cause symptoms similar to hot flashes, so laboratory tests may be needed to confirm that menopause is the culprit if your suspected hot flashes do not follow a typical menopause pattern.

Estrogen hormone treatment is effective in stopping menopause hot flashes but the actual cause of flashes is not known. The brain centers responsible for regulation of body temperature, however, are located near the centers responsible for hormone regulation.

Flushes are usually most bothersome immediately before and after cessation of menstrual periods. They tend to subside in frequency and severity as the body adjusts to decreased hormone levels. Occasional flushes can occur even decades after menopause, but it is unusual for women to report serious problems with flushes after the first few years.

Vaginal Dryness and Urethral Changes. The lining of the vagina is a specialized mucous membrane similar to the lining of the mouth. It is very elastic and its lining cells exude lubrication during sexual arousal. The vaginal walls and the skin of the vulva and urinary opening (urethra) respond directly to estrogen stimulation. When estrogen is low the vaginal lining becomes thinner and loses some of its elasticity and lubricant-producing capability. These changes, called atrophy, often result in vaginal dryness that is especially noticeable during intercourse. Dryness can result in greater susceptibility to injury, vaginal irritation, and infection.

Similar changes occur in the lining of the urethra and bladder and may result in irritation and the loss of elastic support of the urethral muscles. These changes can cause persistent urinary frequency and urgency (needing to urinate often and needing to hurry to the bathroom as soon as the urge begins), and can aggravate problems with bladder control, such as involuntary urine loss with coughing or sneezing. Unlike hot flashes, the onset of vaginal and urethral changes is usually gradual and often persists, becoming more severe throughout the menopausal years.

Changes in Sexual Functioning. In addition to the vaginal changes described above, aging, hormone levels, and frequency of intercourse all are believed to influence changes in sexual functioning during the second half of life. For both women and men, the arousal response tends to become slower with age. For many women this is an advantage, and can allow more ample time for effective stimulation and arousal before attempting intercourse.

Physical changes linked to aging include a loss of fat and supporting tissues that reduces the size of the vaginal lips. Labial swelling that occurs with arousal is less evident. The length and width of the vagina decrease with age, and the cervix and uterus also become smaller. Changes in sensations during arousal or lovemaking may result, and new ways to achieve effective sexual pleasure may be needed. Exercises to maintain or strengthen the muscles that surround the vaginal and anal openings may also be helpful, because strong muscles may facilitate achieving arousal and orgasm. Kegel's exercises, excellent for this purpose, are described later in this chapter.

Sexual desire is affected by hormones as well as many other factors. Male hormones such as testosterone generally increase sexual desire, and may also help maintain muscle strength. So for women, the small amount of testosterone produced by the ovaries before and after menopause may be important.

Birth Control. As menopause approaches, pregnancy is less and less likely. Nevertheless, you will probably want to continue with birth control until you can be certain that menopause has occurred. A woman who has had fairly regular menstrual periods in the past, who is having other symptoms of menopause such as hot flashes, and who is in the menopause age range (45 to 55) can reasonably assume that she is no longer fertile when six months have elapsed since her last menstrual period. If you are not certain about menopause and want to stop using birth control, then your clinician can arrange a blood test for FSH. A high FSH level indicates that your ovaries are no longer producing eggs.

Bone Strength Loss. Osteoporosis, literally porous bones, is a common and important health problem for women after menopause. Gradual loss of bone density is a normal aging change and begins 10 or 20 years before menopause. Density loss, however, is accelerated when estrogen levels drop.

Loss of bone density results in fragile bones and an increased risk of fracture. Fractures commonly occur in the spine (vertebrae), and can cause decreasing height and vertebral deformity, the "dowager's hump." Fractures of the wrist are very common. An increased risk for hip fracture is especially important because serious or even fatal complications are linked to hip fracture. Recommendations for preserving healthy bones are discussed later in this chapter.

Other Problems. It is not known whether nervousness, depression, headache, anxiety, and memory loss can be caused or aggravated by decreasing hormone levels. Treating these problems with estrogen has produced no better results than has treatment with a placebo (tablets that contain no drugs); therefore, estrogen deficiency per se probably is not the sole cause of these problems. It is possible, however, that hormone changes may contribute. Hormone changes that occur at puberty and recur cyclically throughout the reproductive years are known to influence emotional equilibrium. Also, symptoms that definitely are caused by hormone deficiency, such as hot flashes and vaginal discomfort with intercourse, may secondarily cause significant psychic stress. Sleep disturbed every night by hot flashes or relationship problems because of sex difficulties can be real and serious sources of anxiety and depression, and hormone treatment that corrects these problems is likely to result in an improved sense of well-being.

Stress at home or at work, or difficulties resulting from a partner's adjustment to transitions in his own life cycle, can also affect emotional well-being profoundly. Cultural values about aging likewise have an influence on emotional health.

A reasonable conclusion is that the **emotional problems attributed to hormone deficiency probably stem from a combination of factors**: hormonal, personal, and cultural. Most women feel the effects of at least some of these factors, but the majority are able to cope smoothly with the transition to the postreproductive years and require little or no assistance. It is extremely rare to encounter serious psychiatric disability associated with menopause in a woman who has not had previous psychiatric disease and does not have other personal or situational factors likely to cause severe emotional stress.

I only had hot flashes for a few months. Our sex life was fine once I started using vaginal lubricant so I wouldn't be so dry. I think you have to be philosophical about getting older. What was it Maurice Chevalier said? "It isn't so bad when you consider the alternatives"? That's really true, I think.

If you enjoy being alive—and I do—it is a little saddening to look in the mirror and realize you are aging. But since nothing is going to turn back the clock, I concentrate on the good things: more time for my own projects now that the children are grown; a sense of my own hard-won wisdom. The last few years I have felt quite peaceful and contented. I think life's unavoidable changes are much harder when you resist them.

—WOMAN, 62

Maintaining Strong Bones

Bone density and strength are at their peak during the young adult years. Gradual loss of bone density occurs for both men and women beginning at about age 40. Whether

TABLE 34-1

HIP FRACTURES: NUMBER EACH YEAR FOR 100,000 (WHITE) WOMEN AND MEN

AGE	WOMEN	MEN
30–39	4	14
40–49	28	24
50–59	70	33
60–69	195	92
70+	1,087	463

SOURCE: Adapted from Farmer ME, White, LR, Brody JA, et al: Race and sex differences in hip fracture incidence. *American Journal of Public Health* 74:1374–1380, 1984.

or not osteoporosis will result depends on the rate of loss and on the maximum bone mass the individual has initially. Men, and also black women, have relatively greater initial bone mass than do nonblack women. For them, osteoporosis is much less common, and not likely to be significant until the 70s or 80s. The rate of loss depends on many factors including hormones, diet, exercise, smoking habits, heredity, and kidney function.

Osteoporosis means that bone density is so low and bone structure so porous that the bones are fragile, and can fracture or crush under conditions of normal skeletal stress. A minor bump or fall may be enough to break a bone in the arm or leg; vertebral bones supporting the spinal column may even crush spontaneously.

Because low estrogen levels are an important cause of rapid bone strength loss, women after menopause are the victims of a disproportionate share of fractures. Hip fractures are especially serious. Complications of hip fractures often lead to permanent disability, and death rates within the first year are at least 15% and may be as high as 50% for older age groups or women with additional medical problems. Table 34-1 shows hip fracture risks for women and men.

Spine compression fractures, shown in Illustration 34-1, are even more common; as many as 25% of white women have at least some compression by age 60. A minor vertebral compression fracture can occur silently, with no noticeable symptoms except gradual loss of height. When a more extensive vertebral compression fracture occurs, back pain is likely to be the primary symptom. Typically, pain is initially severe in the mid-lower back, and increases with bending over. Then it subsides gradually after four to six weeks unless or until additional fractures occur.

Normal bone remodeling is out of balance in osteoporosis. Low estrogen leads to increased bone resorption, and the formation of new bone mineral is not sufficient to

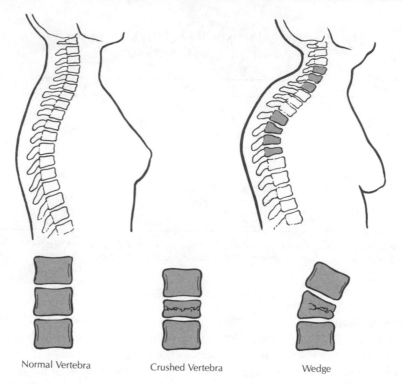

Normal Vertebra   Crushed Vertebra   Wedge

ILLUSTRATION 34-1   As vertebral bones crush or fracture to a wedge shape, a permanent curved deformity of the spine develops and height is lost. Multiple fractures result in dowager's hump.

keep up. The outer dimensions and cell structure of the bone remain normal unless fractures occur, but without enough calcium bone mineral, bone tissue is porous and fragile.

CALCIUM BALANCE

Throughout life new calcium is deposited in bone and, at the same time, calcium is resorbed from bone into the bloodstream. This is a continuous process, governed by hormones and many other factors including the amount of calcium available and the bones' own response to weight bearing or stress that stimulates bone-building cells.

Calcium-controlling hormones, principally calcitonin and parathyroid hormone, are responsible for maintaining a steady level of calcium in the bloodstream. A correct blood calcium level is essential for proper function of all body cells. If the amount of calcium entering the body through absorption in the gut is not sufficient to maintain normal calcium blood levels, then bone resorption is increased to provide the necessary bloodstream calcium. Bones are robbed of calcium to meet the needs of the rest of the body. If dietary calcium intake is greater than calcium need, the excess calcium is eliminated in the stool and urine. Measurement of the blood calcium level, therefore, is not helpful in assessing overall calcium balance or bone health. Blood and urine tests to measure calcium level may be needed, however, to determine whether parathyroid hormone function is normal.

Aging and low estrogen levels are believed to affect calcium balance in several ways. Calcium absorption in the intestine may be impaired and loss through the urine increased; estrogen may also act directly to increase calcitonin hormone release and inhibit bone resorption. When estrogen levels are low, bone resorption is more rapid than bone rebuilding and a gradual overall loss in bone strength results. The dietary intake of calcium also tends to be low for older women, and exposure to sunlight is often limited. About 15 to 30 minutes of sunlight daily is needed for production of vitamin D in the skin which is essential for calcium absorption. Calcium robbers include a diet high in protein, or sodium (salt), and caffeine, nicotine, and aluminum-containing antacids.

After menopause, women require approximately 1,500 mg of calcium daily to maintain calcium balance (1,000 mg for women who are taking estrogen) (3). Surveys show that a typical diet for women this age contains only 400 to 600 mg of calcium. Bone loss is inevitable unless this discrepancy is corrected by increasing dietary calcium or by taking calcium supplements.

Dairy products are the main source of calcium in a typical American diet. Milk contains approximately 300 mg of calcium per 8-ounce cup and "fortified" milk also provides 100 International Units (IU) of vitamin D per cup. Sufficient milk to meet daily calcium needs, five 8-ounce glasses, is likely to mean more calories devoted to dairy products than most women can tolerate, so nonfat milk is a preferable option. Intolerance to dairy products, caused by a deficiency in lactase enzyme, which is essential for digestion of milk, is a common problem. If you have lactase deficiency, you are likely to experience diarrhea, cramps, and gas after eating dairy products. Finding other food sources of calcium is one option (see Table 34-2). For most women, however, taking calcium supplements may be the simplest way to meet calcium needs. Supplements are available without prescription (see Table 34-3). Be sure to spread out your calcium throughout the day and take one of your doses at bedtime to help counteract loss during sleep. Calcium supplements at a dose of 1,000 to 1,500 mg daily are safe unless you have serious kidney disease or rare parathyroid gland problems. If you have any doubts, or are taking other medications already, talk to your clinician before you begin.

EXERCISE

Regular exercise that exerts forceful movement, pull, or stress on your body's long bones is essential for bone health. Bone-building cells are stimulated by exercise, and even temporary immobilization causes significant temporary bone density loss. Re-

TABLE 34-2
CALCIUM IN COMMON FOODS

FOOD	CALCIUM (MG)	FOOD	CALCIUM (MG)
Nonfat milk, 1 cup	300	Broccoli, 1 stalk	150
Cheddar cheese, 1-in. cube	130	Spinach, 1 cup	200
Yogurt, 1 cup	300	Turnip greens, 1 cup	250
Ice cream, 1 cup	200	Most other vegetables, 1 cup	40–80
Beef, chicken, fish, 6 oz.	30–80	Apricots, dried, 1 cup	100
Canned salmon, 3 oz.	170	Dates, pitted, 1 cup	100
Bread, grains, rice, 1 cup	20–50	Rhubarb, 1 cup	200
Tofu (soybean curd), 4 oz.	150	Most other fruits, 1 cup	20–70
Almonds, 1/2 cup	160		
Walnuts, 1/2 cup	50		

SOURCE: Adapted from Notelovitz M, Ware M: *Stand Tall! Every Woman's Guide to Preventing Osteoporosis*. New York: Bantam Books, 1984.

searchers were able to detect bone loss for astronauts after just a few days in space where they were deprived of the force of gravity. **Walking, jogging, bicycling, jumping rope, and weight training (or exercise machines)** are all excellent choices for bone health; swimming is not as effective in stimulating bone cells. Combined with sufficient calcium intake, exercise may even help improve bone density for women who already have osteoporosis (4).

Can adequate calcium intake and a faithful exercise program entirely prevent osteoporosis? The answer to this question is not clear, but researchers suspect that for some women the effects of genetic predisposition and hormones are so important that bone loss will occur despite their best efforts. One example is bone loss recently documented for young women athletes. Extensive athletic training (for example, marathon running) can suppress hormone production for some women enough to stop menstrual periods. Bone density studies of women athletes experiencing amenorrhea have found serious bone loss, in some cases to osteoporosis levels. In one study of runners, calcium supplements did not correct the problem for those women who had persistently low estrogen hormones (5). Maintaining high calcium intake also does not appear to protect bone density after menopause. Researchers studying menopausal women using calcium supplements found bone mineral loss even when the daily intake was 2,000 mg of calcium (6). **So for some women at least, calcium and exercise probably are not sufficient,** although both are necessary for bone health.

TABLE 34-3
CALCIUM SUPPLEMENTS

TYPE OF CALCIUM PRODUCT NAME	CALCIUM (MG) IN ONE TABLET	NO. OF TABLETS FOR 1,000 MG
CALCIUM CARBONATE		
Cal-Supp 600	600	2 (1,200 mg)
Caltrate 600	600	2 (1,200 mg)
Suplical	600	2 (1,200 mg)
BioCal	500	2
Os-Cal 500 (oyster shell)	500	2
Theracal	334	3
Cal-Supp 300	300	4 (1,200 mg)
Calcium Carbonate (Lilly)	260	4 (1,040 mg)
BioCal	250	4
[a]Alka-2 Chewable Antacid	200	5
[a]Tums Antacid	200	5
CALCIUM PHOSPHATE		
Posture (Ayerst)	600	2 (1,200 mg)
CALCIUM LACTATE	80–100	10–13
CALCIUM GLUCONATE	50–60	17–20
CHELATED CALCIUM	50–150	7–20
BONE MEAL DOLOMITE	These products are not recommended because of U.S. Food and Drug Administration warnings about possible lead contamination.	

[a]For women at risk of bone loss who also need antacids, calcium antacids are preferable to aluminum-containing products such as Di-Gel, Gaviscon, Gelusil, Maalox, Mylanta, and Riopan. Aluminum may interfere with intestinal absorption of calcium.

SOURCE: Adapted from: Osteoporosis. *Consumer Reports* 49:576–580, 1984.

RISK FACTORS FOR OSTEOPOROSIS

The most important risk factors for osteoporosis are age, sex (being a woman), and race (being nonblack). Ethnic and genetic factors are important, as are medical problems that affect hormone balance, or calcium absorption, or cause physical immobilization. Some medications can induce or aggravate osteoporosis. Risk factors, including specific diseases and medications, are listed in Table 34-4. In some cases

TABLE 34-4
OSTEOPOROSIS RISK FACTORS

HEREDITARY FACTORS

Being female
Being nonblack
Northern-European ancestry
Fair complexion, sparse hair
Slender
Small (5'2" or less)

LIFESTYLE FACTORS

High-protein diet
Outdoor sunlight less than
  3 hours/week
Low calcium intake
High caffeine and/or phosphate
  intake
High vitamin A or vitamin D intake

MEDICATIONS

Antacids containing aluminum
Thyroid (3 grains or more daily, or
  levothyroxine 300 mg or more)
Steroid (cortisone)
Dilantin (prolonged treatment)
Heparin
Furosemide (diuretic)

MEDICAL PROBLEMS

Early or premature menopause
Amenorrhea (absence of menses)
Abnormal sex chromosomes
Elevated prolactin levels
Anorexia nervosa
Hyperthyroidism (excessive thyroid)
Kidney disease or stones
Diabetes
Gastrectomy (stomach removed
  surgically)
Lactase deficiency (milk intolerance)
Intestinal malabsorption
Bowel disease (colitis, ileitis)
Alcoholism
Bed rest or immobilization longer
  than 3 weeks
Polio or paralysis
Rheumatoid arthritis
Spondylitis
Parkinson's disease

medications can be reduced or alternatives substituted; in other cases the danger of bone loss must be accepted because medical treatment is essential. Women who are at high risk for osteoporosis, however, need to be even more conscientious about calcium balance and exercise, and should seriously consider hormone treatment and routine osteoporosis testing.

TESTING FOR OSTEOPOROSIS

Osteoporosis screening ideally should identify specific women at highest risk for bone strength loss before the loss occurs. Unfortunately, known risk factors are so broad that they are often unhelpful, and there is no simple, inexpensive way to predict with certainty which women will be affected. Routine x-rays are likely to identify osteoporosis only after 30% or more of normal bone density is lost. Blood calcium levels remain

TABLE 34-5
FRACTURE RISK AND HEEL BONE MINERAL CONTENT

HEEL BONE PERCENTILE[a]	RELATIVE RISK OF BONE FRACTURE
100	1
80	2
60	4
40	8
20	10

[a]A percentile score of 80 means that 80% of women have this much bone mineral or less, 20% have more; a score of 100 means that a woman is at the very top of the bone mineral range.

SOURCE: Adapted from Wasnich RD, Ross PD, Heilbrun LK, et al: Prediction of postmenopausal fracture risk with use of bone mineral measurements. *American Journal of Obstetrics and Gynecology* 153:745–751, 1985.

normal even in the face of severe osteoporosis unless parathyroid or kidney problems are present as well.

Women who have lower than average bone mineral as they reach menopause are at high risk for osteoporosis problems, and so are women who lose bone mineral more rapidly than average during the early menopausal years. Three techniques are now being used to measure bone mineral so that a woman's bone status can be compared to average values for other women her age. An initial test result can also be compared to a later test to determine a woman's rate of bone mineral loss. Because these techniques are fairly new, long-term research to determine their precise usefulness in predicting future fracture risk is limited. Also, each of the three techniques has its own technical advantages and limitations, and experts do not all agree on who should be tested with which test, or on the meaning of test results.

Single Photon Absorptiometry.   This techniques measures the absorption of photon radiation to determine bone density in the arm (radius) or heel (os calcis). The equipment required is fairly simple and testing requires only a few minutes, so this approach is suitable for a medical office. It is being used for routine screening in many communities.

A woman who has decreased bone mineral in her heel or arm has a greater risk for fracture than does a woman with a high bone mineral measurement (see Table 34-5). A low score, therefore, may be a good warning that aggressive attention to osteoporosis prevention is needed. A normal result, however, is less helpful.

Dual Photon Absorptiometry.   This technique can be used to measure bone density in the spine. The equipment required is elaborate and the test is therefore costly, although it, too, can be done in just a few minutes.

Spine bone strength is of obvious importance in relation to the fractures that cause vertebral deformity and dowager's hump. Dual photon absorptiometry can be quite a precise technique, but spine measurements do not always accurately predict risk for other kinds of fracture such as hip fracture.

CAT Scan.   With CAT (computerized axial tomography) scans, x-ray and computer equipment are used to construct a precise picture of a cross section of bone. Some researchers believe that a CAT scan of the spine or hip bone provides the most accurate assessment of bone strength available. Others, however, believe that equally accurate testing is possible with dual photon absorptiometry (7). A CAT scan is more expensive than absorptiometry and more time-consuming; it also involves substantially more radiation exposure. Even so, it is definitely a reasonable option when osteoporosis is suspected. In that case a CAT scan or dual photon absorptiometry will be needed for diagnosis (rather than routine screening) and it is important to determine how aggressive medical treatment of osteoporosis should be. The best choice in your own community may depend on the resources available. Both options may not be available, and it may be wise to choose the technique that your local expert is most experienced with. If you are being tested for osteoporosis, you will also need follow-up CAT scans or absorptiometry tests to help determine whether your treatment has been sufficient to slow or stop bone loss.

Evaluation is also appropriate for any woman whose measured height decreases, or who experiences a fracture. Other causes for bone density loss or bone fragility also should be considered. Excessive thyroid or parathyroid hormone production and tumor growth, for example, can result in fragile bones.

RECOMMENDATIONS: PROTECTING YOUR BONES

• **Be sure your calcium intake is sufficient throughout life:**
  800 to 1,000 mg daily—children and young adults
  1,000 mg daily—adults and women taking estrogen (0.625 mg daily or more) after menopause
  1,300 to 1,500 mg daily—pregnant and breastfeeding women
  1,500 mg daily—women not taking estrogen (or taking less than 0.625 mg daily) after menopause
• **Be sure your vitamin D intake is adequate:** 400 International Units daily or sunlight, 15 to 30 minutes on your skin daily. (Avoid excess vitamin D which can impair calcium balance.)
• **Minimize calcium robbers** such as excessive sodium, a high-protein diet, caffeine, smoking, and excess vitamin D or A
• Whenever possible, **avoid drugs that adversely affect calcium balance,** including aluminum antacids (see Table 34-4)

- When medical problems or treatment such as **bed rest or immobilization** may jeopardize your bone health, **discuss steps to minimize this effect** with your clinician
- **Record your measured height** at least once a year. If your height decreases, see your clinician for osteoporosis evaluation.
- **Assess your risk for osteoporosis** as you near menopause. A family history of osteoporosis, and your own lifestyle factors such as diet and exercise, are probably most important. If you are at high risk for osteoporosis, consider carefully the personal pros and cons of hormone treatment. If you decide not to begin hormone treatment, consider osteoporosis screening tests during the first few years after menopause.
- See your clinician promptly to correct any medical problems such as dizzy spells that **increase your risks for falling or accidents.** Likewise, if medications you are taking cause side effects like light-headedness or loss of coordination, work with your clinician to solve the problem. A significantly increased risk for hip fracture has been documented for patients taking certain sleeping pills, tranquilizers, and anti-anxiety drugs including Dalmane, Valium (diazepam), Libritabs (chlordiazepoxide), amitriptyline (Elavil, Etrafon, Triavil), doxepin (Adapin, Sinequan), imipramine (Janimine, Tofranil), thioridazine (Mellaril), Haldol, and chlorpromazine (Thorazine) (8).
- **Accident-proof your home** to reduce your risk of falling. Poor lighting, scatter rugs, poor stairway guardrails, and other hazards need to be eliminated.
- If you have **back pain** that lasts longer than a few days, or fracture a bone, ask your clinician to arrange for osteoporosis evaluation

TREATING OSTEOPOROSIS

If you have significant osteoporosis, then you will need to be cared for by an orthopedist, internist, gynecologist, or endocrinologist experienced in this area. Calcium balance, gentle exercise, and menopause hormone treatment may be prescribed, or you may need additional medications such as fluoride or calcitonin hormone. Progestin and testosterone may also be considered, especially if you are not able to take estrogen. Laboratory tests to monitor the effects of treatment on your calcium balance will be needed, and bone density evaluation will be done periodically to determine whether your treatment is effective.

Deciding About Hormone Treatment

Estrogen hormones have been studied more intensively than perhaps any other drug. Nevertheless, knowledge about the benefits and risks of estrogen is not yet complete, and the subject is confusing. It is not so complex, however, that a thoughtful woman will have trouble understanding the issues. For women at menopause, the main health issues involved in a decision about hormones are shown in Illustration 34-2. The relative importance of each of these issues is quite individual. Depending on a personal

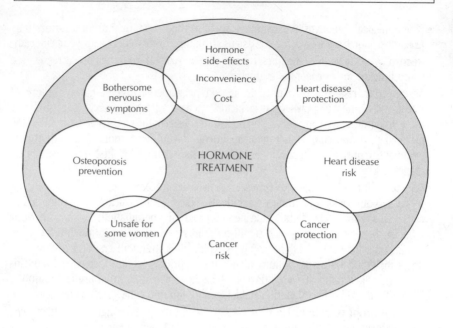

health history and medical risk factors, as well as lifestyle and individual preference, two women may reasonably assess their own personal pros and cons and come to quite different conclusions.

It makes good sense for you to **assume responsibility yourself** for deciding about hormone treatment. Talking to your clinician may be very helpful, but you really are the final decision maker.

Menopause is a good time to evaluate hormone treatment. Except in unusual circumstances, hormone treatment is not recommended until menopause has occurred, but **the bone protection benefit of hormone treatment is greatest if it is started within the first three years after menopause.** A woman 65, 70, or 75 may still reasonably consider starting hormone treatment, though, especially if she is having problems because of bone loss.

HISTORY

During the 1950s and 1960s, great public and medical enthusiasm was generated for the routine use of estrogen after menopause. Menopause was viewed as an estrogen deficiency disease. The use of estrogen drugs intended for this purpose tripled between 1962 and 1975.

Enthusiasm for estrogen replacement therapy was based on encouraging research regarding bone metabolism and on hopes that estrogen would delay or prevent other changes associated with aging, and would preserve a youthful psyche, libido, and skin appearance. In addition, the risk of heart disease and stroke was known to be lower for premenopausal women than for males of the same age. Physicians hoped to extend protection from cardiovascular disease by providing estrogen treatment once natural estrogen production had declined.

Then, in 1975 and 1976, three separate medical researchers **linked the risk of uterine cancer to long-term menopausal estrogen therapy.** These studies compared cancer rates in groups of women who had received estrogen to rates for similar women who were not treated and found that long-term estrogen users were 4.5 to 8 times more likely to develop uterine cancer. Subsequent studies, and overall increases observed in the number of uterine cancer cases in geographic areas where estrogen use was high, confirmed the link.

The uterine cancer connection led to an abrupt drop in estrogen prescriptions. Professional organizations and, in 1976, the FDA (Food and Drug Administration) adopted conservative guidelines. Routine long-term use of estrogen for osteoporosis prevention was not included on the list of approved estrogen uses. Most clinicians, and the previous edition of this book, recommended estrogen treatment for women with premature menopause or definite osteoporosis, but otherwise only for short-term treatment of severe and disabling menopause symptoms. A conservative, and generally negative, climate for hormone treatment persisted from 1976 through the early 1980s.

As additional research data have been published, however, a simple "anti-estrogen" attitude has become less and less reasonable. Newer research has focused on combination hormone treatment: estrogen with progesterone added during the last two weeks or so of each estrogen cycle. Research data from multiple studies now provide convincing evidence that progesterone is effective in preventing uterine cancer. **Women who use combination hormone treatment after menopause have lower rates for uterine cancer than do women who take no hormones at all** (9). Fear of uterine cancer, therefore, is no longer a persuasive reason to withhold hormone treatment. Combination treatment actually reduces risks for this disease, just as birth control Pills have been shown to reduce uterine cancer rates for younger women.

At the same time, there has been increasing medical emphasis on osteoporosis problems. As the age distribution of our population has shifted, the health problems of aging are more and more apparent, and the seriousness of hip fracture especially has commanded public health attention. Hip fracture usually requires surgery, and an average hospital stay of 24 days; the annual cost in the United States for this health problem is more than 7 billion dollars.

So in the mid 1980s, another shift in medical opinion began. Hormone treatment is being considered earlier, and more seriously, by many patients and clinicians, and official policy recommendations are again changing. At a 1984 Consensus Panel sponsored by the National Institutes of Health, **long-term estrogen treatment was approved as an acceptable option for osteoporosis prevention in white women as long as no specific estrogen contraindications were present** (see the section entitled "Contraindications to Hormone Treatment" later in this chapter) (10).

Because the best medical judgment at any point in time is based on **knowledge at that time,** it is not surprising that judgment should shift as new knowledge is acquired. The field of hormone interactions, and especially those involving estrogen, is being intensively studied with hundreds of research studies reported every year. So as you read more about hormones pay close attention to the **date** of the book or article, and the dates of any references cited. You are likely to find that the author's conclusions are strongly influenced by the research evidence and prevailing opinion at that particular time.

Another source of information you are likely to encounter is the package insert provided with every estrogen-containing medication. The insert is required by the FDA, which also specifies the information it must contain. It is intended to cover **all possible risks** and complications of estrogen therapy, but not necessarily all possible benefits. So as you read it, don't be surprised that it conveys overall a somewhat negative view. You are expected to know already the positive reasons for considering estrogen—they are presumably the reasons for which you received the prescription and therefore the package insert!

Guessing about the future is hazardous. **It seems likely, though, that the current hormone revival will continue, and that more and more women will seriously consider long-term treatment.** Their clinicians will probably encourage them. As the number of women over 50 increases in the next decades, osteoporosis will become increasingly important.

At the same time, women are also becoming more and more aware of calcium needs, as well as exercise and diet. The power of a healthier lifestyle has already been shown by reductions in the overall heart disease toll among U.S. men. As we all change to better diets and begin a commitment to exercise, the dire predictions for future heart and bone problems among older women may be averted, or at least curbed. This will probably be true regardless of women's decisions about estrogen.

HORMONE TREATMENT EFFECTS

Menopause Symptoms.   Hot flashes are almost sure to be eliminated within a few days by estrogen oral tablets. For most women, 0.625 mg of conjugated estrogen daily is sufficient, although some women require a higher dose. Hot flashes may reappear during the five to seven hormone-free days of cyclic treatment each month, and are very likely to recur if estrogen treatment is stopped. Vaginal atrophy (thin and dry lining) and atrophy of the urethra are also effectively reversed by oral estrogen at the same dose. Many women, however, find that a smaller dose of estrogen, in the form of estrogen vaginal cream, is also effective for atrophy problems.

Some women find that hormone treatment has other, less clear-cut effects. Loss of sleep because of hot flashes can cause problems like irritability, depression, and fatigue. This may explain the improved sense of well-being that some women report with hormone treatment. Hormones also may affect sex drive directly, or indirectly as vaginal discomfort during sex is improved.

BONE DENSITY CHANGES WITH AND WITHOUT HORMONE TREATMENT

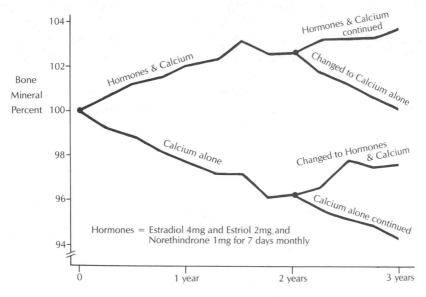

ILLUSTRATION 34-3   Half the women in this study began with calcium alone and half began with calcium plus cyclic hormones; at the end of two years treatments were switched for half the women in each group.

Osteoporosis.   Women who take estrogen after menopause are protected against osteoporosis. Multiple studies have shown that loss of bone density is arrested when a woman begins estrogen, and that the risk of fractures is reduced. Bone strength is protected most effectively when treatment is begun within three years after menopause. An estrogen dose of 0.625 mg of conjugated estrogen daily or its equivalent provides excellent protection, a dose of 0.45 mg daily is sufficient for about 50% of women, and lower doses such as 0.3 mg may be sufficient if calcium supplementation of 1,500 mg is also provided (10). Adequate calcium intake is also necessary, but doses of calcium so far studied (as high as supplements of 800 mg daily) do not reduce bone loss as effectively as estrogen. Illustration 34-3 shows bone density changes over three years for women receiving hormone treatment and calcium compared to women taking only calcium. Results of this study show that calcium alone (500-mg supplements) was not sufficient to prevent loss of bone mineral. Women receiving calcium and hormone treatment (cyclic estrogen and progesterone) gained slightly in bone mineral content, and this effect occurred even when treatment was not started until treatment groups were switched at the end of two years. For women who initially took hormones and then changed to calcium only, bone mineral loss started as soon as hormones were stopped. This study also provides reassurance that the addition of progesterone to hormone treatment does not block the bone preserving effect of estrogen. Estrogen taken alone prevents bone loss, combination treatment with estrogen and progesterone prevents bone loss, and so does treatment with progesterone alone (12).

Some researchers believe that bone loss is greatest during the first few months and years after menopause, and that the loss subsequently slows down. If this proves to be true, then higher rates of loss might also be anticipated when hormone treatment is stopped. The steep loss, 2% per year, observed in the study previously described would tend to substantiate this concern. If stopping treatment does result in a period of rapid loss, a woman who starts and stops treatment several times conceivably might experience greater bone loss overall than she would have had with no treatment at all. Therefore, **intermittent treatment should be avoided** if possible until further research clarifies this issue.

Uterine Cancer.   Treatment with estrogen oral tablets after menopause increases a woman's risk for developing precancerous abnormalities of the uterine lining (adenomatous hyperplasia) and also her risk for cancer. Risks are higher when high doses of estrogen (equivalent to 2.5 mg conjugated estrogen) are used and when treatment is prolonged (five to ten years or more). Some researchers estimate that as many as 10% of women taking oral estrogen alone will develop adenomatous hyperplasia, and 8 cases of endometrial cancer caused by estrogen will occur each year for every 1,000 women using oral estrogen alone for ten years or more (13). Other researchers feel that these estimates are too high (9). Accurate risk comparison is complex because several factors, including obesity, also increase uterine cancer risks. Women who have higher than average natural estrogen production, because of infrequent ovulation or polycystic ovary disease, also are at higher risk for uterine cancer. (See Chapter 41 for more information on uterine cancer.)

Progesterone counteracts the effects of estrogen on uterine lining cells. Synthetic progestins are used to treat endometrial adenomatous hyperplasia when it occurs spontaneously, and **women who take progestin cyclically along with estrogen are effectively protected against the risks of hyperplasia and uterine cancer**. One of the largest studies of menopause hormone treatment found that women receiving progestin for ten days each month along with estrogen had lower rates for uterine cancer than did women receiving no hormones at all (see Table 34-6). The duration of progesterone treatment each month is very important: treatment for at least 10 days each month is essential, and treatment for 14 days may provide more effective suppression of uterine hyperplasia. The optimal dose of progesterone is not known. Typically used progesterones (such as Provera, 10 mg daily) provide effective protection, but there is some evidence that lower doses would also be effective (13).

Abnormal bleeding can be an early symptom of uterine hyperplasia or cancer. **Any bleeding that occurs after menopause must be evaluated promptly if you are not taking hormones or are taking estrogen alone.** Women using combined estrogen and progesterone are likely to have a short bleeding episode after each progesterone batch. Bleeding that occurs any other time, however, demands evaluation.

TABLE 34-6
UTERINE CANCER RATES:
WITH AND WITHOUT HORMONE TREATMENT

HORMONE USED	NUMBER OF UTERINE CANCERS PER 100,000 WOMEN PER YEAR
Estrogen (oral)	434
Estrogen and progesterone (oral)	71
No hormones	242

SOURCE: Gambrell RD: Clinical use of progestins in the menopausal patient: Dosage and duration. *Journal of Reproductive Medicine* 27:531–538, 1982.

Breast Cancer.   Numerous studies have assessed the effect of estrogen on breast cancer risk. Most studies have found no difference in breast cancer rates between women who were taking estrogen and those who did not (14). A few studies have found a protective effect for estrogen, and a very few have found increased risks (9). Estrogen has been linked to breast cancer in some animal species, and when breast cancer is already present, estrogen can stimulate tumor growth if the tumor cells are a type that is estrogen sensitive.

Some researchers believe that treatment with progesterone may have a protective effect against breast cancer, and one researcher has reported lower breast cancer rates for women receiving combined hormones than for women taking no hormones (15). Other experts, however, doubt these results, and do not believe there is a physiologic reason that progesterone would help. Research data to give a definite answer are lacking.

In any case caution about hormones is prudent, especially for women at high risk for breast cancer because of family history and for women who have abnormal mammograms or develop benign breast disease (cysts or lumps, for example) while taking hormones.

Heart Disease.   Heart disease, stroke, high blood pressure, high blood lipid levels (cholesterol and others), and arteriosclerosis (fatty deposits in the lining of arteries) are intertwined problems that are the most significant causes of serious illness and death for women over 50. Even a small change in rates for these problems, positive or negative, is of great public health significance and would overshadow the importance of all the cancer effects combined.

Researchers are justifiably worried about hormone effects on heart disease because early studies of birth control Pill users found that women who used Pills had an increased risk of heart attack and stroke, especially if they used high-dose Pills or were smokers over the age of 35. Like combination menopause hormone treatment, birth control Pills contain estrogen and synthetic progesterone, although the Pill hormone dose is substantially higher, and the specific synthetic hormones used in birth control Pills are somewhat different.

Because of the known risks of birth control Pills, articles on menopause treatment have stressed possible heart disease risks and warned against use of hormones for women who have cardiovascular disease problems or are at high risk because of diabetes or their family medical history.

Estrogen and progesterone both influence cardiovascular disease factors in several distinct ways. Estrogen can directly influence the body's blood clotting mechanism, and the high estrogen level in birth control Pills used twenty years ago was responsible for an increased risk of **blood clot problems such as thrombophlebitis** (clotted, inflamed veins, usually in the legs) and embolism. An embolism is part or all of an abnormal blood clot that has traveled to the lung or brain; embolism is a serious threat and can result in stroke, brain damage, or death. Blood clot effects depend on the dose and type of estrogen involved, and rates for serious blood clot problems have dropped dramatically for birth control Pill users as the overall estrogen dose in Pills has been reduced. The estrogen dose involved in menopause hormone treatment is significantly lower than that in birth control Pills, and most experts believe that their effect on blood clotting is very small or even negligible. Several large studies of menopause hormone users have found no evidence of increased risk for clotting problems or stroke (16); an increased risk for stroke, however, was documented in one study involving 300 menopause hormone users compared to 900 nonusers in Framingham (17).

Some women taking birth control Pills have an increase in **blood pressure**, and some show significant alteration in **glucose tolerance** similar to that in diabetes. These problems are rare, particularly with lower dose birth control Pills, but may be a reason for discontinuing treatment. Studies of menopause hormone users have not found blood pressure or glucose problems (16). Blood pressure may even be decreased slightly for most menopause hormone users although significant blood pressure increase can occur in rare cases (18). For this reason, regular blood pressure checks may be especially important for menopause hormone users. A woman who has high blood pressure or diabetes should have careful monitoring to detect any change in these conditions if she chooses to use hormones.

Estrogen and progesterone both influence **blood lipid patterns**. This is probably their most important cardiovascular disease effect because **blood lipid patterns impact heart attack risk**. Adverse lipid patterns are responsible for atherosclerosis, the deposit of fatty plaques on the inner lining of the body's arteries. When plaques cause narrowing or blockage in the arteries of the heart, or coronary artery disease, heart attack is likely. Estrogen plays a generally protective role, causing a relative reduction in low-density lipids (the bad lipids) and relative increase in high-density lipids (the good lipids). The estrogen–lipid effect is probably the reason that women are protected naturally against

TABLE 34-7
HEART ATTACK RISK FACTORS

RISK FACTOR	APPROXIMATE RISK CAUSED BY THIS FACTOR ("NORMAL" RISK = 1.00)
Previous stroke, high blood pressure, angina (heart pain) or diabetes before age 65	2.2 – 2.6
Previous heart attack	3.9 – 7.3
Cholesterol of 300 mg/dl or more	1.3 – 3.0
Conjugated estrogen treatment	0.4 – 0.6

SOURCE: Adapted from Ross RK, Paganini-Hill A: Menopausal oestrogen therapy and protection from death from ischaemic heart disease. *Lancet* 1:858–860, 1981.

heart disease until menopause; after menopause the heart attack risk for women increases dramatically. Synthetic progestins, especially those found in birth control Pills, somewhat counteract this effect, and cause a relative increase in low-density lipids.

Depending on the balance between estrogen effect and progestin effect, the overall result of taking both hormones together may be an improved lipid pattern, no net change, or a more adverse lipid pattern. This is the reason that the progestin dose in birth control Pills has been progressively reduced over time, and it is also the reason for caution in determining the best dose of progesterone for use after menopause. Also, the effects of different forms of estrogen and progesterone differ somewhat, so that each type and dose requires separate evaluation. Research so far indicates that "natural" estrogen such as equine (horse) estrogen, estrone, or conjugated estrogens are among the most favorable in lipid effects, and that medroxyprogesterone acetate (Provera) may be preferable to other synthetic progestins in this respect (19).

Studies of overall death rates and heart disease deaths for women on the whole provide reassurance about hormone treatment effects. One study has documented higher heart attack rates for estrogen users, particularly those who were smokers (17), but most have found a protective effect, and these include several major studies involving larger populations of women (20). One study of heart attack deaths (see Table 34-7) found that women taking estrogen were about half as likely to die of heart attack compared to "normal" women their age not taking estrogen. Another large study (see Table 34-8) found that overall death rates adjusted for age were significantly lower for women taking estrogen. Lower death rates have even been documented for women who developed uterine cancer while taking estrogen compared to women with uterine cancer who were not estrogen users (21).

TABLE 34-8
OVERALL DEATH RATES: DEATHS FROM ALL CAUSES

	NUMBER OF DEATHS PER 1,000 WOMEN PER YEAR		
	WOMEN WITH UTERUS AND OVARIES IN PLACE	WOMEN WITH PREVIOUS HYSTERECTOMY	WOMEN WITH PREVIOUS OOPHORECTOMY[a]
Women using estrogen	4.9	2.8	1.4
Women not using estrogen	9.0	8.2	11.8
All women	8.2	5.7	7.2

[a]Oophorectomy means surgical removal of a woman's ovaries. Many of these women also had hysterectomy (surgery to remove the uterus).

SOURCE: Adapted from Bush TL, et al: Estrogen use and all-cause mortality: Preliminary results from the Lipid Research Clinics Program follow-up study. *Journal of the American Medical Association* 249:903–906, 1983.

Estrogen use in most of the studies reported through the mid 1980s is statistically linked to lower risks for heart attack and death. Research, however, does not prove that estrogen itself is the sole reason for the protection observed. Women who take estrogen also are likely to have good access to medical care, and may differ from nonusers in other ways that are important to health. It may be, for example, that women who use estrogen also have better financial and information resources that enable them to have a healthier diet and lifestyle than women in the no-estrogen comparison groups. But if further research does substantiate the benefits these studies suggest, then prevention of heart disease will become the most important reason for women to consider postmenopausal hormone replacement.

Despite the reassurance that these studies provide, **women who already have heart disease, or other serious risk factors such as smoking, high blood pressure, diabetes, or high cholesterol, must be cautious.** If hormone treatment is needed, careful surveillance is reasonable to help detect any adverse effects of hormones as soon as possible. Also, **a woman who has already had a stroke, a lung blood clot, or other serious clotting problems should not use hormones.** These disorders are often fatal, so even though there is no clear evidence that menopause hormones increase the risk, it is wise simply to avoid hormones.

Other Risks and Side Effects.   **Gallbladder disease** risk is increased by estrogen use after menopause. About 22 estrogen users out of 10,000 will have gallbladder problems compared to 9 nonusers. Estrogen can also cause problems for women with **uterine fibroid tumors,** or benign leiomyomas. Tumor growth can be stimulated by estrogen, and even the low dose involved in menopause treatment is enough to cause tumor enlargement for some women. **Endometriosis** tissue, also, is responsive to hormone stimulation, but the disease is unlikely to worsen with menopause treatment.

Almost all women under age 60 who take combination estrogen and progesterone treatment (97%) **have bleeding after each progesterone cycle.** Bleeding tends to subside over time, but about 60% of women 65 and older do continue to have monthly bleeding episodes.

The most common hormone treatment side effects are **breast tenderness** and **nausea.** Both of these problems usually subside within the first few months of treatment. A change in estrogen and/or progesterone dose may be helpful. Overall, less than 10% of women experience the side effects listed in Table 34-9.

Progesterone Effects. Treatment with progesterone oral tablets or shots (without estrogen) is moderately effective in relieving hot flashes, but does not combat vaginal dryness or urinary tract problems. Progesterone alone also protects against bone density loss (12).

The interrelated roles of estrogen and progesterone with regard to uterine cancer, breast cancer, and heart disease are described in previous sections in this chapter. The use of progesterone alone, however, is so limited that research on its singular effects is sparse. Many of the possible side effects and risks officially recorded for progesterone are derived from studies of women taking oral contraceptives. Whether these same problems also occur with use of progesterone for menopause treatment is not known. Reported progesterone side effects are listed in Table 34-9.

The most common problems women taking cyclic menopause treatment are likely to notice during the progesterone interval each month are **fluid retention** and **bloating,** possibly accompanied by mild depression and **irritability** similar to the premenstrual syndrome (PMS). As with PMS, these symptoms often improve with a low-sodium diet and exercise. If problems are severe or persistent, however, reducing the progesterone dose may be a reasonable option.

CONTRAINDICATIONS TO HORMONE TREATMENT

A contraindication is a medical condition that renders inadvisable or unsafe a course of treatment that otherwise might be recommended.

Women who have had serious problems with estrogen or progestin in the past, or who have medical problems that might be aggravated by these hormones, should avoid them. Also, if there is any chance you might be pregnant, hormone treatment should be delayed until you have a pregnancy test to be sure you are not.

Many of the following contraindications apply to both estrogen and progestin (marked **); others apply only to estrogen (marked *).

TABLE 34-9
POSSIBLE HORMONE SIDE EFFECTS

PROBLEMS CAUSED BY BOTH ESTROGEN AND PROGESTERONE

Nausea
Fluid retention (which can aggravate epilepsy, migraine, heart and
  kidney disease)
Breast tenderness, breast fluid secretion
Depression
Jaundice (yellow skin)
Loss of scalp hair
Increased hair growth on face
Skin allergy reaction (rash, itching)

PROBLEMS CAUSED BY ESTROGEN

Vomiting
Breast enlargement
Growth of uterine fibroids
Abdominal cramps, bloating
Susceptibility to vaginal yeast infection
Urinary frequency and urgency
Red patches or lumps on skin (legs)
Chloasma (pigment patches on face)
Contact lens intolerance
Increase in curvature of the cornea
Headaches, migraine headaches, dizziness
Weight gain or loss
Diminished sugar tolerance
Increase or decrease in sex drive
Increase in porphyria, chorea

PROBLEMS CAUSED BY PROGESTERONE

Abnormal vaginal bleeding
Acne
Edema (swelling)
Difficulty sleeping or excessive sleepiness
Fever (allergy reaction)

Absolute Contraindications.   (Do not use hormone treatment.)

** Current or past blood-clotting disorders including pulmonary embolism (lung clot) and phlebitis (leg clots)
** Stroke
** Undiagnosed abnormal vaginal bleeding
** Cancer of the breast, uterus, or ovary
** Impaired liver function

Relative Contraindications.   (Avoid hormone treatment, or use only with careful surveillance.) Not all experts or reviewers of this chapter include the conditions marked with an [a], but to the authors their inclusion seems plausible and appropriate.

** Liver disease
** Heart disease
** Kidney disease
** Diabetes
* Gallbladder disease
* Hypertension (high blood pressure)
* Breast disease (atypical hyperplasia) or abnormal mammogram[a]
* Sickle cell disease[a]
* Elective surgery planned in the next four weeks[a]
* Fibroid tumors of the uterus
** Epilepsy
** Asthma
* Severe depression
* Severe migraine headaches

Also, remember that estrogens can interact with other medications you may be taking for unrelated problems, such as anticoagulants, insulin, promazine, meperidine, and with tuberculin skin tests. Discuss this issue with your clinician, and be sure that any clinician you see is aware that you are using hormones.

WEIGHING THE PROS AND CONS

As you consider hormone treatment, you may find it helpful to summarize your personal advantages and disadvantages. Table 34-10 was adapted from a rating scale developed by Sadja Greenwood, M.D., in her book *Menopause Naturally* (see "Suggested Reading"). Use this personal summary to assess each issue depending on its importance to you. You will notice that uterine cancer risk is not included in the summary. The use of progesterone along with estrogen protects so effectively against uterine cancer that this summary assumes it will not be a risk for you. Review the preceding sections of this chapter to assess the importance of factors in your personal or family health history as you decide on your scores.

Your decision about hormone treatment may be a clear-cut no if you have one or

TABLE 34-10
PERSONAL SUMMARY: HORMONE PROS AND CONS

Personal Score					Likely Hormone Benefits
+2	+1	0	–1	–2	Hot flashes eliminated
+2	+1	0	–1	–2	Vaginal/urinary atrophy reversed
+2	+1	0	–1	–2	Osteoporosis prevented
					Benefit/Risk Uncertain
+2	+1	0	–1	–2	Heart disease and stroke
+2	+1	0	–1	–2	Breast cancer
+2	+1	0	–1	–2	Other personal factors (sex drive, mood . . .)
					Possible Hormone Risks/Disadvantages
+2	+1	0	–1	–2	Gallbladder disease risk
+2	+1	0	–1	–2	Growth of uterine fibroids
+2	+1	0	–1	–2	Continuing monthly bleeding
+2	+1	0	–1	–2	Hormone side effects
+2	+1	0	–1	–2	Costs and medical visits

+2 Very significant benefit
 0 Not a significant factor either way
–2 Very significant risk or disadvantage
SOURCE: Adapted from Greenwood S: *Menopause Naturally: Preparing for the Second Half of Life.*
San Francisco: Volcano Press, 1984.

more of the absolute contraindications to treatment. Or it may be an obvious yes because of extremely severe menopause symptoms or a very high risk for osteoporosis. For most women, though, the decision is more complicated. Unfortunately, there are no clear medical guidelines for average women. **Hormone treatment is definitely indicated for women who undergo menopause before age 45,** either spontaneously or as a result of surgery; it is also likely to be recommended for a woman who already has evidence of osteoporosis or has a low bone density discovered by osteoporosis screening tests. And many clinicians today feel that treatment is reasonable for nonblack women strictly as a preventive measure to protect bone, as long as no serious contraindications are present. At the same time, a decision not to take hormones is also reasonable. Either decision, of course, can be reassessed periodically. It is quite likely that medical recommendations will become clearer in the next few years as research findings accumulate.

If you decide not to begin hormone treatment, then attention to calcium, exercise, and tests to evaluate bone loss are especially important; if your bone density is low, or drops sharply, you may want to reconsider. If you are not taking hormone treatment, your clinician may also recommend that you take one batch of progesterone tablets for seven to ten days to see whether your own natural estrogen level is high enough to allow uterine bleeding. This process is called a progestin challenge test. If you have bleeding after taking progesterone tablets, some clinicians would recommend monthly treatment with progesterone to reduce your risk for developing uterine cancer because of high natural estrogen exposure. Taking progesterone, however, may have disadvantages for blood lipids, and there is no conclusive research evidence to determine whether advantages outweigh possible risks.

If you decide to take oral hormone treatment, it makes sense to take an estrogen dose large enough to provide reliable bone protection (see the next section in this chapter). Progesterone along with estrogen is important if you have not had a hysterectomy. The decision about progesterone is less clear-cut, however, if you do not have a uterus. It is possible that progesterone may reduce breast cancer risk; on the other hand, it may adversely affect blood lipids and heart disease risk. Discuss these issues with your clinician. The best choice should become clearer as additional research is reported. There is also no clear-cut rule for how long hormone treatment should be continued. Bone protection persists as long as hormones are taken, but stops when a woman discontinues treatment. So if bone protection is the main medical reason for treatment, then hormones will need to be continued indefinitely. Hormones taken for even a few years, however, are beneficial for bone strength since the onset of bone loss will be delayed.

Hormone treatment can reasonably be started, or stopped, any time during the menopausal years, but intermittent treatment is probably undesirable. Read the section on stopping hormone treatment later in this chapter for more specific information on stopping hormones.

USING HORMONE TREATMENT

Brand names and the chemical composition of commonly available hormone products are listed in Table 34-11, along with the minimum doses needed to provide osteoporosis protection. Although oral tablets are most commonly used, hormone treatment can also be administered by injection or via vaginal cream. The newest form of estrogen for menopause treatment is an adhesive patch that allows hormone absorption through the skin. Hormones in pill form are absorbed through the lining of the stomach and intestines into blood vessels that travel directly to the liver before entering the general circulation. The liver is thus exposed to high concentrations of hormones (or any other medication) taken by mouth. Effects on the liver are probably responsible for the altered clotting factors that can occur with hormones, so the skin patches, which allow direct absorption into the general circulation, may prove to be preferable in this respect. Skin patches, however, may not have the same favorable effects on lipid patterns as oral estrogen, and there is no long-term research to show whether the potentially beneficial effects of oral estrogen on heart disease will be duplicated with skin patch administration (22, 23).

Before beginning hormone treatment you will need a routine annual exam (see Chapter 7) including breast exam, pelvic exam, and blood pressure. A recent mammogram to be sure you do not have unsuspected breast problems, and fasting blood tests for sugar and lipids, are also reasonable. These steps should be repeated annually while you are taking hormones; they are also recommended for women who are not taking hormones.

If you have not had a hysterectomy and decide to take estrogen alone, your clinician will probably recommend an endometrial biopsy before beginning treatment and once a year thereafter.

Hormone Shots.   Injections are often used to control severe menopause symptoms immediately after surgery when removal of the ovaries is necessary in a premenopausal woman. For ongoing treatment, though, oral tablets are less expensive and probably safer. High hormone blood levels are reached within a short time after an injection, and then fall gradually until the next injection, days or weeks later, so continuing treatment by injection exposes the woman to intermittent, and probably undesirable, high hormone levels. Also, there is no evidence that hormone shots, or shots combining hormones and vitamins, are any more effective in controlling menopause symptoms than are simple oral tablets.

Vaginal Estrogen Cream.   Treatment with vaginal estrogen cream is often effective in reversing vaginal dryness problems with a lower overall dose of estrogen than oral treatment. Estrogen from vaginal cream, however, is absorbed into the bloodstream and can reach levels comparable to oral treatment when the vaginal dose is large. This effect appears to be minimal when the vaginal dose is equivalent to 0.3 mg of conjugated estrogen or less daily (24), and 0.3 mg is usually sufficient to correct vaginal dryness. Your clinician will prescribe the specific dosage. Increased uterine cancer risks have not been documented for vaginal estrogen users, even though this treatment does involve exposure to estrogen without progesterone. It is possible that the doses typical for vaginal estrogen users are low enough to avoid uterine cancer risk.

Typical vaginal hormone treatment might involve applications of cream every day for the first ten days or so, then once every two or three days thereafter. Symptoms should improve within five to seven days. A calibrated applicator comes with vaginal cream. Using the Premarin applicator, one whole applicator (4 grams) is a dose of 2.5 mg of hormone. To measure 0.3 mg, only one eighth of the applicator should be filled (one half of the way to the 1-gram mark).

Oral Estrogen and Progesterone Tablets.   Conjugated estrogen tablets (Premarin) and progesterone in the form of medroxyprogesterone acetate (Amen, Curretab, Provera) are the most commonly prescribed menopause treatment hormones in the United States and much of the research data described earlier in this chapter reflects use of these specific products. Effects of other estrogens and progestins are likely to be

TABLE 34-11 DRUGS COMMONLY PRESCRIBED FOR HORMONE TREATMENT

GENERIC HORMONE	BRAND NAME	DOSES AVAILABLE	DAILY DOSE (MG) NEEDED TO PROTECT BONE DENSITY[a]
ESTROGEN			
Conjugated estrogen	(generic)	0.3, 0.625, 1.25, 2.5 mg	0.625
	Premarin	0.3, 0.625, 0.9 1.25, 2.5 mg	0.625
Esterified estrogen	Estratab	0.3, 0.625, 1.25, 2.5 mg	0.625
Estropipate (piperazine estrone)	Ogen	0.625, 1.25, 2.5, 5.0 mg	0.625
Estradiol	Estrace	1 mg, 2 mg	1
	Estrace Cycle Pack	1 mg, 2 mg 25 tablets in one-month plastic pack	1
	Estraderm (skin patch)	0.05, 0.1 mg patch change patch twice each week	0.05
Ethinyl estradiol	Estinyl	0.02, 0.05, 0.5 mg	0.01 (1/2 tablet of 0.02-mg strength)
Quinestrol (long acting)	Estrovis (taken once a week)	100 mg	Unknown
COMBINATION ESTROGEN/TESTOSTERONE		These products are not recommended for long-term use.	
Conjugated estrogen/ methyltestosterone (MT)[b]	Premarin-MT	0.625 + 5 mg MT 1.25 + 10 mg MT	0.625
Esterified estrogen/ methyltestosterone (MT)[b]	Estratest	0.625 + 1.25 mg MT 1.25 + 2.5 mg MT	0.625

[a]A daily dose of 0.3 mg conjugated estrogen or its equivalent may be sufficient to protect bone density for women who also insure a daily calcium intake of 1,500 mg to 2,500 mg through diet and supplementation.

GENERIC HORMONE	BRAND NAME	DOSES AVAILABLE	DAILY DOSE (MG) NEEDED TO PROTECT BONE DENSITY[a] / TYPICAL CREAM DOSE NEEDED 1-3 TIMES WEEKLY TO CONTROL VAGINAL DISCOMFORT
ESTROGEN VAGINAL CREAM[c]			
Conjugated estrogen	Premarin Vaginal Cream	0.625 mg per gram	About 1/2 gram (1/8 applicator)
Estropipate	Ogen Vaginal Cream	1.5 mg per gram	About 1/4 gram (1/16 applicator)
Estradiol	Estrace Vaginal Cream	0.1 mg per gram	About 5 grams (1 applicator)
Dienestrol	DV Ortho Dienestrol	0.1 mg per gram	About 6 grams (1 applicator)

			TYPICAL DOSE (10-14 DAYS EACH MONTH)
PROGESTIN			
Medroxyprogesterone acetate (MPA)[d]	Amen	10 mg (scored)	10
	Curretab	10 mg (scored)	10
	Provera	2.5, 5, 10 mg	10
Norethindrone acetate[e]	Aygestin	5 mg (scored)	2.5 (1/2 tablet)
	Norlutate	5 mg (scored)	2.5 (1/2 tablet)
Norethindrone[e]	Norlutin	5 mg (scored)	2.5 (1/2 tablet)

Products that combine estrogen hormone with a tranquilizer or amphetamine (PMB-200, PMB-400, Menrium, and Mediatric) are not recommended. These additives can be habit forming and are not of demonstrated value in treating menopause symptoms.

[b]Methyltestosterone can cause masculine changes such as growth of coarse dark body hair, scalp hair loss (balding), deepened voice, and increased sex drive; risks for developing liver tumor may also be increased.
[c]Vaginal estrogen absorption results in somewhat lower blood estrogen levels than the same dose given orally. Notice that Estrace and Dienestrol cream contain a smaller amount of estrogen than do the other products available. To use a low vaginal estrogen dose (equivalent to 0.3 mg conjugated estrogen vaginally) measure 1/8 of an applicator of Premarin, or 1/16 of an applicator of Ogen, or a whole applicator of Estrace or Dienestrol.
[d]A lower dose, equivalent to MPA 2.5 to 5 mg, may prove to be sufficient in preventing uterine cancer.
[e]These synthetic progestins may be less desirable than medroxyprogesterone acetate because of blood lipid effects.

CYCLIC HORMONE TREATMENT

S	M	T	W	T	F	S
1 estrogen	2 estrogen	3 estrogen	4 estrogen	5 estrogen	6 estrogen	7 estrogen
8 estrogen	9 estrogen	10 estrogen	11 estrogen	12 estrogen (progestin)	13 estrogen (progestin)	14 estrogen (progestin)
15 estrogen (progestin)	16 estrogen progestin	17 estrogen progestin	18 estrogen progestin	19 estrogen progestin	20 estrogen progestin	21 estrogen progestin
22 estrogen progestin	23 estrogen progestin	24 estrogen progestin	25 estrogen progestin	26	27	28
29	30					

ILLUSTRATION 34-4 Estrogen is usually prescribed for 25 days of each month. To prevent uterine cancer, progesterone is needed for 10 to 14 days each month. This woman begins taking progesterone along with estrogen on the 12th of each month, and begins again with estrogen on the 1st of the next month.

similar, although not necessarily identical. Some experts believe that estrone (estropipate or piperazine estrone, Ogen) may be preferable to other estrogen alternatives. Limited research suggests that estrone causes less alteration in the body chemicals that regulate blood pressure, and yet provides excellent control of menopause symptoms (18). If side effects with estrogen are bothersome, changing to an alternative may be helpful. If progesterone side effects are a problem, reducing the dose may be reasonable. The main progesterone benefit, protection against uterine cancer, is most dependent on the duration of progesterone therapy each month. Using a smaller dose of progesterone for 12 to 14 days is a better choice than using the higher dose for fewer days or omitting progesterone.

A typical pattern for cyclic treatment with estrogen and progesterone is shown in Illustration 34-4. There is nothing "magic" about beginning each cycle on the first of the month, but it makes your calculations easier. If you want to change the timing of your hormone cycle, to avoid bleeding while on vacation, for example, you can add or subtract as many as seven estrogen-only days.

Although most clinicians in the United States recommend cycles of 25 days or so on hormones followed by 5 days off, there is no research evidence to show whether a longer cycle, or even continuous hormones, would make any difference. Treatment with estrogen taken continuously (every day, no interruptions) and progesterone added for 14 days monthly is used in some other countries. With this approach, bleeding occurs a few days after progesterone tablets are finished each month. Another approach may be estrogen and progesterone both taken every day continuously. The continuous schedule may help women who have menopause symptoms during days off hormones in a cyclic pattern, and may put an end to monthly bleeding, at least for some (25).

34:5   HORMONE TREATMENT DANGER SIGNS
A   Abdominal pain (severe) C   Chest pain, shortness of breath, cough H   Headache (severe), dizziness, weakness, numbness E   Eye problems (vision loss or blurring), speech problems S   Severe leg pain (calf or thigh) Stop taking hormone medication and see your clinician at once if you have any of these problems, or if you develop depression, jaundice, a breast lump, or abnormal vaginal bleeding.

No matter what combined hormone cycle pattern you are using, **bleeding should occur only in conjunction with each progesterone batch.** Bleeding usually occurs during the last day or two of progesterone or after each batch, and is usually light to moderate. It should last no more than three to seven days. Mild cramping may accompany bleeding for some women. **If bleeding occurs at any other time during treatment, be sure to contact your clinician.** Further evaluation, including endometrial biopsy, will probably be needed.

And remember calcium balance. Even though you are taking hormones, adequate calcium is still essential for bone health.

While you are taking hormones you should also watch for the possible danger signs of hormone treatment shown in Illustration 34-5. Contact your clinician immediately, and stop hormones in the meantime, if you have any of these symptoms.

STOPPING HORMONE TREATMENT

Women who have taken estrogen for long periods are often surprised to find that they can stop without any noticeable impact. Some women do experience a return of hot flashes if pills are stopped abruptly and may prefer to decrease the dose gradually over a period of months.

Bone loss is likely to resume as soon as estrogen is discontinued, and some researchers believe that loss is especially rapid during the transition from high to low estrogen levels. For this reason it makes sense to avoid **intermittent** hormone treatment whenever possible. Be sure, for example, to arrange your prescription refills on time. If you need to stop because of problems, or you decide to discontinue hormones, then by all means do so. Remember, though, that **your own preventive health efforts with calcium balance and exercise will be even more important.**

ALTERNATIVES TO ESTROGEN TREATMENT

Numerous drugs, diets, vitamins, and therapies have been suggested as alternatives to estrogen for management of menopause problems. Although none has achieved the uniformly high success rate of estrogen for controlling hot flashes and vaginal problems, one or more of these alternatives may prove helpful to you:

Progesterone Treatment. If hot flashes are a severe problem but estrogen is not safe for you, daily progesterone pills or periodic progesterone shots may be helpful. Progesterone, too, is a hormone normally produced by the ovary prior to menopause, but its effects are more limited than those of estrogen (see the section on Minipills—progestin-only pills for birth control—in Chapter 13 for more discussion of complications and contraindications for this hormone).

Progesterone oral tablets at relatively high doses (equivalent to 20 mg of medroxyprogesterone acetate daily) are highly effective in relieving hot flashes. At this dose level, however, adverse effects on blood lipids may occur. Lower doses (10 mg), with little or no demonstrated lipid effect, are effective against hot flashes for some women. Typical treatment might involve oral tablets taken every day, with no interruptions. Injections of slowly absorbed progesterone, called depo-medroxyprogesterone acetate, may also reduce hot flashes. Doses of 150 mg every three months would be typical. Treatment with progesterone alone can cause complications including abnormal bleeding, depression, and weight gain.

Vaginal Hormone Cream. Vaginal cream containing estrogen may be an option for some women even though they have serious contraindications and cannot take oral estrogen tablets. Discuss these alternatives with your clinician. A very small vaginal estrogen dose may be sufficient to relieve vaginal symptoms. Vaginal creams containing the male hormone testosterone are also available. Testosterone (1% or 2%) cream relieves soreness, and is commonly used to treat other vulvar skin disorders (see Chapter 39). Testosterone from the cream is absorbed into the bloodstream, and in large doses may cause masculinizing effects such as growth of facial hair and increased sex drive.

Vitamins. Bioflavonoids and vitamin C have been suggested for treatment of hot flashes. Research evidence for their effectiveness is limited, but one published study reporting use of this combination (a drug called Peridin-C) did document some response to treatment (26). On the whole, though, miracle remedies should be viewed with skepticism. Many herbal remedies and megadose vitamins do have significant effects on body chemistry; that is why they "work" for some people. But very little is known about their potential complications or danger signs. It doesn't make sense to reject a "strong" drug like estrogen because of its known risks only to take another strong drug in the form of herbs whose risks are unknown. Ginseng, for example, can cause blood pressure elevation.

If you are taking vitamins, check to be sure that your daily total for vitamin D is no more than 400 International Units, and for vitamin A no more than 15,000 International Units. Excessive B vitamins, more than 100 mg or so daily, can also cause serious toxicity.

Antispasmodics and Tranquilizers.　　Antispasmodics and tranquilizers are widely used for menopausal symptoms. Some combination drugs like Bellergal that produce general relaxation of smooth muscle may be effective for managing flushes. Many clinicians believe, however, that the primary effect of these drugs and tranquilizers such as Valium and Librium is psychotropic. They blunt the emotional impact of symptoms, along with other life experiences as well. **Tranquilizers are not of any demonstrated value for ameliorating menopausal symptoms.** Tranquilizers may have significant side effects and are also potentially addictive. Nonchemical approaches for improving psychic equilibrium, such as aerobic exercise, meaningful work, psychotherapy, yoga, or meditation, are almost always preferable.

Practical Remedies.　　Feel free to experiment with practical alterations in your daily routine that may help minimize the inconvenience or discomfort of symptoms that you do have. Wardrobe planning that allows you to remove a jacket or sweater may be all you will need during the first year or two when hot flashes are likely to be most severe. You may find that 30 minutes of vigorous exercise every day helps more with insomnia than sleeping pills. Some women find that an immediate drink of ice water can stop a flush reaction. A thermos of ice water on your desk or on the bedside table may be helpful.

Hot flashes tend to be most frequent and severe in hot weather, and some women find that they are triggered by hot foods, hot drinks, caffeine, alcohol, and stress. Avoiding these triggers may help. Also, biofeedback training may be helpful.

Many women use extra lubrication to protect against irritation during intercourse. You can purchase water-soluble lubricants without a prescription. Common brands are Personal Lubricant (Ortho) and K-Y Jelly (Johnson & Johnson). Lubricating suppositories (Lubrin, Upsher-Smith), also containing water-soluble lubricant, may make vaginal placement easier. Some women prefer to use a vegetable oil or unscented cream for lubrication because their lubricating effect persists longer.

Kegel's Muscle Tone Exercises.　　Kegel's exercises are often helpful for women who are having problems with bladder control because of loss of muscle tone. Kegel's exercises are intended to strengthen the pubococcygeus muscles that surround the vagina and anus. In addition to bladder support, these muscles are also important during sexual intercourse. Women with strong muscles and good voluntary control of the pubococcygeus may find arousal and orgasm easier to achieve.

Bladder problems commonly result from muscle tone loss and low estrogen is often the underlying culprit. Evaluation, though, is essential to be sure that you do not have some other cause such as infection. Estrogen treatment may be very helpful, and may help you avoid the necessity for bladder repair surgery. With or without estrogen you may also be able to improve your control through exercise. If so, you will need to continue your exercises regularly and indefinitely or your symptoms are likely to return.

To do Kegel's exercises, try squeezing the muscles of your vagina as you would to stop a stream of urine. Squeeze and continue squeezing as you count to five, and then relax for a count of five. For another exercise, squeeze and relax five times as rapidly as you can. Gradually increase your exercises until you are able to repeat them 50 to 100 times daily. You can do exercises whenever you have a few minutes, while you are waiting in line or stopped at a traffic light, for example.

PREMATURE MENOPAUSE

Estrogen replacement is almost always recommended for women who undergo surgical removal of the ovaries because of infection or other benign disease before age 50. Often such surgery involves hysterectomy as well, so concerns about uterine cancer are not applicable. The very abrupt hormone drop that occurs after such surgery commonly causes severe hot flashes and other menopausal symptoms. Recommendations vary as to the duration of estrogen therapy in such cases, but most clinicians believe that estrogen replacement should be continued until at least age 50, and many would suggest age 55 or 60.

Spontaneous menopause before the age of 40 to 45 is rare, but would also be a strong reason for considering hormone treatment. Women who have low estrogen levels early in life, because of surgery or premature menopause, are at very high risk for osteoporosis and also for premature heart disease. The diagnosis of premature menopause would be based on high blood FSH (follicle-stimulating hormone) levels accompanied by low estrogen production. A woman would be likely to seek evaluation because of absent menstrual periods (amenorrhea) and possibly hot flashes. These are the primary symptoms of premature menopause, which is also called ovarian failure.

Finding Postmenopausal Zest (PMZ)

Finding PMZ may require looking, and possibly changes in daily life. There are several reasons, though, why so many women do succeed. Menopause is often a natural time of change for your family and home situation as well as for your body. For many women the changes have very positive benefits, and may mean time and personal energy to explore activities, talents, or desires that were not feasible earlier in life. More time and energy are also available for personal health improvement.

Lifestyle changes may also seem easier because the rewards are immediate and obvious. At age 50, you are likely to notice how much better you feel with even a small improvement in your exercise or diet; younger women may find the difference less noticeable. And the perspective and wisdom gained through years of managing somehow are helpful. Remembering traumas overcome in the past can help keep present-day anxieties or terrors in perspective.

In **Menopause Naturally**, Sadja Greenwood reviews helpful steps toward PMZ in detail. Reading her book, and others as well, is a good starting point for a serious PMZ seeker. Dr. Greenwood's recommendations include:

- Take time to explore your own feelings about aging; identify negative beliefs and myths that you may be harboring unawares; strengthen your positive mental picture of aging
- Stay (or become) involved with other people, and with constructive, ongoing human tasks
- Learn healthy ways to help yourself relax and calm down. Stress is a normal part of life; stress-reduction techniques like meditation or relaxation exercises are much healthier than alcohol, tranquilizers, or stewing. Practice stress reduction for minor, everyday stresses, and you will have a weapon available when big stresses do occur.
- Find ways to make exercise a reliable and pleasurable part of everyday life. Include both aerobic exercise to benefit your heart and bones and stretching exercises to help with relaxation and flexibility.
- Learn about nutrition and make healthy food a high priority. For women after 50, a diet high in complex carbohydrates and vegetables, moderate to low in protein, and low in fat has many health benefits. Plenty of calcium, and not much sugar and salt, are also good rules.
- Tackle toxins. Menopause is an excellent time to quit smoking, reduce or eliminate caffeine intake, or cope with alcohol problems.
- Be sure you have the help you need. Take the time to find an excellent clinician—competent, committed to preventive health, and able to communicate with you. And if you are suffering because of depression or problems at home, for example, ask for help.

Let **yourself** be your own number one priority. It is entirely fair and reasonable to do so, but if you are like many women, this will be quite a new experience.

SUGGESTED READING

Brecher, Edward M., and editors of Consumers Report Books: *Love, Sex and Aging.* Mount Vernon, N.Y.: Consumers Union, 1984.

Budoff, Penny W.: *No More Hot Flashes and Other Good News.* New York: G.P. Putnam's Sons, 1983.

Cutler, Winnifred B., Garcia, Celso-Ramon; and Edwards, David A.: *Menopause: A Guide for Women and Men Who Love Them.* New York: W.W. Norton & Co., 1983.

Greenwood, Sadja: *Menopause Naturally: Preparing for the Second Half of Life.* San Francisco: Volcano Press, 1984.

Notelovitz, Morris, and Ware, Marsha: *Stand Tall! Every Woman's Guide to Preventing Osteoporosis.* New York: Bantam Books, 1984.

Sarrel, Lorna J., and Sarrel, Philip M.: *Sexual Turning Points—The Seven Stages of Adult Sexuality.* New York: Macmillan, 1984.

REFERENCES

1. Jensen J, Christiansen C, Rodbro P: Cigarette smoking, serum estrogens, and bone loss during hormone-replacement therapy early after menopause. *New England Journal of Medicine* 313:973–975, 1985.
2. Scott JZ, Cumming DC: The menopause. *Current Problems in Obstetrics, Gynecology and Fertility* 8:1–58, 1985.
3. Avioli LV: *The Osteoporotic Syndrome—Detection, Prevention, and Treatment.* New York: Grune & Stratton, 1983.
4. Aloia JF: Exercise and skeletal health. *Journal of the American Geriatrics Society* 29:104–107, 1981.
5. Lindberg JS, Powell MR, Hunt MM, et al: Increased vertebral bone mineral in response to reduced exercise in amenorrheic runners. *Western Journal of Medicine* 146:39–42, 1987.
6. Riis B, Thomsen K, Christiansen C: Does calcium supplementation prevent post menopausal bone loss? *New England Journal of Medicine* 316:173–177, 1987.
7. Health and Public Policy Committee, American College of Physicians: Radiologic methods to evaluate bone mineral content. *Annals of Internal Medicine* 100:908–911, 1984.
8. Ray WA, Griffin MR, Schaffner W: Psychotropic drug use and the risk of hip fracture. *New England Journal of Medicine* 316:363–369, 1987.
9. Cutler WB, Garcia C-R: *The Medical Management of Menopause and Premenopause.* Philadelphia: J.B. Lippincott Co., 1984.
10. National Institutes of Health: Osteoporosis. *National Institutes of Health Consensus Development Conference Statement,* Vol 5, No 3, 1984.
11. Ettinger B, Genant HK, Cann CE: Postmenopausal bone loss is prevented by treatment with low-dosage estrogen with calcium. *Annals of Internal Medicine* 106:40–45, 1987.
12. Abdalla HI, Hart DM, Lindsay R, et al: Prevention of bone mineral loss in postmenopausal women by norethisterone. *Obstetrics and Gynecology* 66:789–792, 1985.
13. Whitehead M, Lane G, Siddle N, et al: Avoidance of endometrial hyperstimulation in estrogen-treated postmenopausal women. *Seminars in Reproductive Endocrinology* 1:41–54, 1983.
14. Wingo PA, Layde PM, Lee NC: The risk of breast cancer in postmenopausal women who have used estrogen replacement therapy. *Journal of the American Medical Association* 245:209–215, 1987.
15. Whitehead MI: Controversies concerning the safety of estrogen replacement therapy. *American Journal of Obstetrics and Gynecology* 156:1313–1322, 1987.
16. Ross RK, Paganini-Hill A: Estrogen replacement therapy and coronary heart disease. *Seminars in Reproductive Endocrinology* 1:19–26, 1983.
17. Wilson PWF, Garrison RJ, Castelli WP: Postmenopausal estrogen use, cigarette smoking, and cardiovascular morbidity in women over 50. The Framingham study. *New England Journal of Medicine* 313:1038–1043, 1985.
18. Mashchak CA, Lobo RA: Estrogen replacement therapy and hypertension. *Journal of Reproductive Medicine* 30:805–810, 1985.
19. Lane G, Siddle NC, Ryder TA, et al: Is Provera the ideal progestogen for addition to postmenopausal estrogen therapy? *Fertility and Sterility* 45:345–352, 1986.

20. Stampfer MJ, Willett WC, Colditz GA, et al: A prospective study of postmenopausal estrogen therapy and coronary heart disease. *New England Journal of Medicine* 313:1044–1049, 1985.
21. Chu J, Schweid AI, Weiss NS: Survival among women with endometrial cancer: A comparison of estrogen users and nonusers. *American Journal of Obstetrics and Gynecology* 143:569–573, 1982.
22. Chetkowski RJ, Meldrum DR, Steingold KA: Biologic effects of transdermal estradiol. *New England Journal of Medicine* 314:1615–1620, 1986.
23. Judd H: Efficacy of transdermal estradiol. *American Journal of Obstetrics and Gynecology* 156:1326–1331, 1987.
24. Deutsch S, Ossowski R, Benjamin I: Comparison between degree of systemic absorption of vaginally and orally administered estrogens at different dose levels in postmenopausal women. *American Journal of Obstetrics and Gynecology* 139:967–970, 1981.
25. Weinstein L: Efficacy of a continuous estrogen–progestin regimen in the menopausal patient. *Obstetrics and Gynecology* 69:929–932, 1987.
26. Smith CJ: Non-hormonal control of vaso-motor flushing in menopausal patients. *Chicago Medicine* 67:193–195, 1964.

35

❖

Abnormal Pap Smear Results

Cervical cancer is almost certainly a sexually transmitted disease (STD). Research evidence now strongly suggests that the wart virus, called human papillomavirus, or HPV, is the key culprit (1,2,3). The HPV family includes many slightly different virus strains, and only certain specific HPV strains are linked to cervical cancer. These same strains are also linked to penile cancer. In addition to HPV, other factors such as smoking and infection with herpes virus may also play a role in cervical cancer—possibly as cancer cofactors. Prolonged use of birth control Pills and exposure during fetal life to DES (diethylstilbestrol—DES daughters) may also affect risk, possibly by impacting susceptibility to wart virus infection.

A woman who has precancerous or cancerous cell changes on the surface of her cervix has been exposed to human papillomavirus from a sex partner's penis (4). Because wart virus is slow-growing and often inconspicuous, it may be months or even years before a problem becomes evident, but if you are at risk for any STD, you are at risk for this one as well.

As with other STDs, this one is preventable to some degree. Limit your total number of sex partners and use condoms and/or other barrier contraceptives when you say yes to sex.

And be thankful to the Greek physician/cytologist George Nicolas Papanicolaou. At about mid-century he developed the Pap smear; with this tool, cervical cell changes can be detected and therefore treated, early, well before cancer appears.

The primary purpose of a Pap smear is to detect the presence of abnormal cells on the surface of your cervix. It is a fairly sensitive and reliable test that reveals early precancerous cell changes, as well as true cervical cancer. Regular Pap tests are important, for abnormalities that are detected **early** can be treated easily and very effectively. Usually the earliest precancer cell changes evolve to true cancer over a period of years, so an annual Pap smear is likely to give you and your clinician plenty of treatment time.

The Pap test does not reliably detect cancer of the uterus, vagina, or ovaries. It can detect cervical or vaginal infection in some cases, and can provide a general idea of your estrogen levels. Being faithful about a routine Pap smear schedule is important for all women who have had sexual intercourse. **Pap tests at least once a year are absolutely essential for any woman who has one or more of the following risk factors for cervical cancer:**

• Previous CIN (cervical intraepithelial neoplasia, also called dysplasia; see discussion later in this chapter)
• Infection with HPV (genital warts)
• Previous sexually transmitted infection such as herpes or gonorrhea
• Previous vulvar or vaginal cancer
• Exposure to a male whose previous partner had CIN or cervical cancer
• Exposure to a sexual partner with penile cancer
• Exposure to more than one male sexual partner (lifetime)
• Smoking cigarettes
• DES daughter
• Use of birth control Pills
• First intercourse before age 18 to 20
• First pregnancy before age 18 to 20

To prepare a Pap test your clinician gently rotates a slender wooden or plastic spatula over the surface of your cervix. This is a painless procedure completed in a few seconds during the speculum examination part of a routine pelvic exam. Your clinician spreads cells from the spatula across a glass slide and then sprays the slide or immerses it in a fixative. The slide is sent from your clinician's office to a laboratory to be stained and examined under the microscope by a specially trained technician (cytotechnician) or physician laboratory specialist (pathologist).

The pathologist or cytotechnician who examines your Pap smear slide looks at the shape, size, and structure of the cells; next she/he checks the number of cells of each type to assign a "reading" to your smear. If all the cells on your slide are types of cells that are present on the surface of a normal cervix, then your test result is normal. If abnormal cells are present, your Pap test report will show the type and degree of abnormality.

There are several different schemes for classifying Pap test abnormalities. One of the oldest and most common schemes divides Pap results into five classes: Class I is normal, and Class II designates abnormal infection cells (Class II abnormalities are

TABLE 35-1
PAP SMEAR CLASSIFICATIONS

TERM USED IN THIS CHAPTER	CLASS	OTHER TERMS
Normal	I	Benign, normal Metaplasia Squamous metaplasia
Inflammatory	II	Inflammation Inflammation with atypia Atypia Warty atypia Koilocytotic warty atypia
Mild CIN[a] Moderate CIN[a]	III	Mild dysplasia Moderate dysplasia
Severe CIN[a]	IV	Severe dysplasia Carcinoma in situ
Cancer	V	Invasive cancer

[a]"CIN" means cervical intraepithelial neoplasia.

not precancerous). Class III and Class IV indicate mild to severe precancerous cell changes, and Class V is true cervical cancer.

A newer scheme, preferred by most experts in this field, divides Pap tests into three major categories:

• Benign: no evidence of cancer or of cancer precursors
• CIN (cervical intraepithelial neoplasia): precancerous cell abnormalities are present
• Malignant: cervical cancer cells are present

These schemes are confusing, the names are complicated, and it is not important to memorize them. To make this chapter simpler, only the "CIN system" terminology will be used. If your clinician uses a different scheme or different terms, you can substitute according to Table 35-1. The important point to understand about these schemes and grading systems is that cervical cell changes are a very gradual continuum. If you have CIN, it does not mean that you have cancer. It does mean that you need further evaluation and treatment, however.

Understanding Your Pap Smear Result

An older friend told me she was 40 years old when she had her first Pap smear, when they were *the* hot new test. To me it's unimaginable that there haven't always been Pap smears! Just think how really sick women must have been back then before they had any warning symptoms to send them to the doctor. . . . We're lucky!

—WOMAN, 39

The principle of the Pap test is that cells collected from the surface of your cervix for study will accurately reflect what the surface of your cervix is like. During a woman's reproductive years, the surface (epithelium) of the cervix is composed of about ten cell layers. There is constant cell growth within the cervical epithelium; new cells are produced at the bottom layer, then gradually mature and move up to the top surface as old cells are shed from the top. The Pap test scraper collects cells that are loose and ready to be shed from the top surface layer.

When precancerous cell abnormalities occur, the cell maturation process is disturbed and immature cells move closer to the surface. Unusually large or distorted cells are present, so an **increased proportion** of immature and distorted cells will appear on your Pap smear.

Precancerous abnormalities almost invariably arise at the junction between the multilayered, smooth squamous epithelium that covers the outer surface of the cervix and the velvety, columnar epithelium that lines the cervical canal. The location of this junction, called the SCJ, or squamocolumnar junction, changes with age. Early in the reproductive years, columnar epithelium extends from the cervical canal out onto the surface of the cervix (see Illustration 35-1). The SCJ is located some distance away from the cervical canal opening, and columnar epithelium is clearly visible. Dark pink, velvety columnar epithelium surrounding the cervical opening is also called *ectropion*. The columnar epithelium on the outer surface of the cervix is gradually replaced by squamous epithelium over the first 10 or 15 years after puberty. The replacement process, called **squamous metaplasia**, is entirely normal. At its conclusion, the entire cervical surface is covered by pale, shiny squamous epithelium and the SCJ is located at or inside the cervical opening. Cell patterns suggesting squamous metaplasia are often apparent on a Pap smear. After menopause the cervical epithelium becomes thinner, and may contain only a few cell layers. Cell multiplication and growth are also slowed.

For accurate Pap smear results a good sample from the area of the squamocolumnar junction is essential. Other factors as well can influence Pap smear accuracy.

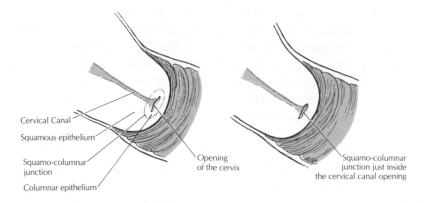

ILLUSTRATION 35-1 Precancerous abnormalities and cervical cancer are most likely to arise at the border between the squamous epithelium that covers the surface of the cervix and the columnar epithelium that lines the cervical canal. The border, called the squamocolumnar junction (SCJ), is located near the opening of the cervical canal.

PAP SMEAR ACCURACY

No medical test is 100% accurate, and that certainly includes Pap smear results. An incorrect diagnosis can be made if you use tampons or douche just before your exam, if the sample is improperly collected, or if the laboratory technician makes an error in reading the smear.

The time interval between Pap smears may also be a factor. After one Pap smear scraping removes the superficial shedding cells from the cervix, time is required for a representative collection of new shedding cells to accumulate. A second Pap smear taken less than four weeks later is not as accurate, so results could be falsely negative.

A false-negative test result, in this case a normal Pap smear report despite abnormal cell patterns actually present on your cervix, is potentially harmful, because both you and your clinician may be misled by the normal report and delay in identifying and treating your problem. As many as 20% of patients with invasive cervical cancer have two or more negative Pap smears during the three years preceding their cancer diagnosis (5). Many of these false-negatives are caused by problems in obtaining and preparing the slide, but in one large study laboratory misdiagnosis led to false-negative reports for 7.5% of the Pap smears that actually showed moderate CIN, severe CIN, or cancer (6). False-positive Pap test reading errors are less common, about 3% in the same study, and may involve less potential danger. Nevertheless, a good rule to follow is never to permit any surgical treatment solely on the basis of one abnormal Pap smear.

Despite inherent accuracy problems, Pap testing is definitely worthwhile. Cervical cancer rates are 200% to 400% higher for women who have not had Pap testing than for women who have had testing; when Pap testing is done, precancerous abnormalities are found and treated so **cancer is prevented.**

For an individual woman, Pap test accuracy problems mean that one Pap test is not enough. **Your best protection against the possible danger of a false-negative Pap smear is your own faithfulness about a regular Pap smear schedule.** If you have three normal Pap smears, for example, over a three-year interval, the chance that a serious abnormality is being missed is exceedingly small. Annual Pap smears thereafter insure that any new abnormalities that develop will be detected at the earliest possible stage.

For ideal Pap smear conditions, schedule your exam midway between menstrual periods, and avoid putting anything into your vagina beforehand. That means no tampons, douching, contraceptive products, or intercourse for one or two days before your test. If conditions are not ideal, however, it may be essential to have a Pap smear anyway. Your Pap smear should not be delayed just because of bleeding, for example. Abnormal bleeding could be due to cervical cancer, and delay would cost you valuable treatment time.

NORMAL PAP SMEAR RESULTS

All the cells at the top layer of normal cervical epithelium are older, fully matured cells with a flat, geometric "pancake" shape and a small nucleus. Your Pap smear slide contains only mature cells if it is normal.

A normal Pap smear report also means that the slide contained a sufficient number of cells for diagnosis, and that slide preparation was satisfactory. Otherwise the report diagnosis should be "insufficient specimen," and you would need a repeat Pap smear at least four weeks later.

The report may also note apparent estrogen effect, low or average, as well as the presence of endometrial cells from the uterine lining. Endometrial cells are not normally found on Pap smears for women after menopause unless the smear specimen was collected close to the time of monthly bleeding related to hormone treatment. If you are postmenopausal and endometrial cells are found, further evaluation for uterine hyperplasia or uterine cancer may be needed (see Chapters 40 and 41).

Your Pap test result is quite likely to be normal. Overall, about 95% of Pap smears are benign, with no evidence of cancer or precancerous abnormalities.

INFLAMMATORY PAP SMEAR RESULTS

When you have a cervical infection or when your cervix is in the process of healing after infection or injury, the surface is disrupted by swelling, and many inflammatory cells—infection-fighting white blood cells—are present among normal mature cells. Inflammation would be expected after a cervical biopsy or for several months after your cervix has been treated with cryosurgery or laser, as described in the section of this chapter entitled "Treatment for CIN." Infectious bacteria may also be present.

Inflammation of the cervix (cervicitis) is commonly caused by infection. Your Pap test is likely to reflect cervicitis no matter what is causing your inflammation. If you have a severe vaginal infection such as trichomonas, your vaginal discharge may contain inflammatory cells and bacteria; these cells may be evident on your Pap smear even if infection has not truly invaded your cervix.

Inflammatory cell changes are not precancerous and do not progress to cancer. Inflammatory smears are undesirable because the presence of a large number of inflammatory cells can obscure the changes in cervical cells that your Pap smear is meant to detect; they interfere with accurate evaluation of your smear. Be sure that you have another Pap smear three to six months after an inflammatory result, once your cervicitis or vaginitis has been treated and cured.

In some cases the possible cause of inflammation is identified in the Pap smear report. Yeast cells or trichomonas organisms present on a Pap slide are a good clue that you may have a vaginal infection (see Chapter 23), but a pelvic exam to be certain is probably reasonable before treatment. You may have a mixed infection, and optimal treatment depends on accurate identification of all your pathogens.

Some women show unexplained inflammatory cells in their Pap smears that persist for long periods, and these women "routinely" have abnormal, inflammatory Pap test reports. This condition is not serious, and it is not an indication of cancer. It is inconvenient, because frequent Pap tests are required.

Atypia or Inflammation with Atypia. When the surface layers are disrupted by infection, immature cells may reach the surface and appear on your Pap smear. These are called **atypical** cells (see Illustration 35-2). The pathologist may also use the term atypia when your Pap smear slide shows just a very few abnormal-appearing cells, too few to assign a definite CIN classification. And in some cases the Pap smear shows large surface cells that have a pale area around the nucleus at the center of the cell. These are called koilocytes, cells infected with wart virus. In this situation the pathologist may report **warty atypia** or **koilocytotic warty atypia.**

Colposcopy evaluation (described later in this chapter) and careful follow-up with **repeat Pap testing every three to six months is essential if your Pap smear shows atypia. Just repeating your Pap smear alone is not safe.** Pap smears can be falsely negative (see "Pap Smear Accuracy" earlier in this chapter), especially if the abnormal area is small in size, and colposcopy may reveal that true CIN, or in very rare cases, true cancer, is already present (7). Atypia may have been the only clue, with no Pap smear evidence of more advanced problems. You and your clinician must assume that a Pap smear report of atypia means **possible CIN,** even though the report is classified as benign.

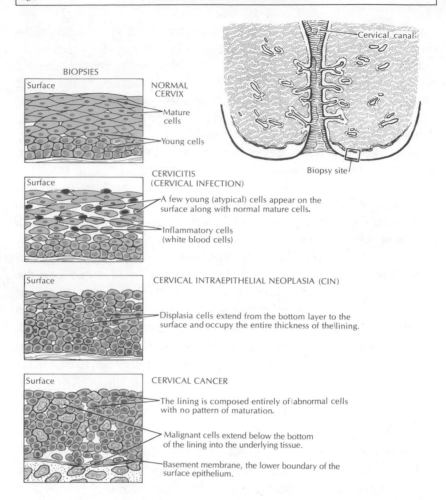

BIOPSIES

Surface — NORMAL CERVIX

Mature cells

Young cells

Cervical canal

Biopsy site

Surface — CERVICITIS (CERVICAL INFECTION)

A few young (atypical) cells appear on the surface along with normal mature cells.

Inflammatory cells (white blood cells)

Surface — CERVICAL INTRAEPITHELIAL NEOPLASIA (CIN)

Displasia cells extend from the bottom layer to the surface and occupy the entire thickness of the lining.

Surface — CERVICAL CANCER

The lining is composed entirely of abnormal cells with no pattern of maturation.

Malignant cells extend below the bottom of the lining into the underlying tissue.

Basement membrane, the lower boundary of the surface epithelium.

ILLUSTRATION 35-2   **The Pap smear detects abnormal cells present on the surface of the cervix. A cervical biopsy provides a sample of tissue with cell layers *intact*.**

Studies of women with Pap smear evidence of atypia show that 10% to 20% already have definite CIN detectable with colposcopy and biopsy, and that as many as 33% of the remainder will develop CIN within the next 12 months (8,9,10). The rate for CIN is even higher, about 50%, for women who have evidence of atypia on repeated Pap smears. On the other hand, women with definite CIN, proven by biopsy, may have one or more repeat smears reported as negative. This finding occurred for 10% of CIN patients in one study (9).

If you have a Pap smear result showing atypia, and your colposcopy and repeat Pap smear are normal, you can breathe a sigh of relief, at least for the time being. It may be that your problem will solve itself; perhaps you had a temporary cervical infection that healed on its own, or perhaps the first Pap smear was not accurate. Being faithful about your follow-up Pap smears, however, is essential. You need to be absolutely certain that atypia signs do not reappear.

CIN (CERVICAL INTRAEPITHELIAL NEOPLASIA)

When CIN is present, part or all of the squamous epithelial layers are made up of dysplastic or abnormal cells ("dys" means abnormal, "plasia" means growth) as shown in Illustration 35-2. These cells multiply more rapidly than normal squamous cells, and are apparent on a Pap smear because of their large, irregular central cell nucleus. At the severe end of this progression, the entire thickness of the surface epithelium is composed of dysplastic cells, and no normal mature squamous cells are present. CIN cell changes are restricted to the epithelium (surface) of the cervix, and usually to only a small area of the surface. **The abnormal cells of CIN do not invade other tissues.**

CIN is precancerous, or potentially cancerous. In 30% to 50% of **untreated** cases, abnormal cell development would gradually become more severe and would eventually result in true cancer of the cervix, which can invade other tissues. The time for progression from an initial precancerous Pap result to true cervical cancer is not predictable. Reported time ranges vary from less than a year to ten years. In some cases Pap smear results may return to normal after an initial abnormal smear, and only later reappear as a more severe precancerous abnormality or even invasive cancer (11). **Faithful and frequent follow-up exams and Pap smears are essential for any woman who has had one precancerous Pap result, even if her initial evaluation is normal, and her Pap results have returned to normal.**

With proper treatment CIN can be cured in nearly all cases, and cervical cancer will be prevented.

CIN AND WART VIRUS INFECTION

Human papillomavirus (HPV) is a large virus family with more than 40 distinct strains. Some HPV strains cause warts on the hands, others on the feet, and some primarily affect the genital skin. Several strains choose the cervix, vulva, vagina, and penis, and these are transmitted by sexual intercourse. Some HPV strains cause rough, protruding warts. The strains linked to cervical (and penile) cancer, however, may cause flat warts that are quite inconspicuous and produce no noticeable symptoms. They may not even be visible to the eye without special staining and magnification.

Evidence of human papillomavirus infection is found in 2% to 10% of Pap smears from women under age 30 (3). Cervical cells infected with HPV are abnormal in appearance and the Pap smear may be reported as **warty atypia** or **koilocytotic warty atypia**. In some cases dysplastic cells are present as well, and the Pap smear reading may be reported as CIN. **Further evaluation and treatment is essential for warty atypia, just as it would be for CIN.**

Researchers have been able to demonstrate the link between HPV and cervical cancer only recently. High-tech laboratory methods have allowed researchers to identify different strains of HPV and to find evidence that HPV is present inside cells from CIN or cancer tissue (12). Other cancer risk factors may be involved as well, but the primary importance of HPV in causing CIN and cervical cancer is firmly established.

A woman or man who has genital warts may or may not be infected with the specific HPV strains that can cause cancer. Unfortunately, HPV cannot be grown in culture and there is no practical way to determine which HPV strains an individual does have without elaborate research laboratory investigation. When warts are evident, therefore, you will need very careful evaluation for cervical abnormalities. Colposcopy and a Pap smear are essential, and you will need a biopsy if suspicious areas are seen on your cervix. The procedures are described in the next section. Men with genital warts, too, require careful evaluation (see the last section in this chapter).

Evaluation and Treatment

If your Pap test shows CIN or atypia, the first step is to be sure that the diagnosis is accurate. The goal in evaluation is to verify that the Pap smear findings are not in error, and to be sure that you do not have invasive cervical cancer.

CERVICAL BIOPSY

The Pap smear, a sample of shedding cells from the surface of the cervical epithelium, provides a reflection of cervical abnormalities, but for complete and accurate diagnosis the pathologist must evaluate the **layered structure** of cells that make up the surface. A biopsy provides the pathologist an actual tissue sample **with all the cell layers intact,** as shown in Illustration 35-2. **Cervical biopsy,** to remove a shallow 1/16-by-1/16-inch piece of tissue from the outer surface of the cervix, is a simple office procedure. You may have a short cramping sensation just as the biopsy is done, but it should stop within a few seconds and a local anesthetic usually is not necessary. **Endocervical curettage (ECC),** to provide biopsy samples from the lining of the cervical canal, may also be needed. For ECC your clinician will use a very narrow metal scraper called a curet to remove a shallow strand of cervical lining tissue as the curet is scraped downward inside your cervical canal. ECC is also likely to cause cramping that lasts a minute or two. If your Pap result is CIN or cancer, your clinician is almost certain to recommend biopsy.

Biopsy sites are best chosen by careful examination of the cervix with a colposcope (see Chapter 4). This procedure is painless. The colposcope looks like binoculars mounted on a tripod or moveable arm; for colposcopy your clinician looks through the colposcope to see the surface of your cervix magnified 10 to 20 times normal size. The colposcope does not touch you, but you will have to lie still with a speculum in place in your vagina for as long as 10 or 20 minutes for the exam. Also, your clinician will use dilute vinegar solution, mopped over your cervix with a cotton swab, to remove mucus and make the surface features more distinct and you may notice a mild stinging sensation from the vinegar.

The magnification provided by colposcopy will help your clinician determine exactly where the abnormal area is. Biopsy specimens can then be taken from the most abnormal area(s). Also, your clinician will look for abnormal blood vessel patterns visible with colposcopy that may indicate an area of more severe CIN or invasive cancer. The ECC specimens are needed to check for any abnormalities hidden from view up inside the cervical canal.

Complications after biopsy or ECC are rare. You should avoid intercourse, douching, and tampons for about a week so that your cervix can heal, and watch for signs of infection such as pain, fever, or abnormal vaginal discharge. Contact your clinician if you have any of these signs or if you have heavy bleeding. It is normal to have some spotting or very light bleeding after biopsy.

If your clinician is able to see the entire abnormal area with colposcopy and your biopsy report confirms CIN, then you have the information you need to assess your treatment options. If there is any doubt about colposcopy findings, if your biopsy report does not agree with your Pap smear, or if your ECC shows evidence of CIN, then your clinician will probably recommend conization surgery to remove a major part of your cervical surface.

CERVICAL CONIZATION SURGERY

Before colposcopy became widely available, conization surgery was a routine recommendation for a woman with mild CIN, moderate CIN, and in some cases severe CIN. Today, conization is recommended only for selected patients who have CIN, but who cannot be evaluated fully with the colposcope because the abnormal area extends up into the cervical canal beyond the view of the colposcope. If the entire extent of the abnormal area is not visible, it is impossible for a clinician to be certain, with colposcopy alone, that biopsy specimens represent the worst areas of abnormality. Conization surgery in this situation provides the information that colposcopically directed biopsies are otherwise able to provide: the assurance that CIN alone, and not cancer, is responsible for abnormal Pap smear results. Conization is also appropriate if biopsy results are not conclusive.

Because the entire surface epithelium around the cervical opening and the lining of the cervical canal are removed in conization surgery, it may serve to eradicate the abnormal areas, thus providing treatment for CIN as well as diagnosis. Conization, however, would not be advised when treatment alone is the goal. Serious complications

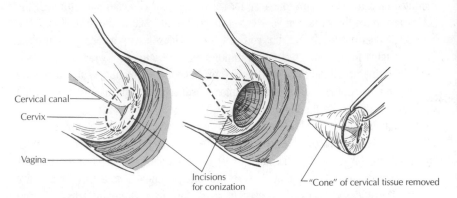

Cervical canal

Cervix

Vagina

Incisions
for conization

"Cone" of cervical tissue removed

ILLUSTRATION 35-3   Conization of the cervix is a major surgical procedure
that may be necessary when CIN is present and the abnormal area extends
up into the cervical canal beyond the view of the colposcope.

are more common with conization than they are with cryosurgery or laser treatment,
the other options for eradicating CIN. Also, conization surgery requires general
anesthesia and is performed in a hospital or surgical center setting.

For a conization procedure you are given general anesthesia and then positioned as
for a pelvic examination. The surgeon uses a vaginal speculum to see your cervix. After
she/he places stitches on each side of your cervix to stabilize it and to diminish
bleeding, she/he makes a circular incision through the surface of the cervix so that the
entire abnormal area is included within the portion to be removed (see Illustration
35-3). The incision is extended deep into your cervix in a cone shape so that the lower
portion of the cervical canal is removed along with the outer surface of the cervix. After
the center cone of cervix is removed, the cut edges of the cervix are stitched.

Heavy bleeding is a common complication of conization that can occur during or
immediately after surgery or about ten days later when the cervical stitches are
absorbed. One patient in ten may require treatment, including transfusion, hospitalization, and/or further surgery, because of hemorrhage. Infection and perforation of the
uterus are other immediate complications that can occur with conization, but they are
uncommon.

Long-term effects of conization can also be serious. Cervical incompetence, leading
to premature delivery in subsequent pregnancies, sometimes occurs. Inadequate cervical
mucus production after conization (which removes a substantial portion of the cervical
tissue that contains mucus glands) may be a cause of impaired fertility. Conization
can also cause scarring of the cervical canal. If the cervical canal is blocked,
menstrual blood may be trapped inside the uterus. Cervical scarring can also interfere
with proper cervical dilation during labor and delivery in later pregnancies.

TREATMENT FOR CIN

The goal of CIN treatment is to eradicate the abnormal cells. If conization surgery has been necessary for diagnosis, then no further treatment may be necessary. Hysterectomy would also eliminate the abnormal cells, for the uterus and cervix would be completely removed (see Chapter 49). **In most cases, however, either cryosurgery or laser treatment will be recommended.**

You and your clinician will want to consider several factors as you decide on treatment for CIN. Your feelings about future pregnancies are one factor, as well as your age and other medical problems you may have. Another factor is the size and location of the abnormal area on your cervix. The severity of your CIN is another factor, although research evidence now indicates that overall size may be more important than severity in determining treatment success (13). Even if you have **severe CIN (carcinoma in situ)**, most experts (14) believe that it is reasonable and safe to choose cryosurgery or laser treatment, and this would be a completely appropriate choice if you desire future pregnancies.

Hysterectomy.   Hysterectomy may be a reasonable choice if future pregnancy is not a consideration for you and you have other significant gynecologic problems that could also warrant surgery. Problems with pain or bleeding because of benign uterine fibroids might be an example. The likelihood that CIN would recur after hysterectomy is remote, but you will still need to be faithful about follow-up exams.

Cyrosurgery.   If your area of CIN is not too extensive, then cryosurgery will probably be your treatment choice. Cryosurgery is a five- or ten-minute office procedure that allows your clinician to freeze the surface of your cervix; cryosurgery is almost painless and is extremely effective in eradicating CIN. Overall, CIN is cured with a single cryosurgical treatment in about 90% of cases; when persisting CIN is treated a second time with cryosurgery, the cure rate reaches 98% (15).

Complications after cryosurgery are not common. Narrowing or scarring of the cervical canal can occur, however, and may be of special concern when a DES daughter requires CIN treatment (see Chapter 42). Destruction of mucous glands by cryosurgery can also reduce cervical mucus secretion and impair future fertility in rare cases, although in other cases cervical mucus quality and fertility are improved (16).

Complications are less common with cryosurgery and laser treatment than they are with any of the other CIN treatment options. Hysterectomy and conization involve the risks of major surgery, and fertility problems after conization surgery are not uncommon. Complications are also higher for cautery, used in the past to treat early CIN; cautery with heat or electric current is no longer a preferred option because the extent of tissue destruction is more difficult to control and pain during treatment is more severe than is the case with cryosurgery or laser treatment.

Laser Treatment. A carbon dioxide laser beam, guided by a colposcopic view of your cervix, can be used with great precision to evaporate a shallow area of the surface epithelium. Laser treatment is especially helpful when the abnormal CIN area is geographically large. With one or more laser treatment appointments, a wide area can be safely and effectively eradicated. Healing after laser treatment is likely to be more rapid, and the area of destruction more precisely controlled, than is the case with cryosurgery. Laser may also be better suited for treating areas higher up in the cervical canal where effective freezing is difficult to achieve, or when treatment with cryosurgery has failed to eradicate CIN. Laser treatment success rates are similar to rates for cryosurgery. CIN can be eradicated in at least 98% of patients, but approximately 10% require more than one treatment (17).

Laser treatment does not usually cause severe pain, and can be done without general anesthesia in most cases. The treatment is time-consuming, however, and laser equipment is expensive. It is not commonly available in office practice, so outpatient treatment at a hospital may be necessary. As a result, laser treatment is likely to be more expensive than cryosurgery.

FOLLOW-UP AFTER TREATMENT

No matter what your treatment is for CIN, faithfulness about follow-up exams is essential. With cryosurgery or laser treatment, frequent exams and Pap smears during the first six to twelve months are needed to determine whether treatment has been successful. A reasonable follow-up plan might include repeat Pap tests 3 to 4 months after treatment, again at 6 to 8 months, and again at 12 to 15 months. Repeat colposcopy may also be recommended. The purpose of intensive follow-up is to detect any persisting abnormality as soon as possible. Following this schedule, with colposcopy repeated at the time of the first follow-up visit, researchers in one study were able to detect 98% of persisting abnormalities at the first visit (18). After conization surgery, follow-up Pap smears are also essential to be certain that all of the abnormal epithelium has been removed. If your Pap smears show CIN again, you will need further treatment.

While your cervix is healing after cryosurgery, laser, or conization, you will be strongly advised to use condoms. Healing will require at least six to eight weeks, but continuing with condoms at least until your follow-up Pap smear results are normal is a wise precaution.

Women who use birth control Pills have a slightly higher than average risk for developing CIN. Whether or not using birth control Pills has any effect on the progression of CIN or healing after treatment, however, is not known. The results of one small study provide some reassurance. The rate of progression from mild to more severe CIN was no faster for Pill users than it was for women using other birth control methods (19).

You will need good birth control protection during your healing phase. **Pregnancy must be delayed until you are sure that CIN has been eradicated.** Ideally, you should wait until you have had three normal Pap smear results at follow-up exams at least one month apart.

In the months and years after CIN treatment your clinician will also watch carefully for vaginal or vulvar abnormalities. Cancer and cancer precursors involving the vagina and vulva are also linked to human papillomavirus, so the fact that you have had CIN means you are at risk for these problems as well. Your risk for developing CIN of the cervix again in the future is probably also higher than average. See Chapter 41 for more information on risk factors and symptoms of vulvar and vaginal cancer.

MINIMIZING YOUR RISKS FOR CIN

I was floored when I found that having dysplasia is no different from having gonorrhea, at least in one respect: You get it from a sex partner! "Nuns don't get cervical dysplasia," my doctor says. Why didn't anybody tell me sooner?

—WOMAN, 28

Since CIN is a sexually transmitted disease linked to HPV (human papillomavirus) infection, **the most important preventive measures are those that decrease your risk of exposure to sexually transmitted infection,** or reduce the risk of acquiring infection if exposure does occur. Barrier methods of birth control such as condoms or a diaphragm help prevent infection, and using them significantly reduces a woman's risk for cervical cancer. Increased infection susceptibility may also be a factor in cervical cancer risk for some groups of women. Very young women, DES daughters, and women who use birth control Pills all tend to have a larger area of velvety columnar epithelium on the surface of the cervix. Clinicians call this ectropion. These same groups also have somewhat higher cervical cancer risks than average. It is possible that ectropion tissue makes a woman more susceptible to acquiring virus infection, and if this is true, the risk increase observed would make sense. Some researchers, however, feel that the risk for birth control Pill users and DES daughters is actually related to slight differences in their numbers of sexual partners.

Smoking cigarettes is also statistically linked to CIN; whether smoking acts as a cocarcinogen or whether women who smoke differ in other ways that might affect CIN risk from women who do not smoke is not known. It is also possible that additional factors such as diet may play a role in cervical cancer risk (see Chapter 41). One small study has documented lower vitamin C levels in women with CIN compared to women with normal Pap results (20).

If you have CIN you might consider switching from birth control Pills to condoms, and increasing your intake of vitamin C, beta carotene, and possibly folic acid. There isn't any definite proof that these precautions would help, but they certainly won't be harmful, especially if the extra inconvenience and cost aren't an issue.

An epidemic of wart virus is now occurring. The number of people being treated for genital warts has increased 400% to 500% in the last decade, and like all sexually transmitted diseases, warts are especially common among young people. Recognized warts are more common than herpes, and even more people actually have wart virus infection but are unaware of it because they do not have obvious, visible warts.

To minimize your risk for acquiring CIN, avoid intercourse or use condoms faithfully if:

• You are very young (less than 18 to 20 years of age)
• You (or your partner) have more than one current partner
• You suspect for any reason that your partner may have a sexually transmitted infection
• Your partner has penile warts or penile cancer
• Your partner has had a previous partner with CIN or cervical cancer

It makes sense to consider CIN risk as you make decisions about your relationships: the more lifetime partners you have, the greater your risk will be. Using condoms for the first three to six months of any new relationship is another reasonable option. This will help allow time for any previously acquired infection to become apparent and be treated before it is spread further—to you! Using condoms as a routine practice all the time is also an entirely reasonable idea.

Human papillomavirus infection in males is often inapparent. Flat warts caused by the CIN-producing virus strains may be very inconspicuous and may not even be detected by medical exams in some cases. If you have CIN, or warts, however, evaluation for your partner is essential. A meticulous search may be necessary, with at least six-power magnification using a magnifying lens or colposcope. Thorough swabbing of the penis with 5% vinegar solution is also essential to make skin areas infected with wart virus appear white so they contrast with normal skin. Your clinician, a urologist, or a dermatologist may be good choices for your partner's exam. Warts (condyloma) may be found in 50% to 90% of male partners of women with CIN or warts (21,22). Your partner's warts should be treated, and he will need faithful follow-up because of his risk for developing penile cancer, also linked to HPV infection.

REFERENCES

1. Crum CP, Ikenberg H, Richart RM, et al: Human papillomavirus type 16 and early cervical neoplasia. *New England Journal of Medicine* 310:880–883, 1984.

2. Guijon FB, Paraskevas M, Brunham R: The association of sexually transmitted diseases with cervical intraepithelial neoplasia. A case-control study. *American Journal of Obstetrics and Gynecology* 151:185–190, 1985.

3. Genital warts, human papillomaviruses, and cervical cancer. *Lancet* 1:1045–1046, 1985.

4. Campion MJ, Singer A, Clarkson PK: Increased risk of cervical neoplasia in consorts of men with penile condylomata acuminata. *Lancet* 1:943–946, 1985.

5. Morell ND, Taylor JR, Snyder RN, et al: False-negative cytology rates in patients in whom invasive cervical cancer subsequently developed. *Obstetrics and Gynecology* 60:41–45, 1982.

6. Yobs AR, Swanson RA, Lamotte Jr LC: Laboratory reliability of the Papanicolaou smear. *Obstetrics and Gynecology* 65:235–244, 1985.

7. Jones WB, Saigo PE: The "atypical" Papanicolaou smear. *Ca—A Cancer Journal for Clinicians* 36:237–242, 1986.

8. Reiter RC: Management of initial atypical cervical cytology: A randomized, prospective study. *Obstetrics and Gynecology* 68:237–240, 1986.

9. Davis GL, Hernandez E, Davis JL, et al: Atypical squamous cells in Papanicolaou smears. *Obstetrics and Gynecology* 69:43–46, 1987.

10. Nash JD, Burke TW, Hoskins WJ: Biologic course of cervical human papillomavirus infection. *Obstetrics and Gynecology* 69:160–162, 1987.

11. Dunn JE Jr, Crocker DW, Rube IF, et al: Cervical cancer occurrence in Memphis and Shelby County, Tennessee, during 25 years of its cervical cytology screening program. *American Journal of Obstetrics and Gynecology* 150:861–864, 1984.

12. Burk RD, Kadish AS, Calderin S, et al: Human papillomavirus infection of the cervix detected by cervicovaginal lavage and molecular hybridization: Correlation with biopsy results and Papanicolaou smear. *American Journal of Obstetrics and Gynecology* 154:982–989, 1986.

13. Richart RM, Townsend DE: Outpatient therapy of cervical intraepithelial neoplasia with cryotherapy or CO_2 laser, in Osofsky HJ (ed): *Advances in Clinical Obstetrics and Gynecology*, Vol 1. Baltimore: Williams & Wilkins, 1982.

14. Nelson JH Jr, Averette HE, Richart RM: Dysplasia, carcinoma in situ, and early invasive cervical carcinoma. *Ca—A Cancer Journal for Clinicians* 34:306–327, 1984.

15. Bryson SCP, Lenehan P, Lickrish GM: The treatment of grade 3 cervical intraepithelial neoplasia with cryotherapy: An 11-year experience. *American Journal of Obstetrics and Gynecology* 151:201–206, 1985.

16. Baram A, Paz GF, Peyser MR, et al: Treatment of cervical ectropion by cryosurgery: Effect on cervical mucus characteristics. *Fertility and Sterility* 43:86–89, 1985.

17. Stein DS, Ulrich SA, Hasiuk AS: Laser vaporization in the treatment of cervical intraepithelial neoplasia. *Journal of Reproductive Medicine* 30:179–183, 1985.

18. Falcone T, Ferenczy A: Cervical intraepithelial neoplasia and condyloma: An analysis of diagnostic accuracy of posttreatment follow-up methods. *American Journal of Obstetrics and Gynecology* 154:260–264, 1986.

19. Bamford PN, Forbes-Smith PA, Rose GL, et al: An analysis of factors responsible for progression or regression of mild and moderate cervical dyskaryosis. *British Journal of Family Planning* 11:5–8, 1985.

20. Romney SL, Duttagupta C, Basu J, et al: Plasma vitamin C and uterine cervical dysplasia. *American Journal of Obstetrics and Gynecology* 151:976–980, 1985.
21. Levine RU, Crum CP, Herman E, et al: Cervical papillomavirus infection and intraepithelial neoplasia: A study of male sexual partners. *Obstetrics and Gynecology* 64:16–20, 1984.
22. Sedlacek TV, Cunnane M, Carpiniello V: Colposcopy in the diagnosis of penile condyloma. *American Journal of Obstetrics and Gynecology* 154:494–496, 1986.

36

Endometriosis

You are likely to read about an endometriosis epidemic, especially among affluent women who pursue education and career plans and along the way suffer increasingly with its symptoms, or who discover a serious endometriosis problem when they try to become pregnant late in their reproductive years. Actually, no one knows for sure whether an epidemic is indeed occurring or whether the disease always was common but wasn't correctly diagnosed. Laparoscopy, surgery that allows a surgeon to inspect the pelvic organs through an illuminated tube, has greatly facilitated the diagnosis of endometriosis. Before laparoscopy, a clinician might suspect endometriosis because of the symptoms but could not confirm the diagnosis without major abdominal surgery. Laparoscopy is now commonly used for evaluation of pain problems and fertility problems, and endometriosis is a common finding—sometimes suspected beforehand, and sometimes completely unsuspected.

For women in the reproductive years endometriosis is likely to get worse, not better, over time. If you know you have endometriosis and you know you want childbearing in your future, consider amending your personal timetable. Try to arrange for childbearing early, before endometriosis has a chance to (literally) gum up the works.

The lining of the uterine cavity is called the endometrium. The term "endometriosis" is used when areas of endometrial tissue are found **outside** the uterine cavity. Endometriosis areas may be tiny, barely visible clusters of deep pink endometrial cells, or large clumps the size of a silver dollar or even larger. The most common locations

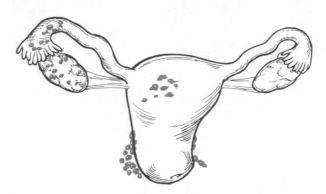

ILLUSTRATION 36-1   Common sites for endometriosis.

for endometriosis implants—the outside surface of the uterus, the surface of the fallopian tubes, the ovaries, the surface of the bladder, the rectum, and the ligaments behind the uterus—are shown in Illustration 36-1.

Closely related to endometriosis is a condition called adenomyosis. This term is used when endometrial lining tissue invades the inner wall of the uterus, extending downward from the surface of the uterine cavity into the fibrous and muscle layers beneath. The symptoms of adenomyosis are similar to those of endometriosis, and the two may coexist.

No one knows exactly what causes endometriosis. One theory is that during menstruation, endometrial cells from the uterine lining are carried out through the ends of the fallopian tubes into the abdomen, where they implant and grow to form endometriosis patches. This process is called retrograde menstruation. Another theory is that endometriosis patches originate from primitive cells that have been present in the abdomen since fetal development and undergo transformation into endometrial cells in the adolescent or young adult years.

Despite a decade of extensive research, the disease remains an enigma, and researchers suspect that endometriosis may not be a single disorder. It may be that the symptoms and abnormal tissue implants now classified as one disease actually arise as the end result of several quite different disorders. Subtle alterations in the normal immune system response to menstrual debris may be significant, as may prostaglandin hormone levels. Also, electron microscope study of endometriosis tissue suggests that it is not identical to normal endometrial lining tissue, at least in its response to hormone stimulation, so the concept of endometriosis as simply misplaced uterine lining tissue may not be accurate (1).

Many risk factors, including quite unflattering psychological characteristics, have been hypothesized for endometriosis. Little or no persuasive research data, however, support these hypotheses. The research dilemma is that endometriosis diagnosis rates are strongly influenced by laparoscopy rates. Laparoscopy, in turn, is much more likely to be undertaken by women who have fertility problems, have delayed childbearing, and have socioeconomic resources that assure access to sophisticated medical care, than it is by women who are economically disadvantaged or have already completed a successful pregnancy. Laparoscopy probably is also more common among women who have the skills and assertiveness to follow through with the evaluation of a problem such as pelvic pain. So it should not be surprising that endometriosis **diagnosis** is less common among socioeconomically disadvantaged women (2). **Whether or not the disease is less common remains to be determined.**

It is possible, of course, that endometriosis is a disease of affluence, or of limited childbearing. Pregnancy provides a nine-month interruption of cyclic menstrual hormones, and the total number of lifetime cycles is reduced for a woman who has multiple pregnancies.

Hereditary factors may also be significant. **Endometriosis rates for mothers and sisters with endometriosis were roughly two to three times higher** than rates for comparison groups in one study, and the hereditary pattern followed the maternal line (mother, grandmother) rather than the paternal line (father, grandfather) in 80% or more of cases (3).

Researchers estimate that 5% to 15% of women in the reproductive age range have endometriosis. It is a very common, but often unsuspected, incidental finding at the time of surgery performed for some other reason. Symptoms are absent or fairly minor in most cases, but endometriosis can cause severe problems that are disabling, and in very rare cases, a serious health threat.

Symptoms

Endometriosis is three days of pain every cycle. Every month I vow it won't rule my life, and every month beads of sweat line my upper lip and my secretary asks what's wrong and I run up the white flag. It's a sort of tyranny.

—WOMAN, 27

The most common symptom with endometriosis is pain, especially excessive menstrual cramps. Endometriosis patches respond to changes in the hormone cycle with cell growth and shedding similar to what occurs in normal uterine lining inside the uterus. Bleeding from endometriosis patches may cause painful irritation of the peritoneum that lines the abdominal cavity. Also, the release of excessive prostaglandin hormone from shedding endometriosis cells may stimulate smooth muscle spasm so that uterine cramps and intestinal contractions that result in diarrhea and/or nausea are both intensified.

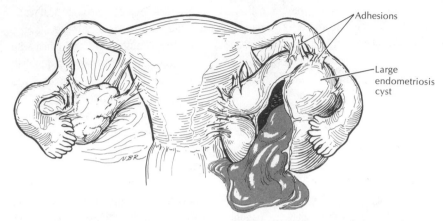

ILLUSTRATION 36-2   Large "chocolate" cyst of endometriosis. The ovary is almost completely covered by an endometriosis cyst; old, dark blood is leaking out of the cyst.

Endometriosis patches may be tender to touch or pressure. Implants or clumps behind the uterus or on its surface may be responsible for pain during intercourse, especially with deep penetration, and pain during bowel movements. Intestinal pain can also result from endometriosis patches on the wall of the intestine or colon.

Endometriosis is sometimes associated with irregular menstrual bleeding patterns, but precisely how endometriosis may affect cyclic hormone patterns is not known. Severe endometriosis involving the ovaries could directly alter ovary function, but other hormone effects may be involved as well. Adenomyosis often causes very heavy menstrual bleeding and/or bleeding at abnormal times.

Bleeding from endometriosis sites inside the abdomen can cause scar tissue that obstructs the fallopian tubes, or an accumulation of endometriosis tissue can cover part of one or both ovaries and interfere with the escape of eggs. Either action can impair fertility. Bleeding can sometimes occur within a mass of endometrial cells so that a blood-filled cyst gradually forms. This is called an endometrial or "chocolate" cyst and is a fairly common cause of enlarged ovaries (see Illustration 36-2). It is called a "chocolate" cyst because the accumulated blood turns to a chocolate brown color over time.

Endometriosis symptoms may begin at puberty, but more commonly they start several years after menstrual periods begin. The symptoms tend to increase gradually over the years as the endometriosis areas increase in size.

Endometriosis symptoms tend to become worse over time until menopause occurs and cyclic hormone stimulation stops. After menopause, the abnormal implants shrink away and the symptoms subside. Hormone replacement therapy after menopause, however, may cause continuing endometriosis problems in some cases (2).

In rare cases endometriosis implants are found at such remote locations as the lung or kidney, where they might cause episodes of coughing blood or blood in the urine that coincide with menstrual periods. In very rare cases endometriosis implants can invade vital structures such as the bowel or bladder wall and become a serious threat to health. In this situation aggressive treatment with medication and/or surgery may be necessary to prevent life-threatening complications such as bowel perforation.

FERTILITY PROBLEMS WITH ENDOMETRIOSIS

Extensive endometriosis, with scarring and structural damage involving the tubes and ovaries, is an understandable cause of fertility problems. How moderate endometriosis with no evidence of structural blockage may affect fertility is less clear. It is possible that chemical, immunologic, or hormone alterations caused by endometriosis patches could alter fertility, but no specific hypotheses have been definitely proven.

Unsuspected mild or moderate endometriosis is a common finding among infertile women, and rates for fertility problems are higher (30% to 40%) among women with endometriosis than among couples in the general population (15%) (2).

For patients with severe endometriosis, treatment may be the only hope for restoring fertility. Overall pregnancy success after surgery for women with **severe** endometriosis is only about 40%, but surgical treatment is generally accepted as the best approach available (4). For patients with **mild or moderate** disease, however, research findings are contradictory. Endometriosis treatment is followed by excellent pregnancy success rates. Pregnancy rates, however, are also excellent for similar patients who **do not** receive treatment, and statistical analysis in some studies shows no definite advantage for treatment (5).

There is no doubt that endometriosis **can be** a cause of impaired fertility. On the other hand, most patients with endometriosis do not experience fertility problems, and even when endometriosis is present the main culprit in fertility impairment may be some other factor entirely.

An increased risk of pregnancy loss through miscarriage has also been suggested in some studies of women with endometriosis. A 1986 study, however, found that miscarriage rates were not as high as previously reported, and were no higher than the rate for the general population (6).

Diagnosis

Your clinician may suspect endometriosis on the basis of your symptoms and a pelvic exam. The history of your symptoms **over time** is particularly important because it is unusual for severe symptoms to appear suddenly with endometriosis. Your exam may be entirely normal, or your clinician may be able to feel one or more nodules on the surface of your uterus or in the area between your uterus and rectum; you may notice tenderness as your endometriosis nodules are bumped during an exam.

A history and an exam cannot provide a definite diagnosis, however. Other common problems such as pelvic infection and benign uterine tumors called leiomyomas or fibroids can cause similar symptoms and exam findings. And unfortunately, there are no specific laboratory tests that can confirm endometriosis. A blood test for endometriosis may be possible in the future, however. Researchers have found that women with endometriosis have elevated levels of CA-125, a normal cell protein in uterine tissue, and tests to detect it may be feasible for diagnosis in the future.

If your symptoms are not severe, a definite diagnosis may not be necessary. If you are having severe problems, however, and aggressive endometriosis treatment is being considered, then a definite diagnosis is essential.

Laparoscopy or exploratory surgery (see Chapter 48) will permit your surgeon to see your pelvic organs; one of these procedures is almost always necessary for a definite diagnosis of endometriosis, and also allows your surgeon to determine how extensive it is in your case.

ENDOMETRIOSIS STAGES

Your clinician uses stages to describe the precise severity of endometriosis. Minimal or mild endometriosis means that implants are 1 inch or less in size, are not widespread, and extensive scar tissue is not present. Moderate endometriosis means that larger implants and/or deeper penetration into ovary tissue or more extensive scar tissue is present. With severe endometriosis large implant size and penetration or extensive scar tissue are present (7). By using a standard scoring system, your gynecologist can make a meaningful comparison between your situation and the treatment results reported for other women with similar disease.

Symptoms do not always correlate with endometriosis severity. Some women with extensive endometriosis have minimal symptoms, and some women with minimal endometriosis have severe symptoms.

Treatment

If endometriosis symptoms are mild, you may not need treatment of any kind, or perhaps your clinician will recommend prescription medication to use during painful menstrual periods. Antiprostaglandin medications such as ibuprofen (Motrin, Advil, Nuprin) are often effective in relieving endometriosis pain (see Chapter 31). A regular cyclic schedule of birth control Pills may be recommended, especially if you need contraceptive protection. The growth of uterine lining tissue is diminished for a woman taking birth control Pills so endometriosis problems may be diminished as well.

If your symptoms are severe, if you have heavy internal bleeding, or if you are having difficulty becoming pregnant, then a definite diagnosis and treatment specifically for endometriosis will be needed. A gynecologist experienced in the management of endometriosis is the most appropriate choice for your initial laparoscopy or laparotomy surgery, and to help you assess treatment options after that. Treatment may also be recommended if your endometriosis involves the bowel or bladder, even if your symptoms are not severe. Your two basic treatment options include surgery to remove endometriosis implants, or hormone suppression to allow an opportunity for implants to shrink on their own. In deciding between treatment options you and your gynecologist will want to consider your current and future desires for pregnancy, the extent of your endometriosis, and any personal medical factors that might make one choice or the other unwise.

HORMONE SUPPRESSION TREATMENT

Hormone medication can be used to suppress your natural hormone cycles and stop the cyclic growth of endometriosis patches. Treatment for at least three to nine months is likely to be recommended to give your patches a chance to shrink or even disappear. Hormone treatment is most effective when the implants are small.

Your clinician may prescribe synthetic progestin alone, a combination of estrogen and progestin such as birth control Pills, or a synthetic male hormone (androgen) called danazol (Danocrine). Another alternative, available in some centers conducting research on endometriosis treatment, is a synthetic pituitary hormone blocker called gonadotropin-releasing hormone agonist or GnRH agonist. This treatment stops ovary hormone production by blocking pituitary gland hormones that normally stimulate ovary cycles.

Continuous Progestin or Birth Control Pills. With progestin alone, such as injectable Depo-Provera (medroxyprogesterone) or oral Provera (medroxyprogesterone acetate) or Norlutate (norethindrone acetate), or a combination of estrogen and progestin such as found in birth control Pills, you will need fairly high doses of hormones to stop your menstrual periods for such a long period of time. If you use birth control Pills, you will take the Pills continuously with no days off, and you will probably have to increase your Pill dose or take additional estrogen along with your Pills over the months of treatment in order to prevent bleeding episodes. By the end of a nine-month suppression treatment you may be taking two, three, or more Pills each day. Because this treatment involves a fairly high hormone dose, you are likely to have side effects such as nausea, breast tenderness, weight gain, and fluid retention. You cannot use birth control Pills for endometriosis if you have contraindications to the use of Pills. (Read Chapter 13 for Pill contraindications.)

Continuous progestin or birth control Pill treatment is called pseudopregnancy because it involves steady exposure to progestin, which also occurs in pregnancy. This treatment results in relief of pain for at least 80% of women (1). Pregnancy rates following pseudopregnancy treatment, however, are lower than rates reported for danazol treatment. The relative effectiveness of these two treatments has not been extensively documented in careful comparison studies, but danazol has become a more common treatment choice (1).

Danazol (Danocrine) Treatment. Danazol is a synthetic hormone in the androgen (male hormone) family. Taking danazol blocks pituitary gland release of FSH (follicle-stimulating hormone) and LH (luteinizing hormone) and also acts directly on the ovary to interfere with the production of estrogen and progesterone (8). Symptoms are improved for 80% to 90% of patients taking danazol, and the size and extent of implants are also reduced (1). Danazol works best for mild to moderate endometriosis; large clumps of tissue in severe endometriosis are not likely to resolve, and it cannot correct scar tissue already present. Recurrence after treatment is common: as many as 50% of women experience renewed symptoms within a year after treatment (9).

I found the idea of taking male hormones fairly upsetting. I was *not* interested in acquiring a hairy chest and becoming a baritone! But I sure did want a baby, and it worked! (No horrible side effects, either!)

—WOMAN, 32

Side effects with danazol are quite common, and are not surprising, since the purpose of treatment is to alter your hormone pattern temporarily. Some side effects are the result of the low estrogen and progesterone levels caused by the drug, and some reflect its androgenic (male hormone) effects. About 80% of women have at least some of the effects listed in Table 36-1, but 90% of women are able to continue the drug despite these problems. Most side effects stop when treatment is stopped, but male hormone effects such as changes in hair and voice may not be reversible. Serious medical complications with danazol are not common. It can cause liver problems in rare cases, so any signs of liver impairment such as jaundice (yellow skin and eyes) should be reported immediately to your gynecologist. Also, your gynecologist may recommend periodic blood tests to check for liver impairment while you are taking danazol, especially if you are having very prolonged or repeated treatment. Fluid retention caused by danazol may be a special hazard for a woman who already has other significant medical problems. Danazol treatment is also unwise if there is any chance that a woman is already pregnant, because a female fetus exposed accidentally to its male hormone effects may have abnormal development of the genital organs. Pregnancy is not likely while a woman is taking danazol, but it is not safe to count on

TABLE 36-1
POSSIBLE SIDE EFFECTS OF DANAZOL TREATMENT

SIDE EFFECTS RELATED TO ANDROGEN	SIDE EFFECTS RELATED TO LOW ESTROGEN
Acne	Hot flashes
Fluid retention (edema)	Sweating
Mild hirsutism	Vaginal dryness, burning, itching
Decreased breast size	Vaginal bleeding
Deepening of voice	Nervousness
Oily skin and/or hair	Mood swings
Weight gain	
Enlarged clitoris (rare)	

OTHER EFFECTS REPORTED (DANAZOL'S ROLE AS THE CAUSE IS UNCERTAIN)

Skin rash	Irritated stomach and/or intestine
Nasal congestion	Nausea
Dizziness	Vomiting
Headache	Constipation
Sleep disturbance	Muscle cramps or spasms
Tiredness	Joint swelling, immobility
Tremor	Pain in back, neck, or legs
Tingling in arms or legs	Pelvic pain
Vision problems	Blood in urine
Anxiety	Loss of hair
Depression	Change in sex drive
Change in appetite	Abnormal sugar tolerance
Chills	Increased blood pressure

SIGNIFICANT MEDICAL EFFECTS

Liver impairment with jaundice (yellow skin), elevated liver enzymes on
   blood test (Report jaundice promptly to your gynecologist)
Altered insulin requirement for women with diabetes
Altered response to anticoagulant (blood-thinning) medication
Altered blood cholesterol and lipid levels

SOURCES: *Physicians' Desk Reference* (ed 40). Oradell, N.J.: Medical Economics Co., 1986.
Speroff L, Glass RH, Kase NG: *Clinical Gynecologic Endocrinology and Infertility* (ed 3). Baltimore: Williams & Wilkins, 1983.

danazol for effective birth control. Faithful use of a barrier birth control method such as a diaphragm or condoms throughout danazol treatment is essential.

A contraindication is a medical situation or problem that renders inadvisable or unsafe a course of treatment that might otherwise be recommended. Contraindications to danazol treatment are (9):

- Pregnancy or breastfeeding
- Abnormal vaginal bleeding whose cause is not known
- Significant liver disease
- Serious heart disease
- Serious kidney disease

If you have epilepsy or migraine headaches, or less severe heart or kidney disease, treatment may be possible with close surveillance. If fluid retention aggravates these problems, it may be necessary for you to stop taking danazol.

Overall, most women treated with danazol find it very helpful and beneficial. It is not likely to be recommended unless your symptoms are substantial or fertility problems require treatment; in these situations its benefits are likely to outweigh the problems caused by side effects. Danazol treatment can be used alone or before or after surgery. Danazol treatment can also be repeated, or prolonged treatment used, to control problems for a woman who has severe symptoms but is not trying to become pregnant.

Typical danazol treatment is 400 mg to 800 mg daily taken in two to four doses. The higher dose is likely to be recommended if fertility problems are the main reason for treatment. A lower dose may cause fewer side effects, however, and is less expensive. Reducing the dose after the first few months of treatment may be an option, and very low doses of 100 mg daily or less may be sufficient to control symptoms in some cases (8).

Taking danazol is likely to cause amenorrhea—absence of menstrual periods— especially if higher doses are used and/or treatment is prolonged.

GnRH Agonist (Gonadotropin-Releasing Hormone Blocker). This drug causes profound, temporary ovary suppression so that natural estrogen and progesterone production are halted almost entirely. Initial research reports show encouraging results for effective control of endometriosis symptoms. Approximately 80% of 400 patients treated with GnRH agonist in one study had significant improvement in the extent of endometriosis documented by laparoscopy before and after treatment (10). Follow-up studies of fertility after treatment and of recurrence rates are not yet available. From the women's point of view, GnRH agonist treatment is like temporary menopause, and its side effects are predictable menopause symptoms such as hot flashes and vaginal dryness (1). More serious side effects such as bone mineral loss and adverse changes in lipid metabolism may also be possible, so further study will be necessary to determine how the benefits and risks of GnRH treatment compare to those of other endometriosis treatment options.

SURGICAL TREATMENT

Your clinician may recommend surgery if your endometriosis is extensive, if your symptoms are severe, if you have a large mass of endometrial tissue, or if you have a greatly enlarged ovary. Surgery is also a reasonable choice when endometriosis is causing fertility problems. Surgery is probably more effective than hormone treatment in restoring fertility when endometriosis is moderate or severe, and surgery avoids the six to nine months of delay necessary with hormone treatment before conception can be attempted. In some cases hormone suppression treatment is recommended before surgery or for the first few months after surgery, particularly for a woman who anticipates that surgery will be needed but does not want to conceive immediately.

Pregnancy rates are highest during the first year after surgery. After that, the recurrence of endometriosis may interfere with pregnancy success. Your surgeon will probably advise that you begin trying to conceive soon after recovering from surgery.

The goal with endometriosis repair surgery (also called conservative surgery) is to remove scar tissue or adhesions and as much endometriosis tissue as possible without risking damage to pelvic structures. Such damage might trigger further scar tissue formation after surgery. **If at all possible your surgeon should leave both ovaries in place, as well as both tubes and your uterus.** Repair surgery is likely to be most successful if your surgeon is experienced with fertility reconstruction such as tuboplasty and has the training necessary to use precision microsurgery techniques. The specific surgical steps required in your case will depend on the damage found at surgery. Lumps of endometriosis tissue may be surgically removed, and similar patches destroyed by electric cautery. Scar tissue will be removed in a procedure called lysis of adhesions, and your tubes and ovaries will be restored as nearly as possible to normal position. Fertility surgery is described in detail in Chapter 10.

This type of repair is major abdominal surgery called laparotomy. It is performed in a hospital with general anesthesia, and requires a four- to six-day hospital stay and a six-week period of convalescence at home. An incision approximately 5 inches long will be necessary across your lower abdomen just above the pubic hairline, or in the midline starting several inches below your navel and extending downward to your pubic bone (see Chapter 48 for more detailed information on laparotomy).

If you don't plan any future pregnancies, your surgeon may recommend hysterectomy, or, if your ovaries are badly damaged, hysterectomy and removal of your ovaries (see Chapter 49). Hysterectomy and oophorectomy (ovary removal) may be the best way to end your problems with endometriosis. **Approximately 15% of women who have conservative repair surgery have later recurrences that require a second surgery** within 10 years (11). If your ovaries are not severely affected and your endometriosis does not extensively invade organs other than the uterus, then hysterectomy alone, with the ovaries preserved, may be reasonable. Your ovaries, however, will continue to produce the hormones that stimulate endometriosis if they are left in place, so future problems are possible even after hysterectomy unless your ovaries are removed at the same time.

New Laparoscopy Techniques.   Surgical treatment with laparoscopy instead of full abdominal surgery can be performed at an outpatient surgical center and involves a much briefer recovery period. A 1-inch incision for the laparoscope and one or two additional tiny incisions for instruments are all that is required. In some cases it may be possible for your surgeon to use electric cautery to eradicate small areas of endometriosis during routine laparoscopy. New techniques utilizing surgical laser during laparoscopy are also being developed, and with laser it may be possible to vaporize abnormal endometriosis tissue so precisely that neighboring normal tissue is not affected and more extensive surgery can be safely performed. Laser with laparoscopy involves a shorter time for convalescence, and internal healing also may be expedited because bleeding and tissue damage are minimized. The risk of infection following surgery also may be reduced when a larger abdominal incision is not necessary. This is a very new technique, however, and few surgeons have had extensive experience performing the procedure. Research statistics to compare the overall safety and success rates of laser surgery with other treatment options are not available. If you are considering laser laparoscopy, it is entirely reasonable to ask your surgeon how many times she/he has performed the procedure, and what treatment problems have occurred.

Laparoscopy treatment is possible only if the surgeon can see pelvic structures clearly through the laparoscope. If extensive scar tissue blocks the laparoscope view, then full abdominal surgery is the only surgical option.

ASSESSING TREATMENT OPTIONS

Patience and good, clear communication are essential for both you and your gynecologist if you have endometriosis problems. Despite the many research studies reported, **there are no clear-cut rules for treatment.** Also, appropriate treatment for you may change over time depending on what happens with your endometriosis and with your own personal priorities.

In general, endometriosis tends to be a continuing and progressive problem, but you may experience ups and downs. Your symptoms may be severe for several months and then abate even without treatment, perhaps to return later.

As you and your gynecologist weigh treatment choices, be sure to discuss your plans and hopes about future pregnancy, including the time line you have in mind. **If future pregnancy is a definite part of your life plan, then active treatment such as hormone suppression may seem worthwhile even if your current symptoms are not severe.** Alternatively, you may want to consider using birth control Pills for contraception in the meantime to gain their possible benefit for your endometriosis.

Your gynecologist may even encourage you to consider pregnancy earlier than you originally planned. Pregnancy, with its long menstruation-free interval, may help your endometriosis, and if you delay pregnancy you may find that you have impaired fertility.

If future pregnancy is not an issue, then treatment decisions will depend mainly on your symptoms. If you have a mass of tissue in the area of the ovary, surgery may be medically necessary to be sure it is not a tumor. Aggressive treatment or surgery may also be necessary if endometriosis involves a vital structure such as your bowel. Otherwise it will be up to you to decide whether your pain is severe enough to require treatment.

RESOURCES

The Endometriosis Association
A U.S.–Canadian nonprofit organization devoted to support for women with endometriosis, education about endometriosis, and research into the causes and cure for this puzzling disease. The national office publishes a bimonthly newsletter, and distributes brochures and an information packet. Local chapters throughout the country serve as support and self-help groups for members. For more information, write to: The Endometriosis Association U.S.–Canadian Headquarters, P.O. Box 92187, Milwaukee, Wis. 53202.

REFERENCES

1. Schmidt CL: Endometriosis: A reappraisal of pathogenesis and treatment. *Fertility and Sterility* 44:157–173, 1985.
2. Molgaard CA, Golbeck AL, Gresham L: Current concepts in endometriosis. *Western Journal of Medicine* 143:42–46, 1985.
3. Lamb K, Hoffmann RG, Nichols TR: Family trait analysis: A case-control study of 43 women with endometriosis and their best friends. *American Journal of Obstetrics and Gynecology* 154:596–601, 1986.
4. American College of Obstetricians and Gynecologists: Management of endometriosis. *ACOG Technical Bulletin* No 85, May 1985.
5. Olive DL, Lee KL: Analysis of sequential treatment protocols for endometriosis-associated infertility. *American Journal of Obstetrics and Gynecology* 154:613–619, 1986.
6. Metzger DA, Olive DL, Stohs GF, et al: Association of endometriosis and spontaneous abortion: Effect of control group selection. *Fertility and Sterility* 45:18–22, 1986.
7. The American Fertility Society: Revised American Fertility Society classification of endometriosis: 1985. *Fertility and Sterility* 43:351–352, 1985.
8. Speroff L, Glass RH, Kase NG: *Clinical Gynecologic Endocrinology and Infertility* (ed 3). Baltimore: Williams & Wilkins, 1983.
9. *Physicians' Desk Reference* (ed 40). Oradell, N.J.: Medical Economics Co., 1986.
10. LHRH analogues in endometriosis. *Lancet* 2:1016, 1986.
11. Malinak LR, Wheeler JM: Association of endometriosis with spontaneous abortion, prognosis for pregnancy, and risk for recurrence. *Seminars in Reproductive Endocrinology* 3:361–369, 1985.

37

❖

Breast Problems

Breast lumps are very common, and few things are more frightening for a woman. Other breast problems like pain or tenderness are also common. Many women, in fact, believe they have a breast disease—fibrocystic "disease"—because this term was often used in the past for more-tender-than-average, dense breasts. Experts now delete the word "disease," although symptoms, of course, remain.

Less common breast problems include abnormal nipple discharge, infection, and injury. This chapter addresses each of these problems, and the last section is a brief review of plastic surgery for breast augmentation or reduction.

One breast change that you need not worry about is the relatively sudden appearance of a breast bud in a young adolescent. As the first stage of female breast development begins, a firm, round, movable, painless lump develops directly underneath the nipple; buds usually occur in both breasts at about the same time. A breast bud does feel like a lump; so if you are not certain, see your clinician.

And even if your problem is a real breast lump, take heart. Statistics are on your side, and it is quite likely that the lump will turn out to be benign (noncancerous). Remember, too, that **a breast lump is not the only sign you need to be watching for.** Be aware of all the breast cancer danger signs in Illustration 37-1, and see your clinician promptly if you have any questions.

When you call for an appointment, explain that a breast lump or other danger sign is your concern. Your clinician should see you within just a few days, and if this is not possible because she/he is on vacation, for example, ask to be referred to another clinician who can see you promptly.

What to Expect
If You Have a Breast Lump

I found a lump in my right breast; a hard place, in the upper, outer part, that should have been soft. All morning and afternoon I pretended I hadn't found it; then I felt it again in bed. Still there.

Not Betty Ford this time, or Ann Jillian. Me. I tried to remember the statistics: "Most lumps aren't cancer," but how many is *most*? "Only your doctor can tell for sure," but I didn't want to see a doctor. I wanted the lump not to be there.

Next morning I called my doctor. He found my lump, too. He said, "There's almost no chance this is anything but benign, but it should come out, just to be sure." He scheduled me for a needle aspiration biopsy. I went straight from his office to the library and read about the statistics, but I couldn't connect myself with any of the numbers.

All I did was worry. I told my friend Lynn, who said, "Don't worry," and then asked if I wanted her to keep my cat, "just in case." I decided not to tell anyone else.

I tried not to touch the lump, but I did, over and over. Especially at night, I found myself touching it unconsciously. Was it bigger? smaller? I realized I *loved* my breast. It was part of me, and I cried when I thought about losing it. But I didn't think I would die, not even at three in the morning.

The needle aspiration didn't work, so they scheduled me for a regular incisional biopsy. On biopsy day, I *didn't* water the plants, and I left enough cat food for a day. Positive thinking. Nurses ran tests, and my surgeon talked to me about the surgery consent form. I wrote "only" next to Breast Biopsy—even though he had already agreed we would do *no more surgery immediately*, no matter what the initial lab report showed. "It's very important to me to have time to think," I said, even though I was *sure* I would agree to more surgery if it was cancer.

No breakfast on biopsy day. I got shots instead, and tried a few feeble wisecracks with the nurses. I remember being wheeled down a hall, masked faces, and someone saying, "This may sting a little." I recognized my surgeon and smiled at him. The rest is sort of a blur, even though I was awake.

Later, I heard, "You're okay. It wasn't cancer."

Lynn drove me home and I slept all day.

ADAPTED FROM *CAROL COMER, "THE COLD WAR BETWEEN ME AND THE TUMOR."*
ATLANTA JOURNAL AND CONSTITUTION SUNDAY MAGAZINE, November 20, 1977. Used with permission of the author. Her story has been slightly modified to reflect typical clinical practice in the 1980s.

37:1   BREAST CANCER DANGER SIGNS

Breast lump
Lump in underarm or above collarbone
Persistent skin rash, flaking, or eruption near the nipple
Dimpling, pulling, or retraction in one area of the breast
Nipple discharge
Sudden change in nipple position (such as inversion)

See your clinician at once if you have any of these signs.

Most stories have happy endings like this woman's, because 75% to 95% of breast lumps that are biopsied are benign. Read Chapter 5 to learn about mammography, how to examine your breasts, and what kind of breast changes to look for.

Even if you are tempted to wait and see if a lump will go away, call your personal physician or go to a clinic at once. **There is absolutely nothing to be gained by waiting.**

STEPS IN EVALUATION

Your clinician will **examine your breast** to confirm your findings. Careful examination of your other breast, and also your axilla (the technical term for your underarm) on each side, is important. Your clinician will also check for enlarged lymph nodes above your collarbones.

If you are under 30 and the lump feels like breast gland tissue, your clinician may recommend that you wait about one month (one menstrual cycle) to see if the lump goes away. If the lump persists after a cycle, you will definitely need further evaluation.

Mammography may also be recommended, depending on your age and other cancer risk factors in your case. If you are 40 years old or older, mammography is quite likely to be recommended before biopsy, and quite unlikely if you are 30 or younger. The decision in between is based on assessment of your specific situation. Mammography, an x-ray of your breast tissue, can help identify the exact location and size of the lump, and give some indication of the likelihood that cancer may be found. Your x-ray will also be checked carefully for any other suspicious areas in either breast that need further evaluation. **Mammography is helpful, but cannot give a final diagnosis. In some cases a lump that is easily felt cannot be seen on x-ray.** So unless you are very young, your clinician will recommend biopsy even if your lump appears to be entirely benign in your x-ray.

Ultrasound evaluation may also be helpful in some cases. Using sonar (sound waves), it may be possible to determine whether your lump is a solid mass or a fluid-filled cyst.

If your clinician suspects your lump is a fluid-filled cyst, it may be possible to remove (**aspirate**) the fluid with a syringe, a simple office procedure. Aspiration is vaguely painful but quick, and if the lump vanishes and the fluid is clear, your entire problem is solved. If the fluid is bloody, it must be sent to a pathologist, and microscope slides prepared for evaluation. Clear fluid may also be submitted for microscopic evaluation if your clinician feels this is needed. If fluid is not found, or the cyst recurs, then your clinician will probably recommend **biopsy**.

In most areas, general surgeons usually assume responsibility for breast evaluation and perform breast biopsies and surgery. In some cities, however, gynecologists assume this role. Your clinician will undoubtedly be able to recommend a surgeon; otherwise you might consult a breast screening clinic, your local National Organization for Women, a Planned Parenthood clinic, or a surgical nurse friend for suggestions.

BREAST BIOPSY

A breast biopsy is the surest and most common procedure for dealing with a breast lump. It is a surgical procedure in which abnormal tissue, usually the entire lump, is removed and sent to a pathologist for microscopic examination.

Breast biopsy may also be needed when there isn't a lump, for example, when mammography has identified a suspicious area in the breast. If the abnormality is not a lump, or the lump is too small to feel, special x-ray procedures to pinpoint the correct area for biopsy may be done just prior to surgery. With dye localization, for example, the dye placement is checked on x-ray so the surgeon can be certain the biopsy is accurate.

Needle Biopsy. In some situations needle biopsy to obtain tiny samples of a lump through a needle may be a reasonable option. This procedure does not require an incision and can be done as an office procedure. Needle biopsy is not likely to be successful unless the lump is fairly good-sized. It may be recommended when the likelihood of cancer is fairly high in order to speed up diagnostic time. Your surgeon may perform the needle biopsy or you may be referred to a pathologist for this procedure.

For needle biopsy, your surgeon or pathologist will use a local anesthetic to deaden a small patch of skin, and then insert the biopsy needle into your breast lump. Several samples, with needle insertions from several angles, will probably be needed. The procedure may be slightly uncomfortable but takes only a few minutes, and healing of your biopsy site is much faster than healing after an incision. Needle biopsy samples are evaluated microscopically by a pathologist. If there is any doubt about the biopsy results, or if this approach fails to provide an adequate sample, then a surgical biopsy will be needed.

Surgical Biopsy. Surgical breast biopsy is usually done in a hospital or surgical center. In some cases general anesthesia may be needed, but local anesthesia is usually

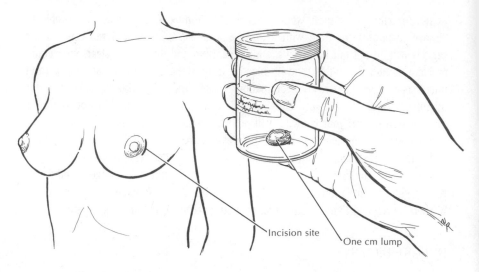

ILLUSTRATION 37-2   Breast biopsy incision site and biopsy specimen for evaluation. The entire lump is usually removed.

an option. Many women choose to have a biopsy with local anesthesia when it is feasible in order to save money and to minimize possible risks of anesthesia complications (see Chapter 45).

The surgeon thoroughly cleans the breast skin over the lump. Next, local anesthetic solution is injected into the skin and underlying tissue to deaden sensation temporarily in the area of the lump. She/he makes an incision, removes the lump, and then closes the incision with stitches. The incision is usually 1 or 2 inches long, and the surgeon follows the breast contour if possible so that the healed scar will be as inconspicuous as possible (see Illustration 37-2). If you choose general anesthesia, you will be asleep during the entire procedure and local anesthetic solution will not be used.

Most surgeons and patients now choose to schedule biopsy only, with plans for further treatment deferred until the pathologist's final report is completed. Preparation of optimal microscope slides and evaluation by the pathologist usually require 24 to 48 hours. By waiting for the final report, you may avoid the (rare) likelihood of an incorrect initial reading, and there is no evidence that delay of a few days or even a week or two is harmful even if cancer is found and further surgery is necessary.

In some situations, biopsy followed immediately by further surgery, if necessary, may be a reasonable choice, particularly for women who need to minimize their exposure to general anesthesia because of a health problem. If you have agreed to immediate further surgery, your surgeon will ask the pathologist to evaluate the biopsy tissue **immediately**, while you are still asleep in the operating room. The pathologist can freeze a portion of tissue and examine it within about 15 minutes. **Evaluation of**

TABLE 37-1
BREAST BIOPSY OUTCOME

AGE	% OF BIOPSIES THAT WERE BENIGN (NO CANCER)[a]
35–39	94
40–44	90
45–49	87
50–54	84
55–64	78
65–74	74

[a]The likelihood that a breast lump may be malignant increases with increasing age. Lumps are much more common, however, among younger women.

SOURCE: Baker LH: Breast cancer detection demonstration project: Five-year summary report. *Ca—A Cancer Journal for Clinicians* 32:194–225, 1982.

frozen sections is not as accurate as evaluation after the routine procedure for preparing and examining biopsy tissue, and this is a disadvantage of combined surgery. On the other hand, it may avoid the necessity for two episodes of general anesthesia, a significant advantage in some cases. Be sure to discuss these options with your surgeon before your biopsy is scheduled.

BREAST BIOPSY RESULTS

The vast majority of breast biopsy results are benign. Table 37-1 shows biopsy outcome for 280,000 women enrolled in a breast cancer screening program. The participants received breast exams and mammography and almost 4% required biopsy at the time of their initial screening. Biopsy rates thereafter were lower, about 2% each year (1). The likelihood that a breast biopsy will reveal cancer increases with age. The likelihood that cancer will be found also depends on other breast cancer risk factors in your particular case, and breast cancer risk factors and treatment options are discussed in detail in Chapter 41. Your breast biopsy is most likely to show one (or more) of the following common breast problems.

Fibrocystic "Disease." This term encompasses a range of findings including small or large cysts and benign hyperplasia ("hyper" means excessive, "plasia" means growth) of the breast gland tissue. An old term for this problem was chronic cystic mastitis. "Disease" is printed in quotations here because experts now feel that fibrocystic breast characteristics do not really indicate disease: at least 60% to 90% of all women have them to some degree. Read about fibrocystic breast problems in the next section of this chapter.

Fibroadenoma.   This is the most common of the benign breast tumors. It is likely to arise as a solitary, firm, distinct lump, and is composed mostly of fibrous tissue. A fibroadenoma is usually rubbery and freely movable. Fibroadenoma is most often discovered in women between the ages of 14 and 40, and the appearance of a second fibroadenoma months or years after the first is also common.

Fat Necrosis.   After breast injury a lump may form as white blood cells invade the area and injured fat cells are encapsulated by fibrous tissue. Fat necrosis may also occur spontaneously with no recognized trauma. The lump is likely to be small, distinct, and tender. Fat necrosis is a rare cause of breast lumps.

Papilloma.   The structure of a papilloma tumor is delicate, so as it develops within a breast duct, it can bleed, and bloody or cloudy discharge is quite likely. Nipple discharge, rather than a mass, is usually its first sign. A papilloma can also develop within a breast cyst, and malignant papillomas also occur. Papilloma is quite uncommon in women less than 50 years old.

Mastitis.   "Mastitis" means inflammation of breast tissue. It most commonly occurs during pregnancy or breastfeeding when bacteria invade one or more areas of breast gland tissue and cause infection. This infection can be treated effectively with antibiotics in most cases, and the mass will resolve completely. In some cases surgery may be needed to drain infectious fluid that has accumulated in a pocket (abscess) to facilitate recovery. Occasionally, unsuspected mastitis will be discovered when a breast mass is removed at biopsy.

Other Breast Problems

Problems associated with fibrocystic breast characteristics are even more common than breast lumps. Often the two are linked, and fibrocystic characteristics are also responsible for most of the tenderness, pain, and cyclic fluctuation in breast size that women experience. These interrelated issues are discussed in the first part of this section. Other problems, described in the sections following, are much less common.

FIBROCYSTIC BREASTS

Is it reasonable to use the term "disease" for a process that occurs in as many as 60% to 90% of women? Probably not, and experts now stress the importance of more precise diagnosis so that the relationships between different types of benign breast disease and future cancer risks can be more meaningfully assessed. From the woman's point of view, however, the symptoms are still the same even though the word "disease" may be eliminated from her clinician's diagnosis.

A few days before my period my breasts get so sore the pain wakes me up when I turn over at night. They feel like rubbery, gobby blobs, especially in the outer half. I don't let my lover near them during that time.

—WOMAN, 30

Symptoms.   Symptoms range from mild to severe and are often intermittent. Many women notice monthly cyclic patterns, with symptoms most severe just before each menstrual period. Fibrocystic breast problems usually subside after menopause. Common symptoms, and exam signs you or your clinician are likely to notice, are:

• Tenderness in one or both breasts with pressure or touch
• Breast pain
• An intermittent or persistent sense of breast engorgement associated with dull, heavy pain and tenderness
• Intermittent appearance of cysts or lumps that form and then resolve within a few weeks
• A dense, pebbly consistency to breast tissue, often most noticeable in the outer quadrants
• Formation of persistent cysts or lumps that require aspiration or biopsy

Causes.   The cause of fibrocystic breasts is not known, but the symptoms and signs are linked to a woman's hormone patterns. Estrogen stimulates the growth of breast gland cells; progesterone modulates the estrogen effect and allows gland cells to arrange themselves into structurally mature glands. Hormone changes during normal menstrual cycles induce cyclic changes in breast symptoms, and so can hormone medications.

Many women who take birth control Pills or hormone treatment after menopause notice breast swelling and tenderness during the first few days or weeks of treatment. In most cases this effect subsides quickly, however. Exposure to a consistent, steady level of estrogen probably signals the breast tissue to reduce its response to estrogen. Women using Pills for ongoing birth control are **much less likely** to have fibrocystic breasts than are comparable women not taking Pills. The consistent, low hormone content of Pills decreases fibrocystic symptoms.

Why some women with entirely normal estrogen and progesterone cycles develop severe symptoms and others do not is not known, but researchers suspect that hereditary as well as dietary and other factors influence how breast tissue responds to normal hormone stimuli.

Diagnosis.   You and your clinician may make the diagnosis of fibrocystic breast characteristics on the basis of your symptoms and your breast exam. If you have mammography, the tissue may appear more dense than average. Precise diagnosis, however, is not possible unless you have a biopsy. Biopsy will be needed if you have a persistent lump, or worrisome exam findings, and the pathologist should be able to determine the specific kind or kinds of abnormalities present in your case.

From the pathologist's point of view, the venerable term "fibrocystic breast disease" was a term used to encompass a wide range of microscopic tissue abnormalities. An even older term was "chronic cystic mastitis." The pathologist might see excessive fibrous tissue between the breast glands or cyst formation within the glands.

Excessive growth of the gland tissue lining—a condition called hyperplasia—might also be observed, ranging from a mildly increased number of lining cells, retaining normal patterns of structure and maturation, to more excessive and abnormal growth. In extreme cases, hyperplasia might be quite similar to early cancer, with loss of normal cell maturation patterns and atypical cells present.

Overall, about 70% of women whose breast biopsy results are benign fibrocystic "disease" have fibrous tissue or cysts, but no hyperplasia, so **future breast cancer risk is not affected**. About 30% do have evidence of hyperplasia, and their future breast cancer risk is a little more than double the risk for the average woman. **Women who have hyperplasia with abnormal cells present have a fivefold increase in risk** (2). Your biopsy pathology report is likely to use the term "atypia" to describe hyperplasia with abnormal cells present.

Treatment.   No effective medical treatment to reverse fibrocystic breast characteristics is known. Changes in diet may be helpful, and medication to combat symptoms may be a reasonable option in severe cases.

Excessive dietary fat may be an important causative factor. In a small study of women suffering pain with fibrocystic breasts, researchers found that reducing daily fat intake to about 25% of daily calories also reduced their breast pain. Hormone studies for these women showed significant decreases in estrogen hormone and in prolactin hormone levels. Prolactin, released by the pituitary gland, is normally responsible for stimulating breast gland activity. The change in diet for these women had other desirable effects as well: daily calorie intake was reduced slightly and the average weight loss was 3% in the first three months (3).

This study was too small to be accepted as proof that a high-fat diet is the culprit in fibrocystic breast problems. Of course, reducing dietary fat has its own rewards and no known adverse consequences, and is certainly worth trying if breast problems are bothersome.

The possible role of **methylxanthines** in breast symptoms is controversial. Methylxanthines include:

• Caffeine in coffee, cola, and other products
• Theophylline in tea
• Theobromine in chocolate and cocoa

Several small studies have documented significant improvement in symptoms and in breast exam findings within two to six months after eliminating methylxanthines from the diet (4). Researchers studying biopsy results, however, did not find any difference in microscopic pathology results between women who consumed little or no coffee and those drinking four or more cups daily (5). Caffeine is not a health-enhancing substance, any more than high dietary fat is, so reducing total intake of methylxanthines has many other potential benefits.

Withdrawal symptoms such as headache are quite likely if caffeine consumption is abruptly stopped. Decreasing caffeine gradually over several weeks may circumvent this problem, or you may prefer to put up with headaches for the first few days knowing that it will soon end.

Vitamin E, alpha-tocopherol, has also been used successfully to relieve breast symptoms. Researchers believe that vitamin E may favorably alter blood lipid (fat) constituents and indirectly influence hormone levels as well. In two small studies, 60% to 80% of women taking vitamin E, 300 International Units twice daily, had improvement in breast symptoms within one to three months (6). Other researchers have recommended vitamin E (400 to 1,200 International Units daily) in conjunction with hormone treatment for breast problems (7).

Danazol, a synthetic androgen that inhibits release of the pituitary hormones governing estrogen and progesterone production in the ovary, is approved by the FDA for treatment of fibrocystic breast problems. This drug is also used for treatment of endometriosis. Depending on the dose used, danazol (trade name Danocrine) may reduce the effect of hormones on breast tissue or block ovulation and stop menstrual cycles altogether. Most women using danazol notice improvement in their symptoms as soon as one or two months after beginning treatment. Side effects, however, are also quite common, especially if the dose required is high. Danazol can cause fluid retention and typical androgenic effects such as hair growth and male hair distribution patterns. When treatment is stopped, normal menstrual cycles and hormone patterns usually resume promptly, but androgen side effects may not be reversible in some cases. Recommended doses for danazol treatment of breast problems range from 50-mg, to 200-mg tablets taken twice a day for three to six months.

Another drug that affects pituitary hormone release, **bromocriptine**, has also been used for fibrocystic breast problems. Bromocriptine reduces prolactin release, and is commonly used to treat infertility or the absence of menstrual periods caused by excessive prolactin. It can also be used to suppress breast milk production after pregnancy or to treat galactorrhea, inappropriate breast milk production. Treatment with low-dose bromocriptine (2.5 mg daily) was effective in reducing fibrocystic breast symptoms for about half the patients in one study (8). Side effects with bromocriptine include nausea, headache, dizziness, fatigue, and low blood pressure causing faintness with sudden change in posture. As many as 30% of patients experience side effects (see Chapter 10, Table 10-7), and they may be severe enough to interfere with normal activities.

Treatment with **progesterone** pills or shots, or with evening primrose oil capsules, has also been suggested for fibrocystic breast problems (8). Progesterone treatment is probably less effective than the alternatives described above, and research data to document possible risks or adverse effects for primrose oil are not available.

Prognosis.   If fibrocystic breast problems diminish as a result of lowered dietary fat, methylxanthine elimination, and increased vitamin E, the benefit is likely to persist as long as the diet changes are maintained. Recurrence of symptoms after drug treatment, however, is common, and more than one course of treatment may be needed.

The prognosis for future breast cancer risk depends on the underlying microscopic abnormalities involved (read the section entitled "Diagnosis" above). **Most fibrocystic symptom sufferers, however, are not at high risk.**

Special care with breast self-exam and faithfulness about annual exams and periodic mammography are essential. A small lump signaling early cancer may be less obvious if a woman has dense, irregular breast tissue. Mammography results, also, are harder to interpret when tissue is dense. So extra attention and care will be needed for exams, and biopsy will be essential if you and your clinician have any doubts about a suspicious area.

NIPPLE DISCHARGE

The breast normally manufactures a small amount of clear, sticky, lubricating fluid that can be expressed from the nipple with pressure, and it is entirely normal to see a few drops when the nipple is squeezed.

Secretion of excessive clear fluid, enough to leak spontaneously in small amounts, is not uncommon and may result from sexual breast and nipple stimulation, or from medications including birth control Pills and some tranquilizers.

If nipple discharge is more than a few drops or if it is watery, cloudy, pink, or bloody, further evaluation is essential. Benign and malignant breast tumors can cause discharge, and discharge may be their very first sign. In some cases discharge occurs before the tumor is large enough to feel as a lump, and mammography may be entirely normal. Evaluation is also essential if the discharge is caused by oozing from a skin rash near the nipple that persists. This can also signal an underlying tumor. Tumor, however, is not the most common cause of discharge.

In evaluating discharge, your clinician will review your medical history including any medications you have taken recently and examine your breasts carefully. She/he may prepare a microscope slide with a drop or two of discharge. Evidence of bleeding, such as red blood cells, or in some cases, abnormal tumor cells may be visible on the slide.

If profuse milky discharge is the problem and no breast lump is present, the diagnosis is likely to be galactorrhea, or inappropriate milk production. Steps in evaluation and treatment for this problem are described in the next section. Galactorrhea is likely to involve both breasts. Other kinds of discharge may involve both breasts, or only one. When discharge involves both breasts, the likelihood is low that cancer is responsible.

If you have a breast discharge, your evaluation will follow the same steps described above for managing a lump. Mammography and biopsy will be recommended if your discharge is pink (blood-tinged) or obviously bloody. In rare cases, nipple discharge may occur because of unsuspected breast infection. In this situation, treatment for the infection will resolve the problem.

Multicolored discharge, often bilateral, is likely to be caused by **duct ectasia.** Ectasia is most likely to occur when estrogen hormone levels are low, as they often are after menopause. With ectasia, ducts leading to the nipple become blocked by accumulated, dried breast secretions. Normal body defenses compound the problem by sending white blood cells, and an inflammation reaction results. Bacteria from the skin may also invade the area, causing true infection. Swelling, pain, or itching may occur, and the discharge may be green or multicolored. If a lump is present, often caused by inflammation, then biopsy will be necessary. Otherwise, daily cleansing of the nipple with an antibacterial soap such as hexachlorophene may be sufficient. Hormone treatment to prevent persistent problems may also be reasonable.

Galactorrhea.   Inappropriate breast milk production is not really a breast problem, but is a hormone abnormality originating in the pituitary gland.

Normally, hormone patterns of pregnancy prepare the breast to manufacture milk, and milk production is triggered after pregnancy by high prolactin levels. Prolactin release from the pituitary is stimulated by suckling, and milk appears within a day or two after nursing has begun. Once established, milk production may continue for quite some time even after nursing is stopped. Expression of milk may be possible with nipple stimulation as long as six months later.

Milk production not associated with pregnancy and breastfeeding can occur whenever pituitary prolactin release is persistently elevated for any reason. Sexual breast stimulation can cause elevated prolactin, and so can stimulation of nerves to the thoracic (chest cage) area. Galactorrhea sometimes occurs after surgery or injury involving the chest wall, and may even be caused by prolonged chest and breast stimulation resulting from dedicated athletic training in loose-fitting clothes. Many drugs can cause prolactin abnormalities, including phenothiazine tranquilizers such as Thorazine, some antidepressants, and some high blood pressure medications.

In many cases, galactorrhea is accompanied by prolonged amenorrhea, the absence of menstrual periods. High prolactin levels can block cyclic hormone patterns, so menstrual periods stop. Levels of estrogen and progesterone are likely to be low, so other symptoms such as vaginal dryness may be evident as well.

Evaluation of galactorrhea is likely to start with blood tests to check for elevated prolactin or low thyroid levels. (Low thyroid is a rare cause, but quite easy to treat.) If prolactin is high or galactorrhea persists, x-rays of your head will be needed to be sure that you don't have a tumor in your pituitary gland. Tests should be repeated every six months or so as long as galactorrhea persists.

Bromocriptine is usually effective in treating galactorrhea. Read the section on fibrocystic breast problems for details on bromocriptine treatment and possible side effects.

PLASTIC SURGERY TO ALTER BREAST SIZE

I thought I was the only woman in the world who had breast surgery. When I finally confessed at work why I had used that sick leave, two other women said, "You too?"

—WOMAN, 31

In most cases, the reason for plastic surgery to change breast size (called mammoplasty) is cosmetic. Most commonly, women simply want bigger breasts. Like any other cosmetic procedure, this surgery is entirely elective, and possible complications are stressed because there are no major health benefits to weigh against its potential risks. Unless there are medical indications for surgery, a cosmetic procedure is also likely to be excluded from health insurance coverage, so the decision about surgery may involve a significant financial decision as well. Nevertheless, many women (more than you might guess) decide to undergo mammoplasty, and most are very happy with the result.

Mammoplasty can sometimes be considered therapeutic rather than cosmetic, and may be quite strongly recommended by a surgeon and covered under your health insurance. Such therapeutic mammoplasty might be considered when the goal is:

• To equalize breast size for a woman who has a marked size discrepancy. This is an uncommon and harmless congenital abnormality, but can be very tough to live with.
• To reduce breast size for a woman who has extremely large breasts that are out of proportion with her overall body size
• To reestablish a symmetric appearance after mastectomy

Increasing breast size through augmentation mammoplasty is a simpler procedure than reduction surgery. Augmentation is achieved by placing a soft, correctly shaped prosthesis behind the breast gland tissue. Prostheses are available in a range of sizes and shapes, and are made of inert materials designed to retain their soft, pliable shape permanently. Insertion of the prosthesis involves an incision along the lower edge of each breast or partway around the areola that surrounds the nipple to allow the surgeon to slide the prosthesis between the breast and the muscle layer covering the ribs or just beneath the muscle layer. Prosthesis insertion can usually be accomplished without disrupting the breast tissue, so breast glands and ducts retain their normal structure and function. After surgery, normal breast tissue is located on the surface, over the prosthesis, and your own or your clinician's breast examination should not be impaired. Subsequent breastfeeding is not even likely to be a problem.

Serious complications after augmentation are not common, but do sometimes occur. Breast infection or bleeding immediately after surgery is possible, either of which might necessitate further surgery to remove the prosthesis. Later, less dangerous problems are more common. Gradual formation of fibrous tissue around the implant may make it undesirably stiff, or even cause puckering and pain in nearby normal tissue, and manipulation to break the fibrous tissue may be necessary. Displacement of the prosthesis can also occur, creating an odd or lopsided breast contour. Correcting these problems may involve further surgery. Prostheses now available, however, are much less likely to cause serious problems than were older techniques involving injections or synthetic sponges. It is important to remember that augmentation surgery is surgery, and all surgery has risks. Be certain that increasing your breast size is something you are genuinely doing for yourself and not for someone else before you proceed.

Procedures for augmentation are somewhat more difficult for a woman who has had a mastectomy because space for the prosthesis must be created surgically. Problems with good skin healing are more likely if the skin must be stretched to cover the new breast shape, and loss of skin sensation over the area is likely. If mastectomy has involved removal of the nipple, plastic repair is possible, but cannot truly duplicate a normal nipple in appearance, or in sensitivity.

Local anesthesia, with surgery in an outpatient surgery facility, is usually recommended for breast augmentation. It is a fairly minor procedure, and even if general anesthesia is used, an overnight hospital stay is not likely to be necessary.

Reduction mammoplasty is a major surgical procedure. General anesthesia and hospitalization for several days after surgery will be necessary. Several incisions will probably be required to obtain a normal breast contour and a normal-appearing nipple location. Loss of at least some skin sensation and/or nipple sensation is also quite likely. Reducing breast size involves removing some of the breast gland tissue, so normal breast gland and duct structure is disrupted, and breastfeeding after reduction surgery is likely to be impossible, and will also be discouraged because the infection risk is higher if the breast ducts are not able to drain properly.

Before deciding on breast augmentation or reduction, be sure you understand clearly what benefits you can reasonably expect, and the possible problems as well. The decision is entirely yours, and **no reputable surgeon would want to pressure you** to decide in favor of surgery. Do not hesitate to seek a second or even third opinion as you make your decision. Your surgeon should explain the specific procedure or options that would be best in your particular situation, and should provide a thorough assessment of possible risks and problems as they apply to you.

You will also want to be sure that the surgeon you choose is well trained and experienced in mammoplasty. In most communities, mammoplasty is undertaken by plastic surgeons who are specialists in this area, and perform hundreds of breast surgeries each year.

REFERENCES

1. Baker LH: Breast Cancer Detection Demonstration Project: Five-year summary report. *Ca—A Cancer Journal for Clinicians* 32:194–225, 1982.
2. Love SM, Gelman RS, Silen W: Fibrocystic "disease" of the breast—A nondisease? *New England Journal of Medicine* 307:1010–1014, 1982.
3. Rose DP: Low-fat diet may decrease mastalgia. *Ob-Gyn News,* Vol 20, No 14, July 1985.
4. Brooks PG, Gart S, Heldfond AJ, et al: Measuring the effect of caffeine restriction on fibrocystic breast disease. *Journal of Reproductive Medicine* 26:279–282, 1981.
5. Lubin F, Ron E, Wax Y, et al: A case-control study of caffeine and methylxanthines in benign breast disease. *Journal of the American Medical Association* 253:2388–2392, 1985.
6. Sundaram GS, London R, Manimekalai S, et al: Alpha-tocopherol and serum lipoproteins. *Lipids* 16:223–227, 1981.
7. Vorherr H: Fibrocystic breast disease: Pathophysiology, pathomorphology, clinical picture, and management. *American Journal of Obstetrics and Gynecology* 154:161–179, 1986.
8. Pye JK, Mansel RE, Hughes LE: Clinical experience of drug treatments for mastalgia. *Lancet* 2:373–377, 1985.

38

Bladder and Kidney Problems

Problems involving the urinary tract, which includes your kidneys, bladder, and urethra, are so common among women that you are almost certain to encounter at least one of them sometime during your life. Most common is bladder infection. It is very often linked to sexual intercourse but can arise spontaneously as well. Urethritis, inflammation or infection of the urethra, too, is linked to intercourse. Infections, and steps you can take to minimize your problems with them, are described in the first part of this chapter.

Problems with urine control are also very common, especially during the postmenopausal decades. Most often these problems are caused by structural changes in tissues that support the bladder and urethra, and may be a late-appearing consequence of childbearing. Structural support problems and surgery to correct them are described in Chapter 39. Sometimes urine control problems are the result of other factors, though, and possible causes other than pelvic damage from childbirth are described in this chapter.

Infection/Inflammation

Infections frequently attack the urinary system and can cause problems ranging from mild burning sensations during urination to serious illness or even death. Most urinary infections are caused by bacteria from the vagina or anus that gain access to the urethra and bladder. Infection can sometimes arise spontaneously, but usually occurs

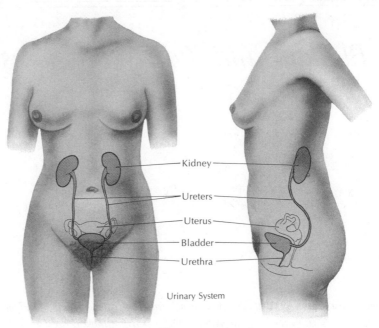

Urinary System

ILLUSTRATION 38-1   **The woman's urinary system.**

after injury or irritation to the external urethral opening caused by vigorous intercourse or by a urine catheter (a rubber tube inserted through the urethra into the bladder to drain urine). Urinary tract infections can also be caused by diseases such as diabetes that diminish resistance to infection, by kidney stones, or by structural abnormalities that obstruct urine flow from the kidneys. Infection can attack the urethra, bladder, or kidneys, or all three sites together (see Illustration 38-1).

The word ending "itis" means inflammation. Inflammation is a normal body defense response that causes an increase in blood flow to the problem area and an influx of infection-fighting white blood cells. Tenderness and swelling in the area result at least partly from these normal defense reactions. In many cases the inflammation response is triggered by infection, an entirely appropriate response to invading foreign organisms. Inflammation, however, can also be triggered by other factors such as chemical irritation or allergy.

URETHRITIS
(INFECTION/INFLAMMATION OF THE URETHRA)

Infection of the urethra, the tube that carries urine from the bladder to the outside of the body, causes burning during urination and/or a urethral discharge. In women the urethra is about an inch long. Urethritis often accompanies a bladder infection (cystitis) and is usually treated with the same medication.

Urethritis can occur without an accompanying bladder infection when it is associated with gonorrhea, chlamydia, herpes, trichomonas, or other vaginal infections (see Chapters 22 and 23). If you have urethritis, then careful evaluation for vaginal infection will be needed, as will tests to detect unsuspected gonorrhea or chlamydia if you are sexually active.

Symptoms of urethritis are also common among postmenopausal women who have low levels of estrogen hormone. This skin and other tissues of the vulva, vagina, and urethra all respond to low estrogen with gradually diminished skin thickness and resilience. These changes make the skin so delicate and sensitive that the trauma of everyday living may be enough to cause small cracks or ulcers and lead to inflammation called atrophic urethritis, vulvitis, or vaginitis.

Nonspecific Urethritis (NSU). Your clinician may use this term for the very frustrating situation that occurs when symptoms of urethritis are present, but no specific cause can be found. Researchers suspect that most cases of NSU actually are caused by infection, but the bacteria involved are so difficult to grow in laboratory conditions that they cannot be identified. Until recently, chlamydia was among the hard-to-document culprits. Tests for chlamydia are now available, and this bacterium is a common cause of NSU for both women and men. It also causes other serious infection problems (see Chapter 25).

Urethral Diverticulum. A rare cause of persisting or recurring urethritis problems is a urethral diverticulum, a tiny pouch attached to the normally straight urethral canal. Urine and bacteria trapped in the pouch predispose you to infection. Urethral diverticulum is an uncommon problem; it can be identified with urethroscopy, examination of the inside of the urethral canal through a tiny lighted tube, and can be surgically corrected.

CYSTITIS (BLADDER INFECTION)

At first I just thought it was odd that I woke up at one-thirty A.M. to go to the bathroom. Then I was up at three and five, and finally I got the picture. Bladder infection! The price I pay when David comes home on leave . . .

—WOMAN, 23

The bladder is a muscular storage bag for urine, the fluid waste products that the kidneys have filtered from the blood. Urine can remain in your bladder for many hours if you don't urinate frequently, and like a stagnant pool anywhere, it can be a prime target for bacterial overgrowth.

Your symptoms might include:

• Feeling of pressure, urgency to urinate
• Burning during urination or urethral discharge
• Frequency of urination; urinating in small amounts
• Having to get up at night to urinate
• Cramping and pain in the center of your lower abdomen after urinating
• Urine that has an unusual odor
• Urine that is cloudy or bloody (red or pink)

Bladder infections (cystitis) are much more common in women than in men, since bacteria have to travel only about an inch or two to reach a woman's bladder from the outside of her body, compared to the 6 inches or more bacteria must travel to reach a man's bladder.

Sexual intercourse is such a common trigger for bladder infection that it is sometimes called "honeymoon cystitis." Bacteria present in the woman's vagina or on genital skin gain access to the bladder with the forceful movements and common mild to moderate tissue trauma of intercourse.

Symptoms with cystitis may be fairly subtle and persistent or they may begin suddenly and increase in severity so rapidly that a woman is immobilized within just a few hours. Cystitis can be miserable, but it is not usually a serious health threat. If infection spreads upward from the bladder to involve the kidneys as well, however, the consequences can be serious.

PYELONEPHRITIS
(INFECTION OF THE KIDNEY)

Infection of the kidney is called pyelonephritis. Symptoms include fever, chills, and pain in the back at or just above waist level on one side or the other. The back pain is likely to be more persistent than simple muscular backache, and you may feel really sick. Symptoms of bladder infection may be present as well. Pyelonephritis can be a very serious infection and requires prompt, aggressive antibiotic treatment and a thorough evaluation of the source of infection. Kidney infections are most common during pregnancy and can cause premature delivery.

LABORATORY EVALUATION AND DIAGNOSIS

Your clinician may be able to diagnose urethritis or cystitis on the basis of your symptoms and a simple microscopic examination of your urine. She/he will find that your urethra and/or bladder are tender to pressure during your pelvic exam (see Illustration 38-1), and microscopic examination of your urine will show bacteria and white blood cells, neither of which are present in normal urine. If you are having your first attack, and the onset and symptoms you have are just right for cystitis, your clinician may feel it is reasonable to treat you with prescription antibiotics on the basis of a phone call only. An exam and further tests will definitely be needed, however, if you think there is any chance of a sexually transmitted infection, or if factors in your medical history such as drug allergy, pregnancy, or significant medical problems might make cystitis more dangerous, or treatment more difficult, for you.

In addition to a pelvic exam to check for tenderness, your clinician will look for evidence of vaginal infection. A wet smear (see Chapter 4) to check for yeast and trichomonas and laboratory tests for gonorrhea and chlamydia may be needed. All of these can cause urethritis and cystitis. Your clinician may also order a urine culture and sensitivity test to determine what specific bacterium is causing your infection and which antibiotics will be most effective. Culture and sensitivity results will not be available for about 48 hours, so your clinician will begin your treatment immediately with an antibiotic that is usually effective and change it after the test results come back if necessary.

Your culture results may or may not be clear-cut. If the report shows 100,000 colonies or more of one bacterial species, your diagnosis is settled. Unfortunately, in as many as 30% to 50% of cases culture results are not so definitive (1). Results that show several different organisms present or a smaller number of bacterial colonies are common, and hard to interpret. The specimen may have been contaminated by bacteria from the skin, so results may not be meaningful. Or the culture may show no growth at all because your infection is being caused by an organism that requires more elaborate laboratory culture techniques. In these situations your treatment may have to be based on good clinical guesses.

Microscopic urine evaluation may also be hard to interpret. Bacteria are not always visible, and blood cells may be present for other reasons. Bleeding, and red blood cells visible in urine under the microscope, are common findings with infection. Red blood cells in urine may also mean a kidney stone or other less common bladder or kidney problems. If bleeding is your primary symptom, your clinician is likely to recommend additional tests to make an accurate diagnosis.

Asymptomatic Infections.   Unsuspected bacteria are found in the urine of 4% to 7% of pregnant women tested, and a small percentage of healthy nonpregnant women as well. This condition is called asymptomatic bacteriuria, and despite the absence of symptoms, treatment to eradicate the infection is wise. Pyelonephritis could occur as a result and cause serious problems, especially if the woman is pregnant.

TREATMENT

Sulfa medications such as Gantrisin (sulfisoxazole) and broad-spectrum antibiotics such as tetracycline or ampicillin are commonly used to treat cystitis. (If you have certain kinds of hereditary anemia, you should not use sulfa drugs. Be sure to discuss this with your clinician.) There are several different treatment schedules that may be possibilities.

Single-Dose Treatment.   For a woman who is not pregnant and has an initial attack of cystitis with no evidence of kidney infection, treatment with one (large) dose of an antibiotic such as amoxicillin, tetracycline, or trimethoprim-sulfamethoxazole (Bactrim, Cotrin, or Septra) may be sufficient to cure the infection. Cure rates for this approach have been as high as cure rates for 14-day treatment in some studies, although a recent study found somewhat less satisfactory success rates (2). Follow-up testing to be sure your infection is cured is important with this approach.

Intermediate (Traditional) Treatment.   Treatment maintained for a full seven to ten days is traditional. Some experts feel, however, that treatment for three or four days is sufficient, and side effects are less likely. Also, you are less likely to develop yeast vaginitis with short-term treatment (see Chapter 23). More prolonged treatment will be needed if infection involves the kidneys, persists or recurs despite treatment, or if a sexually transmitted disease is suspected. Effective treatment for chlamydia will require seven full days of tetracycline or doxycycline taken very faithfully; both you and your partner must be treated.

Suppression Treatment.   Low-dose antibiotic treatment continued for weeks or months may be recommended for a woman who has persistent problems with recurring infection. For some women, a preferable alternative may be low-dose antibiotics taken each time intercourse occurs or at the first sign of infection symptoms (3). Typical treatment might be Bactrim or Septra, one half of a regular strength tablet each night at bedtime, or with intercourse, or four regular strength tablets at the first onset of painful urination or frequency.

Whichever medication schedule you and your clinician choose, be sure to take all the medication prescribed, even if your symptoms subside soon after treatment is started. Insufficient treatment can lead to development of antibiotic-resistant bacterial strains, and you may be more likely to have problems with persisting or recurring infection. Also, don't try to treat yourself with old antibiotics you may have at home; your urine culture may be inaccurate if you have recently taken antibiotics. If gonorrhea, chlamydia, or trichomonas is causing your infection, a short course of antibiotics is not sufficient; you need the full recommended treatment. Also, your partner will need to be treated at the same time you are.

I've had several bladder infections, and my worst symptom is usually just plain old pain. My doctor said it was from bladder spasm. The Pyridium works for that though, and I don't mind the "designer urine" color.

—WOMAN, 31

If you are having severe bladder spasm and frequency of urination, your clinician may prescribe Pyridium (phenazopyridine hydrochloride) to soothe your bladder and urethra temporarily until the infection begins to subside. Pyridium may turn your urine dark orange, a harmless, temporary effect. If urinating burns badly, urinate in a bathtub full of warm water. Avoid tea, coffee, and alcohol. **Be sure to drink plenty of water** while you are recovering from infection to decrease the concentration of bacteria in your urine and help flush out your bladder. Cranberry juice or ascorbic acid may help because they make your urine acidic. Avoid or at least decrease the frequency of intercourse.

Follow-up Care. Your clinician is likely to recommend a urine culture about two weeks after you have finished taking your medication to confirm that the bacteria that caused your infection have been eradicated. If bacteria or symptoms are still present, further treatment will be needed.

If you have had a serious kidney infection or repeated episodes of cystitis, your clinician will probably recommend a series of tests to evaluate your entire urinary system. She/he may test you for diabetes and may recommend an intravenous pyelogram (IVP), an x-ray evaluation of the urinary system. The radiologist injects dye into your arm vein and then takes a series of x-rays that would reveal any obstruction in the flow of urine from your kidneys to your bladder. You may be referred to a urologist for further evaluation, and you may need cystoscopy, an office procedure that permits your clinician to see the inside of your urethra and bladder through a thin, lighted tube called a cystoscope.

If you use a diaphragm and have recurring bouts of cystitis, be sure to see your clinician for a change in diaphragm size or rim type. You may even need to change to a different method of birth control (see Chapter 12). Diaphragm users in one recent study were about three times as likely to develop bladder infection as users of birth control Pills (4). Pressure from the rim of your diaphragm against the urethra and bladder could interfere with complete emptying of the bladder and predispose you to infection. Using a slightly smaller diaphragm that exerts less pressure may be an option, and you will want to be sure to urinate before and after intercourse, and frequently and completely while you are wearing your diaphragm. Removing the diaphragm promptly after its six to eight hours or alternating use of the diaphragm with condoms might be reasonable. If bladder infection problems persist despite these measures, however, it may be best to change entirely to another contraceptive method.

Preventing Urinary Infection: Suggestions

Many women find that infection crops up when they have very frequent and vigorous intercourse, especially after a long period of little or no intercourse. A clear and strong link between sexual intercourse and both urethritis and bladder infection is documented statistically (4). Other factors such as diet, hygiene, and urination habits may play a role as well. Research evidence for these factors, however, is very limited. The following suggestions include factors with research-documented significance (5) shown with an asterisk (*), as well as commonly accepted hygiene measures to minimize the likelihood of bacterial contamination. You may be able to stave off infection if you follow these suggestions:

• Do everything you can to minimize your risk of exposure to sexually transmitted diseases; many STD organisms can cause urinary tract infections as well as other terrible problems
• Make sure you have plenty of lubrication during intercourse; if natural lubrication is limited, try a water-soluble lubricant such as K-Y Jelly or birth control foam
• Change intercourse positions frequently; rear entry and side-by-side positions may decrease friction on your urethral opening. Avoid anal intercourse to decrease the likelihood of contaminating your vagina and urethral opening with bacteria from the rectum.
• Stop having intercourse if you begin to feel sore or tender
• Make sure you are drinking plenty of healthy fluids (such as water and fruit juice), and that you urinate frequently and completely
• Urinate after intercourse, within 15 to 30 minutes if possible*
• Shower carefully every day, and ask your partner to do the same
• Wipe from front to back after using the toilet; the goal is to avoid the transfer of bacteria from the rectum to the vulva or urethra
• Avoid deodorant soap, hygiene sprays, and deodorant sanitary pads*
• Minimize your use of tampons*
• Avoid wearing tight jeans*
• Avoid tea*
• Avoid cola soft drinks*
• Minimize coffee and soda pop in your diet*
• Minimize beer, wine, and liquor in your diet*

Women who wore pantyhose or underwear made of synthetic fabrics in the study cited above did not have significantly higher risks for urinary tract infection.

Problems with Urine Control

Normal urine control requires proper functioning of brain and spinal cord centers that coordinate urination reflexes, normal autonomic nervous system responses, normal muscle response in the bladder wall and in the sphincters (valves) of the bladder and urethra, and normal bladder and urethral structure. Loss of control, called incontinence, can occur for many different reasons. It is more common among elderly people, and more common among women than men. Bladder size and resilience decrease with age, as do urine flow rate and the ability to empty the bladder completely. For women, structural damage from childbirth and the effects of low estrogen hormone levels after menopause on genital tissues are very common causes of incontinence, and may compound other incontinence problems as well.

Incontinence symptoms range from mild to severe. For women, occasional involuntary loss of a few drops of urine under predictable circumstances is extremely common. A forceful cough or sneeze with a very full bladder, for example, is likely to provoke urine loss even for a healthy young woman. If incontinence is a regular occurrence or is severe enough that frequent visits to the toilet or daily sanitary pads are needed, then evaluation to determine its cause is entirely reasonable.

POSSIBLE CAUSES OF INCONTINENCE

Temporary incontinence problems are quite common with urinary tract infection. Other symptoms are likely to be present, but in some cases loss of control is the first evidence of a problem. Severe constipation with impacted stools, or activity restriction such as bed rest, may also cause temporary incontinence. Many drugs, including some sedatives, sleeping pills, tranquilizers and antidepressants, some diuretics, and drugs used for heart problems or gastrointestinal spasm, may also impair urine control (6).

Neurologic problems including peripheral nerve damage from diabetes or spinal disc disease can cause urine retention that distends the bladder and leads to frequent or continuous urine leakage as urine overflows from a maximally stretched bladder whose muscles cannot function effectively. Neurologic problems can also cause intermittent bladder emptying with loss of voluntary control and no warning of imminent urination. In this situation the reflexes controlling urination may be normal but no longer under voluntary control.

Bladder wall muscle that is hyperactive causes episodes of incontinence preceded by a warning. The urge to urinate is followed a few seconds or minutes later by another involuntary bladder contraction. This is a fairly common type of incontinence and can result from temporary problems such as urinary infection, bladder irritation from radiation treatment or tumor, or neurologic problems.

Stress incontinence, urine loss that occurs only with stress such as coughing or physical exertion that temporarily increases pressure inside the abdomen, is especially common among postmenopausal women. Increased urine loss occurs with stress in other types of incontinence as well, so distinguishing between the different types may not be easy. Incontinence can be caused by hyperactive bladder wall muscles that contract in response to stress. Commonly, though, stress incontinence results from loss of pelvic support for the bladder and urethra. It is often linked to pelvic relaxation and damage from childbirth, and these problems are described in Chapter 39. Surgery to restore more normal pelvic structure is one possibility. For many women, however, exercises to improve pelvic muscle tone (Kegel's exercises, see Chapter 39) will be effective. Also, hormone treatment to counteract atrophy (thin and fragile skin and subcutaneous tissue) may be helpful.

A **fistula** from the bladder or urethra is an uncommon cause of incontinence for women. A fistula—an abnormal passage—can occur with severe childbirth injury or after radiation treatment for cancer. The most common cause in the United States is injury during hysterectomy surgery (see Chapter 49). A fistula is likely to cause persistent, watery vaginal discharge.

EVALUATION AND TREATMENT

Incontinence is a frustrating and inconvenient problem; in some cases it is also medically significant. Impaired urinary control that is accompanied by incomplete bladder emptying may increase risks for bladder infection and for serious kidney infection; it may also be a danger sign for significant medical or neurologic problems. Thorough evaluation is definitely needed. Also, once the cause or causes are found, it is usually possible to treat the problem effectively so symptoms are cured or at least substantially improved (6).

Evaluation is likely to begin with a thorough, general medical evaluation, including neurologic assessment and tests for unsuspected medical disorders such as diabetes. Specialized evaluation of the bladder and urethra may also be needed and you may be referred to a urologist.

Treatment naturally depends on the underlying cause(s) found. Even if the cause cannot be corrected, however, treatment with medications that alter bladder function may be a possibility. You can reasonably expect treatment to be helpful.

REFERENCES

1. Latham RH, Wong ES, Larson A, et al: Laboratory diagnosis of urinary tract infection in ambulatory women. *Journal of the American Medical Association* 254:3333–3336, 1985.
2. Hooton TM, Running K, Stamm WE: Single-dose therapy for cystitis in women. *Journal of the American Medical Association* 253:387–390, 1985.
3. Wong ES, McKevitt M, Running K, et al: Management of recurrent urinary tract infections with patient-administered single-dose therapy. *Annals of Internal Medicine* 102:302–307, 1985.

4. Foxman B, Frerichs RR: Epidemiology of urinary tract infection: I. Diaphragm use and sexual intercourse. *American Journal of Public Health* 75:1308–1313, 1985.
5. Foxman B, Frerichs RR: Epidemiology of urinary tract infection: II. Diet, clothing, and urination habits. *American Journal of Public Health* 75:1314–1317, 1985.
6. Resnick NM, Yalla SV: Management of incontinence in the elderly. *New England Journal of Medicine* 313:800–805, 1985.

Problems of
the Vulva and Vagina

The vulva, vaginal lips, and vagina itself are the locus of suffering for some of women's most common afflictions. Vaginitis, herpes, and warts can attack these sensitive tissues and are so important and prevalent that they have chapters of their own (Chapter 23, "Vaginitis"; Chapter 26, "Herpes"; Chapter 27, "Genital Warts"). Other vulvar and vaginal disorders, fortunately, are not as common.

This chapter begins with a brief discussion of vaginal and vulvar hygiene, including information about douching, because so many women have questions about these issues. The second section is devoted to skin disorders that affect the vulva, and the final section to benign (noncancerous) vaginal problems including prolapse, cystocele, and rectocele. Vulvar and vaginal cancers are not common; risk factors, danger signs, and treatment are discussed in Chapter 41.

VAGINAL HYGIENE

The normal, healthy vagina cleanses itself every day. Slight discharge from the cervix and vaginal walls keeps the vagina moist, and the downward flow of moisture carries old cells, menstrual blood, and other matter out of the vagina quite effectively. Normal vaginal discharge is scant, sticky, and clear or white on most days. For several days around the time of ovulation in each cycle, discharge becomes abundant, clear, and slippery. A normal discharge has a characteristic mild odor and dries to a yellowish color on underclothes.

My grandmother said a woman isn't clean until she's douched. My
mother said douching a couple of times a month makes her feel better, whatever better means. My doctor said don't do it. Once in a while
I do, though. If I feel itchy or maybe I smell funny to myself I douche,
kind of to head off vaginitis. I have no idea whether it does any good.

—WOMAN, 36

Almost all clinicians agree that **there are no health benefits whatsoever to be gained
from routine douching.** (In some cases, clinicians do recommend douching as a
temporary adjunct to treatment for certain vaginal infections.) **In fact, douching and
hygiene sprays may even be harmful,** especially if you use these products incorrectly.

Some researchers suspect that douching **may encourage the spread of infection** from
the vagina up into the uterus and tubes. The force of the douching liquid may actually
push infection-contaminated liquid up into the uterus. Or perhaps douching washes
away the protective mucous plug in the cervical canal, and so makes it easier for
bacteria and other organisms to travel up the cervical canal into the uterus. In one
study, 90% of women being treated for PID (pelvic inflammatory disease) reported that
they douched more than once a week; only half as many healthy women in the
comparison group reported douching that often. **Another study has linked tubal ectopic
pregnancy to douching.** Women who douched at least once a week were twice as likely
as women who never douched to have an ectopic pregnancy. Women who used
commercial douche products at least once a week had four times the ectopic pregnancy
risk (1). Ectopic pregnancy risk is also linked to previous pelvic infections, so the
results of these two studies corroborate each other.

These research results do not prove that douching caused the infection risk. It is
possible, for example, that the women in the studies who douched frequently did so
because of subtle changes in vaginal odor or discharge that were disturbing to them; in
other words, the pelvic infection caused discharge abnormalities which in turn caused
douching. Or perhaps the women douched because they felt a need to wash away their
partner's sperm before having intercourse with another partner, so multiple partners
was the cause of infection risk.

**On the other hand, it is entirely possible that douching itself did contribute to
infection risk in these studies.** And in any case, douching does not appear to be a
medically safe practice. If you feel a need to douche, listen instead to whatever subtle
symptoms or personal concerns are making you feel the need. If your vaginal
secretions seem peculiar or unpleasant, see your clinician to make sure you don't
already have an infection. And if your sexual lifestyle makes you feel the need to
douche, do your very best to change it. Serious health risks (see Chapters 22, 25, and
28) are at stake.

If you choose to douche nevertheless, follow these suggestions for using douche products as safely as possible.

Do not rely on douching as a method of birth control. Even if you douche immediately after intercourse, some sperm will still have time to enter the cervical canal, where they won't be washed away by the douching liquid.

Use gentle water pressure. If you use a bulb syringe, squeeze gently. If you use a hanging bag, don't hang it more than 2 or 3 feet above your body.

Use plain warm water only and don't douche more often than once a week. Water cleans just about as well as commercial douching products and is less likely to be irritating. If you choose to use commercial products, use half the strength recommended on the label. If you use vinegar and water douches, use only 1 or 2 tablespoons of vinegar to each quart of water.

Avoid douching if you suspect you have an infection. Don't risk spreading infection up into your uterus. Also, your clinician cannot diagnose an infection if all the evidence has been washed away.

Avoid douching and tampons for three days before a pelvic exam. Pap smear results may be less accurate if your cervix has recently been rinsed or rubbed, and your clinician will want to see your typical discharge.

Vaginal sprays are no more necessary for good hygiene than is douching. If you do choose to use a vaginal deodorant spray, follow label instructions carefully. Don't spray more frequently than the manufacturer recommends, and hold the can at least 6 inches away from your skin. Most important, don't spread your labia apart to spray directly into the entrance to your vagina. Stop using sprays if you develop signs of irritation such as itching, swelling, redness, or tenderness.

VULVAR HYGIENE

Just like skin anywhere on the body, vulvar skin is happiest and most likely to stay healthy when it is kept clean and dry. Bathing or showering once a day or so is all that is necessary under normal circumstances. Use mild bath soap to wash the skin area, rinse thoroughly with water, and dry gently. Plain water with no soap is fine for the delicate mucous membrane lining just inside the vulva, around the urinary opening and vaginal entrance, if you are sensitive to soap or other irritants.

Vulvar problems are most likely to occur whenever the area is exposed to persistent moisture or even dampness. Moisture breaks down the skin surface (remember how sickly skin under a Band-Aid looks?) and promotes the growth of bacteria and yeast organisms as well. Tight clothing, panty hose, and bathing suits can cause dampness, and so can the folds of extra tissue that occur with obesity.

Extra care with vulvar hygiene may be needed when you are combatting the skin problems described in the next section. Your clinician may recommend one or more of the following do-it-yourself intensive care steps for vulvar healing.

• Wet dressings or soaks with Burow's (generic) or Domeboro (trade name) solution. Applying gauze soaked in one of these mildly astringent solutions provides immediately soothing relief for ulceration or open sores, and helps the damaged area to dry and heal after treatment. Use Burow's solution diluted to one-tenth, one-twentieth, or one-fortieth strength or Domeboro solution prepared according to directions on the powder packet. Both are available without a prescription in the drugstore. Store the solution in the refrigerator for an even more soothing and cooling treatment. Leave the wet compress in place for up to 30 minutes, adding more solution as necessary to keep the compress wet. Treatment can be repeated several times daily. Allow your vulva to dry thoroughly after each treatment.

• Sitz baths are simply frequent soaks in warm water, and are often recommended for temporary relief of discomfort with any vulvar skin irritation. Soaks may also speed healing of a boil or skin infection. Use 6 or 8 inches of plain warm water in the tub for each sitz bath, and soak for 10 or 15 minutes. Then allow the vulva to dry thoroughly. Sitz baths may be repeated several times daily, and a soothing additive such as baking soda may be recommended.

• Wash the vulvar skin gently twice each day with a mild soap-free cleanser such as Aveeno Bar and dry thoroughly with a soft towel. (The main ingredient in this cleanser is colloidal oatmeal.)

• Thorough drying of vulvar skin after bathing or soaking may be easier with a hair dryer set on warm (not hot) at low speed

• Wear all-cotton underpants to help absorb moisture and keep the skin surface dry. During intensive care you should avoid nylon or polyester clothing in the vulvar area, and forgo panty hose as well.

• Do not use perfumed douches, sprays, bath powder, or deodorant in the vulvar area

• Use plain white toilet paper, not perfumed or printed

• Use mild laundry soap and very thorough rinsing for laundering underclothes. Avoid fabric softeners, including tissue strips in the dryer.

• Anti-bacterial soap such as Betadine Skin Cleanser, Dial, or Safeguard may be recommended to reduce bacteria on the skin for a woman who has repeated problems with vulvar pimples and boils. Keeping skin dry is also important in overcoming this problem.

• Avoid using anything greasy on your vulva. Petroleum jelly (such as Vaseline) and medications in **ointment** form leave a greasy layer on the skin and trap moisture against the skin surface. Over time, these can make the situation worse, and could even impede healing. Ointment containing medication may be necessary for treatment in some cases, so be sure your skin is thoroughly dry before applying it, use a small amount, and massage the ointment in thoroughly to avoid leaving a greasy film.

VULVAR SKIN DISORDERS

Vulvar skin is subject to many skin problems that affect other body areas such as eczema, moles (called nevi), dermatitis, and even psoriasis. In addition, vulvar skin is uniquely subject to a localized, persistent skin disorder called vulvar dystrophy.

I don't know whether other women have bumps or clogged glands or any of these things I get. We don't exactly talk about vulvar skin at the health club. But my husband sees that skin. I want it to look absolutely perfect.

—WOMAN, 48

Common Vulvar Skin Problems. Women are often concerned about **lumps and bumps** that appear on vulvar skin. In some cases, a bump can be the signal of genital warts, a sexually transmitted affliction. In most cases, though, the bump will prove to be a localized skin infection or clogged sebaceous gland similar to pimples and skin problems that occur elsewhere on the body. Vulvar skin contains hair follicles and good-sized sebaceous glands that produce thick, oily, yellow secretions. It also contains both eccrine and apocrine sweat glands. Eccrine glands are part of the body's temperature regulation system, and are widespread over the whole body. Apocrine glands respond to emotional and adrenaline stimuli by secreting a milky white fluid. Bacteria on the skin interact with apocrine secretions to release a pungent, characteristic odor. Skin near the vulva and in the underarm area are rich in aprocrine glands.

A clogged and infected hair follicle or sweat gland may form a large pimple or boil in the vulvar area. Careful attention to hygiene (see above) may be all that is needed, but antibiotics can be prescribed if the infection is severe. Recurring infection in vulvar sweat glands, called **hidradenitis suppurativa,** is a serious problem for some women; sweat glands under the arms may also be involved. Treatment with antibiotics or even surgery to remove scarred glands may be needed.

Bartholin's Gland Infection. A Bartholin's gland, located just under the surface of the labia majora, can be the cause of a vulvar lump. Infection trapped inside the gland results in an extremely tender, swollen vulva, usually on just one side (see Illustration 39-1).

When active infection is present, your clinician will probably recommend oral antibiotics such as tetracycline or ampicillin and frequent hot soaks. In most cases, the infection will resolve more quickly if the gland is also drained. Your clinician may be able to drain the gland by puncturing it with a needle and withdrawing the fluid into a syringe. This technique resulted in prompt relief of pain and complete healing for 85% of patients in one small study (2). The appearance of the fluid and infection tests can determine the cause of the infection so that appropriate antibiotic treatment can be prescribed. Alternatively, your clinician may use a local anesthetic and perform an incision and drainage (I&D) in the office, or she/he may recommend that the procedure be performed with general anesthesia in a hospital or surgical clinic. Incision and drainage simply means making an incision through the skin into the pus

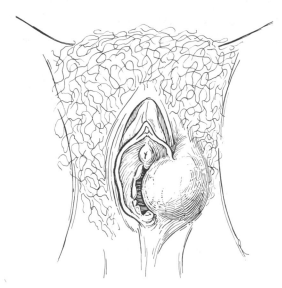

ILLUSTRATION 39-1   An infected Bartholin's gland or cyst can cause a huge lump in one (or both) vulva. If active infection is present, the area is likely to be red, hot, and very tender.

collection in the gland, thus allowing the pus to escape. A gauze wick is usually placed in the incision so that it will remain open for several days to allow complete drainage.

Some clinicians recommend marsupialization rather than simple I&D for treatment of an infected gland. The goal of marsupialization is to create a permanent drainage route for the gland. An incision is made through the skin into the gland, and the edges of the incision are stitched so that it will heal with a fairly large opening. In effect, the gland is converted into a pouch (hence, marsupial). Marsupialization often is successful in preventing later, repeated episodes of infection or formation of a cyst. General anesthesia may be recommended for marsupialization.

Removal of the entire Bartholin's gland may be recommended if a cyst forms, but there is no active infection. The enlarged gland cyst is cut free from its attachments to the vulva, and removed through a 1- or 2-inch incision in the vulvar skin. General anesthesia is usually recommended for cyst removal (cystectomy).

Recovery after Bartholin's gland surgery is rapid except for localized pain, tenderness, and swelling, which may last for two or three weeks. Complications of surgery are unlikely, but bleeding at the incision site or into the tissue around the gland, or damage to nearby structures such as the rectum, is possible.

Vestibular Adenitis.   This is an uncommon problem whose cause is not known. Women with vestibular adenitis often have a history of past yeast infections, and repeated visits to their clinicians to try to cure persistent vulvar irritation. The area of irritation is very localized to one or more spots just outside the hymen, and the spots appear red and are exquisitely tender to touch. A vulvar biopsy is necessary to be sure the persistent spots are not vulvar cancer. There is no known medical treatment, but symptoms can be stopped by surgically removing the area of skin tissue involved.

Atrophic Vulvovaginitis.   Loss of estrogen hormone at menopause may also cause symptoms of itching and burning. This condition, called atrophic vulvovaginitis, causes vaginal and vulvar skin to become thin and dry. When estrogen levels are low, the vaginal lining gradually becomes thinner and less resilient. Normal vaginal secretions that provide lubrication during intercourse are also reduced, so the tissue is more susceptible to trauma. Using additional lubrication may help prevent this problem, or it can be treated with replacement estrogen vaginal cream or pills (see Chapter 34).

Scratch–Itch Syndrome.   Burning and/or itching of the vulvar skin can be an extremely frustrating problem, and often leads to a vicious cycle. Scratching causes the skin to thicken and become stiff and leathery; cracks in thickened skin, in turn, cause more itching and burning. To break the cycle your clinician will try to identify and eliminate the culprit responsible for your initial symptoms, and at the same time, use treatment to reduce itching so scratching will stop.

Discharge from a vaginal infection, especially a yeast infection, may cause burning and itching of vulvar skin. Vaginal infections are discussed in Chapter 23. Exposure to bacteria-laden urine during a bladder infection can cause vulvar irritation. Another common cause is skin sensitivity to irritating chemicals or skin allergy; vulvar skin is particularly sensitive and may be the only area of your skin that shows an allergic reaction. Contraceptive products, lubricants, detergent or fabric softener used in laundering underwear, menstrual products, dye or chemicals in toilet paper, or medications applied to the vulva can all cause allergic reactions. Vulvar skin that is thin and delicate because of low estrogen hormone levels, after menopause for example, may be especially sensitive. After the initial scratch–itch problem is overcome, long-term treatment with estrogen vaginal cream or pills may help prevent recurrence.

After eliminating any infection, possible irritating agents, or hormone problems, treatment to stop the scratch–itch cycle is likely to involve cortisone and scrupulous attention to vulvar hygiene. Cortisone is extremely effective in relieving itching. Typical treatment might be a potent prescription cortisone such as betamethasone ointment, called Valisone 0.1%, usually applied four times daily. Eurax cream (crotamiton, used also for treating scabies) is also helpful in reducing itching, but like all cream preparations contains alcohol and may cause burning. To avoid burning, initial treatment with cortisone may be needed before beginning Eurax cream or estrogen vaginal cream. Weeks or even months of treatment may be required if skin thickening is severe. If treatment is not successful in reversing your symptoms, however, your clinician will recommend further evaluation including biopsy to be sure that you don't have skin cancer, and to check for vulvar dystrophy.

Vulvar Dystrophy.   The initial signs of vulvar dystrophy are likely to be one or more patches of dry, thickened skin, often accompanied by persistent itching. The patch may be red and swollen at first, but later becomes opaque white. As the condition progresses, the abnormal, white skin area expands to cover all or most of the vulva. Thickened, dry skin may form tiny cracks that burn and itch, or the skin may become glossy, and very thin. Loss of normal vulvar elasticity may narrow the vaginal opening. The fat layer just under the vulvar skin may be lost, so that the outer labia are flat and shrunken.

Biopsy will be necessary to distinguish between vulvar dystrophy and more ominous precancerous or cancerous vulvar abnormalities. All of these can be similar in appearance. Your clinician is likely to recommend colposcopy to pinpoint the best area(s) for biopsy. With colposcopy, the surface of the skin can be examined with magnification (see Chapter 4). Your clinician will identify the most severely affected or abnormal areas for biopsy.

Vulvar biopsy is a simple office procedure. A local anesthetic is used to deaden a small patch of skin temporarily, and a tiny circle of skin is removed for study by a pathologist. The spot should heal quickly, and stitches probably will not even be necessary.

The pathologist's main task will be to determine whether vulvar skin cancer is present. Otherwise, the pathology report is likely to show chronic inflammation (microscopic evidence of inflammation that has been present for months or even years) with either excessive growth (hypertrophy) or insufficient growth (atrophy) of surface skin layers. Older terms used for these problems were **leukoplakia** and **lichen sclerosis**.

Treatment with ointment or cream containing testosterone (such as testosterone propionate 2%) is likely to help reduce symptoms of vulvar dystrophy. The cause of this disorder is not known, and likewise no real cure is available. It is likely to be persistent, requiring continuous treatment to keep symptoms at bay, and may gradually progress in severity over time.

VAGINAL PROBLEMS

The vagina itself is made of remarkably resilient tissue. It is likely to heal completely, leaving no permanent evidence of a past problem, after even the most severe vaginal infection (see Chapter 23). And likewise, after childbirth, it returns pretty much to its previous shape and size. The vagina causes few problems on its own.

Structural Abnormalities.   Minor disruptions during fetal development can lead to abnormalities such as a septum in the vagina, or even two separate vaginas. Remnants of glands present during fetal development may later form small cysts in the vaginal wall, called Gartner's duct cysts. These abnormalities are all entirely benign, and plastic surgery to correct them is possible if their presence causes problems.

Normal vaginal openings, like other body parts, come in a wide range of sizes and shapes. For most women, the opening is large enough and the tissue surrounding the opening (called hymen tissue) is elastic enough that it will be able to stretch for insertion of a tampon or penis without any danger of serious tearing. If the opening is too small to allow the flow of menstrual blood, or the tissue is extremely thick and tight, then minor plastic surgery repair to enlarge the opening may be needed.

A vaginal opening that is too large is quite unlikely to cause problems. Tearing (called laceration) during childbirth may result in a widened opening, particularly if the tear(s) is not repaired at the time of delivery. Later plastic surgery is an option if the woman feels her new architecture interferes with sexual functioning, or experiences other problems with bladder and bowel control. In many cases, though, Kegel's exercises (see next section) to strengthen the underlying muscle support for the vagina are effective in counteracting these problems.

Overall vaginal depth and width, too, have quite a wide normal range. Because the vaginal lining is elastic, problems in accommodating a penis are very rare, even for women who are petite. Similarly, generous vaginal size is unlikely to be a problem as long as underlying muscle tone is adequate to allow the woman voluntary control over muscles that contract the area.

Problems with inadequate vaginal dimensions can occur as a result of surgery or cancer treatment. Technical problems can occur during hysterectomy surgery that interfere with the surgeon's ability to preserve sufficient vaginal tissue as the cervix is cut free from the top of the vagina. Similarly, radiation treatment for cancer of the pelvic organs can cause vaginal problems if it induces scarring or fibrous tissue formation that interferes with elasticity.

VAGINAL PROLAPSE, CYSTOCELE, AND RECTOCELE

We personally support the entire panty shield industry, I and all the other moms in the world who wet their pants with every sneeze or cough! Better panty shields than surgery, I say. Maybe if they're in the area for something else some day, they can fix that too. Not before.

—WOMAN, 39

Prolapse, cystocele, and rectocele are not actually vaginal problems. The vaginal tissue is quite normal, but vaginal architecture is altered because the **underlying muscle and fibrous tissues** that should support the bladder, rectum, and uterus have been damaged in childbirth. As a result, the bladder may bulge against the roof of the vagina (cystocele), the rectum may push the floor of the vagina upward (rectocele), and the cervix may sag low in the vagina (prolapse), sometimes even reaching the vaginal opening (see Illustrations 39-2 and 39-3). The culprit is **pelvic relaxation**, a global

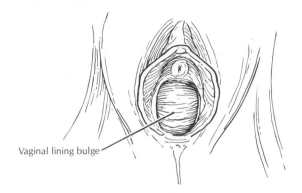

Vaginal lining bulge

ILLUSTRATION 39-2 A woman who has a cystocele may notice a bulge of the vaginal roof just inside the vaginal opening when she is standing, or when she coughs or sneezes. Problems with bladder control may also accompany this otherwise harmless condition.

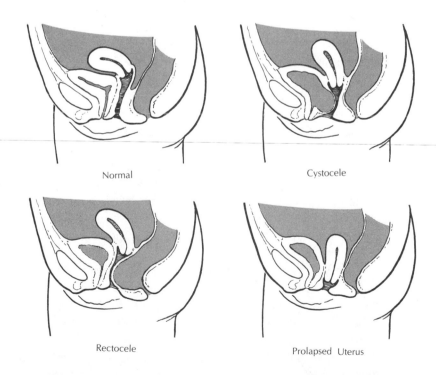

Normal

Cystocele

Rectocele

Prolapsed Uterus

ILLUSTRATION 39-3 Rectocele, cystocele, and prolapse occur when fibrous and elastic tissues that support the bladder, uterus, and rectum become lax. The bladder or rectum can cause a bulge in the roof or floor of the vagina, or the uterus and cervix can sag close to the vaginal opening.

term used for all three of these problems, each of which is caused by excessive stretching during vaginal delivery. Muscle and fibrous pelvic support tissue is less elastic than vaginal lining tissue. It is almost certain to be altered permanently by childbirth, and most women notice at least some changes after delivery. Severe problems with pelvic relaxation, however, are most likely to emerge years or even decades later as aging and hormone changes cause further loss of tissue integrity in a woman who has had multiple childbirth injuries. Pelvic relaxation problems were common in the past among women who bore many pregnancies and quite likely experienced at least some arduous deliveries. These problems are much less common now with average childbearing at one, two, or three pregnancies, and with cesarean section intervention as an alternative to vaginal delivery when the baby is too large, or its position severely unfavorable.

Vaginal bulges, in themselves, are not harmful unless the vaginal lining actually protrudes to the outside through the vaginal opening. This is extremely rare, but can create problems as exposure to air and friction may wear through the delicate vaginal lining. If the bulges stay inside, they are likely to be painless, and usually do not interfere with normal vaginal functioning.

A woman may be quite unaware that bulges are present, even during intercourse or tampon insertion. In most cases, surgery to repair cystocele or rectocele is undertaken because of problems controlling urine flow, or problems in defecating. The bladder bulge means that the base of the bladder has dropped, and the change in its position relative to the urethra may interfere with proper functioning of the muscular valves responsible for blocking urine flow.

Problems with bowel function result if strong contractions of the gut propel stool into a dead-end rectal bulge rather than out through the anal opening. Once trapped in the bulge, intestinal pressure cannot effectively move the stool further along unless the woman uses her fingers inside her vagina to provide a firm roof for the bowel pathway.

Your clinician should be able to make the diagnosis of rectocele or cystocele on the basis of symptoms you report and a simple pelvic exam. The bulges should be evident as you hold your breath and bear down to increase the pressure inside your abdomen. Whether or not surgery is needed, however, and whether repair surgery would be likely to correct bladder problems in particular, are more difficult questions.

The mere presence of cystocele and/or rectocele does not necessarily mean that surgery is needed. It is true that bladder and/or bowel problems may develop later, and are more likely if you already have evidence of pelvic support damage, and that surgery later may be riskier. You will be older and therefore more likely to have other medical problems. On the other hand, you may be one of the many women who do not ever develop problems. Surgery in the absence of compelling symptoms is truly elective. The decision is really up to you, and you may want to consider a second opinion before making a choice.

If surgery is being considered because of bladder control problems, then **careful and thorough bladder evaluation prior to surgery is essential.** It may not be possible to determine for certain whether surgery will help, and what kind of repair would be best, on the basis of your symptoms and pelvic exam alone. If you have typical symptoms of stress incontinence, such as urine loss when you cough, sneeze, or jump, your clinician will definitely suspect that a drooping bladder base is responsible. But you may need actual measurements of bladder pressure, size, and muscle response, and possibly even x-ray dye studies of bladder structure, to be sure that some other problem altogether is not causing your symptoms. These studies are called urodynamic evaluation, and you may be referred to a specialist in this specific area for your testing.

Many common problems, unrelated to pelvic architecture, can influence bladder function temporarily or cause persistent problems. Urinary tract infection and irritation of the urethra because of infection or low hormone levels after menopause are examples. Many medications, including some sedatives, tranquilizers, antihistamines, antispasmodics used for intestinal problems, and certain heart medications, can also affect bladder function. So can diabetes and neurologic disorders.

If you have low estrogen hormone levels because of natural or surgical menopause, and/or lax muscle tone, then treatment to correct these problems might be a reasonable first step before making a definite decision about surgery. Estrogen hormone vaginal cream or oral hormone treatment may help restore a more normal, resilient vaginal and urethral lining, and improved bladder control may result.

Simple exercises to strengthen the muscular supports for the vagina and urethra, called Kegel's exercises, should result in improvement within a month or so if this approach is going to be helpful in your case. These same exercises may also be recommended after surgical repair to help maintain the improved function. **Kegel's exercises are intended to strengthen the pubococcygeus muscle.** You can practice finding your pubococcygeus muscles by using them to stop the flow of your urine stream. The two basic Kegel's exercises are:

• Squeeze (contract) the muscles firmly, count to 3, then relax completely
• Squeeze and relax five times as rapidly as you can

Kegel's exercises can be done almost anywhere, while waiting in line for example. Begin with 5 to 10 repetitions of each kind and increase gradually to at least 100 of each daily.

As Kegel's exercises build muscle strength, bladder control may improve, and your ability to experience effective penile stimulation during intercourse may improve as well. To maintain progress, however, you probably will need to continue a regular Kegel's exercise program indefinitely. Biofeedback techniques to teach Kegel's exercises have been developed (3) and a self-treatment instrument to deliver a mild electric current that triggers muscle contractions is also available. The instrument, called Vagitone, is manufactured by Gyn-O-Tek, Inc., P.O. Box 29017, Portland, Oregon 97229, and can be purchased only with a prescription from your doctor.

Another alternative to surgery is the **vaginal pessary.** A pessary is a firm latex device, something like a contraceptive diaphragm without the rubber dome, placed inside the vagina to provide additional support to the bladder and uterus. Pessaries are available in a range of sizes and shapes, and may be an especially reasonable choice for a woman who has significant symptoms with pelvic relaxation but is not a good candidate for surgery because of other medical problems.

If bladder or bowel problems are severe, or persist despite exercises, then pelvic repair surgery may be a life-enhancing choice. Surgery to reposition the base of the bladder and the urethra, such as the Marshall-Marchetti-Krantz procedure, involves an abdominal incision similar to any laparotomy (see Chapter 48). Surgery may involve hysterectomy to remove the uterus (see Chapter 49) and vaginal repair as well. Surgery to correct cystocele and rectocele is called A&P (anterior and posterior) repair. Even with surgery, however, **success in restoring normal bladder function cannot be guaranteed.** Depending on the problems involved, 15% or more of women who undergo surgery find that symptoms persist, or recur in the first few years after surgery. A second attempt at surgery repair may be needed, or further evaluation may uncover other factors involved.

Pelvic repair is major surgery that requires general anesthesia and hospitalization for several days. Possible risks for anesthesia and major surgery are described in Chapter 45, as well as preoperative precautions and postoperative danger signs you will need to watch for.

REFERENCES

1. Chow W-H, Daling JR, Weiss NS, et al: Vaginal douching as a potential risk factor for tubal ectopic pregnancy. *American Journal of Obstetrics and Gynecology* 153:727–729, 1985.
2. Cheetham DR: Bartholin's cyst: Marsupialization or aspiration? *American Journal of Obstetrics and Gynecology* 152:569–570, 1985.
3. Burgio KL, Robinson JC, Engel BT: The role of biofeedback in Kegel exercise training for stress urinary incontinence. *American Journal of Obstetrics and Gynecology* 154:58–64, 1986.

CHAPTER
40

❖

Disorders of the Cervix, Uterus, Tubes, and Ovaries

Problems involving the reproductive organs account for a disproportionate share of all medical visits for women, especially during the reproductive years. These problems can be as frightening as cancer (see Chapter 41), or as troublesome and persistent as infection (see Chapters 22 to 29). Less serious problems, however, are very common, and almost every woman is likely to encounter one or more of the afflictions described in this chapter.

Cervix

CERVICITIS

Inflammation of the cervix, called **cervicitis**, is most often caused by infection (see Chapter 22), but exposure to chemicals in vaginal hygiene or contraceptive products may be the offender in some cases. Inflammation is the result of normal body defenses: white blood cells are mobilized to enter the affected area, local blood circulation is increased, and the cervix becomes swollen and red.

If you have mild cervicitis, you may not notice any symptoms at all. However, cervicitis can cause profuse, pus-like vaginal discharge with a foul odor that persists throughout your cycle. Discharge is often thin or of a mucous consistency, and gray white or yellow in color. Cervicitis may cause pain during intercourse or when you touch your cervix, spotting or bleeding after intercourse, or even abdominal pain and back pain. **Remember that pain and abnormal discharge can be signs of serious pelvic infection.**

Your clinician may suspect cervicitis on the basis of your symptoms, the appearance of your cervix, or an abnormal Pap smear that shows inflammatory cells (see Chapter 35). **Tests for gonorrhea and chlamydia are essential if you have cervicitis.** These bacteria are frequent causes of cervical infection, and cannot be detected without special laboratory procedures (see Chapter 22). Your clinician may also prepare a wet smear (see Chapter 4) right in the office to look for trichomonas organisms or abnormal vaginal bacteria.

If your cervix surface appears abnormal, a Pap smear is essential and your clinician may use a colposcope to distinguish between a simple inflammatory reaction and cancerous ulceration. Biopsy of abnormal areas may be necessary in making a precise diagnosis. These procedures are described in Chapter 4.

If your clinician finds that you have an infection, she/he will treat it; if a chemical irritant is causing cervicitis, your clinician will advise you to avoid it.

Treatment for your partner is crucial if your cervicitis is caused by gonorrhea, chlamydia, or trichomonas infection, and you will be advised to avoid intercourse until your cervicitis is cured. If you do have intercourse, ask your partner to use condoms until your inflammation is gone and your treatment is completed.

Chronic cervicitis—inflammation that persists for months or even years—is a problem for some women, and can cause abnormal discharge and persistent inflammatory Pap smear results. Cultures can provide assurance that gonorrhea or chlamydia is **not** present, but it may not be possible to determine what specific type(s) of bacteria is indeed responsible for your trouble. Your clinician may treat this kind of cervicitis with "nonspecific" medication, such as sulfa vaginal cream or douches that kill bacteria in the vagina and cervix. As the general bacterial population is reduced, your body defenses may be more able to overcome your cervical infection. Your clinician may also recommend vaginal creams or douches to promote an optimal acid–alkaline balance in your vagina.

Prolonged or repeated problems with cervicitis may lead you to consider cryosurgery, which is described in Chapter 4. Cervicitis may make it difficult or impossible for you to become pregnant, because abnormal cervical mucus production interferes with sperm's ability to penetrate your cervical canal.

You may decrease your likelihood of developing cervicitis if you minimize your exposure to sexually transmitted infection, so see Chapter 22 for suggestions that can reduce infection risk. Avoid chemical irritants in douching products and deodorized tampons, and seek treatment promptly for vaginal infections so that organisms don't have a chance to invade your cervix.

ECTROPION, EROSION, AND ULCERATION

The outer surface of the cervix is normally pale pink and smooth. The surface is made up of several layers of flat, shiny cells called **squamous** epithelium. The normal lining of the cervical canal is a single layer of tall, red, velvety cells and a rich supply of

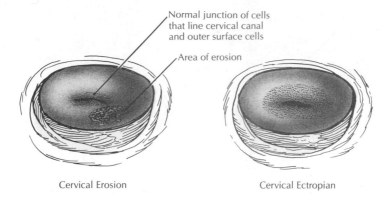

Cervical Erosion   Cervical Ectropian

ILLUSTRATION 40-1   Velvety, red, cervical canal lining tissue may extend from the canal out onto the surface of the cervix in a circular area around the opening of the canal. Your clinician calls this area ectropion; it is entirely normal, and is especially common in young women.

mucus glands and is called **columnar** epithelium. The junction between the squamous cells and the columnar cells is normally located very near the opening of the cervical canal.

Ectropion, also called eversion, means that columnar cells spread from the normal junction close to the cervical opening out over the surface of your cervix (see Illustration 40-1). In some cases, columnar cells can spread to cover a large part of the cervix. Ectropion may be more extensive during pregnancy and in DES daughters, women who take birth control Pills, and young, never-pregnant women. With ectropion you may have a heavy mucous discharge, because you have a larger than average number of mucus-secreting glands. Eversion increases your risk of infection, because bacteria are more likely to thrive in these delicate mucus-secreting tissues.

Erosion or ulceration of the cervix can be caused by infection, trauma, or chemicals. Erosion means that the cervical surface layer is partially or completely absent in one area. An eroded area looks raw and red and may cause spotting. Erosion is more common when columnar cells extend onto the surface of the cervix because columnar cells are less hardy than squamous cells. Cervical injury from intercourse, tampon insertion, or speculum insertion can lead to erosion. Herpes infection, early syphilis, and cervical cancer can cause ulceration on the surface of the cervix. If an ulcer is present, careful evaluation for all these problems is essential. A Pap smear, colposcopy, and biopsy (see Chapter 4) may be necessary for an accurate diagnosis.

CERVICAL POLYPS

A polyp, any protruding growth attached by a stem, can arise from mucous membrane lining almost anywhere in the body, such as the nose or intestine, for example.

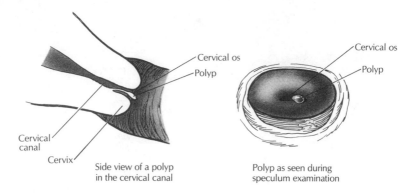

ILLUSTRATION 40-2   A cervical polyp may cause abnormal bleeding or spotting.

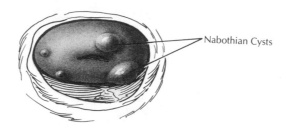

ILLUSTRATION 40-3   Two nabothian cysts, large enough to feel with a fingertip, are present on this cervix. The cervical opening is somewhat irregular in shape because of a tear during childbirth. After healing, a larger than average area of canal lining is visible on the surface of the cervix. Neither of these abnormalities is likely to cause future problems, however.

Cervical polyps are very common, and almost always benign (not malignant). Polyps may be single or multiple, tiny or quite large. They are composed of epithelial tissue usually originating from the surface lining of the cervical canal, and are attached by a stalk to the canal lining (see Illustration 40-2). Polyps contain a rich blood vessel supply and are quite fragile, so bleeding after intercourse or between menstrual periods is a common symptom. Polyps often are discovered incidentally during routine pelvic examination.

Polyp removal is usually a simple and painless office procedure. Your clinician can grasp the polyp with a small clamp near its base and twist it free, or scrape the canal lining with a tiny curet (an instrument with a sharp scraper at one end) to free a polyp at its base. Manipulation of your cervix may trigger brief cramping, but the polyp itself is not likely to be pain-sensitive. After removal, the polyp will be evaluated microscopically by a pathologist for any evidence of cancer or precancerous abnormalities. Regrowth of polyps is quite common.

NABOTHIAN CYSTS

When the opening of a cervical mucous gland becomes blocked, trapped secretions can form a smooth round lump just under the surface of the cervix. As secretions accumulate, the lump can become large enough to see or feel with a fingertip, and is called a nabothian cyst (see Illustration 40-3). Nabothian cysts are very common, and unlikely to cause any problem whatsoever. No treatment is required.

CERVICAL STRUCTURE

A cervical canal that is abnormally narrow, a condition called cervical stenosis, may interfere with the flow of menstrual blood from the uterus and may even impair fertility. Complete blockage is very rare, but should be considered especially for a young woman who fails to start menstruating but does have cyclic menstrual symptoms such as cramps. Cervical stenosis may also occur later in life after cone biopsy surgery or cryosurgery (see Chapter 35) or after a D&C, an abortion, or a severe infection. Stenosis following cervical surgery appears to be especially likely for DES daughters (see Chapter 42).

Stenosis can usually be corrected by cervical dilation. Slender metal rods of gradually increasing diameter may be inserted to stretch the cervical canal, or dilation with laminaria or a synthetic dilating rod may be used. Laminaria or rod dilation involves insertion of a small rod that gradually swells as it absorbs fluid from the cervix and vagina (see Chapter 18). The rod is removed after several hours. In most cases cervical dilation can be carried out with local anesthesia as a simple office procedure.

Cervical incompetence is the term used when a cervix stretches too easily during pregnancy and allows the cervical opening to dilate before the pregnancy has reached full term. The result is premature labor and delivery, in some cases before the fetus is able to survive outside the uterus. Painless cervical dilation and miscarriage after the first three months of pregnancy are possible signs of cervical incompetence.

When cervical incompetence is suspected, frequent exams to check for early dilation will be needed during the first few months of pregnancy, and ultrasound may be used to watch for internal changes in your cervix. Cerclage, surgery to place a strong suture tie around the cervix and hold it shut, may be recommended after the first 12 to 14 weeks of pregnancy are completed. Your cerclage procedure will probably be done in a hospital or surgical center under general anesthesia. The tie is left in place until active labor starts or pregnancy reaches full term.

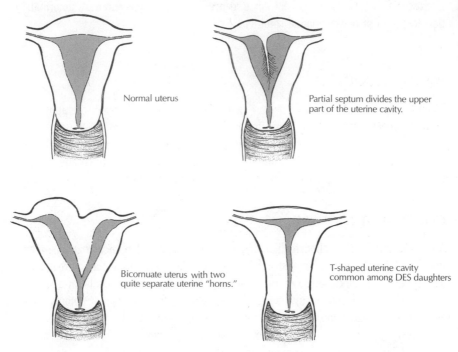

Normal uterus

Partial septum divides the upper part of the uterine cavity.

Bicornuate uterus with two quite separate uterine "horns."

T-shaped uterine cavity common among DES daughters

ILLUSTRATION 40-4   Minor abnormalities in uterine architecture are quite common, and often cannot be detected with routine pelvic examination. They may become evident when the uterus enlarges during pregnancy, or may be detected incidentally at the time of surgery performed for some other reason.

Uterus

UTERINE STRUCTURE

During fetal development a woman's reproductive organs are formed from two parallel cords of embryonic tissue that fuse to form one central uterus, cervix, and vagina. If fusion is incomplete or slightly disrupted, it is easy to understand how the common birth defects of double or partially double uterus might arise (see Illustration 40-4). In rare cases a woman might even have two quite separate uteri, each with its own cervix and vagina. DES daughters (see Chapter 42) have a somewhat higher than average incidence of structural abnormalities.

Congenital abnormalities in uterine shape are unlikely to cause any noticeable symptoms. They may be discovered incidentally at the time of surgery such as D&C (dilation and uterine scraping) or abortion, or during fertility evaluation. In some cases these abnormalities do interfere with pregnancy success. If the uterine cavity is divided by a septum, a pregnancy that implants may be unable to establish a good blood supply or may have insufficient room for growth, so pregnancy repeatedly ends in miscarriage. Surgery to correct the uterine abnormality may be recommended if this occurs.

Whenever congenital abnormalities in the reproductive tract are discovered, **evaluation of the urinary tract will also be needed.** The kidneys and urinary tract develop at about the same time in fetal life as the reproductive organs and simultaneous abnormalities in both systems are common. IVP (intravenous pyelogram), an x-ray dye test to outline the kidneys, bladder, and ureters leading from the kidneys, should reveal any structural problems that are present.

When I was 20 and just engaged I had my first pelvic exam. The doctor told me I had an infantile uterus. I worried about sex and about getting pregnant for three years. When I did become pregnant my obstetrician set my mind at ease. What a dreadful, pejorative term!

—WOMAN, 58

Variations in uterine size are not considered abnormal. Like noses, normal uteri come in a wide range of sizes from quite small to quite large. Terms like "infantile" or "juvenile" uterus have no scientific meaning, and no place in gynecology diagnosis. A small uterus is just as good as an average or large one, and can be expected to perform entirely normally for purposes of conception and pregnancy. Similarly, uterine position is unlikely to affect function. A **"tipped"** or **retroflexed** uterus (see illustration in Chapter 3) does mean that the cervical opening is likely to be near the roof of the vagina rather than the floor, and that deep downward thrusting during intercourse is likely to bump the uterus and may be uncomfortable. When pregnancy occurs, however, uterine enlargement after about 10 to 12 weeks of pregnancy makes a previously tipped uterus indistinguishable from any other uterus. After pregnancy, it may return to a tipped or retroflexed position, or it may become an anterior uterus instead.

Prolapse. A falling or dropping uterus is properly named uterine prolapse. This problem most commonly occurs after menopause when diminished hormones and aging changes bring loss of elasticity and strength to the fibrous and muscle tissue that supports the uterus, accentuating previous damage to uterine support that occurred during pregnancy and childbirth. Prolapse is not really an abnormality of the uterus itself, and the most common problems caused by prolapse are disruptions in bladder capacity and control of uterine flow. These are discussed in Chapters 38 and 39.

TABLE 40-1
CAUSES OF ABNORMAL BLEEDING AFTER MENOPAUSE

PROBLEM FOUND	% OF PATIENTS WITH BLEEDING
No abnormality found	23
Estrogen medication	27
Atrophic vaginitis	10
Cervical polyp	7
Uterine polyp	7
Uterine hyperplasia	3
Uterine cancer	13
Cervical cancer	4
Other cancer	3
Other (leiomyoma, etc.)	4

SOURCE: Adapted from Morrow CP, Townsend DE: *Synopsis of Gynecologic Oncology* (ed 2). New York: John Wiley & Sons, 1981.

ABNORMAL UTERINE BLEEDING

Abnormal bleeding is one of the most common gynecology problems, and virtually every woman is likely to encounter it. Abnormal bleeding often originates from the uterus, but can also arise from other sources such as the vagina and cervix. Uterine bleeding may occur when an entirely normal uterus responds in a normal way to abnormal hormone patterns originating outside the uterus. Possible causes and management of abnormal bleeding are described in Chapter 32.

Abnormal uterine bleeding before menopause is most likely to be caused by temporary hormone disruption, and may be associated with a benign ovary cyst or with polycystic ovary disease (described later in this chapter). Uterine fibroids (also described later in this chapter) can be another cause of abnormal bleeding. Evaluation is essential, though, to be sure that unsuspected infection is not the cause and that bleeding is not a sign of early pregnancy problems. **After menopause, abnormal bleeding is less common and prompt evaluation for uterine cancer will be essential.** Table 40-1 shows the final diagnosis for 330 women who were evaluated for bleeding after menopause. Cancer was not the leading diagnosis. Cancer likelihood, though, does increase with age, and also increases somewhat if bleeding persists six or more days. Cancer will be found in about 30% of women who have bleeding after age 70 (1).

Pregnancy, uterine cancer, infection, and endometriosis, all of which can cause abnormal bleeding, are discussed in Chapters 8, 41, 22, and 36. Other common uterine causes of abnormal bleeding are described in the sections in this chapter on polyps, hyperplasia, and fibroid tumors.

UTERINE POLYPS

Like cervical polyps, polyps arising from the lining of the uterine cavity are quite common. Your clinician may call this problem endometrial polyps; the technical name for uterine lining is endometrium. Most uterine polyps are composed of normal uterine lining tissue and are not malignant. Uterine cancer can grow in a polyp shape, however, as can a fibroid tumor (see the section on fibroids).

Your clinician may suspect uterine polyps because of abnormal uterine bleeding patterns or excessively heavy menstrual flow. In rare cases, the stalk of a uterine polyp is long enough that the polyp can be seen protruding through the cervical canal. In most cases uterine polyps are identified during a D&C (uterine scraping) or hysteroscopy performed to determine the cause of abnormal bleeding. Polyp problems are likely to be cured at least temporarily by D&C. The fragile polyps can be scraped away or removed with polyp forceps during D&C in most cases, so the bleeding problems they previously caused are cured unless polyp formation occurs again.

The excessive growth and heaping up of endometrial lining tissue that occurs in the formation of a polyp is quite similar to the excessive lining growth that occurs with uterine hyperplasia. Often hyperplasia and polyps coexist, and both are linked to increased risks for uterine cancer in the future. A woman who has had uterine polyps has about nine times the average risk for developing uterine cancer later in life (2).

UTERINE HYPERPLASIA

Hyperplasia means excessive growth ("hyper" means excessive, "plasia" means growth). Stimulation of the uterine lining by prolonged and/or high levels of estrogen hormone can lead to hyperplasia as a normal response of normal uterine lining tissue to abnormal hormone patterns. In this case, hormone medications or problems in the ovary or pituitary gland are responsible for the problem. Persistent estrogen excess does predispose a woman to eventual development of precancerous abnormalities in the uterine lining and uterine cancer. For some women, abnormalities in the uterine lining may also contribute to hyperplasia problems. If parts of the uterine lining tissue lack normal sensitivity to progesterone hormone, they may fail to undergo the maturation normally triggered by progesterone exposure during the last half of each menstrual cycle.

When the pathologist examines samples of uterine lining obtained by endometrial biopsy or D&C for a woman with hyperplasia, she/he will see uterine lining that is thicker than normal, with an abnormally large number of both lining cells and underlying tissue cells. She/he will be looking carefully to determine whether the cells are organized in a normal pattern of layers and whether or not grossly immature or abnormally shaped cells are present.

Abnormal cells and an abnormal layer arrangement are signs that precancerous changes are occurring in the uterine lining. When this type of hyperplasia, called adenomatous or atypical hyperplasia, is found, more aggressive treatment will be needed (see Chapter 41).

Hyperplasia can be reversed in most cases with oral progesterone. Another D&C or thorough office biopsy to be sure the hyperplasia is entirely eradicated will be needed after initial treatment. After that, progesterone treatment for 14 days or so each month may be needed if the abnormal hormone patterns that caused hyperplasia continue in the future. A prolonged abnormal hormone pattern is quite likely since failure to ovulate in a regular cyclic pattern is often a persistent or recurring problem.

Any woman who has had hyperplasia will need careful surveillance for uterine cancer thereafter. Your cancer risk is higher than average for the rest of your life unless your uterus is removed for some other reason. Routine annual endometrial biopsies beginning around menopause, when uterine cancer is most common, may be a reasonable precaution for a woman who has had hyperplasia. Treatment with progesterone for 10 to 14 days may be recommended to determine whether you are exposed to a high level of natural estrogen. If you are, you most likely are producing a uterine lining thick enough to bleed after 10 to 14 days of progesterone. This regimen, called a progesterone challenge test, may help identify women who need to take progesterone treatment each month in an effort to counteract persistent estrogen exposure. Your clinician may recommend routine monthly progesterone even without a progesterone challenge test.

FIBROID TUMORS
(UTERINE LEIOMYOMAS)

A fibroid tumor, or leiomyoma, is a noncancerous tumor that arises from uterine muscle and connective tissue. Other names your clinician may use are fibromyoma or myoma. About 99.5% of fibroid tumors are benign. In less than 5 cases out of 1,000, a leiomyoma is found to be malignant (2). Leiomyomas are very common; 20% of women over 30 have at least some evidence of leiomyoma. The tumors are most often discovered among women in their 30s and 40s, but can occur in young women as well. They are much more common among black women than they are among white women; the reason for this difference is not known.

Leiomyomas are usually firm, spherical lumps that often occur in groups (see Illustration 40-5). The presence of leiomyomas is likely to increase the overall size of the uterus. The size of individual tumors varies widely; they can be as small as a pea or as large as an apple or even a cantaloupe. Leiomyomas that grow near the outer surface of the uterus create a firm protruding bump or knob that can be detected during a pelvic examination. Leiomyomas near the inner lining of the uterus, however, may not be evident during pelvic examination. Leiomyomas sometimes extend from the outer surface of the uterus on a stalk; these are called **pedunculated** leiomyomas and may be difficult to distinguish from an enlarged ovary.

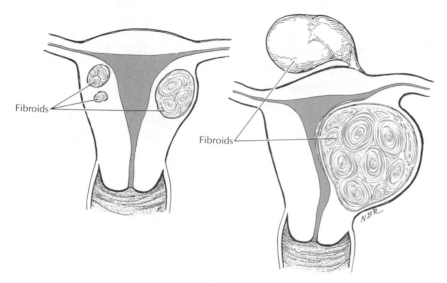

ILLUSTRATION 40-5   The uterus on the left has three small leiomyomas. On the right is an enlarged uterus with a large leiomyoma and one leiomyoma on a stalk (called a pedunculated leiomyoma).

Most women who have leiomyomas have no symptoms at all; their tumors are first discovered during routine pelvic examination. If symptoms do occur, they may include lower abdominal pain, a feeling of fullness and pressure in the lower abdomen, frequent urination caused by tumor pressure on the bladder, and in rare cases swelling of the lower abdomen. Leiomyomas can cause heavy menstrual periods, bleeding in between periods, and severe menstrual cramps. If a leiomyoma grows rapidly, it can outstrip its nutritional supply from nearby blood vessels, with the result that oxygen-deprived tissue degenerates and dies, causing abdominal pain. Rapid increase in tumor size is common in pregnancy, when high estrogen levels stimulate tumor growth. Birth control Pills and estrogen medication taken after menopause can also accelerate tumor growth.

In some cases leiomyomas can interfere with implantation of an embryo and cause impaired fertility, and leiomyomas may also interfere with successful growth of an early pregnancy and lead to miscarriage. If you have leiomyomas, it makes sense to avoid long delays in your plans for childbearing. Your fibroids may get worse.

Evaluation.   Your symptoms and your pelvic examination are the basis for diagnosing leiomyomas. If your clinician finds that your uterus is lumpy, enlarged, or irregular in shape, she/he may suspect leiomyomas even if you have not had any symptoms.

A sonogram (see Chapter 4) can detect an irregular uterine shape and uterine enlargement. In some cases, a sonogram can also distinguish between an enlarged

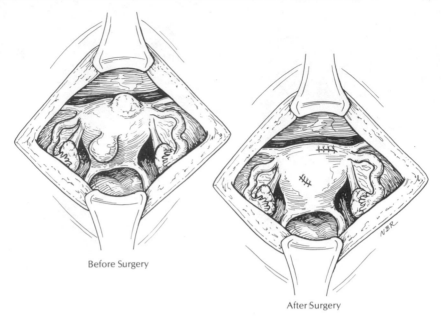

Before Surgery

After Surgery

ILLUSTRATION 40-6   Surgical removal of fibroid tumors is called myomectomy.

ovary and a leiomyoma. A pelvic x-ray sometimes reveals calcium deposits typical of fibroids in the area of a suspected leiomyoma tumor. Your clinician may advise a D&C (see Chapter 47) or a hysteroscopy (see Chapter 46) if you have had abnormal bleeding, and may be able to feel bumps inside your uterus during a D&C if leiomyomas are present. She/he will also be able to examine you more thoroughly when you are anesthetized, because your abdominal muscles will be fully relaxed.

Treatment.   When your clinician first diagnoses small leiomyomas, it is unlikely that you will need immediate surgery. Unless you have severe hemorrhage (bleeding) or unbearable pain, it will be safe for you to take time to think about your alternatives.

The first step is to be certain that leiomyomas are the cause of your symptoms or abnormalities. If you are having irregular bleeding or your uterus is enlarged, your clinician will probably recommend a D&C without delay to be certain that you don't have an unrelated malignancy, or a simple problem like uterine polyps. Similarly, prompt evaluation will be necessary if your clinician feels a mass in the area of your ovary. The mass is likely to be a leiomyoma if you have other leiomyomas on your uterus as well, but it is essential to be sure that unsuspected ovarian cancer is not present.

Once your diagnosis is confirmed, treatment options for fibroid tumors are:

• Wait; have frequent pelvic exams to detect rapid or excessive growth

- Have myomectomy surgery to remove only the leiomyoma(s) and repair the uterus as much as possible (see Illustration 40-6)
- Have a hysterectomy (see Chapter 49)
- Consider drug treatment to induce temporary menopause (available in research programs)

Leiomyomas are unlikely to shrink or disappear on their own until after menopause. **After menopause, no new leiomyomas are likely to develop, and those already present usually shrink in size.** If symptoms have not been a problem before menopause, they rarely will be after menopause.

Before menopause, it is more likely that your leiomyomas will continue to grow and that you will gradually notice more and more symptoms. In the premenopausal years, leiomyomas usually do not improve with time; nor is there any simple medical treatment.

Research on experimental drugs that block pituitary hormone stimulation to the ovaries has shown promising results for some patients. By inducing a temporary drop in estrogen level similar to menopause, this treatment produced dramatic tumor shrinkage for about half of the patients in one small research study (3). This approach may be of particular importance for a woman who has very large fibroids and wishes to preserve future fertility. Tumor shrinkage prior to surgery could improve the likelihood that uterine repair will be successful.

Leiomyomas that are more than 5 inches (12 cm) in diameter—grapefruit size—are more likely than smaller ones to cause significant medical problems. Small leiomyomas may remain unchanged for years with no serious symptoms at all. Once menopause occurs, tumors typically shrink in size so that they no longer can be detected even during pelvic examination.

The only risk with small leiomyomas is the very rare instance of a leiomyoma that is cancerous. Surgery is the only reliable way to distinguish a malignant tumor from one that is benign. Malignancy is almost always detected at the time of surgery to remove what was assumed to be a benign leiomyoma. The risk of malignancy is small, and surgery should not be recommended solely because of cancer risk.

If your uterus and tumors are less than grapefruit size overall and your symptoms are not severe, then it is reasonable to delay surgery, especially if you expect menopause soon. Even if your tumors are larger, delay still may be reasonable. There is nothing intrinsically harmful about leiomyomas, so it is reasonable to base your decision on your own assessment of how important your symptoms are. If you are not having severe problems with bleeding and pain, then just living with your tumors is a reasonable option.

If you would like to become pregnant in the future, you may want to consider myomectomy. Myomectomy may also be recommended if your clinician suspects that leiomyomas are causing infertility or repeated miscarriage. New laser techniques for myomectomy utilizing laser surgery are now available in some communities, and laser can be used in conjunction with traditional surgery (laparotomy, see Chapter 48) to decrease uterine bleeding as each leiomyoma is cut free from the uterine wall (4). Some types of fibroids can be located and removed with a hysteroscope and cautery (see Chapter 46).

In most cases, though, myomectomy surgery involves a standard 5-inch abdominal incision and postoperative recovery similar to that for abdominal hysterectomy. Your surgeon is likely to ask for your consent to possible hysterectomy when you plan myomectomy surgery. In some cases the location and size of the leiomyomas makes uterine repair technically difficult or even impossible, so hysterectomy may be necessary. **Be sure to discuss this issue with your surgeon beforehand.**

If myomectomy surgery and uterine repair has required one or more incisions through the wall of your uterus, then your clinician is likely to recommend that any subsequent pregnancy be delivered by planned cesarean section. Your healed myomectomy incision might weaken and separate during labor contractions, which could lead to very serious bleeding or even stillbirth.

If future pregnancy is not a consideration, **hysterectomy** is usually a better surgery option than myomectomy. Hysterectomy ends your problem with leiomyomas, whereas myomectomy may be only a temporary solution. It is often impossible to remove all traces of tumor during myomectomy, and tumor remnants may continue to grow and new tumors may develop as well. Approximately 25% of women who have myomectomy surgery eventually undergo hysterectomy because of continuing problems with leiomyomas (5).

Surgery for leiomyomas is elective surgery in almost all cases. In other words, there is no absolute medical necessity or rush in deciding about surgery unless bleeding is extremely heavy and cannot be controlled any other way or pain is unbearable. Surgery is likely to be recommended, and is a reasonable option, when:

• Your uterus, or one or more of your tumors, is larger than grapefruit size
• Tumor growth is rapid
• You have a mass in the area of your ovary that is probably a leiomyoma on a stalk, but surgery is necessary to be sure it is not an ovarian tumor
• You are having bleeding heavy enough to cause anemia or severe pain
• Your uterus is large and growing and you wish to preserve future fertility, so you choose to have myomectomy early when good repair is most likely to be successful
• You have had difficulty becoming pregnant or have had several miscarriages and your clinician suspects that leiomyomas may be responsible for these problems

Fallopian Tubes

Infection and endometriosis commonly cause problems involving the fallopian tubes. Either can lead to such severe damage that essential tubal function is irreversibly destroyed, or fertility is at least severely impaired. Scarring from infection or endometriosis can also produce massive swelling in one or both tubes and can trigger formation of adhesions, strands of scar tissue that stretch from the tubes to nearby structures such as the bladder, bowel, and uterine ligaments. Adhesions can be dense enough to enshroud a tube or ovary completely, or to bind the tube in an abnormal position. When tubal damage or adhesion formation is causing fertility problems, surgery to repair the tubes or remove adhesions (called lysis of adhesions) may be possible; these procedures are discussed in Chapter 10.

If fertility is not an issue and repeated infection attacks or endometriosis are causing severe pain, surgery to remove the uterus and tubes, called hysterectomy with salpingectomy, may be a better option. Treatment for tubal infection is discussed in Chapter 25 and endometriosis in Chapter 36.

Problems **originating** in the fallopian tubes are quite rare. Tumors, both benign and malignant, are possible but extremely uncommon. Tumor symptoms such as abnormal bleeding or a lump or mass in the tube are much more likely to be caused by other more common gynecological problems, so most fallopian tube tumors are discovered unexpectedly in the process of evaluating bleeding or a mass.

Birth defects resulting from faulty development of the reproductive organs can lead to the absence of one tube, or to formation of one or more fluid-filled cysts that arise from tiny remnants of fetal tube precursor tissue. Such cysts are called **paraovarian cysts**. They are fairly common, and are not malignant. Paraovarian cysts are most often discovered incidentally at the time of surgery for some other reason.

A thin sheet of fibrous connective tissue called the broad ligament drapes over each fallopian tube. Large veins draining the uterine blood supply pass through the broad ligament, and formation of varicosities in these veins is not uncommon, particularly after a pregnancy. When varicosities are present, the involved vein contains areas that are widely dilated, and may follow a meandering path, so that blood flow through the varicose area is slow. Spontaneous formation of large clots inside the vein is possible; if a clot breaks off and travels to the lung (embolizes), very serious lung problems or even sudden death may result. This condition, called **pelvic vein thrombosis**, is most likely to occur when inflammation (thrombophlebitis) is present because of infection after full-term pregnancy, abortion, or another cause, or after pelvic surgery.

Ovaries

Almost every woman can expect to have at least one encounter with an ovarian cyst sometime during her reproductive years. Ovarian tumors are much less common. Ovary problems can also arise because of infection or endometriosis (see Chapters 22 and 36), or because of persistent hormone abnormalities. When the normal hormone patterns of ovulation are blocked, the ovaries may become enlarged and cystic as egg follicles form and grow but fail to complete their maturation. This problem, commonly called polycystic ovary disease, is discussed in a later section of this chapter.

OVARIAN CYSTS AND TUMORS

Symptoms.   A cyst is a fluid-filled sac, and a tumor is a solid mass of cells. An ovarian cyst or tumor can develop with no symptoms at all, or you may notice a sensation of fullness in your lower abdomen, some discomfort, or pain during intercourse. You are most likely to find out about a cyst or tumor during a pelvic exam when your clinician detects an enlarged ovary.

Ovarian cysts occasionally cause sudden, severe pain if the cyst ruptures, causes internal bleeding, or becomes twisted. Pain can even be mistaken for appendicitis, and you may also have weakness, nausea, and vomiting. Your clinician might admit you to a hospital because of the severity of pain alone.

Infection in your uterus and tubes can cause similar symptoms, so if you are having pain and cramps, be sure to take your temperature at home, and tell your clinician if you have fever (a temperature of 100.4 degrees Fahrenheit or higher by mouth) or unusual vaginal discharge, or if you suspect that you have been exposed to chlamydia or gonorrhea.

Ectopic (tubal) pregnancy can also mimic ovarian cysts or tumors. If you have pregnancy symptoms or think for any reason that you might be pregnant (see Chapter 8 for signs of pregnancy), be sure to tell your clinician.

Evaluation.   If you have an enlarged ovary, your clinician will consider your age, your medical history, your family history, your symptoms, and the size of your ovary as she/he determines what is causing your problem.

Cancerous ovarian tumors are very rare in women under 30. Cysts that arise from an egg follicle or a corpus luteum (called functional or retention cysts) during a normal hormone cycle are very common among women under 30, and your clinician may simply recommend that you return for a second examination several weeks later to determine whether your ovary has returned to normal size. Most functional cysts simply disappear, and they are usually harmless.

Hormone suppression is sometimes recommended for a young woman who has an enlarged ovary less than 2 inches in size. (A normal ovary is about 1.5 to 1.75 inches in size.) If your ovarian enlargement is caused by a functional cyst, hormone treatment with birth control Pills to suppress your natural hormone cycle should cause your cyst to shrink and disappear. Your clinician will examine you after you have completed one or two cycles of Pills to see if your ovary has returned to normal size. If your ovary remains enlarged after hormone medication, you probably don't have a functional cyst, and you may need surgery to determine the cause of your ovarian enlargement. Hormone medication is not recommended for women over 40 because of the possibility of ovarian cancer.

If your ovary is larger than 2 inches (5 cm) in size, or if you are over 40, or if you are having bothersome pain, your clinician may recommend laboratory and x-ray tests or even exploratory surgery. Evaluation will also be needed if your ovary has remained enlarged despite hormone suppression. Tests that may be recommended include:

• A sonogram (see Chapter 4) to provide a precise measurement of the size of your ovaries, and to determine whether the enlargement is caused by a cyst or a tumor
• A pregnancy test to be sure that you are not pregnant
• An abdominal x-ray to look for calcium or fatty deposits within your ovary that are common with certain types of tumors. Small cysts usually are not visible on an x-ray; sometimes a large cyst can be identified because it displaces other nearby structures that are usually visible.
• Hormone blood tests to check for polycystic ovary disease

It is usually impossible for your clinician to tell exactly what kind of cyst or tumor you have without surgery. Surgery allows your clinician to examine your ovary directly and remove a small piece of ovarian tissue for microscopic evaluation. She/he will determine what further surgery you immediately need, if any, on the basis of the appearance of your ovary and, if necessary, a microscopic evaluation of a frozen section of tissue by the pathologist.

In some cases, laparoscopy may be an option for initial evaluation. Laparoscopy is a fairly simple surgical procedure that permits the surgeon to look at your ovaries through a lighted tube inserted through a 1-inch incision just below your navel. Laparoscopy would be reasonable if your clinician suspects that a problem such as endometriosis rather than a tumor is the cause of ovary enlargement. Endometriosis can sometimes cause a large, blood-filled cyst, called a chocolate cyst, to form on or near the ovary (see Chapter 36). If a sample of ovarian tissue is needed for analysis, your surgeon may attempt an aspiration or biopsy through the laparoscope or you may need exploratory surgery (laparotomy) with a 5-inch abdominal incision.

FUNCTIONAL OVARIAN CYSTS

Functional cysts or retention cysts are responsible for ovarian enlargement in more than half the cases, and you probably won't need any extensive tests or surgery if you have a functional cyst. There are many other kinds of ovarian cysts and tumors, and overall about 75% to 85% are benign (not cancerous).

A normal egg follicle is a small cavity that contains an egg and follicle fluid. After ovulation, the follicle cells rearrange themselves to form a corpus luteum. The corpus luteum often contains fluid surrounded by a layer of luteal cells. If an egg follicle is abnormally large, then it is by definition a cyst, a fluid-filled sac. An abnormally large fluid-filled corpus luteum is also a cyst.

Follicular cysts and corpus luteum cysts are called "functional" cysts because they are the result of normal ovary functions.

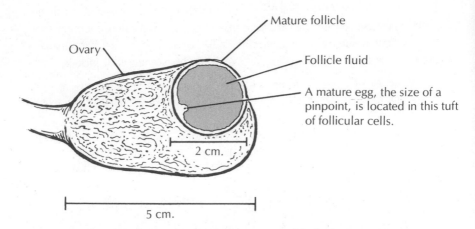

Mature follicle

Ovary

Follicle fluid

A mature egg, the size of a pinpoint, is located in this tuft of follicular cells.

2 cm.

5 cm.

ILLUSTRATION 40-7   This normal ovary (shown actual size) is approximately 5 cm in length. The normal follicle developing near the surface is 2 cm in diameter. This follicle is mature, and will rupture within a few hours, to release its fluid and egg. Fluid and a few drops of blood may spill on the lining of the abdominal cavity and cause irritation and pain for a few hours.

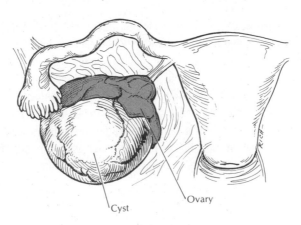

Cyst   Ovary

ILLUSTRATION 40-8   Large corpus luteum cyst.

Follicle cysts are quite common. Many women notice pain at the time of ovulation that is caused by rupture of a normal egg follicle as it releases the egg (see Illustration 40-7). If you have sudden, one-sided pain that occurs about halfway between two menstrual periods and is gone within 24 hours, chances are that you had a follicle cyst rupture.

Corpus luteum cysts are even more common. You will most likely have at least one sometime during your reproductive years. Illustration 40-8 shows a large corpus luteum cyst that formed spontaneously during the second half of an otherwise normal

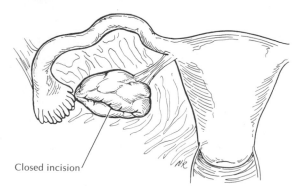

ILLUSTRATION 40-9   A cyst is removed, and the ovary is repaired with sutures.

cycle. You may notice an abnormally light or short period or irregular bleeding if you have a corpus luteum cyst, and you and your clinician may be worried about the possibility of pregnancy or ectopic pregnancy. You may need to have a pregnancy test sensitive enough to detect very early pregnancy or ectopic pregnancy (see Chapter 8). If there is any doubt about pregnancy, your clinician might recommend a sonogram or laparoscopy.

If you have really severe pain with a functional cyst, your clinician may recommend hospital observation. Internal bleeding can occur with a large functional cyst, and in rare cases surgery may be necessary to stop bleeding. It is almost always possible for your surgeon to remove the cyst and repair your ovary by stitching over the area of the cyst (see Illustration 40-9).

Functional cysts are rare in women who take birth control Pills on a regular schedule. If you are using Pills regularly when your clinician discovers an enlarged ovary, you will need further evaluation. Similarly, if your ovarian enlargement persists, or a cyst fails to resolve after one or two months, then a functional cyst is probably not the diagnosis. You may have a benign ovarian tumor, ovarian cancer, or ovarian enlargement caused by endometriosis, infection, or polycystic ovary disease.

BENIGN OVARIAN TUMORS

Some of the many types of benign ovarian tumors are entirely solid and some can form cystic (fluid-filled) areas within the tumor. One common type, called a **dermoid cyst** or **teratoma**, can develop hair or even teeth within the tumor. (The dermoid cyst arises from germ cells that ordinarily make eggs, and these cells are capable of differentiating into many different types of tissue.) An x-ray that shows teeth may permit your clinician to diagnose a dermoid even before surgery. About 99% of dermoid cysts are benign, but as with other ovarian tumors, careful microscopic evaluation by the pathologist is necessary for a complete diagnosis. In rare cases areas of malignancy can be found inside the tumor.

TABLE 40-2
OVARIAN TUMOR DIAGNOSIS BY AGE

AGE	% OF TUMORS THAT ARE BENIGN (NONCANCEROUS)
29 or less	98
30–39	90
40–49	71
50 or older	50

SOURCE: Adapted from MacKay EV, Beischer NA, Cox LW, et al: *Illustrated Textbook of Gynaecology*. Sydney, Australia: W.B. Saunders Company, 1983.

Some types of ovarian tumors tend to be bilateral, that is, both ovaries are affected. In some cases tumors are initially found in both ovaries, and in others, a second tumor develops later. Dermoid cysts are bilateral in 15% to 20% of patients (2).

Surgery and microscopic analysis of removed tumor tissue are necessary to distinguish between a benign ovarian tumor and ovarian cancer. The likelihood that a tumor is malignant increases with age, as shown in Table 40-2. Whenever ovarian cancer is a possibility, special evaluation before surgery will be needed, including a chest x-ray and intravenous pyelogram (IVP), an x-ray study to outline the position of the kidneys, ureters (the tubes leading from the kidneys to the bladder), and the bladder. Additional tests may be recommended if bowel or other symptoms are present (see Chapter 41).

After surgery, be sure you know what type of tumor was found and whether you are likely to have another tumor in the future. You might want to ask your surgeon to give you a copy of your surgery and pathology reports to keep in your personal medical records. These reports may be helpful to a clinician caring for you in the future.

If you have ovarian cancer, your surgeon will probably remove the tumor, both ovaries, and your uterus and tubes as well. Chapter 41 presents more detailed information about different types of ovarian cancer and their treatment.

If your tumor is benign, it may be possible for your surgeon to remove just the tumor and leave your ovary in place. Even if your surgeon has to remove one ovary, your remaining ovary is usually able to maintain your normal hormone levels, and one ovary is usually sufficient for fertility.

Be sure that you understand any recommendations your clinician may have for special surveillance in the future. If your tumor type is one that tends to recur or involve both ovaries, then faithfulness about follow-up and routine pelvic exams in the future will be important.

POLYCYSTIC OVARY DISEASE

Polycystic ovary disease (PCO) is not a single medical disorder. PCO is a group of symptoms linked together that can result when ovulation is blocked for a prolonged period of time. Stein-Leventhal syndrome is another name used in the past to describe this problem. The symptoms of PCO are:

• Persistent absence of ovulation
• Persistent production of estrogen and higher than normal production of androgens (male hormones)
• Higher than normal production of the pituitary hormone LH (luteinizing hormone) with low or average production of FSH (follicle-stimulating hormone)
• Thickened, enlarged ovaries—often twice normal size
• Abnormal menstrual patterns: absence of menstrual periods (affects 50%) or irregular heavy bleeding (affects 25%)
• Excessive growth of hair and masculine hair texture and distribution (affects 70%)

All of these symptoms are the result of disrupted hormone patterns. For most PCO patients, the abnormal patterns, once established, are quite persistent and may mean that ovulation occurs only rarely or not at all during the reproductive years. Without regular ovulation fertility is severely impaired, so pregnancy is unlikely unless the problem is treated. PCO patients also tend to be obese. Some researchers feel obesity is a consequence of the hormone abnormalities that cause PCO, and others feel it is a factor that contributes to causing PCO.

The initial cause(s) of PCO are not entirely understood. For some patients, a hereditary predisposition to PCO has been identified, transmitted through the father's family line only to female offspring. This indicates that the problem may be carried on the female sex chromosome (X chromosome). For most patients, though, a clear cause is not yet understood.

PCO symptoms develop as a consequence of persistent ovulation failure. The hormone abnormalities of ovulation failure reinforce and perpetuate the symptoms because of the changes in ovarian structure they cause. In other words, once started, PCO disease continues and progresses as a vicious cycle.

In simplified form, the steps in the cycle are:

• FSH release by the pituitary is normal or low, but sufficient to initiate new follicles in the ovary just as it would during the early part of a normal cycle
• As the follicles develop, their cells release estrogen hormone, as they normally would
• Ovulation signs normally provided by the pituitary fail to occur at midcycle
• Ovary follicles therefore fail to undergo final maturation and egg release, and fail to transform into a corpus luteum
• With no corpus luteum formation, the ovaries fail to produce progesterone; instead, estrogen production continues

- The follicles initially stimulated by FSH persist, and additional follicles begin development due to continuing FSH stimulation
- Gradually the ovaries enlarge, with formation of more and more follicles; total estrogen production is too high and persists continuously
- Persistent estrogen production at a steady level blocks pituitary gland release of cyclic surges of FSH and LH, so ovulation is not triggered
- The follicles release male hormones and hormone precursors along with estrogen, as they normally would. Because too many follicles are active, male hormone levels are abnormally high.

Diagnosis.   Your clinician is likely to suspect PCO on the basis of your symptoms, but tests may be needed to be sure that you do not have some other problem. Your evaluation will depend on the specific symptoms you are having.

If you are having **no menstrual bleeding at all** (amenorrhea), then the evaluation described in Chapter 33 will be necessary to be sure you do not have problems such as a pituitary gland tumor, premature menopause, or severe thyroid abnormality.

If you are having **irregular bleeding patterns,** then endometrial biopsy or D&C surgery (see Chapters 4 and 47) may be needed to obtain shreds of uterine lining tissue that can be evaluated microscopically by a pathologist. Abnormal bleeding can be caused by abnormal precancerous growth of uterine lining tissue (hyperplasia) or by uterine cancer, so evaluation is especially important if you are over 35. **Rates for uterine cancer and precancerous abnormalities are higher than normal for women who have persistent absence of ovulation with PCO.** Breast cancer risks may also be higher than average.

Evaluation may also be needed to make sure that **enlargement of your ovaries** is caused by PCO and not by a tumor. Steps for diagnosis of enlarged ovaries are described earlier in this chapter.

Excessive hair growth is a common problem with PCO, and evaluation and treatment for hirsutism is discussed in the last part of this section.

Once other serious possibilities are excluded, the diagnosis of PCO does not require extensive testing for confirmation. Your clinician may recommend a blood test for LH and FSH; low or normal FSH and elevated LH levels confirm the diagnosis, although 10% to 20% of PCO patients do not have elevated LH because their male hormone production is high enough to suppress LH release (6).

Treatment.   The goals in treating PCO disease are to protect you from the adverse long-term effects that persistent estrogen exposure in the absence of ovulation may have on your uterus and breasts, and to help control the specific symptoms you may be having. These goals can be accomplished by:

- Treatment to induce ovulation
- Hormone medication to suppress ovary production of estrogen and male hormones

• Intermittent treatment with progesterone hormone to interrupt the effects of steady estrogen exposure

If you want to be pregnant, then **ovulation induction** is the obvious choice. Treatment with clomiphene is successful in inducing ovulation for approximately 80% of patients (7), and if clomiphene is unsuccessful, injections of human menopausal gonadotropin may be a reasonable option. Ovulation induction is described in detail in Chapter 10. Surgery to remove a portion of one ovary, called **wedge resection,** may be considered if medical treatment to induce ovulation fails. Wedge resection was more commonly used before sophisticated medical methods for inducing ovulation were developed. After wedge resection surgery, there is an immediate drop in the production of male hormones that may allow ovulation to resume spontaneously. The effect is often temporary, however.

All of the treatments designed to induce ovulation involve fairly intensive medical supervision and significant medication costs, so although ovulation is the real "cure" for PCO problems, these treatments are not recommended unless you are actively trying to conceive.

Hormone treatment to **suppress ovarian activity** is a reasonable choice if you do not want to conceive now, and are having problems with excessive hair growth. This treatment also provides the added benefit of contraceptive protection. Regular birth control Pills effectively suppress ovarian hormone production, but if birth control Pills are unwise or contraindicated because of other medical problems, then similar suppression can be achieved with daily progesterone tablets or long-acting progesterone injections. Typical treatment options prescribed by your clinician might be Provera, 30 mg daily, or Depo-Provera, 150 mg by injection every three months.

Intermittent progesterone treatment is a reasonable choice if you are not trying to conceive, do not need birth control protection, and are not having hair problems. Progesterone tablets such as Provera, 10 mg taken for 10 to 14 days once every four weeks, can protect against the development of precancerous uterine lining abnormalities, could reverse abnormalities already present, and should also control problems with irregular bleeding. You can expect to have bleeding after each batch of progesterone tablets. If bleeding occurs at any other time, it may indicate that you have had a normal spontaneous ovulation cycle and your clinician may recommend that you stop progesterone to see if normal cycles will persist. Otherwise you may need to be evaluated for other causes of abnormal bleeding (see "Abnormal Uterine Bleeding" earlier in this chapter).

Hirsutism and Signs of Excessive Male Hormone. For many women with persistent absence of ovulation, problems with hair growth and other effects of excessive male hormone levels are the most troublesome part of the PCO syndrome. Symptoms of excessive androgens (male hormones) depend on the level of hormone present; symptoms may include:

• Excessive hair growth on the face
• Excessive body hair
• Hair that is dark and coarse
• Male pattern of hair distribution (face, lower abdomen, thighs, chest, breasts)
• Oily skin and acne
• Increase in libido
• Loss of scalp hair (male pattern baldness)
• Deepening of the voice
• Enlargement of the clitoris
• Change in body shape (wider shoulders, narrower hips)

Changes in hair and skin are most common; severe forms of masculinization (virilization) are quite rare.

Women who have hair problems but no disturbance in menstrual cycle patterns are not likely to have any serious hormone problem as the cause of hair growth. In most cases their hair growth is entirely normal and is a hereditary characteristic much like height and body shape. Treatment to suppress ovary hormone production, or treatment with spironolactone (described in the next section), may nevertheless be helpful in some cases. Male hormone levels produced by the ovary are almost certain to be normal in this situation, but the hair follicles may be more sensitive than usual to whatever male hormone is present, so treatment to decrease the level of male hormone may result in reduced stimulation of hair growth.

If menstrual abnormalities are present, or if the change in hair or skin occurs rapidly over a period of months, then further evaluation for hormone abnormalities is reasonable. In addition to persistent absence of ovulation with polycystic ovary syndrome, which is fairly common, rare problems that can cause hirsutism include (6):

• Ovarian tumor that secretes male hormones
• Adrenal tumor or hyperplasia (excessive adrenal gland tissue growth)
• Cushing's syndrome (excessive adrenal hormone production)
• Brain injury (trauma)
• Multiple sclerosis
• Medications such as testosterone, Dilantin, danazol, Nilevar, Anavar

Laboratory studies may be needed to measure blood testosterone level, the hormone precursor DHAS (dihydroepiandrosterone sulfate), prolactin, thyroid, and cortisol (adrenal gland hormone).

If DHAS, prolactin, thyroid, and cortisol levels are normal, then the ovary is the source of excessive male hormone production. All of the problems listed above are rare or extremely rare; if one is found, however, then further treatment for that specific problem will be needed.

Hormones and Hair Growth.   Hair growth, hair shaft thickness, and dark color are all stimulated by male hormones. Estrogen, on the other hand, retards hair growth, decreases shaft width, and reduces pigmentation. Hair growth **cycles** are also influenced by hormones. Normally, each hair follicle follows its own pattern of growth, resting, and shedding, and follicles are not in synchrony, so some are growing while others are shedding. Follicle development tends to become synchronized when estrogen and progesterone levels are both high, as in pregnancy. When this occurs, all the follicles may grow and then shed together, resulting in disconcerting (but temporary) hair loss.

Hormone patterns are key in hair growth, but unfortunately, hormone treatment does not provide a rapid cure. Once hair growth cycles in a follicle have been initiated, they will continue indefinitely with the hair shaft size and color determined at the time growth was started. Hormone treatment that reduces ovary production of male hormones will prevent stimulation of new follicles, but hairs already established will keep on growing. Plucking, tweezing, waxing, shaving, and depilatories do not stop follicle growth cycles. Only electrolysis, which destroys the individual hair follicle, can reduce the amount of hair already present.

Patience is required. Hormone suppression can be achieved with birth control Pills or with progesterone, but improvement in the apparent rate of hair growth may not be evident for as long as 6 to 12 months. Electrolysis can be done at the time treatment is initiated if cosmetic problems are severe, but may need to be repeated after six months of treatment. Follicles already initiated prior to hormone suppression will have continued in their growth cycles.

Nothing has *ever* assaulted my image of myself as a woman as profoundly as having a *beard* on my chin! I was terribly self-conscious whenever I was close to anyone. It was definitely the worst thing about PCO disease for me. Praise the dear Lord for electrolysis.

—WOMAN, 32

Treatment for Hirsutism.   Treatment to suppress ovary production of male hormones for women with persistent absence of ovulation is described earlier in this chapter. Unwanted hair is one of the most common, and reasonable, motives for choosing this treatment. For women who cannot or should not take birth control Pills or progesterone medications, several other approaches are possible.

Spironolactone, a diuretic, and cimetidine, a drug used mainly for ulcer disease, have both shown promising results in the treatment of hirsutism (6). Spironolactone decreases male hormone production and also blocks its effect on hair follicles. Cimetidine is effective without altering male hormone levels. It may block the effect of hormones on hair follicles. Cimetidine also decreases production of stomach acid; side effects are not common but can include diarrhea, dizziness, sleepiness, rash, and headache, as well as rare but more serious problems. Decreased sex drive and temporary breast enlargement may also occur. The effects of spironolactone on fluid balance and other possible side effects are discussed in Chapter 30.

Precautions for PCO Patients.   Persistent absence of ovulation is linked to several serious medical problems. If you have PCO, you will need to be faithful about routine exams, and you may need special surveillance for:

• Precancerous abnormalities in the uterine lining
• Uterine cancer
• Breast cancer
• Coronary heart disease

The hormone patterns associated with PCO mean, in theory, that your risk for these problems may be higher than average, but except for uterine cancer, research is not yet available to determine whether risks are indeed increased, and if so, how much. One study of blood lipid levels did find that women with PCO had higher than normal levels of triglycerides and the undesirable very low-density lipids, as well as higher blood pressures. All of these are statistically linked to increased risk for heart disease (8).

Pelvic Pain and Pain During Intercourse

It got so bad I didn't know if I dreaded sex because it hurt or if it hurt because I dreaded it. Not an easy situation for a six-month-old relationship!

—WOMAN, 24

Lower abdominal pain and pain during intercourse (dyspareunia) are very common, and often the two are linked: pelvic pain may be triggered or aggravated by intercourse, and pain that you first notice during intercourse can bother you at other times as well. Your clinician will ask you to describe what your pain is like, when it occurs, how it is related to your menstrual cycle and your daily activities, how long you have had it, and how it has changed since it first began. She/he will examine you to try to determine exactly where your pain is originating, and will evaluate you for any medical problems that may be related to your pain.

PAIN AROUND THE ENTRANCE TO THE VAGINA

Vaginal infection is the most common cause of burning, itching pain near the entrance to the vagina and on nearby skin areas. You are likely to notice pain first soon after intercourse because inflamed tissue is sensitive to any kind of friction or pressure. Read about the causes and treatment of vaginitis in Chapter 23.

Another common cause of discomfort during intercourse is friction. If you and your partner begin intercourse before you are fully aroused, your normal lubricating response with arousal may not have a chance to moisten your vagina thoroughly. Intercourse may feel uncomfortable, and friction can irritate the entrance to your vagina and the vaginal walls as well. Your lubrication response may be diminished if your estrogen levels are low, such as immediately after a full-term pregnancy, when you are nursing, or after menopause. It may also be diminished by antihistamines and some other medications. Allowing time for your lubrication response may take care of the problem, or you may want to use extra lubrication such as contraceptive jelly, cream, or foam, a lanolin-based moisturizer such as Lubriderm, or a nonprescription, water-soluble lubricant such as K-Y Jelly. Hormone treatment makes sense to counteract thinning and drying of the vaginal lining after menopause or in the immediate postpartum period (see Chapter 34).

Pain or tenderness in the area of your urinary opening (urethra) during intercourse can be caused by inflammation from a vaginal infection, by a bladder or urethral infection, or by a pocket (diverticulum) that forms in the wall of the urethra. Estrogen deficiency after menopause can cause the urethra to become dry and fragile (see Chapter 34). See your clinician so that she/he can treat any infection and make sure your urethra is normal.

The clitoris is normally an exquisitely sensitive area. Many women find that direct clitoral stimulation is distinctly painful, even when the clitoris is perfectly healthy.

Painful spasm of vaginal muscles when intercourse or a pelvic exam is attempted is a problem that seems to be associated with traumatic sexual experiences or painful medical experiences in the past. Counseling and conditioning exercises at home can help you gradually become accustomed to vaginal manipulation and penetration. Vaginismus, pain or muscle tightness severe enough to make intercourse impossible, is rare, but often resolves with treatment. Pain with attempted intercourse can be caused by a small, rigid hymen opening which can easily be corrected by exercises, or in extreme cases, by a minor surgical procedure.

PAIN DEEP IN THE VAGINA OR ABDOMEN

Pain deep in the vagina or lower abdomen can arise from the cervix, uterus, tubes, or ovaries, or from nearby intestines or the bladder, and often a diagnostic laparoscopy helps solve the puzzle. Pain originating from any of these structures can feel quite similar. Often pelvic pain is diffuse, and may be accompanied by lower back pain. In some cases pain originating inside the pelvis can radiate down the inner or front part of the thighs. Nerves that are responsible for communicating pain sensations inside the abdomen exit from the spinal cord in the lower back and are not as precise in localizing their pain message as are nerves to the skin; that means that when pain messages are transmitted they may be hazier in location, so nearby nerves to the back and legs may be included in the message.

Most of the problems that cause deep pain can also cause pain during intercourse, especially with deep penetration or thrusting when your partner's penis bumps a tender cervix or jars your pelvic organs. If your problem is restricted to a small area, such as a cyst on one ovary, you may have pain with some intercourse positions but not with others. A generalized problem, such as infection in your uterus and both tubes, is likely to cause pain with any intercourse position. Deep pelvic pain and pain during intercourse can be caused by pelvic infection, cervical infection, bladder infection, ovary cysts, scar tissue, endometriosis, benign or malignant tumors, or narrowing and shortening of the vagina after hysterectomy. (All of these problems are discussed in detail in other parts of this book.) Appendicitis, infection in an intestinal pocket (diverticulitis), and inflammatory intestinal disease (ulcerative colitis and ileitis) can also cause pelvic pain.

UNEXPLAINED PELVIC PAIN

Pelvic pain can be a devastating problem that interferes with normal activities and sexual functioning. Usually, your clinician will be able to identify the cause of your pain and can plan appropriate treatment, but sometimes not. In some cases laparoscopy surgery, which allows your surgeon to see your pelvic organs (see Chapter 48), may be an appropriate step for evaluation of pain. You might want to seek a second clinician's opinion, or try evaluation by a specialist in intestinal problems.

Surgery to remove "offending" pelvic organs may seem like an attractive idea when pain is really bothersome, but surgery probably is not a reasonable option. **If the cause of your pain cannot be determined, and your laparoscopy results are normal, there is no real reason to believe that surgery will cure it.**

In the past, medical textbooks have linked complaints of pelvic pain with psychological problems. This link is probably unjustified in most cases, because pelvic pain is usually caused by real disease. In some cases, however, pelvic pain may indeed be related to psychological or social stress, and some women may benefit more from counseling than they would from surgery or repeated evaluations. There is no reason to exempt the pelvis from the list of human body parts that react to stress.

REFERENCES

1. Morrow CP, Townsend DE: *Synopsis of Gynecologic Oncology* (ed 2). New York: John Wiley & Sons, 1981.
2. Novak ER, Woodruff JD: *Novak's Gynecologic and Obstetric Pathology with Clinical and Endocrine Relations* (ed 8). Philadelphia: W.B. Saunders Co., 1979.
3. Maheux R, Guilloteau C, Lemay A, et al: Luteinizing hormone-releasing hormone agonist and uterine leiomyoma: A pilot study. *American Journal of Obstetrics and Gynecology* 152:1034–1037, 1985.
4. McLaughlin DS: Metroplasty and myomectomy with the CO_2 laser for maximizing the preservation of normal tissue and minimizing blood loss. *Journal of Reproductive Medicine* 30:1–9, 1985.
5. Mattingly RF, Thompson JD: *Te Linde's Operative Gynecology* (ed 6). Philadelphia: J.B. Lippincott Co., 1985.
6. Speroff L, Glass RH, Kase NG: *Clinical Gynecologic Endocrinology & Infertility* (ed 3). Baltimore: Williams & Wilkins, 1983.
7. Schriock E, Martin MC, Jaffe RB: Polycystic ovarian disease. *Western Journal of Medicine* 142:519–522, 1985.
8. Mattsson L-A, Cullberg G, Hamberger L, et al: Lipid metabolism in women with polycystic ovary syndrome: Possible implications for an increased risk of coronary heart disease. *Fertility and Sterility* 42:579–584, 1984.

41

❖

Cancer of the Breast and Reproductive Organs

It is hard not to worry about cancer, and cancer of the reproductive organs is a major health threat for women. Most cancers of the reproductive organs are cured if they are detected and treated early. Your own healthy lifestyle decisions, annual pelvic exams, Pap tests, and monthly breast self-examinations, together with prompt attention to cancer danger signs, are your insurance policies against the risks of reproductive system cancer.

If you or someone close to you has breast or reproductive tract cancer, this chapter will not tell you all you need and want to know, but it is a place to begin. It includes statistics on survival rates for each of the cancers discussed, and there is more good news than bad. However, predictions aren't for everyone. If you choose not to read outcome statistics, don't read this chapter or skip the sections entitled "Treatment."

Personal and medical steps to protect yourself from cancer are covered in Chapter 7. Our greatest challenge is to free our air, water, and food from the profound chemical assault that makes the cancer fight a tougher one than it ought to be.

The warning signs that you and your clinician need to watch for are:

Breast Cancer
• Breast lump
• Lump in underarm or above collarbone

- Persistent skin rash, flaking, or eruption near the nipple
- Dimpling, pulling, or retraction in one area of the breast
- Nipple discharge
- Sudden change in nipple position (such as inversion)

Skin Cancer on the Vulva
- Persistent sore or warty growth on the skin of the vulva
- Persistent itching, pale areas, redness, or thickening of vulvar skin

Cervical Cancer
- Pap test results that show precancerous cell changes
- Persistent ulcer or growth on the cervix
- Abnormal bleeding or spotting
- Abnormal vaginal discharge
- Bleeding after intercourse

Uterine Cancer
- Abnormal bleeding in an irregular pattern or any bleeding after menopause
- Enlarged or growing uterus, especially after menopause
- Heavy mucus discharge
- Pap test results that show uterine cancer cells (Pap tests are not reliable for detecting uterine cancer)

Ovarian Cancer
- Enlarged ovary
- After menopause, an ovary that is large enough to be felt during routine pelvic examination
- Abdominal bloating, fullness or discomfort, or bladder or rectum pressure from an enlarged ovary
- Pap test results that show ovarian cancer cells (Pap tests are not reliable for detecting ovarian cancer)

Vaginal Cancer (very rare)
- Abnormal bleeding
- Lump, thickening, or persistent ulcer in the vaginal wall

Fallopian Tube Cancer (very rare)
- Profuse, watery, vaginal discharge
- Abnormal bleeding
- Enlarged fallopian tube

Many of these signs can be caused by problems other than cancer, but the warning signs do mean that you need careful evaluation without delay.

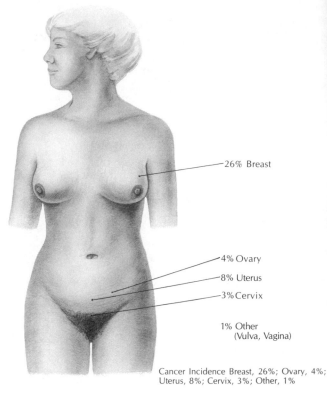

26% Breast

4% Ovary

8% Uterus

3% Cervix

1% Other
(Vulva, Vagina)

Cancer Incidence Breast, 26%; Ovary, 4%;
Uterus, 8%; Cervix, 3%; Other, 1%

ILLUSTRATION 41-1   Reproductive tract cancer sites in women. Approximately 465,000 new cases of cancer are reported for women each year nationwide. Of these, 41% involve the reproductive organs. Overall about 218,500 cancer deaths among women are reported annually.

Reproductive tract cancers account for less than 30% of cancer deaths; cure rates for reproductive cancers are higher overall than rates for many other kinds of cancer. Lung cancer is now the leading cause of cancer deaths for women as well as men. Statistics do not include minor skin cancers or preinvasive cancer of the cervix. (Silverberg E: Cancer statistics, 1986. Ca—A Cancer Journal for Clinicians 36:26–41, 1986.)

Almost half of all cancers that occur in women involve the reproductive organs (see Illustration 41-1). Your age and many other factors influence your own cancer risk. For example, if you are 22 years old, the likelihood that an enlarged ovary is due to cancer is very low; it is much higher if you are 72 years old. Similarly, breast cancer is extremely rare before the age of 25 but is a leading cause of death for women aged 40 to 44. Other factors that influence cancer risk, descriptions of symptoms you might have, and the evaluation and treatment your clinician is likely to recommend for each of the cancers listed above are discussed in this chapter.

Basic Facts About Cancer

The American Cancer Society reports annual statistics on the 35 or so most important types of cancer, and there are dozens of other rare types as well. Each cancer has its own specific characteristics. Different cancers may have entirely different causes, risk factors, and patterns of growth and spread, and quite different health consequences. Some are almost always cured, and so pose less threat to health than common problems such as high blood pressure or diabetes.

All cancers do share two characteristics, though, to earn their name. Malignant cells that compose the cancer have lost the control mechanisms that normally regulate cell growth and multiplication. Unchecked cell growth may be quite slow in some cancers, faster in others, but continues at the expense of normal tissue or overall body needs. Malignant cells also have the ability to spread or invade. Cancer cells originating at one location can cross the boundaries that normally separate one type of tissue from another, or one organ from another. Cancer spread through lymph nodes often involves nearby structures first, but can also spread through the bloodstream to distant body structures. A colony of cancer cells growing outside the site of cancer origin is called a metastasis. Metastatic cancer colonies are often responsible for cancer's most serious health effects. Common sites for metastatic colonies include the lymph nodes, liver, lung, bones, brain, and ovaries; unchecked growth of a tumor colony can interfere with essential functions of the affected organ.

CAUSES OF CANCER

The alterations in cell functions responsible for unchecked cell growth and the ability to spread are not yet known. So the ultimate "cause" of cancer is still a mystery. Risk factors for many types of cancer are known, however, and research has identified specific triggers that are involved in initiating certain kinds of cancer.

Risk Factors. A risk factor is an attribute or condition that is linked statistically to higher than average risk for developing a particular medical problem. Some cancer risk factors, such as smoking cigarettes, directly cause the cancer. Other risk factors, such as obesity in the case of uterine cancer, may not be directly responsible for causing cancer, but a statistical link occurs because obesity is associated with altered hormone patterns that in turn cause cancer. In research, statistics often make it possible to identify risk factors before the reason for their cancer connection is known. Risk factors are important because they can be used to help identify women who need extra careful surveillance.

Except for the poorly understood role virus infection may play in some forms of cancer, there is no evidence that cancer is contagious. Even in the case of possible cancer-associated viruses such as human papillomavirus, it appears that many people may carry the virus, but only a few are destined to develop cancer. The effect of other carcinogens—agents that promote cancer—is similar: only a certain proportion of individuals exposed will actually develop cancer. No one knows what factors determine the outcome, but researchers suspect that the presence or absence of cocarcinogens and the individual's inherent susceptibility may both be important.

Inherent susceptibility may explain why the risk for some forms of cancer is higher when there is a family history of that cancer. For other kinds of cancer, however, hereditary factors are not significant.

Carcinogens.   Exposure to certain chemical substances, drugs, and forms of radiation leads quite reliably to irreversible cell damage and provides the setting for cancer development. Some carcinogens act alone; some in concert with other chemicals called cocarcinogens or promoters. Some are believed to exert their effect by triggering virus activity that leads to cancer, or by interfering with normal body defenses that would otherwise attack and destroy abnormal cells.

Table 41-1 lists some common carcinogens. By far the most important is cigarette smoke. Different carcinogens are linked to different cancers, or groups of cancers, and in most cases their effects are evident only after prolonged exposure. Often cancer does not occur until years later. The time between exposure and subsequent development of cancer, the **latent period**, can be as long as 10, 20, or even 40 years, depending on the type of cancer involved.

A latent period of 15 to 20 years explains why the link between phenacetin and bladder cancer was not discovered until the mid 1970s. A slight increase in this rare cancer, previously almost unheard of among young women, was traced to use of phenacetin in amounts large enough to reach a total of a kilogram or more. Prior to this discovery, phenacetin was a common ingredient in nonprescription pain relievers such as APC (aspirin, phenacetin, caffeine), Darvon Compound, Emprazil, Fiorinal, Norgesic, Sinubid, and Synalgos. In 1982 the national Food and Drug Administration (FDA) determined that phenacetin use in over-the-counter and prescription drugs should be stopped, so pain relief products no longer contain phenacetin.

Virus Infection.   A link between virus infection and certain animal cancers has been clearly demonstrated. In humans the evidence is not yet conclusive, but a role for viruses is strongly suspected in cervical, vulvar, vaginal, and penile cancer, and in AIDS (see Chapter 28), and viruses may also be involved in other cancers as well. Virus infection could act as a cocarcinogen along with other factors, could lead to cancer by impairing the body's defenses, or could act directly to alter the nuclear coding responsible for regulating cell growth and multiplication.

Diet and Cancer.   Studies of cancer rates in different population groups have led researchers to suspect that diet may play a role in cancer risk. Colon cancer, for

TABLE 41-1
COMMON CARCINOGENS

CARCINOGEN	TYPE(S) OF CANCER
CIGARETTE SMOKE/TOBACCO	Lung, larynx, mouth, esophagus, bladder, kidney, stomach, prostate, pancreas, cervix, vulva, vagina
CHEMICALS	
Asbestos	Lung, intestinal tract
Petroleum	Nose, larynx, lung, skin, scrotum
Paraffin	Nose, larynx, lung, skin, scrotum
Coal soot/tar	Lung, larynx, skin, scrotum, bladder
Benzene	Leukemia
Vinyl chloride	Liver, brain
Nitrosamine	Stomach, esophagus
Arsenic	Lung, liver, skin
Chromium	Nose, larynx, lung
Iron oxide	Larynx, lung
Nickel	Nose, lung
RADIATION	
Ultraviolet radiation (sunlight)	Skin
Ionizing radiation (x-ray, radioactivity)	Leukemia, lung, skin, uterine sarcoma
MEDICAL TREATMENTS/MEDICATIONS	
Radiation treatment (for cancer)	Leukemia, lung, skin
Some chemotherapy treatment (for cancer)	Leukemia, lymphoma, bladder, lung, skin
Immunosuppressive drugs (for transplant)	Lymphoma, leukemia, liver, lung, skin
Dilantin (for epilepsy)	Lymphoma
Phenacetin (formerly an over-the-counter pain reliever)	Bladder
Estrogen	Uterus
DES (diethylstilbestrol)	Vagina, cervix, breast (?)
Androgen	Liver
Oral contraceptives	Liver, cervix (?)
PUVA (for psoriasis)	Skin

SOURCES: Brody JE, Holleb AI: *You Can Fight Cancer and Win*. New York: McGraw-Hill, 1977. Schottenfeld D: Cancer risk of medical treatment. *Ca—A Cancer Journal for Clinicians* 32:258–279, 1982.

example, is much more common in the United States than it is in many other countries. And, as immigrants come to adopt U.S. dietary habits, their colon cancer rates increase to reach U.S. levels. High dietary fat and low fiber and roughage in the typical U.S. diet are believed to be responsible for this effect. High fat levels in the gut promote growth of bacteria that produce carcinogenic chemical by-products. The intestinal lining is continously exposed to a possible carcinogen, and exposure is increased because lack of fiber results in slower intestinal transit time. A diet high in fat is also believed to increase the risk for breast cancer.

Other suspected diet culprits that increase stomach cancer risk include dried, salted, smoked, broiled, or pickled foods; high-starch diet; and foods containing nitrites, a compound that can be converted in the intestine to the potent carcinogen nitrosamine. Foods high in nitrite include bacon, sausage, hot dogs, and preserved meats. High caffeine intake has been tentatively linked to pancreatic cancer, and excessive alcohol to mouth, throat, esophagus, and liver cancer (1). Breast cancer risk may also be affected by alcohol, even when consumption is moderate (three drinks per week).

Cancer and Vitamins/Minerals.   The role of vitamins in preventing or treating cancer is highly controversial. High-dose vitamin C has been strongly promoted for decades by Dr. Linus Pauling. Results published in 1985 of a carefully designed research trial at the Mayo Clinic, however, showed no benefit with vitamin C treatment for patients who already had cancer (2). This study does not prove, however, that vitamin C is irrelevant to cancer risk. Animal research and studies of dietary differences between people who have developed cancer and similar people who do not have cancer suggest that several vitamins and minerals may play a role in reducing susceptibility to cancer (3). These include vitamin C, vitamin A, or beta carotene, and possibly vitamin E, and folic acid, one of the B complex vitamins. Minerals in this category include calcium and selenium, and possibly iodine and molybdenum.

Human research in this area is limited, and there is no evidence to show whether vitamin or mineral **supplements** would be beneficial, or what dose might be appropriate. Evidence is persuasive enough, however, that beta carotene, 30 mg (milligrams) every other day, was selected for testing in a large, well-designed study involving 22,000 physicians in the United States (4). Researchers suspect that taking beta carotene may reduce rates for lung cancer and cancer overall in the group taking regular supplements. People who eat a diet high in carrots and cruciferous vegetables such as cauliflower and broccoli have lower cancer rates; beta carotene is a nontoxic form of vitamin A.

Excessive intake of vitamin and mineral supplements may have serious toxic effects, so moderation is essential and it's wise to discuss this with your clinician. Fat-soluble vitamins (E and A) can cause adverse effects if taken in high doses, and so can vitamins C and B. Toxic side effects have been documented for daily doses of vitamin A that exceed 25,000 International Units (I.U.), vitamin E more than 1,200 I.U., vitamin C more than 2 to 10 grams, and vitamin B more than 500 mg. Even carrots in excess may have adverse effects. Eating large quantities of carrots (1 pound daily) was responsible for blocked menstrual cycles for young women in one small study (see Chapter 33). **Excessive selenium can be toxic or even fatal.** A total intake of 200 mcg (micrograms) per day should be sufficient, and larger doses (2,500 mcg) may be toxic.

Cancer and Hormones. Hormones play a role in several types of cancer and both natural hormones and hormone medications can potentially affect cancer risks. Some hormone patterns are associated with a reduced cancer risk; others with a risk that is higher than average.

The possible effects of hormone medications on cancer risk have been of particular concern for obvious reasons, but several factors have made research difficult and confusing. Long-term study is required. Cancer development often involves a long latent period, and hormone exposure occurs over years or decades. During that time, a woman's own natural hormone patterns must be considered as well as any hormone medications she has used. The interplay between hormones, the medication dose, and timing are significant. It is not surprising, therefore, that researchers studying one group of women and one kind of hormone medication may find that their results differ from findings of other similar, but not identical, studies.

Adverse effects of DES, the synthetic estrogen diethylstilbestrol, were first discovered more than 20 years after it was approved as a treatment to prevent miscarriage. Use of DES during pregnancy resulted in increased vaginal and cervical cancer rates among DES-exposed daughters and increased breast cancer rates among DES mothers (see Chapter 42).

Fortunately, research findings on the whole are reassuring for the most commonly used hormone medications. Birth control Pill users, for example, have lower than normal rates for cancer of the uterus and ovaries, but may have slightly increased rates for cervical cancer (see Chapter 13).

For both uterine cancer and breast cancer, estrogen and progestin significantly impact cancer risk, but their roles are not yet fully understood. In general, estrogen triggers cell multiplication and growth in breast tissue as it does in the uterine lining. Progesterone, on the other hand, is responsible for the development of mature and orderly gland and duct arrangement in the tissue. Normal tissue growth and structure require both hormones, with proper levels and cyclic timing for each.

Women who take estrogen hormone after menopause have higher than normal uterine cancer rates unless they take progesterone hormone along with the estrogen. Using progesterone results in uterine cancer rates that are lower than normal.

A few researchers have found slightly increased breast cancer risks for some women using birth control Pills and for postmenopausal women taking estrogen drugs. Most studies, however, have not found any increase in breast cancer with these drugs. There is some evidence that progestin used along with estrogen may be protective against breast cancer for postmenopausal hormone users.

"Ideal" hormone patterns, those most protective against breast and reproductive cancer, are not yet precisely known. Nevertheless, women who have natural hormone production patterns that result in high cancer risk should consider treatment that may reduce future risks. Many clinicians now recommend treatment with progestin medication for women who have abnormally high natural estrogen because of obesity or polycystic ovary disease (see Chapter 40).

Personality and Cancer.   Research reports and articles in the lay press have suggested that cancer risks may be linked to specific personality characteristics, especially passiveness, depression, and the inability to express emotions or to relate warmly and affectionately with others. This dreary assessment is reminiscent of the now-debunked speculation 75 years ago that immoral thoughts were the cause of tuberculosis. As the essayist Susan Sontag points out, both of these theories relieve us all of responsibility for a tragic medical problem by blaming the victims.

It is true, however, that emotional factors can affect health profoundly. Your susceptibility to serious illness is high whenever there are major stresses such as the death of a partner, job loss, or a geographic move, so it is conceivable that overall psychic well-being could affect cancer susceptibility as well.

Cancer Precursors.   For some types of cancer, cellular changes preceding the development of true cancer have been identified. Dysplasia on the surface of the cervix (see Chapter 35) and atypical hyperplasia of the uterine lining (see Chapter 40) are two examples of identifiable cancer precursors. A woman with either of these untreated precancerous conditions is much more likely than other women to develop cancer. It is likely that precancerous abnormalities will be found for many (if not all) types of cancer as research and testing methods improve.

Precancerous abnormalities, however, are not cancer. **Abnormal precancerous cells lack both of the essential cancer characteristics: their growth is abnormal but not unchecked, and they are not able to spread or invade beyond normal tissue boundaries.**

In Situ Cancer.   In situ, meaning in place, is a term used to describe very early cancer that has not yet penetrated through the normal boundary of the tissue in which it has arisen. Malignant cells within the cancer are presumably capable of invading into adjacent tissue or spread to other tissues, but have not yet done so. In situ cancer, therefore, is the most advanced stage of precancerous tissue abnormalities.

CANCER DIAGNOSIS

The purpose of cancer **screening** tests such as Pap smear, stool blood, and breast self-exam is to identify individuals who need further evaluation for cancer. Some screening tests are recommended for everyone, others only for individuals with family or medical history risk factors. Recommendations are based on the balance between the costs and risks associated with the test and its effectiveness is leading to earlier detection that saves lives or improves treatment outcome. Chest x-ray for detection of lung cancer was formerly used as a screening test but is no longer recommended because cancer death rates and treatment outcomes were not improved by screening.

The purpose of **diagnostic** testing is quite different. Whenever symptoms (such as persistent cough in the case of lung cancer) are present, or screening tests have pinpointed an individual at risk, then tests designed to find and document the problem are needed. Diagnostic tests such as chest x-ray may help locate the site of the problem, but **a definite cancer diagnosis is based on biopsy.**

Biopsy involves surgical removal of part or all of the tumor, and preparation of microscope slides for evaluation by a pathologist. In some cases, initial slides are prepared by freezing a tissue specimen (frozen section) so the pathologist can provide a tentative diagnosis within a few minutes. This approach may be used during a surgical procedure when the extent of surgery needed will depend on whether or not cancer is found. Frozen section slides, however, are slightly less accurate than permanent slides. The preparation of permanent slides, which requires 24 hours or more, permits the pathologist to make a final diagnosis.

When cancer is strongly suspected, or biopsy diagnosis has already been made, then tests to evaluate the extent of the cancer are essential. The proper choice of cancer treatment depends on an accurate assessment of the type of cancer involved and its **stage.** Cancer specialists use staging to describe the tumor size and degree of nearby or distant metastatic spread. Detailed and specific criteria define stages for each type of cancer, and allow the specialists to recommend the treatment that has worked best for other patients with similar cancer.

Determining the extent of cancer may involve sophisticated tests such as CAT scan (computerized axial tomography) or MRI (magnetic resonance imaging), x-ray studies such as barium enema, GI series to outline the intestinal tract, or IVP (intravenous pyelogram) to outline the kidneys and urine drainage system. These diagnostic studies should show whether a tumor is compressing or displacing organs in the abdominal cavity, or has spread to the lungs, liver, or brain. A bone scan or x-rays may be needed to look for evidence of metastic colonies in bone, and blood tests may be used to determine whether metastases in the liver are interfering with its function.

For some types of cancer, specialized tests may be needed. With breast cancer, for example, tumor cells can be tested for their responsiveness to hormones. This test must be arranged at the time of biopsy. Knowing whether or not breast cancer cells are positive for estrogen and progesterone receptors will help in planning optimal treatment.

In the future, blood tests may be used for early detection of some cancers that produce unusual chemicals or abnormally high levels of normal body constituents. Blood tests for such by-products can now be used to monitor treatment response for some cancer patients. In research studies, patients with cancer of the ovary, fallopian tubes, uterus, and cervix have been found to have abnormally high levels of the antigen CA-125. It is possible that a routine blood test for a marker protein such as CA-125 might be feasible for cancer screening in the future (5).

CANCER TREATMENT

The goal in cancer treatment is to rid the body of as many of the malignant cells as possible. The symptoms and serious health effects of a cancer, such as severe weight loss, are directly related to the total number of cancer cells present, sometimes called "tumor burden." Tumor burden also may impair the body's normal immune defenses that would otherwise identify and destroy abnormal cells. And if all, or almost all, of the malignant cells are eradicated, then cure is possible.

Surgery, radiation, and chemotherapy (drug treatment) are the three main weapons in cancer treatment. Often they are used together or in sequence. With surgery, tumor cells are physically removed. In some cases the goal is to remove a major portion of the tumor so that radiation, drugs, and the body's own defenses are better able to combat tumor cells left behind. In other cases, complete removal of the malignant tumor area is feasible. Often, a margin of normal tissue adjacent to the tumor and nearby lymph nodes are removed during cancer surgery to insure that areas of unsuspected malignant spread near the primary site are not left behind. Surgery for cancer often is more extensive and involves removal of considerably more tissue than is surgery for nonmalignant problems, so the term "radical" may be added to the surgery title.

In the past, surgery was the mainstay of cancer treatment. It was the only hope for cure, and radiation and drug treatment were used mainly for treatment of cancer recurrence or inoperable cancer. Tremendous improvements in radiation treatment and chemotherapy methods, however, have changed this pattern. **They are often used as part of initial treatment now, and recommended surgical procedures have become generally less radical. Radiation and/or drugs are used to assist in the initial eradication process.**

Both radiation and chemotherapy work because of their ability to kill cancer cells. Cancer cells grow and multiply rapidly and are therefore more susceptible to the toxic effects of radiation and chemotherapy drugs than are most normal body cells. For success, radiation or chemotherapy must be toxic enough to destroy the maximum possible number of cancer cells, but not so toxic that essential normal tissue is irreversibly damaged.

Radiation treatment is often focused on one (or more) limited areas. Areas of known tumor or likely areas of spread such as nearby lymph nodes can be subjected to high radiation doses, sparing other areas of the body. High-power x-ray or other sources of radiation such as radium, a radioactive element, may be used. In some cases treatment involves temporary implantation of slender rods containing a radioactive material directly into the tumor site. Rods release radiation into the tumor over a period of hours and are then removed. In other cases, x-ray treatment repeated periodically over several weeks or months might be recommended to eradicate stray tumor cells or areas of tumor not accessible to surgery. Radiation may also be used before surgery to shrink the size of a tumor, making surgery easier and more successful.

Chemotherapy drugs travel throughout the body, and therefore have the potential to destroy cancer cells in metastatic colonies anywhere they happen to be located. Many different chemotherapy drugs are now used routinely, and dozens more are under research investigation. Because different drugs exert their toxic effects through different mechanisms, they are often used in combination. One drug, for example, may interfere with cell division, while another blocks production of an essential cell protein. Using a combination drug approach exposes rapidly growing cancer cells to multiple toxic effects while limiting the impact of each separate toxic effect on other normal body cells.

The first reliable cancer cures are credited to chemotherapy. Use of methotrexate, one of the first chemotherapy drugs, made possible the "routine" cure of choriocarcinoma, a uterine cancer that arises from pregnancy (chorionic) tissue. About 90% or more of women with this cancer can now expect to be completely cured through drug treatment. Many other forms of cancer, including children's acute leukemia, Hodgkin's disease, and testicular cancer, are now cured with chemotherapy in a majority of cases (6).

TREATMENT SIDE EFFECTS

Cancer surgery requires recovery from trauma and from the loss of whatever structures have been removed, just as other surgeries do. Because surgery is often extensive and the cancer patient's health at the time of surgery is not optimal, recovery may be slow. Many weeks or even months may be required to regain strength. Fatigue associated with surgical healing is also compounded if radiation or chemotherapy treatment is needed during this time.

Surgery side effects such as severe swelling and restricted muscular motion were common after cancer surgery such as radical mastectomy a decade ago, but are fortunately much less common now. These problems resulted from removal of the lymph drainage system and muscle tissue underneath the breast. This type of radical surgery has been replaced by newer procedures such as modified radical mastectomy that do not cause such severe surgical side effects.

Numbness in the area of surgery is common, and may be permanent or may resolve slowly over months or years. Numbness occurs whenever nerves to the skin and underlying tissues are cut.

In some cases cancer surgery patients also have to accommodate to temporary or permanent disruption in normal body functions. Learning to care for and live with an artificial opening ("ostomy") for bowel or bladder function is one example.

Because they are designed to be toxic, it is not surprising that chemotherapy and radiation treatment commonly cause side effects. In general, their toxic effects have the greatest impact on body tissues that normally grow most rapidly. Cells that line the stomach and intestinal tract, skin and hair cells, and bone marrow cells are in this category. Temporary damage to gastrointestinal tract lining often causes nausea, inability to tolerate food, and sores or ulcerations in the mouth. Loss of hair is also common, although regrowth can be expected once treatment is completed. Bone marrow toxicity can cause a drop in production of normal red and white blood cells, and lead to anemia and impaired infection-fighting capacity. Blood transfusion may be necessary if anemia is severe.

Radiation treatment and chemotherapy may also cause fatigue, and many patients experience a generalized or vague sense of malaise, not feeling well or strong. Depression is also common; treatment may be a direct contributor to depression, but it is also a quite normal response to the stress of the cancer diagnosis itself.

EFFECTS ON REPRODUCTIVE FUNCTION

If surgery needed for cancer involves removal of the uterus, fallopian tubes, and/or ovaries, then reproductive capacity is permanently ended. Radiation treatment and chemotherapy also may affect fertility; ovarian function can be temporarily or permanently blocked.

Disruption of normal cyclic hormone patterns during cancer treatment is common. This can cause abnormal bleeding or, more commonly, absence of menstrual periods. In some cases menstrual function and fertility resume during treatment or after treatment is completed. The likelihood of permanent ovarian failure depends on the type and extent of cancer treatment. If one or both ovaries, for example, can be shielded from radiation or are outside the area of treatment, then it may be possible to preserve future fertility. Ovarian failure, also called premature menopause, is less common among women treated with chemotherapy during childhood than it is for women who have already reached puberty when treatment is begun.

CANCER AND BIRTH CONTROL

Pregnancy during cancer treatment is not desirable. Estrogen and progestin hormone levels are high during pregnancy, and can stimulate growth of some types of cancer. Also, both radiation and chemotherapy can have severe effects on a developing fetus. The risk of fetal damage is highest if exposure occurs during the first 12 weeks of pregnancy. Effective birth control, therefore, is essential for women of reproductive age undergoing cancer treatment.

Barrier methods of birth control such as condoms or the diaphragm are safe choices for most cancer patients. A woman who has a hormone-dependent cancer, such as uterine or breast cancer, should not use birth control Pills. Risks with an IUD (intrauterine device) may also be higher if cancer treatment causes a drop in infection-fighting cells, or if treatment involves the use of steroid drugs such as cortisone. Steroids can impair the body's ability to fight infection and may also reduce the IUD's effectiveness in preventing pregnancy.

Careful planning is needed for recovered cancer patients who decide on pregnancy. Pregnancy does not appear to have adverse effects on a woman who has recovered from many common cancers including leukemia and Hodgkin's disease (7). Pregnancy should not be initiated, however, until treatment is successfully completed, and there is little or no likelihood that additional chemotherapy or radiation would be necessary during the pregnancy.

CHOOSING A SOURCE OF CARE

Cancer treatment is an extremely complex and rapidly changing field, so initial evaluation and treatment are usually undertaken by a cancer specialist or team of specialists. A surgeon or gynecologic surgeon with subspecialty training in cancer surgery, a radiologist with additional training in cancer treatment, and a specialist in internal medicine with subspecialty training in chemotherapy may all be needed. The term "oncology" is added to the specialty title to denote subspecialty training in cancer for these fields, such as gynecologic oncology or oncology surgery, for example.

The American Cancer Society and the National Cancer Institute can provide patients or their physicians with information about treatment alternatives. Referral information is also available to assist the patient or family physician in locating an appropriate cancer center or treatment program, as well as any specialized research treatments that might be appropriate. Often, consultation with several experts, or a second opinion in planning the most favorable treatment, may be recommended. A second opinion is essential whenever the first opinion is that "nothing can be done."

COPING WITH AND BEYOND CANCER

For cancer patients, their families, and their friends, cancer is in some respects like other serious medical problems, but in other respects it is unique. Medical advances have made long-term survival possible for close to 50% of people with cancer, but essential support services during the long and often stressful journey are not as well developed in some areas.

The first weeks and months after the diagnosis of cancer are likely to be dominated by hectic and intensive medical events. Medical visits, diagnostic tests, and the initial phases of treatment consume the patient's time and energies, and often tax the coping strength of family members and friends as well. Important decisions must be made during this phase. The clinician or team of clinicians who will provide treatment must be selected, and in some cases a choice between different treatment options will be necessary.

The initial phase of cancer coping requires an intensive educational effort as the patient, family, and friends learn about the specific type of cancer and its treatments. Many books, pamphlets, and brochures are available through the National Institutes of Health and the American Cancer Society (see "Resources" at the end of this chapter).

It is also essential to understand clearly just what to expect during and after treatment. If surgery is planned, what exactly will be removed? Will changes in other body functions such as bowel and bladder be involved? Will fertility be affected? Often the answers to these questions eliminate needless fears, and being prepared ahead of time almost always makes coping after surgery easier.

During the initial, hectic medical phase both patient and family also must confront the issue of personal mortality. **Fear, anxiety, and depression are absolutely normal aspects of this process.** As with any life-threatening illness or event, the experience of coping with cancer is also likely to be life changing, and some of the changes can be positive. The truly important aspects of life may be clearer, and it may be easier to let go of unimportant or petty problems.

The second phase of cancer coping begins after the initial diagnosis and treatment have been successfully completed. A hectic medical schedule is replaced by periodic exams and tests for evidence of cancer growth or recurrence. Intermittent therapy may also be appropriate during this time. This long phase is powerfully stressful also, with the natural fear of cancer's recurrence and the long, often discouraging, process of regaining strength and finding ways to adapt to home, work, and community. A **support group of other patients and families who are dealing with similar problems may be especially helpful** (8). During this phase, and the years of "permanent survival" quite likely to follow, cancer alumni may continue to face special problems with employment and insurance. Also shared with other cancer alumni is an ongoing need to stay informed about possible long-term effects of cancer treatment.

There are likely to be times that are very tough. Anything that can be done to make life easier is a good idea. Friends enlisted to help with practical chores like grocery shopping, transportation, finding a wig, or household help can make a difference. This may also be a time to consider counseling. Coping as a cancer patient or family member adds to whatever stresses were already present, and therapy can provide added support.

Many cancer patients find that at times people are less sensitive than one might wish them to be. Matter-of-fact or less than kind treatment by medical personnel, particularly, is hard to bear, and this is such a common complaint that it probably reflects the stresses medical people experience as they care every day for cancer patients. The truth is, if they weren't matter-of-fact, they probably couldn't do their job at all; at least not for long.

What cancer patients most need from friends and family is not advice but good listening. Fear of being abandoned and having to face the cancer struggle alone is almost universal. **As a friend, just being there is invaluable.**

Breast Cancer

Breast cancer is a leading cause of death for women age 40 to 44. It is the most common type of cancer in adult women. About 1 in 11 U.S. women who are adults in the mid 1980s will develop breast cancer in their lifetimes. For females who are born in the 1970s and 1980s the risk is slightly higher, about 10 per 100 in whites and 7 per 100 in blacks, perhaps because they will be exposed to more carcinogens in their lifetime (9).

SYMPTOMS

Cancer of the breast usually appears as a solitary lump. Approximately half of all breast cancers begin in the upper, outer quadrant of the breast and feel solid, hard, painless, and nontender. Some breast cancer lumps, however, are tender or painful. Many are irregular in shape and not easily defined. As the cancer becomes advanced, the nipple may draw up into the breast and the skin on the breast may appear dimpled. Tumor growth in the breast can cause thickening and swelling of the overlying skin (like orange peel, called peau d'orange), or retraction and dimpling if the tumor becomes adherent to the skin above it. Some kinds of breast cancer cause dry, flaky skin around the nipple or red or inflamed skin, and some cause watery or bloody nipple discharge. Cancer can also cause a previously everted nipple to become inverted.

Very early breast cancer may be identified by mammography before a lump or mass is large enough to feel during examination. The radiologist may suspect cancer because of a tiny mass visible on x-ray or because of suspicious calcium deposits.

A definite diagnosis of breast cancer is based on biopsy results. Often, the entire lump is removed. The pathologist can provide a preliminary frozen section diagnosis at the time of surgery. The final diagnosis, however, is not possible for 24 to 48 hours. This is the time required for preparation of accurate, permanent microscope slides. Because frozen section slides can be inconclusive or inaccurate in rare cases, most surgeons recommend that further surgery be delayed until the final slides are evaluated. There is no evidence that delay of a few days, or even one or two weeks, affects treatment success. This allows time for a thorough review of treatment options and decision making, and in rare cases, may prevent mastectomy surgery that would have been performed unnecessarily because of a frozen section diagnosis that is revised after evaluation of permanent slides. Breast biopsy procedures are described in Chapter 37.

Laboratory tests to determine whether tumor cells are sensitive to hormones (estrogen and progesterone receptor assays) are essential for breast biopsy. The assay is not necessary if the tumor is benign, but if cancer is found, then the assay must be

TABLE 41-2
BREAST CANCER RISK AND FAMILY HISTORY

FAMILY MEMBER(S) WITH BREAST CANCER HISTORY	RELATIVE RISK
Grandmother and/or aunt	1.5
Mother or sister— diagnosis after age 45	2.1
Mother or sister— diagnosis at or before age 45	3.1
Mother *and* sister	13.6

SOURCE: Sattin RW, Rubin GL, Webster LA, et al: Family history and the risk of breast cancer. *Journal of the American Medical Association* 253:1908–1913, 1985.

done immediately, with fresh biopsy tissue. (In some cases the tumor may be so small that assay is technically impossible.)

RISK FACTORS

The cause(s) of breast cancer is not known, but the risk for development of breast cancer is lower or higher than average for certain groups of women.

Women who begin menstruating after age 17, have menopause before age 45, or have surgery that removes the ovaries before age 40, have a **lower than average** likelihood of breast cancer. Breast cancer is extremely rare before the age of 25 and uncommon before age 35. Some 80% of breast cancers occur in women over 40 (10).

The most important factors associated with a **greater than average risk** for breast cancer are:

• Previous cancer of the breast
• Close family history of breast cancer

A woman whose mother or sister developed breast cancer before age 45 has approximately three times the normal risk for breast cancer. In some families the overall risk of breast cancer among mother and daughters is nearly 50% (see Table 41-2). Other factors as well have been identified by statistics, and may also contribute to breast cancer risk (11). The precise role and importance of these factors, however, is not yet clear.

• Some types of fibrocystic breast disease (hyperplasia, atypical hyperplasia, see Chapter 37)
• Previous radiation treatment or chemotherapy

- Exposure to carcinogens, impaired immune response
- DES exposure in pregnancy (DES mothers) (12)
- High dietary fat intake
- Consumpton of alcoholic beverages
- Menstrual cycles for more than 40 years
- Impaired fertility, no pregnancy, first pregnancy after age 30
- Uterine cancer

If one or more high-risk factors applies in your case, then you should seriously consider routine mammography screening beginning at age 35, and you will need to be particularly conscientious about routine exams by your clinician and your own monthly breast self-exams.

Hormones and Breast Cancer.   The last three risk factors listed above and DES exposure during pregnancy are all related, either as causes or effects, to a woman's hormone patterns throughout life. Women exposed to higher than average levels of natural estrogen hormone appear to have higher than average risks for breast cancer. Natural estrogen levels may also be higher than average for women whose diet is high in fat. Ovulation failure can occur with high or prolonged ovary production of estrogen, and this could explain the statistical link between fertility impairment and cancer. It is possible, however, that the **hormone patterns of pregnancy contribute a protective effect against cancer** development later in life. If this is true, absence of pregnancy rather than high natural estrogen could explain the statistical links that are observed.

Numerous studies have attempted to determine what effects estrogen **medications** may have on breast cancer risk. Study results published in the 1970s were inconsistent: some studies found no effect, and a few studies found an apparent increase in risk. Subsequent researchers, however, have not documented increased risks in larger, well-designed studies of postmenopausal hormone treatment (13), or of birth control Pill use (14). A possible protective effect for progestin has been documented in one large study of postmenopausal women using combined estrogen and progestin treatment. Hormone treatment and breast cancer risk is also discussed in Chapters 13 and 34.

Prolactin hormone, secreted by the pituitary gland, is essential for normal breast function, and may play a role in breast disease as well. Whether or not prolactin is involved in the development and progression of breast cancer, however, is not known. Some researchers have found excessive prolactin production linked to breast cancer risk, while other studies have shown no such effect. Excessive prolactin release can occur because of several different medical disorders (see Chapter 33), and can also be triggered by some medications, including phenothiazine tranquilizers and the high blood pressure drug reserpine.

Precursors.   Although specific precursors for breast cancer have not yet been clearly identified, researchers suspect that certain types of benign breast disease may prove to be precancerous. Statistics in the past have shown that women with benign breast disease and/or lumps are more likely to develop breast cancer than are women who do not have breast disease. More recent research pinpoints a certain type of benign disease, specifically atypical hyperplasia, as the possible precursor. One study found that 70% of women who undergo breast biopsy for benign disease **do not** have a significantly higher breast cancer risk; the remaining 30%, however, have an increased risk because of atypical hyperplasia, or a combination of cystic disease with a family history of breast cancer (15).

Bilateral Breast Cancer. In most cases breast cancer arises as a single tumor in one breast. The risk for developing a second breast cancer in the other breast, however, is **five times greater** than it would be for a woman who did not have previous breast cancer. Overall approximately 13% of premenopausal breast cancer victims and 4% of postmenopausal breast cancer patients will develop cancer in the other breast. The risk is even higher in some situations: approximately 45% of women who develop breast cancer before menopause and have a positive family history are destined to develop a second breast cancer within 20 years. Cancer that arises in the breast gland lobes (rather than in a duct) is already bilateral at the time of initial diagnosis in 30% of cases or more (11).

Careful evaluation of both breasts at the time of initial treatment is crucial because unsuspected bilateral cancer may already be present, and conscientious lifelong screening is absolutely essential for any woman who has had breast cancer. In some situations, bilateral mastectomy to prevent a second cancer may even be a reasonable consideration.

CANCER TYPES AND STAGES

The most common type of breast cancer is **simple infiltrating duct carcinoma**, sometimes called scirrhous carcinoma. It produces a small hard tumor, and originates in the lining of a breast duct. **Intraductal carcinoma**, another type, grows initially as strands or cords inside the cavity of a breast duct. Tumor tissue and secretions may be extruded through the nipple with slight pressure. This type of tumor is uncommon, but has an excellent prognosis for cure. **Medullary carcinoma** and **colloid carcinoma** also arise from breast duct lining but form soft bulky lumps. **Paget's disease** is a cancer similar to intraductal cancer, but often causes redness, cracking, ulceration, and swelling in the skin of the nipple and surrounding areola before a mass can be felt. Cancer called **lobular carcinoma** can also arise from breast gland lobes, although this is uncommon.

The staging of breast cancer is determined by the size of the primary tumor, the degree of infiltration into adjacent skin and muscle, and the presence of malignant cells in nearby lymph nodes or distant sites. Table 41-3 shows criteria for breast cancer stages.

TABLE 41-3
BREAST CANCER STAGES

STAGE	EXTENT OF TUMOR
1	Tumor less than 5 cm in diameter No node involvement
2	Tumor less than 5 cm in diameter Nodes in underarm contain tumor
3	Tumor 5 cm or more in diameter And/or adjacent skin involved And/or tumor in nodes under arm or nearby
4	Metastases present

Tumor spread to underarm lymph nodes and nodes in the chest wall under the breast may occur early, when the primary tumor is only of modest size. Approximately half of all women with breast cancer already have lymph node involvement at the time of diagnosis. The most common sites for distant spread are bones and the lung; other likely sites are the adrenal glands, brain, ovaries, and liver.

TREATMENT

Breast cancer treatment has changed quite dramatically since the mid 1970s. Radical mastectomy was the mainstay of initial treatment for decades, and is now quite uncommon (see Table 41-4). Decisions about initial treatment are based on the size and location of the cancer, and on its stage. Possible surgery options are described in Table 41-5.

A woman whose tumor is 4 cm (about 1.5 inches) or less, and is at stage 1 or 2, may be an appropriate candidate for segmental mastectomy, sometimes called lumpectomy or tylectomy ("tyle" is Greek for lump). If the location of the tumor permits its complete removal and surgery is followed by radiation treatment, with chemotherapy added if positive nodes are found, five-year survival chances are excellent. A large collaborative study documented five-year survival for over 90% of women with negative nodes and 75% for women with positive nodes (16). This approach produced results equal or superior to total mastectomy used alone.

Some centers are now studying radiation implant treatment, with no surgery at all, for small stage 1 tumors.

For larger tumors, or tumors with more extensive local spread, treatment options are likely to be modified radical mastectomy or simple mastectomy, possibly followed by radiation treatment (see Illustration 41-2). Overall ten-year cure rates with these two

TABLE 41-4
CHANGING CHOICES FOR BREAST CANCER SURGERY[a]

	% OF BREAST CANCER PATIENTS			
TYPE OF SURGERY	1972–1974	1975–1977	1978–1980	1981–1982
Partial mastectomy (including lumpectomy)	5.7	7.3	10.5	11.5
Simple mastectomy (removal of breast)	16.6	14.0	11.1	10.4
Modified radical mastectomy (breast and lymph nodes)	29.3	47.6	64.2	72.4
Radical mastectomy (breast, nodes, pectoral muscles)	48.5	31.0	14.2	5.7

[a]Represents percentage of women patients 25 and older discharged from approximately 400 American hospitals.

SOURCE: National Center for Health Statistics.

TABLE 41-5
BREAST CANCER SURGERY OPTIONS

NAME(S)	DESCRIPTION OF TISSUE REMOVED
Partial mastectomy Lumpectomy Segmental mastectomy Tylectomy	Tumor and surrounding margin of normal breast tissue, along with overlying skin
Subcutaneous mastectomy	Lateral breast tissue only (skin and nipple are not removed). Breast tissue close to the nipple cannot be entirely removed with this approach.
Simple mastectomy Mastectomy Total mastectomy	The entire breast and overlying skin, including the fascia (the thin fibrous layer covering the muscles underneath the breast)
Modified radical mastectomy	The entire breast, breast skin, fascia, and lymph nodes in the underarm
Radical mastectomy Halstead mastectomy	The entire breast, breast skin, fascia and underlying pectoral muscle, lymph nodes in the underarm, and deeper lymph node drainage system in the chest wall
Axillary node dissection	Lymph nodes in the underarm

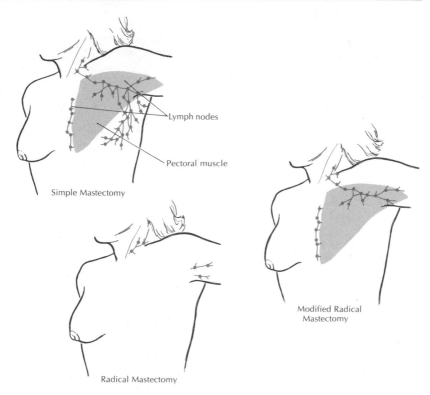

Simple Mastectomy

Lymph nodes

Pectoral muscle

Modified Radical Mastectomy

Radical Mastectomy

ILLUSTRATION 41-2   Only breast tissue is removed in a simple mastectomy. Breast and some lymph nodes are removed in modified radical mastectomy. Breast, underarm nodes, chest nodes, and pectoral muscle are removed in radical mastectomy.

approaches seem to be as good as rates following full radical surgery, and these less extensive procedures are unlikely to cause the problems with skin healing, decreased arm movement, and arm swelling that are common after radical mastectomy. Approximately 75% of patients with no node involvement reach the five-year survival mark no matter which type of mastectomy is chosen, and 75% of the five-year survivors can expect to live ten years. When tumor has already involved underarm nodes the rate is 60% for five-year survival, and 65% for ten-year survival (17). Modified radical mastectomy and simple mastectomy are very similar in healing, cosmetic appearance (see Illustration 41-3), and muscle function. The advantage some surgeons cite of removing underarm lymph nodes is that decisions about further treatment with radiation or drugs may be facilitated when the positive or negative status of underarm nodes is known. If underarm nodes were not obviously enlarged, then leaving them in place did not adversely affect long-term survival in the ten-year study cited above. Some of the patients treated with simple mastectomy had later surgery to remove nodes that became enlarged, but for some, tumor cells present in the

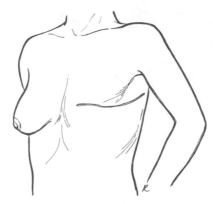

ILLUSTRATION 41-3   Mastectomy incision. Some surgeons use an up-and-down incision instead.

nodes never developed enlarged nodes and their treatment success rates were as good as rates for patients whose nodes were removed (17).

The role of chemotherapy in breast cancer treatment is also changing. In the past, drug treatment was used mainly for recurrent cancer or metastatic tumor growth. Today, chemotherapy is much more likely to be considered as part of initial treatment. The use of tamoxifen, an antiestrogen drug, has shown encouraging results. In one large study tamoxifen begun within eight weeks after surgery and continued for two years reduced breast cancer deaths by 34% during the first five years (18). This study included premenopausal women who had positive underarm nodes and postmenopausal women with and without nodes. Tamoxifen was helpful in all of these subgroups, and for both estrogen-receptor-positive and estrogen-receptor-negative tumors.

Reviewing available research data in 1985, a National Institutes of Health Consensus Conference recommended that **tamoxifen should be used as standard treatment after surgery for postmenopausal women who had positive nodes** at the time of surgery and an estrogen-receptor-positive tumor. The Conference recommended routine chemotherapy treatment after surgery for premenopausal women with positive nodes. For premenopausal women, however, the Conference felt that research data were insufficient to determine what type of chemotherapy would be best, so a variety of drugs and drug combinations are still under investigation.

Tamoxifen is taken in tablet form and blocks the effects of estrogen. Side effects severe enough to discontinue treatment have occurred in 4% of patients. Problems with hot flashes are common, and occur because of the intended antiestrogen effect of the drug. Other possible side effects are loss of appetite, nausea, depression, fatigue, migraine, thrombophlebitis (clot in a vein), neuropathy (nerve problems), and rash or allergic reaction.

AFTER BREAST CANCER

Coping with breast cancer and its treatment involves many of the issues described earlier in this chapter in "Basic Facts About Cancer," and some unique issues as well. Considerable effort and time may be required to regain strength and mobility of your arm on the surgery side, especially if you have had radical mastectomy. Most women are able to resume normal activities within six to eight weeks. Volunteers from the American Cancer Society's Reach to Recovery program may be of help. The program provides a temporary breast form to wear home from the hospital, and its volunteers, recovered mastectomy patients themselves, are likely to be familiar with local resources for breast prostheses, lingerie, and clothing.

Concerns about sexual functioning are common, and entirely understandable. Many women are fearful that their sexual attractiveness has been diminished, and are apprehensive about how their partner will react. Changes in sexual patterns may also be necessary. Other forms of sexual pleasuring may be needed to make up for the loss of breast and nipple tissue that usually is highly responsive to sexual stimulation.

For some women, breast reconstruction surgery may be a reasonable option. Reconstruction cannot truly recreate a breast, but can provide approximate symmetry and greatly reduce problems with clothing. After simple mastectomy or modified radical mastectomy, reconstruction is usually possible and fairly straightforward. A permanent prosthesis is inserted surgically underneath the muscles of the chest wall. Skin grafts can also be used to construct a new nipple if desired. Breast reduction surgery for the other breast may also be considered to balance breast size after reconstruction. Reconstruction after radical mastectomy is much more complex, and is not always feasible. Skin grafts and muscle tissue flaps may be necessary. Reconstruction is usually delayed 6 to 12 months after mastectomy, but in some cases can be done at the time of initial mastectomy.

During the months and years after breast cancer, faithfulness about follow-up exams and tests is necessary. Be sure that you understand exactly what your specialist advises at each phase of follow-up. In addition, careful monitoring will be needed for your remaining breast: mammograms and exams at least once a year for the rest of your life are crucial.

You will also need to remember that hormones may affect breast cancer cell growth. In general, women who have had breast cancer should avoid any medication that contains estrogen hormone.

Cancer of the Vulva and Vagina

Both vulvar and vaginal cancer are quite rare, accounting for less than 1% of all new cancers in women. These two cancers share some of the same risk factors, and as in cervical cancer, exposure to sexually transmitted virus infection probably plays a role. Simultaneous cancer in two or more sites—vulva, vagina, and cervix—can occur (19).

Symptoms of Vulvar Cancer.   Vulvar cancer most often arises on the labia majora (see Chapter 2) as an **ulcer, thickening, or lump.** Other initial sites include the labia minora, clitoris, skin between the vagina and rectum, and vaginal entrance. Early symptoms are likely to be a mass or lump, itching, pain or burning in the skin, bleeding, an ulcer, or burning with urination. Delay in recognizing early vulvar cancer is quite common because it can be similar in appearance to vulvar warts or chronic infection. For this reason, **biopsy is essential whenever a vulvar ulceration, or a growth thought to be a wart, fails to heal despite treatment.** Likewise, burning or itching of vulvar skin that persists more than a few weeks and is not resolved after treatment for any infection that may be present also deserves careful evaluation. Investigation is also needed for any area on the vulva that changes in color, whether the change is brown, white, pink, or gray.

Symptoms of Vaginal Cancer.   **Abnormal bleeding or bloody vaginal discharge** is the most common initial symptom of this rare cancer. The tumor itself is likely to form a thickening or warty growth on the surface of the vaginal lining, most often located in the deep, upper part of the vagina.

Evaluation to detect vulvar or vaginal cancer is likely to involve colposcopy, and may include use of a dilute vinegar solution wash or staining with blue dye that highlights areas suspicious for malignancy. Colposcopy (see Chapter 35) permits your clinician to view the surface of the skin through magnifying binoculars and pinpoint areas where the surface is more dense than normal or where abnormal blood vessel patterns are present.

Biopsy is essential for diagnosis. Both vulvar biopsy and vaginal biopsy are simple procedures that can be done easily with local anesthesia during an office visit (see Chapter 39).

RISK FACTORS

The cause(s) of vulvar and vaginal cancer is not known, but researchers suspect that infection with certain types of human papillomavirus (condyloma or wart virus) is involved in the most common forms of both cancers. Although both occur most often among older women, rates for early vulvar cancer are increasing among younger women. Young women are also the primary victims of vaginal clear cell adenocarcinoma, the very rare cancer that alerted researchers to health risks for DES (diethylstilbestrol) daughters and sons (see Chapter 42).

Risk factors for vulvar cancer include (19,20):
• Previous vulvar cancer precursor (VIN) (see below)
• Previous cervical cancer
• Previous vaginal cancer
• Previous vulvar dystrophy (see below)
• Previous sexually transmitted infection (especially genital wart virus)
• Smoking cigarettes

Risk factors for vaginal cancer are (20):

• Previous vaginal cancer precursor (VAIN) (see below)
• Previous cervical cancer
• Previous vulvar cancer
• Previous radiation therapy such as cervical cancer treatment
• Previous sexually transmitted infection (especially papillomavirus, genital wart virus)
• DES (diethylstilbestrol) exposure during fetal development
• Use of a pessary

Cancer Precursors.   Whether or not vulvar dystrophy, sometimes called lichen sclerosus, leukoplakia, or kraurosis, is a cancer precursor is not known. In appearance this disorder can mimic vulvar cancer, so frequent and careful examinations are necessary to be certain that cancer is not overlooked. Dystrophy is discussed in Chapter 39.

Precancerous abnormalities of the vulvar and vaginal lining and very early cancer that does not yet show evidence of invasion beyond normal lining tissue boundaries have been identified. These problems parallel the sequence from dysplasia to carcinoma in situ to invasive carcinoma found in the development of cervical cancer and are similarly named. Vulvar intraepithelial neoplasia (called VIN) and vaginal intraepithelial neoplasia (called VAIN) are terms for mild dysplasia (VIN 1 and VAIN 1) through severe dysplasia or carcinoma in situ (VIN 3 and VAIN 3).

Hormones.   What role (if any) that hormones have in vulvar and vaginal cancer is not known.

CANCER TYPES AND STAGES

About 90% of all vulvar and vaginal malignancies are squamous cell carcinomas, arising from the surface of the vulvar skin or the mucous membrane lining the vagina. Malignant melanoma, cancer originating in pigmented skin cells, accounts for about 6% of vulvar cancers and cancer originating in a Bartholin's gland accounts for 4%. Tumor arising from glandular tissue accounts for 4% of vaginal cancers. This type of cancer, called adenocarcinoma, includes the rare clear cell tumors linked in

TABLE 41-6
VULVAR AND VAGINAL CANCER STAGES

STAGE	EXTENT OF TUMOR
Vulvar carcinoma in situ	Severe *precancerous* abnormality. Tumor has not penetrated normal vulvar skin layer boundary.
Vulvar Cancer	
1	Tumor 2 cm or less, vulva only
2	Tumor more than 2 cm, vulva only
3	Tumor extends to nearby skin, urethra, anus, and/or enlarged lymph nodes
4	Tumor extends to lining of bladder or rectum and/or nodes fixed or ulcerated and/or distant sites (metastases)
Vaginal carcinoma in situ	Severe *precancerous* abnormality. Tumor has not penetrated normal vaginal lining (mucosa) boundary.
Vaginal Cancer	
1	Tumor involves vaginal wall only
2	Tumor involves vaginal wall and underlying tissue
3	Tumor involves vagina and nearby structures up to the pelvic wall
4	Tumor extends to the lining of bladder or rectum or structures outside the pelvis, or to distant sites (metastases)

some cases to DES exposure. Other types of cancer can occur in the vulva or vagina, but are extremely rare.

Stages for vulvar and vaginal cancer are shown in Table 41-6. Both vulvar and vaginal cancer tend to spread locally to nearby structures and lymph nodes. For vulvar cancer, the presence or absence of lymph node spread is more important than cancer stage in predicting treatment success. A large tumor with no microscopic evidence of cancer in the lymph nodes is less dangerous than a small tumor accompanied by positive nodes. Positive nodes are found in about one third of patients who undergo surgery for vulvar cancer (20).

TREATMENT

For vaginal cancer, initial treatment with radiation is likely to be recommended. Surgery also may be an option depending on the tumor location and size. Thorough evaluation prior to treatment is essential to determine the precise extent of the tumor, and to detect any distant spread.

Careful evaluation to detect simultaneous cervical cancer is essential in evaluation of vaginal cancer, and in vulvar cancer as well.

For extensive vulvar cancer, surgery to remove the vulva, underlying tissue, and lymph nodes in the groin is the most common treatment. This procedure, called radical vulvectomy, is likely to involve two or three weeks in the hospital to allow time for initial healing of skin flaps from the thigh used to reconstruct the area around the vagina. The vagina itself is not removed, although sexual function will be affected by loss of the clitoris, which is removed. If the tumor site is localized to one area, less extensive surgery to remove the tumor along with a margin of adjacent normal tissue rather than the entire vulva will be the recommended approach.

Treatment success with vulvectomy for vulvar cancer is quite encouraging: survival rates at five years are about 65% to 75%. Overall five-year survival rates after treatment for vaginal cancer are about 90% for stage 1, 60% for stage 2, and 40% for stage 3 (20).

Treatment of In Situ Cancer. If vulvar carcinoma in situ (localized within normal tissue margins) affects one discrete skin area, it can be treated by surgical excision of that skin area or by laser treatment (see below). Often, however, a widespread area is involved with multiple patches of in situ carcinoma. In this situation, surgical treatment requires complete "simple" vulvectomy, sometimes called skinning vulvectomy. The term "simple" here is used to distinguish this procedure from radical vulvectomy. From the patient's perspective, however, vulvectomy is not a simple procedure. Skin grafts are required to replace vulvar skin, and interference with sexual function may be significant. The use of laser treatment for in situ cancer has provided an alternative. Laser treatment, often possible as an outpatient procedure, can be used to destroy abnormal areas by evaporating the surface layer of skin. Skin healing occurs without the necessity for skin grafts. Laser treatment may also be recommended for vaginal in situ cancer. Alternatively, treatment with vaginal cream containing a cancer chemotherapy drug may be considered.

AFTER VULVAR OR VAGINAL CANCER

Recurrence of vulvar or vaginal cancer at or near its original site is not uncommon, and this can even occur in skin grafted from elsewhere as part of initial surgery. Also, a woman who has had vulvar or vaginal cancer has higher than average risks for developing cervical cancer as well.

Being faithful about recommended follow-up examinations and Pap smears is crucial. Colposcopy of the cervix, vagina, and vulva to detect early signs of cancer recurrence may also be reasonable.

Cervical Cancer

Invasive cervical cancer is not as common as it used to be, but it is still very much with us: overall 1 or 2 women out of 100 develop this disease during their lifetime. Rates for invasive cervical cancer have fallen dramatically over the last 40 years because testing methods including Pap smears and colposcopy now permit identification of cancer precursors and quite effective treatment in most cases before the disease can progress to an invasive stage.

Treatment for true cervical cancer is, on the whole, successful. If the cancer is detected and treated before there is evident spread beyond the cervix, the five-year survival rate is 80% or more. If malignant cells have spread beyond the cervix but are confined to nearby tissue such as the uterus and vagina, the five-year rate is about 60% (20).

Because early detection makes such a big difference, it is important to have regular Pap tests even if you hate pelvic exams. **Cervical cancer often does not have early symptoms that you would be likely to notice.** It is usually entirely painless in its early stages and might grow undetected for several years if it isn't identified on a Pap test.

When symptoms are present, they are most likely to be abnormal vaginal bleeding or discharge. Bleeding may seem like abnormal menstrual periods: too long, too frequent, or too heavy, or may be triggered by intercourse. Abnormal discharge may be mucus or it may be watery, cloudy, or have a bloody tinge. **Careful evaluation for cervical cancer, including biopsy and/or endocervical curettage (scrapings from the lining of the cervical canal; see Chapter 35), is justified whenever abnormal bleeding or discharge persists and is unexplained.** If other causes such as infection are not found and treatment does not stop the problem, then the possibility of hidden cervical cancer should be considered, even if Pap smears have been normal.

The diagnosis of cervical cancer requires biopsy. Cervical biopsy is a simple office procedure (see Chapter 35). If the abnormal area is located high in the cervical canal, and cannot be seen fully with colposcopy, then cone biopsy will be necessary to determine whether cancer is present (colposcopy and cone biopsy are also described in Chapter 35). Cone biopsy, however, should not be done if cervical cancer has already been identified, because recent cone biopsy surgery may interfere with cancer management.

In some cases, cervical cancer is discovered incidentally because of hysterectomy surgery undertaken for an unrelated problem. This is not desirable because optimal cervical cancer treatment may include use of radiation treatment rods temporarily placed inside the cervical canal and uterus before surgery. Therefore, **careful evaluation for unsuspected cervical cancer is essential prior to any hysterectomy.** Be sure that you have had a recent, and entirely normal, Pap smear and that no abnormal-appearing areas are present on your cervix before surgery is scheduled.

Simultaneous development of vulvar or vaginal cancer along with cervical cancer is much more common than would be expected by chance. Also, the sequence of precancerous abnormalities for vulvar and for vaginal cancer parallels that for cervical cancer, and all three have been linked to human papillomavirus (see "Risk Factors" below). So, if cervical cancer or precursors are found, then careful evaluation to detect vulvar or vaginal disease is needed.

RISK FACTORS

More than 90% of all cervical cancers are squamous cell carcinomas, and researchers believe that this cancer is a sexually transmitted disease.

Numerous risk factors identified in the past, such as early or multiple pregnancies, first intercourse at an early age, or previous herpes, gonorrhea, or syphilis infection, all correlate directly with the overall number of male sexual partners to whom a woman has been exposed. The number of sexual partners, in turn, correlates with the likelihood that the woman has also acquired human papillomavirus (HPV), now believed to be the primary culprit (21). See Chapters 27 and 35 for more information on HPV and its link to cervical cancer and cancer precursors. Other risk factors such as smoking cigarettes or use of birth control Pills may also be involved as independent factors or cofactors in cancer risk, and so may DES exposure during fetal development (DES daughters).

Several factors can reduce the risk of cervical cancer a woman faces. In general, any steps to avoid sexually transmitted infection will reduce cervical cancer risk. Lower than average risk is associated with:

• First intercourse deferred until age 18 to 20 or older
• Intercourse with only one male partner
• Use of condoms
• Use of a diaphragm
• Use of spermicide

Circumcision and Jewish ethnicity, thought in the past to be protective factors, are now known to be unrelated to cancer risk except to the extent that they correlate with sexual monogamy and abstinence before marriage.

Factors associated with **higher than average** cancer risk are:

• Previous CIN (cervical intraepithelial neoplasia, also called dysplasia)
• Genital wart virus infection (some strains)
• Previous vulvar or vaginal cancer
• Exposure to a male whose previous partner(s) had cervical cancer or CIN
• Exposure to a sexual partner who has (or had) penile cancer
• Exposure to more than one male sexual partner (compared to the risk for a woman with one lifetime partner, two partners increase the risk 250%; six partners, 600%) (22)
• Smoking cigarettes
• DES (diethylstilbestrol) exposure during fetal development

• Birth control Pills used four years or more
• Previous herpes, gonorrhea, syphilis, or other sexually transmitted infections
• First intercourse before age 18 to 20
• First pregnancy before age 18 to 20

Cancer Precursors.   A clear sequence of precancerous abnormalities has been identified for cervical cancer. These abnormalities, called dysplasia or CIN (cervical intraepithelial neoplasia), are described in Chapter 35. In most cases, cancer precursors are first suspected because of abnormal Pap smear results. Researchers believe that the development of cervical squamous cell cancer almost always begins with mild dysplasia (CIN 1) and progresses through moderate and severe stages in a predictable way over a period of several years. In some instances, however, more rapid progression may occur, and invasive cancer is found even though Pap smears have not shown progression through each of the intermediate dysplasia steps. For an individual woman the time sequence cannot safely be predicted in advance.

Hormones.   What role hormones may play in the development of cervical cancer is not yet known. DES daughters' rates for dysplasia and CIN are about twice as high as rates for other women (23) and it is likely that future research will document higher rates for true cervical cancer as well. How DES exposure influences risk is not known. It is possible that the presence of ectropion or adenosis, an extensive area of glandular epithelial tissue on the surface of the cervix, which is a common finding among DES daughters, provides a geographically larger setting for the development of dysplasia, or increases susceptibility to sexually transmitted virus infection that in turn causes the problem (23).

Research on the relationship of birth control Pills and cervical cancer is contradictory. Most studies have found no evidence of increased dysplasia or cancer rates among Pill users. A long-term British study, however, found slightly increased cervical dysplasia and cancer rates for women taking Pills longer than four years compared to women using IUDs (24). Whether Pill hormones or other unrelated differences between Pill and IUD users in this study were actually responsible for the difference in cancer rates is not known. Even a small difference in the average number of sexual partners for each group, for example, could have a significant impact on cancer rates. An increased risk of cervical cancer was also documented in a 1985 U.S. study of Pill users, and results in this study were corrected statistically to account for differences in the number of sexual partners reported. The cervical cancer rate for women using Pills five years or more were about two times the rate for comparable women not using Pills. Rates were highest for women using Pills that contained more than 50 mcg of estrogen (25).

Pill users have more ectropion (see above) than do women not using Pills. This characteristic is also normally present in young women during the early reproductive years. Infection susceptibility in ectropion tissue might explain the apparent role of exposure to intercourse at an early age and birth control Pill use in increasing cervical dysplasia and cancer risk.

Pregnancy probably has an adverse effect on cervical cancer. Treatment success rates are lower when cancer is discovered during or soon after pregnancy. The reason for this effect is not known, but it is possible that high hormone levels associated with pregnancy may be significant.

CANCER TYPES AND STAGES

Squamous cell carcinoma, also called epidermoid cancer, accounts for about 90% of cervical cancers. Less common cancers such as adenocarcinoma originating from glandular tissue, make up the balance. Some of the adenocarcinomas are related to papillomavirus or exposure to sexual intercourse, but others are not. Adenocarcinoma is less reliably detected by Pap smear and colposcopy. Treatment success rates are good, however.

Squamous cell cancer arises at the squamocolumnar junction, a transformation zone between the smooth, squamous epithelium that covers the surface of the cervix and the velvety, glandular, columnar epithelium that lines the cervical canal. Initial tumor growth occurs on and into the cervix, and extends to nearby structures including the lower portion of the uterus, along the side of the uterus into the pelvis, and the bladder just in front of the cervix. Spread to lymph nodes in the pelvis is also common. Subsequent tumor growth and tumor recurrence after initial treatment most often occur within the pelvis; metastases to distant sites occur somewhat less often than with other types of cancer. When metastatic spread does occur, the lungs and central bones are the most common sites.

Cervical cancer stages are shown in Table 41-7. **Microinvasive cancer** is a term used for very early cancer, with evidence of spread no more than 3 millimeters (1/8 inch) below the tissue layer boundary. Some cancer experts feel that conservative treatment that preserves future fertility may be an option when cervical cancer is found at this stage. For cervical cancer, both the overall size of the tumor and the stage are important factors in treatment success.

TREATMENT

Initial treatment depends on the extent of tumor and its location, so thorough evaluation beforehand is essential. In addition to biopsy diagnosis and a physical exam, evaluation should include (20):

• Accurate pelvic exam, performed with general anesthesia if necessary
• Chest x-ray
• IVP (x-ray dye study of kidneys, ureters, bladder, and urethra; see Chapter 38)
• Pap smear of uterine tissue to look for malignant cells

TABLE 41-7
CERVICAL CANCER STAGES

STAGE	EXTENT OF TUMOR
Carcinoma in situ (severe dysplasia, CIN 3)	A severe *precancerous* abnormality. Tumor has not penetrated the normal cervical lining boundary.
Cervical Cancer Microinvasive carcinoma (also called stage 1a)	Tumor penetrates no more than 3 mm below cervical lining boundary (no evidence of spread elsewhere)
1b	Tumor involves cervix and uterus only
2	Tumor extends to upper vagina and/or supporting structures along the sides of the uterus
3	Tumor extends to the pelvic wall
4	Tumor extends to the lining of the bladder or rectum, and/or to distant sites (metastases)

• Stool blood test
• Routine blood chemistry panel (blood count, kidney and liver function tests, and blood calcium)

The purpose of several of these tests, including the x-ray studies, is to look for evidence of metastases. Additional tests may be needed if the tumor is large or there is already evidence of spread.

If the tumor is small, and is confined to the cervix and uterus (stage 1 or 2) then surgery (radical hysterectomy) may be recommended for initial treatment. Radical hysterectomy involves removal of the uterus and cervix, upper vagina adjacent to the cervix, and uterine supporting ligaments along with accessible pelvic lymph nodes. The ovaries can be left in place to preserve normal hormone function if the woman has not already reached menopause. Radiation treatment may be recommended after surgery, or in some cases beforehand to reduce tumor size so that surgery can be more successful.

Radiation treatment combined with chemotherapy will be recommended for initial treatment if cervical cancer is more advanced or if the woman's overall health status would make surgery risky. Treatment may involve rods containing a radioactive source temporarily placed inside the cervical canal and uterine cavity, and oval radiation sources, called ovoids, placed in the vagina. These procedures involve a few days' stay in the hospital, but little discomfort. External radiation treatment also is usually recommended to treat a wider area of the pelvis.

Five-year survival rates for cervical cancer are about 80% for stage 1, 60% for stage 2, 30% to 40% for stage 3, and 10% for stage 4 (20).

AFTER CERVICAL CANCER

Careful surveillance for early signs of recurring cancer in the pelvis is essential during the first two years after cervical cancer treatment. Frequent exams and Pap smears every two months will probably be recommended. Recurrence after the first five years is quite unlikely, but exams and Pap smears every six months are a reasonable long-term precaution.

As with a history of any reproductive tract cancer, it may be prudent to avoid medication containing estrogen hormone. Some cancer experts, however, feel that hormones, including birth control Pills, may not be a hazard for women who have been treated successfully for cervical cancer.

Surveillance for subsequent uterine, bladder, vaginal, and skin cancers will also be needed after radiation treatment for cervical cancer. Rates for all of these malignancies are increased after cervical cancer radiation, and they may occur after a latency period as long as 20 years. Vulvar cancer rates may also be higher than average, but research findings so far do not show an increase in ovarian cancer, or in leukemia, lymphoma, or colon cancer (26).

Using condoms routinely for intercourse is a very reasonable idea even if birth control protection is not an issue. Condoms may protect you against further exposure to papillomavirus that could contribute to future problems with vaginal or vulvar cancer. Condoms may also protect your partner against exposure to inapparent papillomavirus infection in your vaginal lining.

Male partners of women with precancerous cervical abnormalities or cervical cancer **are at risk for future penile cancer.** They are also very likely to have evidence of penile wart virus infection (see Chapter 35). Careful and thorough evaluation is essential because penile wart infection is often inconspicuous or even invisible to the naked eye.

Cancer of the Uterus

Uterine or endometrial cancer is the second most common reproductive system cancer, ranked just below breast cancer in incidence. Approximately 3 women out of 100 can expect to develop uterine cancer during their lifetimes (9).

Uterine cancer is rare before the age of 40 and usually occurs after menopause. Most women who develop uterine cancer before age 40 have had clearly abnormal hormone patterns and have failed to ovulate regularly. Excessive ovary estrogen production caused by polycystic ovary disease (see Chapter 40) or, in rare cases, a hormone-producing tumor may be responsible for the problem.

The most common early sign of cancer in the lining of the uterus is **abnormal bleeding**. About 90% of all women with uterine cancer report abnormal bleeding (20), and it is often the very first sign of a problem. **Bleeding after menopause** is the most important uterine cancer sign. Except for bleeding that occurs immediately after each estrogen–progesterone cycle for a woman taking combined hormone treatment, **any bleeding whatsoever after menopause requires immediate and thorough evaluation.** Bleeding can be light and irregular with spotting, or bleeding can be heavy and prolonged. Some women with uterine cancer have **heavy mucus discharge** or blood-tinged discharge.

Later signs of cancer in the uterus include cramping, pelvic discomfort, pressure in the lower abdomen or bladder pressure, bleeding after intercourse, swollen lymph nodes, and lumps in the groin.

In some cases uterine cancer is first suspected because of abnormal cells seen in a Pap smear. **The Pap test, however, is not reliable in detecting uterine cancer**, and a normal Pap smear result does not provide any reassurance about possible cancer inside the uterine cavity.

In most cases, a definite diagnosis of uterine cancer is made when an endometrial biopsy or a D&C (dilation and curettage) is performed to determine the cause of abnormal bleeding. Endometrial biopsy is an office procedure that allows your clinician to obtain several tiny shreds of uterine lining tissue; it is described in Chapter 4. For D&C, general anesthesia in an outpatient surgery facility is likely to be recommended. More extensive scraping of the entire uterine cavity is possible with D&C, and it provides multiple shreds of lining tissue for the pathologist to evaluate. D&C is described in Chapter 47.

Several specialized instruments designed to facilitate endometrial biopsy are available, including some that combine vacuum with a narrow flexible curet or scraper tube (such as Vabra or Vakutage). Rates for accurate diagnosis with these instruments compare favorably to D&C (27). Also, they may be somewhat easier to use and less uncomfortable than the traditional metal endometrial curet when the cervix is narrow, as is often the case after menopause.

Instruments to rinse or flush surface cells from the uterine cavity have also been developed in hopes that uterine lining Pap smears could be used to detect abnormalities before symptoms occur. So far, however, no simple screening test has been shown to be effective.

Complete evaluation for abnormal bleeding can be carried out in the office in most cases. **Evaluation should include a pelvic exam, Pap smear, and scraping from the cervical canal** (called ECC or endocervical curettage) to check for cervical cancer, and **endometrial biopsy** to obtain a reasonable sample of uterine lining tissue. If these procedures are not successful with local anesthesia in the office, then general anesthesia and D&C will be necessary, or hysteroscopy (see Chapter 46) may be recommended. This procedure allows your surgeon to view the inner lining of the uterus through a slender illuminated tube inserted through the cervical canal.

Interpretation of pathology slides from an endometrial biopsy or D&C can be very tricky, and consultation by a pathologist who specializes in gynecologic cancers may be needed to be sure that the final diagnosis is correct. False-positive slide interpretations, that is, an initial diagnosis of cancer or cancer precursor later found to be less serious by an expert pathologist, is especially common (28).

RISK FACTORS

The cause(s) of uterine cancer is not known, but uterine cancer risk is strongly linked to estrogen hormone. Both estrogen medication exposure and abnormal hormone patterns that occur naturally can cause high uterine cancer risk. In general, risk factors associated with higher than average uterine cancer rates are conditions that result in elevated estrogen levels or in prolonged exposure to estrogen without normal cyclic progesterone interruptions. **Taking birth control Pills for at least one year reduces a woman's risk for uterine cancer.** The protective effect lasts for at least ten years. **Uterine cancer risk factors include:**

• Obesity
• Previous uterine adenomatous hyperplasia (see the following "Precursors" section)
• History of abnormal uterine bleeding
• Postmenopausal treatment with estrogen *alone* (without progestin)
• Impaired fertility, or few or no pregnancies
• History of infrequent or absent ovulation
• Polycystic ovary disease
• Uterine polyps
• Previous radiation treatment involving the pelvis
• Diabetes
• Breast, ovary, or bowel cancer
• Menopause after age 52
• High blood pressure
• Family history of uterine cancer
• Hypothyroidism
• Previous use of **sequential** birth control Pills (no longer marketed)

If you have one or more risk factors for uterine cancer, then careful surveillance is especially important. Routine endometrial biopsies every year may be reasonable after menopause or even earlier if your history or symptoms warrant. Your clinician may also recommend a **progesterone challenge test** if you have experienced a lapse in ovulation due to menopause, surgical menopause, or hormonal disturbance. Taking progesterone tablets daily for 10 to 14 days will induce bleeding if your recent estrogen hormone level has been sufficient to stimulate growth of the uterine lining. If you have bleeding in response to a progesterone challenge, some experts believe that progesterone treatment for 10 to 14 days **each month**, or combined hormone treatment with estrogen and progesterone, is a wise precaution. Both of these treatments insure that you have sufficient progesterone exposure to **counteract** the stimulating effects of estrogen on the uterine lining. Taking progesterone for this purpose, however, could have adverse effects such as blood lipid alterations. Research to document overall benefits and risks for this approach is not yet available.

Evaluation for possible hyperplasia or cancer is also indicated for **any woman who continues to have menstrual periods after age 52**. She is at greater risk for cancer, and her bleeding could be originating from cancer and be ignored in the false belief that it is menstrual flow.

Precursors.   As in the case with cervical cancer, researchers suspect that precancerous abnormalities may precede the development of true uterine cancer by months or even years. Abnormal cell maturation patterns in the uterine lining, called **adenomatous hyperplasia**, often cause abnormal bleeding or spotting and are identified when a D&C or endometrial biopsy is performed because of bleeding. In some cases the uterine lining will return to normal after treatment with progestin. If this occurs, a follow-up D&C will show that the lining is normal. If the follow-up evaluation shows persistent hyperplasia, however, surgery to remove the uterus should be seriously considered because of the risk that true uterine cancer might later develop.

Microscopic evaluation of uterine lining tissue allows the pathologist to specify the type of hyperplasia present. Cystic hyperplasia is quite common, and is not a precancer abnormality. It is a normal uterine lining response to relatively high estrogen exposure. **Precancerous hyperplasia is called adenomatous or atypical hyperplasia,** and the diagnosis is based principally on maturation patterns and the presence of abnormal-appearing cells that have an excessively large and irregular central cell nucleus.

Whenever adenomatous or atypical hyperplasia is identified by endometrial biopsy, a D&C is essential to be sure that no areas of cancer are present. Atypical or adenomatous hyperplasia and cancer can coexist.

Hormones.   Despite the clear association between estrogen exposure and uterine cancer, there is as yet no definite understanding of how this effect might occur. Excessive natural estrogen levels and estrogen medications both influence risk.

Estrogen-containing medications most commonly used today, birth control Pills and combined hormone treatment after menopause, **do not cause increased uterine cancer risk.** Both provide progesterone exposure as well as estrogen, and women using them have **lower rates for uterine cancer than women taking no hormones at all.**

The uterine cancer risk, however, was responsible for the abandonment of two types of hormone treatment during the 1970s: sequential birth control Pills and long-term menopausal treatment with estrogen alone. Sequential Pills contained twice the amount of estrogen in other birth control Pills and provided estrogen alone for two weeks out of every three-week pack. They were recalled from sale when uterine cancer was identified among young women using the product for birth control. The occurrence of 20 cases of uterine cancer among such young women was enough to lead researchers to the sequential Pill as the cause.

Uterine cancer was linked to long-term menopause treatment with estrogen alone in 1975 and 1976 when three separate medical researchers found that women receiving this treatment were 4.5 to 8 times more likely to develop uterine cancer than were comparable women not receiving estrogen. This research, later substantiated in other studies as well, led the national Food and Drug Administration (FDA) to warn against routine or long-term estrogen use, and to require that all estrogen drugs be accompanied by a patient leaflet explaining possible risks. **A woman who has used estrogen alone after menopause for a year or longer faces an elevated uterine cancer risk even after estrogen treatment is stopped, and her risk may persist as long as ten years or more (29).**

CANCER TYPES AND STAGES

In about 70% of cases uterine cancer arises in the glands of the uterine lining and is called adenocarcinoma. When areas of squamous epithelium are present, the tumor is called adenoacanthoma (benign squamous areas present) or adenosquamous carcinoma (malignant squamous areas present). Combined tumors are quite common. Uterine tumors composed entirely of squamous cells are very rare, as is clear cell carcinoma of the uterus. Cancer arising in a uterine fibroid (leiomyoma) is also very rare.

Initial cancer growth and spread occurs within the lining of the uterus. The tumor surface is fragile and often leads to abnormal bleeding early in the course of this disease. The cervix and the uterine muscle layer just underneath the endometrium are likely to be invaded as tumor growth progresses, as are nearby lymph nodes. Tumor spread may occur through the wall of the uterus or through the fallopian tubes into the abdominal cavity, and distant spread to the lungs, liver, and bone can occur if tumor cells enter the bloodstream.

Uterine cancer stages are shown in Table 41-8. Treatment success rates depend on the extent of tumor spread and also the microscopic appearance of tumor tissue. The outcome is best when the tumor cells are arranged in an orderly pattern, with identifiable cell layers and glandular patterns. This is called a **well-differentiated** tumor. A tumor with little or no orderly pattern is called **undifferentiated**.

TREATMENT

Initial treatment depends on the extent of tumor and its location, so careful evaluation beforehand is essential. In addition to biopsy diagnosis and a physical exam, evaluation should include:

TABLE 41-8
UTERINE CANCER STAGES

STAGE	EXTENT OF TUMOR
Carcinoma in situ	A severe *precancerous* abnormality. Tumor has not penetrated normal uterine lining layer boundary.
Uterine Cancer	
1a	Tumor involves uterine cavity only; the uterine cavity measures 8 cm or less
1b	Tumor involves uterine cavity only; cavity measures more than 8 cm
2	Tumor involves uterus and cervix
3	Tumor involves uterus and nearby pelvic structures
4	Tumor involves bladder or rectum or structures outside the pelvis, including distant sites (metastases)

• Scrapings from the endocervical canal (called endocervical curettage, or ECC) and accurate pelvic examination
• Chest x-ray
• Routine blood and urine tests
• IVP (x-ray dye study of the kidneys, ureters, bladder, and urethra; see Chapter 38)

These tests are designed to detect tumor spread. If the tumor is undifferentiated, or spread is already suspected, then the following additional studies are needed:

• Scan of liver and spleen
• Cystoscopy (inspection of the inside of the bladder through a narrow lighted tube)
• Barium enema (x-ray dye study of the colon and rectum)
• Bone scan (if bone pain is present)

More than 75% of uterine cancer cases are at stage 1 or 2 when diagnosed, and a combination of surgery and radiation is likely to be recommended for initial treatment. Surgery may be undertaken first, with external high-energy radiation treatment immediately afterward. Alternatively, radiation treatment may be carried out before surgery using rods containing a radioactive source placed temporarily inside the uterine cavity and vagina. Surgery would then be scheduled within the next six weeks.

Surgery will include hysterectomy to remove the uterus and cervix along with the fallopian tubes and the ovaries; pelvic lymph nodes will be removed as well in some cases. Tumor spread to the ovaries is common, so it is not safe to leave them in place. At the time of surgery a careful search is made for any evidence of tumor spread to lymph nodes in the pelvis or to other organs in the abdomen. After surgery the pathologist carefully assesses the extent and depth of tumor in the uterus. If the tumor is well differentiated, has invaded less than one third of the uterine wall thickness, and there is no evidence of spread outside the uterus, then surgery alone may be sufficient. Otherwise, external radiation treatment will be recommended.

For stage 3 cancer, radiation is the primary treatment. If the tumor shrinks after radiation, then hysterectomy may be recommended as well. Treatment with high-dose progesterone hormone is likely to be recommended when distant spread has occurred. Progesterone tablets taken orally, such as medroxyprogesterone acetate or megestrol acetate, produce excellent response rates. Tumor regression occurs in as many as 50% of patients, and treatment causes very few serious side effects.

Five-year survival rates for uterine cancer are about 90% for stage 1, 50% for stage 2, 40% for stage 3, and 10% for stage 4.

AFTER UTERINE CANCER

Most uterine cancer recurrences appear during the first two years after initial treatment, so careful surveillance will be needed. Tumor growth can occur in the vagina or remaining pelvic organs, or at distant sites. In 20% of cases, recurring cancer appears five years or more after initial treatment. Good treatment success, and even cure, may be possible with recurring cancer that appears one or two years after initial diagnosis. Radiation treatment and/or further surgery may be options depending on the location of the recurring tumor.

A woman who has had uterine cancer should avoid medication containing estrogen hormone unless it is used as part of hormone therapy specifically designed for her cancer treatment. Progesterone treatment can be used, and provides protection against osteoporosis problems (see Chapter 34). Progesterone also diminishes hot flashes for most women.

Careful surveillance will also be needed for subsequent bladder, vaginal, and skin cancer if radiation has been used for uterine cancer treatment. Rates for all of these malignancies are increased after pelvic radiation, and they may occur after a latency period as long as 20 years. Vulvar cancer rates also may be higher than average, but studies so far have not shown an increase for leukemia, lymphoma, or colon cancer (25).

Cancer of the Fallopian Tube

Fallopian tube cancer is exceedingly rare; it accounts for about 1 out of 1,000 reproductive tract cancers.

Possible symptoms of fallopian tube cancer are pelvic or abdominal pain and abnormal vaginal bleeding or discharge. Watery vaginal discharge, similar in appearance to urine, can also occur. An enlarged tube or a mass in the area of the tube or ovary may be evident with pelvic examination. Because similar symptoms and exam findings are so common with other gynecologic problems, diagnosis of fallopian tube cancer is very difficult, and it is almost always first discovered when surgery is done to evaluate or treat the symptoms. It is rare before the age of 40 or after the age of 60.

Most fallopian tube cancers arise from the glandular tube lining and are called adenocarcinoma. This cancer is similar in behavior and staging as well as treatment and survival to cancer of the ovary (see the following section). Like ovary cancer, fallopian tube cancer is bilateral in about 15% of cases so surgical treatment will involve removal of both tubes and ovaries as well as the uterus.

Cancer of the Ovary

Ovarian cancer is not common. The chance that a woman will develop it during her lifetime is a little more than 1 in 100 (9). Unfortunately, symptoms of ovarian cancer may be absent entirely or quite mild and vague during early stages of the disease. When symptoms do occur, they are likely to be similar to those with nonmalignant ovarian tumors: abdominal pain or discomfort, swelling or a lump in the abdomen, abnormal vaginal bleeding, and/or urinary and intestinal symptoms are most common.

Cancer may be discovered because ovary enlargement is detected at a routine pelvic exam. Pelvic ultrasound, sound waves (sonar) used to create an image of the soft tissue structures in the pelvis, may identify an enlarged or abnormal ovary. In rare cases, ovarian cancer may be detected because of malignant ovary cells evident on a Pap smear.

Definite diagnosis of ovarian cancer almost always requires laparotomy, major abdominal surgery (see Chapter 48). The entire tumor, or at least some biopsy tissue from the tumor, is necessary for preparation of microscope slides that can show what type of tumor is present and whether or not it is malignant. Immediate results from frozen tissue slides can be used to determine the extent of surgery necessary.

Thorough evaluation prior to surgery is essential whenever ovarian cancer is a possibility. A chest x-ray will be needed to look for lung metastases and an intravenous pyelogram (IVP; see Chapter 38) will also be important to trace the location of the ureters leading from the kidneys to the bladder. X-rays of the bowel with a barium enema are also necessary to assess whether the tumor involves the intestine. Also, a Pap smear, endocervical curettage (scrapings from the lining of the cervical canal), and endometrial biopsy will be needed if symptoms include abnormal bleeding.

Earlier detection of ovarian cancer may be possible in the future with blood tests to identify proteins produced by cancer cells. Researchers have identified several substances, including CA-125 (an antigen present in many ovarian cancer tumor cells), that are linked to ovarian cancer. These blood tests are not yet precise enough to be used for routine cancer screening, but can be helpful in evaluating tumor response to treatment.

RISK FACTORS

The cause(s) of ovarian cancer is not known. Some women have **lower than average** risks. The use of **birth control Pills** for at least one year significantly reduces a woman's risk for developing ovarian cancer during the time she takes them; protection continues for at least ten years thereafter. **Pregnancy** and **breastfeeding** also are protective. **Factors that confer an increased risk of ovarian cancer are** (20,30):

• Family history of ovarian cancer, especially in the mother or a sister
• Previous cancer of the colon or rectum, or hereditary intestinal polyps
• Ovulation for more than 40 years
• Impaired fertility, no pregnancy, first pregnancy after age 30
• Menopause after age 55
• Talcum powder exposure (vaginal area)
• Previous breast cancer or benign breast disease
• Hypothyroidism
• Obesity
• High blood pressure
• Endometriosis
• Asbestos exposure
• Excessive coffee consumption
• Mumps or rubella in childhood/adolescence
• Close family history of uterine cancer (mother, sister)
• Caucasian, especially Jewish, ethnicity

The last ten factors are statistically linked to higher than average ovarian cancer rates, but their significance is not yet clear.

If you have one or more of these risk factors, be especially conscientious about your annual pelvic exams. **More frequent exams and even routine ultrasound scans** may be reasonable, particularly for women at high risk (31,32). Also, **pay attention to any persistent abdominal symptoms even if they are mild.** A vague sense of pressure, bloating or fullness, hazy discomfort, and altered bowel or bladder patterns are all good reasons for a pelvic exam to check for ovary enlargement.

Before menopause, normal ovaries are large enough to be felt during pelvic exam; during the menopausal years the ovaries decrease to about half their previous size. **Careful evaluation for ovarian cancer is essential for any woman three years or more past menopause who has a palpable ovary.**

CANCER TYPES AND STAGES

Approximately 13% of ovarian cancers are classified as **borderline malignancy.** These tumors, also called **proliferative cystadenomas** or tumors of low malignancy potential, are much less aggressive than other ovarian cancers, and treatment prognosis is good.

About half of all ovarian cancers are **serous carcinoma.** This type of tumor often includes both cystic (fluid-filled) and solid components, and involves both ovaries in a third of cases.

Mucinous carcinoma, somewhat less aggressive than serous cancer, and **endometrioid cancer** each account for about 15% of ovarian cancers. Endometrioid carcinoma is similar in appearance to cancer arising in the uterine lining, and occurs with simultaneous uterine cancer in 15% to 30% of cases. Cell patterns in 15% of ovarian cancers are not clear; these tumors are called **undifferentiated.** Many other types of cancer can arise in the ovary, but are rare. Clear cell carcinoma, mixed tumors, and malignant teratoma (dermoid) are some examples. Benign teratomas are quite common, but about 1% are found to contain malignant elements.

Ovarian cancer stages are defined in Table 41-9. Because early ovarian cancer is so silent, cancer is detected at stage 1 in no more than 40% of cases.

Initial spread of ovarian cancer is through the capsule surrounding the ovary and onto its surface. Spread to nearby structures is also common, including the uterus and fallopian tubes, the fatty apron overlying the intestine, called the omentum, and the surface of the intestine. Tumor patches on the surface of the ovary or bowel often cause production of abnormal fluid secretions within the abdominal cavity. This fluid, called ascites, can cause abdominal bloating or swelling. Tumor may also spread to the lymph nodes that drain from the ovaries; these nodes are located behind the abdominal cavity, and are called retroperitoneal nodes. Common sites for metastic spread of ovarian cancer outside the pelvis are the lung, pleura (covering of the lung), liver, and bone.

TREATMENT

The extent of initial surgery for ovarian cancer depends on the extent of the tumor found, and in some cases, the patient's decision about the importance of future fertility. The main goal is to remove as much of the tumor and any areas of local spread as possible. Removal of both ovaries, fallopian tubes, and uterus is likely to be recommended, even if there is no evidence of tumor involvement outside the primary ovary. The chance of coexisting tumor in the other ovary or uterine cancer is fairly

TABLE 41-9
OVARIAN CANCER STAGES

STAGE	EXTENT OF TUMOR
1a	Tumor involves only one ovary. No abdominal fluid is present.
1b	Tumor involves both ovaries
2	Tumor involves ovary(ies) and nearby pelvic structures
3	Tumor involves ovary(ies) and abdominal structures and/or lymph nodes underlying the abdomen
4	Tumor has spread to distant sites (metastases)

high, especially with some types of ovarian cancer. If tumor involvement is extensive at the time of surgery, it may not be possible to remove it. In that situation surgery to reduce the total amount of tumor will be attempted if this is possible without risk of severe damage to the bowel, or other abdominal organs.

Limited surgery to remove only the involved ovary and fallopian tube, thus preserving future fertility, may be a reasonable option for a young woman with stage 1a cancer and a tumor of borderline malignancy or true cancer of a type that is not severely aggressive.

Unless the cancer is very early (stage 1a), additional treatment with radiation and/or chemotherapy is recommended. Radiation may involve use of a radioactive phosphorus solution inside the abdominal cavity, or radiation treatment with x-ray soon after surgery. Treatment with one or a combination of anticancer drugs is likely to begin as soon as radiation is completed.

In some cases, radiation and chemotherapy result in such good tumor shrinkage that surgery is possible for a tumor initially too extensive for removal. Second laparotomy surgery may also be recommended when chemotherapy treatment is being used and the patient has no evidence of remaining cancer. In this situation, surgery is called "second-look" laparotomy, and is undertaken to determine whether chemotherapy treatment can be stopped.

For ovarian cancer, treatment success depends on the stage and also on the specific type of cancer involved (33). Table 41-10 shows survival rates at five years for women with borderline malignancy and overall rates for other ovarian cancers.

TABLE 41-10
OVARIAN CANCER PROGNOSIS

TYPE OF CANCER	STAGE 1	STAGE 2	STAGES 3 AND 4
Borderline malignancy (cystadenoma)—five-year survival rates	95	72	50
Other ovary cancers (all types)—overall survival rates	63	38	7

SOURCE: Morrow CP, Townsend DE: *Synopsis of Gynecologic Oncology* (ed 2). New York: John Wiley & Sons, 1981.

AFTER OVARIAN CANCER

Surgery for ovarian cancer is quite similar to other common types of major abdominal surgery, such as hysterectomy. Recovery after ovarian cancer surgery is likely to be slow, however. A large vertical incision in the middle of the lower abdomen is necessary, and the surgery itself is extensive and lengthy. Also, postoperative treatment with radiation and/or chemotherapy drugs may further slow convalescence.

Continuing surveillance will be needed when ovarian cancer has been successfully treated, particularly for a woman who has had limited surgery to preserve fertility. The risk for cancer later in the remaining ovary is about 5%, so faithful and frequent pelvic exams are essential. Surgery to remove the remaining ovary may be recommended after childbearing is completed.

SUGGESTED READING

Alabaster, Oliver: *What You Can Do to Prevent Cancer.* New York: Simon & Schuster, 1985. Up-to-date and clear information on how diet and lifestyle choices impact cancer risk. Detailed diet recommendations and guidelines are explained.

Brody, Jane E.: *Jane Brody's Nutrition Book.* New York: W.W. Norton & Co., 1981. Detailed and comprehensive nutrition guidelines, carefully documented, to minimize cancer and heart disease risks and promote well-being.

Brody, Jane E., and Hollub, Arthur I.: *You Can Fight Cancer and Win.* New York: McGraw-Hill, 1977. Although this book was written in 1977, and some of the statistics and treatments described are now out of date, the long introductory section on cancer prevention and basic facts about cancer is still one of the best overviews available.

Spletter, Mary: *A Woman's Choice.* Boston: Beacon Press, 1982. A careful and quite technical review of all aspects of breast cancer including decision making about treatment options and personal ramifications of the disease. A must for women with breast cancer and their families who wish to understand the problem in depth.

RESOURCES

American Cancer Society

The national organization and local affiliates provide educational materials as well as patient services and rehabilitation resources. American Cancer Society chapters also sponsor patient and family support groups including CanSurmount, I Can Cope, and Reach to Recovery (for breast cancer patients). Find your local chapter in the telephone book or write to the national headquarters: American Cancer Society, 90 Park Avenue, New York, NY 10016.

Cancer Information Service

This national organization provides information, referral, and pamphlets for people who have cancer and their families. The national office answers telephone inquiries from 8 A.M. to midnight (Eastern Standard Time) every day except Christmas, and local chapters are open 8:30 A.M. to 4:30 P.M. Call 1-800-4-CANCER to reach the nearest CIS office. Other telephone numbers are:

Alaska   1-800-638-6070
Hawaii   1-808-524-1234

American Institute for Cancer Research

This national research and education organization publishes a newsletter and public information pamphlets including a summary of dietary guidelines recommended by the Committee on Diet, Nutrition, and Cancer of the National Academy of Sciences. For a list of publications, write to American Institute for Cancer Research, Washington, D.C. 20069.

Make Today Count

A national organization with many local chapters to provide peer support for cancer patients and their families. Write to Make Today Count, P.O. Box 222, Osage Beach, Mo. 65065.

National Cancer Institute

This branch of the U.S. Public Health Service publishes educational materials helpful for professionals and the public, such as *Eating Hints: Recipes and Tips for Better Nutrition During Cancer Treatment* (NIH Publication No 84-2079). For a publications list and order form write to Office of Cancer Communications, National Cancer Institute, National Institutes of Health, Building 31, Room 10A18, Bethesda, Md. 20205.

Comprehensive Cancer Centers

These centers, designated by the National Cancer Institute, offer comprehensive cancer care and are also active in research and professional training (many other centers, as well, offer high-quality comprehensive cancer care):

Comprehensive Cancer Center
University of Alabama in Birmingham
Birmingham, Alabama

Jonsson Comprehensive Cancer Center
UCLA Medical Center
Los Angeles, California

University of Southern California
Comprehensive Cancer Center
Los Angeles, California

Yale University Comprehensive Care Center
New Haven, Connecticut

Georgetown University/Howard University
Comprehensive Cancer Center
Washington, D.C.

Comprehensive Cancer Center for the State of Florida
University of Miami Hospital and Clinics
Miami, Florida

Northwestern University Cancer Center
Chicago, Illinois

University of Chicago Cancer Research Center
Chicago, Illinois

Johns Hopkins Oncology Center
Baltimore, Maryland

Dana-Farber Cancer Institute
Boston, Massachusetts

Comprehensive Cancer Center of Metropolitan Detroit
Detroit, Michigan

Mayo Clinic/Mayo Comprehensive Cancer Center
Mayo Clinic
Rochester, Minnesota

Memorial Sloan-Kettering Cancer Center
New York, New York

Roswell Park Memorial Institute
Buffalo, New York

Columbia University Cancer Center
New York, New York

Comprehensive Cancer Center
Duke University Medical Center
Durham, North Carolina

Ohio State University Comprehensive Cancer Center
Columbus, Ohio

Fox Chase Cancer Center
Philadelphia, Pennsylvania

University of Texas Health System Cancer Center
MD Anderson Hospital and Tumor Institute
Houston, Texas

Fred Hutchinson Cancer Research Center
Seattle, Washington

University of Wisconsin Clinical Cancer Center
Madison, Wisconsin

REFERENCES

1. Nutrition and cancer: Cause and prevention. An American Cancer Society special report. *Ca—A Cancer Journal for Clinicians* 34:121–126, 1984.
2. Wittes RE: Vitamin C and cancer. *New England Journal of Medicine* 312:178–179, 1985.
3. Boushey HA, Smith LH Jr: Diet and cancer—Should we change what we eat? *Western Journal of Medicine* 146:73–78, 1987.
4. Hennekens CH, Eberlein K: A randomized trial of aspirin and beta-carotene among U.S. physicians. *Preventive Medicine* 14:165–168, 1985.
5. Niloff JM, Klug TL, Schaetzl E, et al: Elevation of serum CA 125 in carcinomas of the fallopian tube, endometrium, and endocervix. *American Journal of Obstetrics and Gynecology* 149:1057–1058, 1984.
6. Cancer Chemotherapy. *Medical Letter on Drugs and Therapeutics* 29:29–36, 1987.
7. Weinstein LS, Katz B: Oncology patients pose challenge in choosing birth control method. *Contraceptive Technology Update* 6:66–67, 1985.
8. Mullan F: Seasons of survival: Reflections of a physician with cancer. *New England Journal of Medicine* 313:270–273, 1985.
9. Seidman H, Mushinski MH, Gelb SK, et al: Probabilities of eventually developing or dying of cancer—United States, 1985. *Ca—A Cancer Journal for Clinicians* 35:36–56, 1985.
10. Council on Scientific Affairs: Early detection of breast cancer. *Journal of the American Medical Association* 252:3008–3011, 1984.

11. Vorherr H: *Breast Cancer: Epidemiology, Endocrinology, Biochemistry, and Pathobiology.* Baltimore-Munich: Urban & Schwarzenberg, 1980.

12. Greenberg ER, Barnes AB, Resseguie L, et al: Breast cancer in mothers given diethylstilbestrol in pregnancy. *New England Journal of Medicine* 311:1393–1398, 1984.

13. Kaufman DW, Miller DR, Rosenberg L, et al: Noncontraceptive estrogen use and the risk of breast cancer. *Journal of the American Medical Association* 252:63–67, 1984.

14. Oral contraceptive use and the risk of breast cancer in young women. *Morbidity and Mortality Weekly Report* 33:353–354, 1984.

15. Dupont WD, Page DL: Risk factors for breast cancer in women with proliferative breast disease. *New England Journal of Medicine* 312:146–151, 1985.

16. Fisher B, Bauer M, Margolese R, et al: Five-year results of a randomized clinical trial comparing total mastectomy and segmental mastectomy with or without radiation in the treatment of breast cancer. *New England Journal of Medicine* 312:665–673, 1985.

17. Fisher B, Redmond C, Fisher ER, et al: Ten-year results of a randomized clinical trial comparing radical mastectomy and total mastectomy with or without radiation. *New England Journal of Medicine* 312:674–681, 1985.

18. Nolvadex Adjuvant Trial Organisation: Controlled trial of tamoxifen as single adjuvant agent in management of early breast cancer. *Lancet* 1:836–839, 1985.

19. Kaufman RH, Freidrich EG Jr (eds): Vulvar disease. *Clinical Obstetrics and Gynecology* 28:121–242, 1985.

20. Morrow CP, Townsend DE: *Synopsis of Gynecologic Oncology* (ed 2). New York: John Wiley & Sons, 1981.

21. Crum CP, Ikenberg H, Richart RM, et al: Human papillomavirus type 16 and early cervical neoplasia. *New England Journal of Medicine* 310:880–883, 1984.

22. Richart M: personal communication, June, 1985.

23. Robboy SJ, Noller KL, O'Brien P, et al: Increased incidence of cervical and vaginal dysplasia in 3,980 diethylstilbestrol-exposed young women. *Journal of the American Medical Association* 252:2979–2983, 1984.

24. Vessey MP, McPherson K, Lawless M, et al: Neoplasia of the cervix uteri and contraception: A possible adverse effect of the pill. *Lancet* 2:930–934, 1983.

25. Britton LA, Huggins GR, Lehman H: Long-term use of oral contraceptives and risk of invasive cervical cancer, presented at Association of Planned Parenthood Professionals, 23rd Annual Meeting, Seattle, Washington, October, 1985.

26. Hoffman M, Roberts WS, Cavanagh D: Second pelvic malignancies following radiation therapy for cervical cancer. *Obstetrical and Gynecological Survey* 40:611–617, 1985.

27. Bibbo M, Kluskens L, Azizi F, et al: Accuracy of three sampling technics for the diagnosis of endometrial cancer and hyperplasias. *Journal of Reproductive Medicine* 27:622–625, 1982.

28. Winkler B, Alvarez S, Richart RM, et al: Pitfalls in the diagnosis of endometrial neoplasia. *Obstetrics and Gynecology* 64:185–194, 1984.

29. Shapiro S, Kelly JP, Rosenberg L, et al: Risk of localized and widespread endometrial cancer in relation to recent and discontinued use of conjugated estrogens. *New England Journal of Medicine* 313:969–972, 1985.

30. Smith LH, Oi RH: Detection of malignant ovarian neoplasms: A review of the literature. I. Detection of the patient at risk: Clinical, radiological and cytological detection. *Obstetrical and Gynecological Survey* 39:313–328, 1984.

31. Ferrucci JT Jr: Screening for ovarian cancer. *Journal of the American Medical Association* 255:3169, 1986.
32. Ganiats TG: Screening for ovarian cancer. *Journal of the American Medical Association* 256:1892, 1986.
33. Swenerton KD, Hislop TG, Spinelli J, et al: Ovarian carcinoma: A multivariate analysis of prognostic factors. *Obstetrics and Gynecology* 65:264–270, 1985.

Exposure to
Diethylstilbestrol (DES)

Diethylstilbestrol (DES), the first synthetic estrogen, became available for medical use in the 1940s. On the basis of an encouraging research report, physicians prescribed DES for some pregnant women in an attempt to prevent miscarriage. Later research showed, however, that DES does not effectively prevent miscarriage (1), and its use declined. The dangers of DES were not documented until the 1970s, when the first study was published that demonstrated the link between DES and vaginal cancer in daughters of women who took DES during pregnancy. In November 1971, the Food and Drug Administration recommended that DES no longer be used during pregnancy. We now know that DES exposure may have harmful effects on daughters, sons, and the DES-treated mothers themselves.

DES and two similar synthetic estrogens, dienestrol and hexestrol, were the main drugs used for estrogen treatment during pregnancy. The term "DES exposure" is used for all three drugs, and they all appear to have had similar harmful effects. Newer synthetic estrogens such as those now used in birth control Pills have a somewhat different chemical structure and have never been extensively used during pregnancy. It is not known whether DES effects are unique for the specific chemical structure of DES, hexestrol, and dienestrol, or whether similar problems would occur if the newer estrogens were used in high doses during pregnancy.

How to Determine DES Exposure

Between 1940 and 1971, about 6 million pregnant women were treated with DES (2). DES treatment was most common between 1950 and 1955, when as many as 5% to 10% of pregnant women who received care at some medical centers were given the drug (3). DES use declined after 1960, but cases of DES exposure as late as 1975 have been reported.

Consider the possibility of exposure if you (or your mother) fit these criteria:

- You were conceived (or were pregnant) between 1940 and 1975, especially between 1950 and 1960
- Your mother (or you) had bleeding during early pregnancy, previous miscarriage, or diabetes
- Your mother (or you) took any oral medicine in tablet form during pregnancy. DES treatment usually started early in pregnancy and continued with increasing doses until about one month before delivery. It was usually given in tablet form, not by injection, and was marketed under many brand names. (See Table 42-1 for common brand names.)

It may be possible to confirm DES exposure by checking medical records from the time of the pregnancy or by identifying abnormalities that are common with DES exposure if you are a DES daughter or son. Even if you cannot find old medical records, if you suspect that you may have taken DES during pregnancy or you are a daughter or son who may have been exposed, then you may need special medical surveillance.

Possible Effects of DES Exposure: Daughters, Sons, and Mothers

As with most drugs, harmful effects on the fetus are more likely if DES exposure occurred early in pregnancy. Daughters exposed to DES during the first five months of fetal life are more likely to have DES problems than are daughters exposed only in the later months.

CLEAR CELL ADENOCARCINOMA OF THE VAGINA OR CERVIX

This particular type of vaginal or cervical cancer is uncommon, even among DES daughters. About 600 cases worldwide have been reported as of the mid 1980s. Experts estimate that less than 1 DES daughter in 1,000 develops this cancer (4). About two

TABLE 42-1
DES-TYPE DRUGS THAT MAY HAVE BEEN PRESCRIBED TO PREGNANT WOMEN

NONSTEROIDAL ESTROGENS

Benzestrol	Estrosyn	
Chlorotrianisene	Fonatol	Palestrol
Comestrol	Gynben	Restrol
Cyren A	Gyneben	Stil-Rol
Cyren B	Hexestrol	Stilbal
Delvinal	Hexoestrol	Stilbestrol
DES	Hi-Bestrol	Stilbestronate
DesPlex	Menocrin	Stilbetin
Diestryl	Meprane	Stilbinol
Dibestil	Mestilbol	Stilboestroform
Dienestrol	Methallenestril	Stilboestrol
Dienoestrol	Microest	Stilboestrol DP
Diethylstilbestrol	Mikarol	Stilestrate
dipalmitate	Mikarol forti	Stilpalmitate
Diethylstilbestrol	Milestrol	Stilphostrol
diphosphate	Monomestrol	Stilronate
Diethylstilbestrol	Neo-Oestranol I	Stilrone
dipropionate	Neo-Oestranol II	Stils
Diethylstilbenediol	Nulabort	Synestrin
Digestil	Oestrogenine	Synestrol
Domestrol	Oestromenin	Synthoestrin
Estilben	Oestromon	Tace
Estrobene	Orestol	Vallestril
Estrobene DP	Pabestrol D	Willestrol

NONSTEROIDAL ESTROGEN-ANDROGEN COMBINATIONS	NONSTEROIDAL ESTROGEN-PROGESTERONE COMBINATIONS
Amperone	Progravidium
Di-Erone	
Estan	VAGINAL CREAM/SUPPOSITORIES WITH NONSTEROIDAL ESTROGENS
Metystil	
Teserene	AVC Cream with Dienestrol
Tylandril	Dienestrol Cream
Tylosterone	

SOURCE: U.S. Department of Health, Education and Welfare, Information for Physicians: *DES Exposure in Utero*. Publication Number (NIH) 76–1119, 1976.

thirds of these cancers are vaginal and one third cervical. The DES daughters who developed clear cell adenocarcinoma were exposed to DES before the 18th week of gestation, and most cancers became apparent when the DES daughters were between the ages of 14 and 33 (3). This cancer can be successfully treated with surgery and radiation, and interim reports have shown that three out of four women who have been treated for vaginal cancer are alive and well (5). Danger signs for clear cell cancer are **abnormal vaginal bleeding and thickening or lumps in the wall of the vagina.**

DYSPLASIA AND SQUAMOUS CELL CANCER OF THE CERVIX

Dysplasia, precancerous cell changes on the surface of the cervix, and carcinoma in situ (CIS), very early cancer that has not invaded other tissues, are substantially more common among DES daughters than among unexposed women (6,7). Researchers in one U.S. study of 744 pairs of exposed and unexposed women examined each of the nearly 1,500 women yearly. The rate of dysplasia and CIS was 15.7 per 1,000 person years of follow-up for DES daughters, compared to 7.9 for unexposed women (7). Rates were higher in exposed women in this study if they had significant squamous metaplasia, which is described in this chapter in the section on adenosis. Since dysplasia and CIS are known to precede development of squamous cell carcinoma, the most common form of cervical cancer, researchers are concerned that DES daughters may prove to have higher than average rates for this cancer. Research may not ever be able to show whether there is a causal link between DES and cervical cancer because other confounding factors that can increase risk for cervical cancer—multiple sex partners or a history of certain sexually transmitted infections, for example—are hard to separate from DES factors. Pap smears are very reliable for detecting dysplasia and cancer of the cervix. Squamous cell carcinoma of the cervix is curable in most cases if it is detected early.

STRUCTURAL ABNORMALITIES OF THE CERVIX AND VAGINA

As many as 60% of DES daughters have alterations in the shape of the cervix (see Illustration 42-1), the vaginal walls, or the uterus. DES exposure abnormalities include cervical stenosis (significant narrowing of the cervical canal) and a uterine cavity with an irregular T shape (8). A T-shaped uterus is illustrated in Chapter 40. Structural abnormalities raise questions about effects on fertility and pregnancy, and these issues are discussed later in the chapter. Surgery involving the cervix, such as cautery, cryosurgery, or conization, seems to be associated with subsequent narrowing of the cervical canal, so some experts advise DES daughters to **avoid** surgery unless it is absolutely essential for treatment of serious cervical problems (9). Treatment to eradicate areas on the cervix or vagina just because they **appear** abnormal is not recommended.

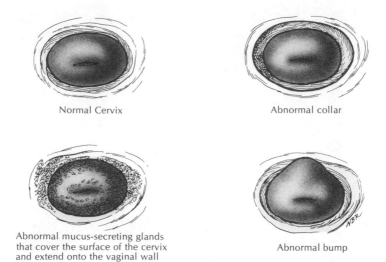

Normal Cervix

Abnormal collar

Abnormal mucus-secreting glands
that cover the surface of the cervix
and extend onto the vaginal wall

Abnormal bump

ILLUSTRATION 42-1 Your clinician may suspect DES exposure if your cervix
has an abnormal shape. (Reproductive Health Resources, Inc. Used with
permission.)

ADENOSIS

The normal surface of the cervix and the vaginal walls is smooth, shiny tissue called squamous epithelium, composed of flat, pancake-shaped cells. The term "adenosis" means that patches of a different type of epithelium appear on the surface of the cervix and/or the walls of the vagina. Adenosis surface cells are tall and velvety columnar epithelium cells, similar to those that line the cervical canal, and adenosis tissue contains a rich supply of mucus-secreting glands (see Illustration 42-2). Adenosis is common among DES daughters. You might have adenosis with no symptoms at all, or you might have a heavy, mucus-like vaginal discharge. Your vagina may not look *at all* unusual to your clinician during your routine pelvic exam. Clinicians use colposcopy and/or iodine staining of the vagina to detect adenosis. The condition sometimes corrects itself as the epithelium matures and columnar epithelium is replaced with normal squamous epithelium. This replacement process is called squamous metaplasia. Adenosis was very uncommon before the era of DES daughters, and its long-term effects are not yet known.

Some researchers are concerned that in addition to clear cell adenocarcinoma risk, a woman with adenosis may have an increased risk for squamous cell carcinoma, which almost always arises from the "transformation zone," a circular area on the surface of a normal cervix where the two types of surface cells meet—the **squamous** cells from the outer surface of the cervix and the **columnar** cells from the lining of the cervical canal. Women with adenosis have a transformation zone that is much larger than normal because columnar, mucus-secreting cells can extend over the whole cervix

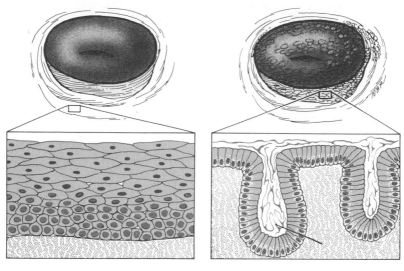

Normal Vaginal Cells   Adenosis

ILLUSTRATION 42-2 Adenosis means that glandular, mucus-secreting cells, normally present only in the cervical canal, extend onto the surface of the cervix and/or vaginal walls. (Reproductive Health Resources, Inc. Used with permission.)

and out onto the vaginal walls. Another concern is that clear cell adenocarcinoma arises from columnar cells. There is as yet no evidence that women with adenosis have an increased risk for cancer, but it makes sense to have Pap smears regularly, including **Pap smears from the vaginal walls** (see routine care recommendations later in this chapter).

PREGNANCY OUTCOME AND INFERTILITY

Studies comparing DES daughters to unexposed women of the same age indicate that DES daughters may be more likely to have ectopic (tubal) pregnancies, miscarriage in the middle trimester of pregnancy, and premature deliveries (10,11). Some studies find that daughters have trouble conceiving, and other studies do not (10,11,12). In one long-term study, 82% of DES daughters who wanted a child have achieved successful pregnancy (4). This percentage is quite similar to the overall pregnancy success rates for all women. For DES daughters, though, the road to success may be longer and more arduous.

HERPES AND GENITAL WART INFECTION

DES daughters in one study had a significantly higher rate for herpes and a slightly higher rate for genital warts, two sexually transmitted viral infections, than did a

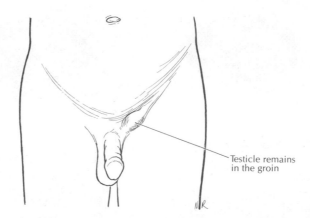

ILLUSTRATION 42-3   An undescended testicle remains in the groin; the scrotum on that side is empty, lacking the firm, round testicle it should contain.

comparison group of unexposed women. Women in both groups had an almost identical number of sexual partners, and the rates for other sexually transmitted diseases were not different (13). It may be that the cervical and vaginal tissue changes sometimes caused by DES—adenosis and subsequent squamous metaplasia—leave a woman's cervix and vagina particularly vulnerable to attack by herpes or wart virus. Researchers believe that wart virus is an important culprit in causing cervical dysplasia, so a propensity for viral infection could explain why dysplasia rates are higher than average among DES daughters. Researchers say it is extremely difficult to distinguish between the influence of viral infection and the influence of DES when dysplasia occurs in a DES daughter. It certainly makes sense to do everything in your power to avoid sexually transmitted infection if you are a DES daughter. Just like all women, you should avoid intercourse when you think there is a risk. Using condoms or another barrier method as a routine practice is also an entirely reasonable idea. Chapter 22 gives advice in detail on avoiding sexual infection.

PROBLEMS OF DES SONS

DES-exposed sons have not yet been studied as extensively as DES daughters, and DES-related problems have only recently been identified and reported for exposed men. To date, there is no evidence of any increased cancer risk for DES sons, but clinicians are concerned. Undescended testicles are an important risk factor for testicular cancer, and DES sons have higher rates of undescended testicles requiring surgical correction than do unexposed men.

More than 30% of DES sons in one study had abnormalities such as testicle cysts, underdeveloped or undescended testicles, or abnormal placement of the urinary opening (see Illustration 42-3). Similar abnormalities were found in only 8% of young men who had not been exposed to DES (14).

In the same study, about 40% of DES sons had low sperm counts and abnormally shaped sperm cells. In half of these young men (20% of all DES sons), sperm production was impaired enough to interfere with fertility. Impaired fertility has not been shown in any large studies, however, so the actual fertility status of DES sons is simply not yet clear (4).

Another study of DES sons did not find any evidence that rates for genitourinary abnormalities were higher in DES sons than in similar men not exposed to DES, nor were infertility problems or testicular cancer more common (5).

PROBLEMS OF DES MOTHERS

In 1985 the federal DES Task Force reported that DES mothers have an increased risk of breast cancer compared to nonexposed women, although an actual cause-and-effect relationship has not been demonstrated (16). The Task Force reviewed two previous studies that followed DES mothers for 20 years; both these studies found that breast cancer rates were about twice as high after 20 years among DES mothers as among nonexposed women. One large U.S. study compared about 3,000 exposed women with about 3,000 unexposed women, and found 118 cases of breast cancer among DES mothers and 80 cases among unexposed women (17). The Task Force was cautious in its interpretation of these study results because of characteristics of the study group of DES mothers and nonexposed women, which may account for some of the difference in disease rates. Further study will be required to confirm these findings and to learn whether DES mothers also have any excess risk for other malignancies.

Guidelines for Medical Care:
DES Daughters, Sons, and Mothers

Whether you are sure about DES exposure or only suspect it, DES daughters, sons, and mothers must be aware of the harmful effects that we now know about, must be faithful about routine examinations, and must be alert for new information about DES problems and any unusual symptoms they may experience.

DES DAUGHTERS

Try to arrange for ongoing routine care with a gynecologist who is experienced with DES problems. Begin having routine exams when your menstrual periods start or at age 14, whichever occurs earlier. Prompt examination is essential if abnormal vaginal bleeding or discharge occurs, even if you are very young. Have a routine exam once a year. If your clinician finds any DES-related abnormalities, you will need more frequent exams. In addition to a routine pelvic exam, your annual examinations should include (2,5):

• A two-slide Pap test: one slide from the cervix and one or more slides from the walls of the vagina
• Colposcopic examination of the cervix and vagina (if Pap test or other findings are abnormal)
• Iodine staining of the cervix and upper vagina (if Pap test results are abnormal)
• Careful palpation (feeling) of the walls of the vagina and cervix to detect thickening, lumps, or roughness
• Biopsy (a tiny tissue fragment removed for microscopic evaluation, see Chapter 4) of any abnormal areas on the cervix or vaginal walls

Routine colposcopy and iodine staining each year for all DES daughters is no longer recommended (5). An initial evaluation should include colposcopy and staining, and subsequent follow-up exam steps depend on whether or not adenosis areas are present in the vagina. If no vaginal adenosis is present, exams once a year with Pap smears are sufficient unless Pap smear results are abnormal or become abnormal in the future. If vaginal adenosis is present, exams and Pap smears should be scheduled every six months, and colposcopy and staining repeated every two years (5).

DES SONS

Make sure that you are evaluated once a year by your clinician. You might try to find a urologist who is specifically interested in and experienced with DES problems. Periodic self-examination to check for lumps or any change in the size or consistency of your testicles is also a reasonable precaution.

DES MOTHERS

See a gynecologist, an internist, or a family physician for your routine care. Your routine exam needs are no different than those of nonexposed women, but it is especially important for you to be very faithful about checkups. Your routine care should include:

• Monthly breast self-examination
• Annual breast exam by your clinician
• Initial mammogram at age 35 to 40, repeated at one- to two-year intervals until age 50, depending on findings and other risk factors, and once a year after age 50
• Annual pelvic exam and Pap smear

Long-term Effects of DES Exposure

The oldest DES mothers are in their 70s, the oldest DES daughters and sons are in their 40s, and researchers still urge more data and more follow-up studies. Older members of both generations are reaching peak years for many types of reproductive tract and other cancers. It is possible that no further harmful effects of DES will be found. On the other hand, DES may be found to increase rates for still more problems. The final answers will not be known for years. In the meantime, you will need to be faithful about routine checkups, and to be sure you are cared for by a clinician with DES experience if problems do occur. Also, you will need to be alert for new research findings that may be relevant for DES-exposed people.

Birth Control Pills and Menopausal Hormones. DES daughters are advised in FDA-approved product labeling that they may use birth control Pills if they are willing to be "monitored with particular care" (18) during and after Pill use, and most clinicians are quite willing to prescribe Pills for their DES patients when no other risk factors are present. Pill product labeling does not specifically mention DES mothers, but most clinicians are willing to prescribe Pills for DES mothers when no Pill risk factors are present and women are willing to be followed carefully, particularly for breast examinations.

Product labeling for menopausal replacement estrogen does not specifically mention DES exposure issues, and most clinicians are willing to prescribe estrogen for exposed daughters or mothers when no risk factors are present and the woman is willing to be followed carefully at frequent examinations.

Legal Issues. More than 1,000 DES lawsuits have been filed in the United States, involving many of the 200 companies that manufactured the drug, as exposed women and their sons and daughters seek remedy for their often substantial medical expenses. DES litigation involves some difficult legal issues, and in the cases that have come to trial, no clear pattern has emerged to reveal how DES lawsuits will be handled. A major legal question is how to decide what companies can be named as defendants when old medical records rarely reveal exactly which one of 200 companies produced the medication a specific woman used, particularly since in many cases DES was marketed generically. Many suits are pending, and the long-term legal outcomes seem no clearer than the long-term medical outcomes (19).

Living with DES. DES can be burdensome to live with for all exposed people, whether or not they experience serious health consequences.

The hardest part is the helpless feeling . . . as though I have no idea what the future will hold for me. Rationally I understand that nobody else on earth actually knows what the future holds, but waiting to see if I get this problem or that problem does make me feel powerless. Sometimes I have to push myself to make plans at all.

—WOMAN, 30

One study of 50 DES daughters and 30 mothers found that the vast majority of women were able to get beyond this major emotional crisis (20). A chance to express and share powerful negative feelings such as helplessness and anger is crucial, and one function of the nationwide DES Action network is to provide such an opportunity for sharing. DES Action addresses are given in the "Resources" section. Joining the organization, and subscribing to its newsletters, may also help you stay informed as new research findings are reported. If you need help coping with your feelings about DES exposure, by all means get in touch with DES Action or a psychotherapist in your area.

RESOURCES

DES ACTION USA
Long Island Jewish Medical Center
New Hyde Park, New York 11040 (516-775-3450)
There are DES Action groups in more than 40 cities. Check your local telephone book or write to the national office. Quarterly newsletters, annual reports, and special publications are available to members. Publications include a 54-page guide entitled *Fertility and Pregnancy Guide for DES Daughters and Sons.* The guide, written in 1983, can be ordered ($6) from the national office.

REFERENCES

1. Food and Drug Administration: DES and breast cancer. *FDA Drug Bulletin* 8:10–11, 1978.
2. Robboy SJ, Noller KL, Kaufman RH, et al: *Prenatal diethylstilbestrol (DES) exposure: Recommendations of the diethylstilbestrol-adenosis (DESAD) project for the identification and management of exposed individuals.* Bethesda, Md.: National Institutes of Health, Publication Number 80-2049, 1980.
3. Herbst AL, Cole P, Colton T, et al: Age-incidence and risk of diethylstilbestrol-related clear cell adenocarcinoma of the vagina and cervix. *American Journal of Obstetrics and Gynecology* 128:43–50, 1977.
4. Melnick S, Cole P, Anderson D, et al: Rates and risks of diethylstilbestrol-related clear-cell adenocarcinoma of the vagina and cervix—an update. *New England Journal of Medicine* 316:514–516, 1987.

5. Morrow CP, Townsend DE: *Synopsis of Gynecologic Oncology* (ed 2). New York: John Wiley & Sons, 1981.

6. Mattingly RF, Stafl A: Cancer risk in diethylstilbestrol-exposed offspring. *American Journal of Obstetrics and Gynecology* 126:543–548, 1976.

7. Robboy SJ, Noller KL, O'Brien P, et al: Increased incidence of cervical and vaginal dysplasia in 3,980 diethylstilbestrol-exposed young women: Experience of the national collaborative diethylstilbestrol adenosis project. *Journal of the American Medical Association* 252:2979–2983, 1984.

8. Stillman RJ: In utero exposure to diethylstilbestrol: Adverse effects on the reproductive tract and reproductive performance in male and female offspring. *American Journal of Obstetrics and Gynecology* 142:905–920, 1982.

9. Haney AF, Hammond MG: Infertility in women exposed to diethylstilbestrol in utero. *Journal of Reproductive Medicine* 28:851–855, 1983.

10. Barnes AB, Colton T, Gundersen J, et al: Fertility and outcome of pregnancy in women exposed in utero to diethylstilbestrol. *New England Journal of Medicine* 302:609–613, 1980.

11. Herbst AL, Hubby MM, Azizi F, et al: Reproductive and gynecologic surgical experience in diethylstilbestrol-exposed daughters. *American Journal of Obstetrics and Gynecology* 141:1019–1028, 1981.

12. Berger MJ, Alper MM: Intractable primary infertility in women exposed to diethylstilbestrol in utero. *Journal of Reproductive Medicine* 31:231–235, 1986.

13. Richart RM, Herbst AL, Kaufman R, et al: Symposium: DES daughters: The risks in their childbearing years. *Contemporary Ob/Gyn* 26:204–232, 1985.

14. Bibbo M, Gill W, Freidoon A, et al: Follow-up study of male and female offspring of DES-exposed mothers. *Obstetrics and Gynecology* 49:1–8, 1977.

15. Leary FJ, Resseguie LJ, Kurland LT: Males exposed in utero to diethylstilbestrol. *Journal of the American Medical Association* 252:2984–2989, 1984.

16. Report of the recommendations of the 1985 DES task force of the U.S. Department of Health and Human Services. *Morbidity and Mortality Weekly Report* 35:155–162, 1986.

17. Greenberg ER, Barnes AB, Resseguie L, et al: Breast cancer in mothers given diethylstilbestrol in pregnancy. *New England Journal of Medicine* 311:1393–1398, 1984.

18. FDA-approved product labeling for oral contraceptives. Manufacturers of oral contraceptives are required to provide a leaflet explaining the benefits, risks, and possible complications of Pills for each patient who fills a Pill prescription. You should be able to obtain a copy of the leaflet, entitled "What You Should Know About Oral Contraceptives," from your physician or pharmacist. Manufacturer's information for physicians as well as the text of the patient leaflet appears in *Physicians' Desk Reference* (ed 40). Oradell, N.J.: Medical Economics Co., 1986.

19. Rymer TA: The diethylstilbestrol dilemma: Who should pay? *Journal of the American Medical Association* 251:3228–3229, 1984.

20. Burke L, Apfel RJ, Fisher S, et al: Observations on the psychological impact of diethylstilbestrol exposure and suggestions on management. *Journal of Reproductive Medicine* 24:99–102, 1980.

CHAPTER

43

Sexual Problems

Almost everyone encounters problems with sexual functioning at some time in life. In many cases, the problem is temporary and the cause is obvious. For many people, however, persistent sexual problems are a source of continuing distress and difficulty. Clinicians who care for women report that sexual problems are extremely common complaints. It is likely that even more women would seek help if they knew how successful treatment approaches for some sexual problems have proven to be.

*In many cases it is appropriate and effective to work on impaired sexual functioning as a problem in its own right. Treatment designed **specifically** to improve sexual functioning can be successful even if overall psychological functioning is not perfect, and other psychological and relationship problems may even improve if sexual functioning is improved. In other cases it may be essential to work on more general psychological or relationship problems. Treatment directed toward improving overall psychological functioning may, as a by-product, help with sexual problems as well.*

Short-term, specific treatment is likely to be successful for a man who has rapid ejaculation problems and for a woman who has been unable to have an orgasm. Specific treatment, by a specialist trained in sexual function, is also a reasonable idea when medical problems are causing sexual impairment. Sophisticated knowledge and experience may be of help.

This chapter is intended as a brief introduction to normal sexual functioning and to some of the common problems and treatment approaches. If you are concerned about a sexual problem, you will probably want to read further. The "Suggested Reading" section at the end of this chapter may be helpful, and your clinician or therapist can also suggest books appropriate for your needs. Don't be surprised, though, if reading fails to solve your problems. Knowledge is essential, and is often helpful, but making personal changes is hard psychological work. If you are suffering, you definitely deserve the help that a counselor can give as you try to make change happen.

Normal Sexual Functioning

It is difficult to describe **normal** sexual functioning, because one hallmark of human sexual behavior is diversity. There is no single normal pattern or even one average pattern. One person may be completely content with a form and frequency of sexual expression that another person finds inadequate or distressing. There are, however, themes of sexual expression that are almost universal, and there are physical responses during sexual activity that occur in predictable patterns for men and for women.

PHYSICAL EVENTS IN HUMAN SEXUAL RESPONSE

In their pioneering book *Human Sexual Response*, Masters and Johnson (1) describe in detail the normal physical changes that occur during sexual activity. This section provides a simplified summary of their observations. They found it helpful to divide the sequence of physical events into four phases: **excitation**, the initial phase of sexual response; **plateau**, a middle phase of sexual response; **orgasm**; and **resolution**, the return to normal. In actual people, of course, the phases blend together and overlap. You may not be able to identify your own phases so precisely.

Excitation Phase.   The initial female response to effective sexual stimulation is engorgement of the blood vessels in the pelvic area; as a result of engorgement, vaginal lubrication soon occurs. Tiny droplets of lubricating fluid appear on the vaginal walls, sometimes as soon as 10 to 30 seconds after excitation begins. Lubrication production continues as excitation continues, and after a few minutes is often noticeable as a distinctly wet sensation at the entrance to the vagina. The initial male response that parallels female lubrication is penile erection. Increased blood flow to the penis results in engorgement of the veins and spongy tissue in the shaft of the penis. Erection may subside partially or completely and then resume as stimulation varies or as distractions intervene.

For a woman, blood vessel engorgement involves the inner vaginal lips (labia minora), as well as the outer lips (labia majora) (see the illustration of external reproductive tract structures in Chapter 2), which spread to uncover the vaginal opening. Engorgement and enlargement of the clitoris, and engorgement of the veins of the breast, occur as well. Nipple erection and an overall increase in breast size may also occur with excitation.

As excitation increases, both men and women may show a generally increased muscle tension, heart rate, and blood pressure; and late in excitation a pink flush may appear that is caused by dilation of blood vessels near the skin surface. The flush appears first on the upper abdomen and spreads upward over the chest, neck, and face. A flush may also occur with orgasm.

Plateau Phase. As sexual arousal increases to the plateau phase the clitoris may retract under the clitoral hood so that it is drawn back somewhat against the pubic bone. This change may make it difficult to see the clitoris itself, which is usually prominent during the initial excitation phase. The clitoris lies close to the muscles of the vaginal outlet and to the junction of the labia, where stimulation of the clitoris by movement of the labia and muscles or by stimulation of the area over the pubic bone is likely to be pleasurable and exciting.

The length and diameter of the upper vagina increase by as much as 1 or 2 inches during the excitation and plateau phases; during the plateau phase, the walls of the outer one third of the vagina—nearest the vaginal opening—become engorged and firm to create a snug sleeve, while the inner two thirds of the vagina remains dilated. Engorgement of the inner and outer lips also increases, and just before orgasm the skin of the inner lips may become deep red or wine colored. The uterus and uterine ligaments may also become engorged, shift forward in position, and increase in overall size.

During the plateau phase, engorgement of the man's testicles may increase their size by as much as 50%, and the testicles and scrotum draw up toward the base of the penis. Some men have nipple erection and breast congestion during this phase as well. Both men and women perceive increased muscle tension and often have a rapid breathing rate late in the plateau phase.

Orgasm. As male orgasm approaches, contraction of the seminal vesicles and prostate gland propels semen into the urethra. This contraction happens before ejaculation and gives the man a sense that ejaculation is imminent. Progression from this point to ejaculation is inevitable. Within moments the muscles of the pelvic floor, urethra, and penis forcefully expel semen (ejaculation) as orgasm contractions occur. Orgasm contractions are rhythmic, occurring every 0.8 second for three or four contractions, followed by less frequent, milder contractions over the next few seconds or minutes.

As female orgasm approaches, the woman's heightened sexual tension may give her a sense that orgasm is imminent, but there does not appear to be a clear-cut preorgasmic phase comparable to the male's preorgasmic release of semen into the urethra. Female orgasm may begin with an initial sustained contraction of the muscles of the vaginal opening that lasts only a few seconds and is followed by a series of rhythmic contractions, or it may begin directly with rhythmic contractions occurring about 0.8 second apart. After an initial series of three to six contractions, the interval between contractions lengthens until a total of perhaps five to ten contractions have occurred.

I get to a point where I feel as if there is no turning back—as if I were not in control anymore, but not in a scary way. At that point I'm not thinking about anything except my own body, and it seems as if nothing could possibly stop my body from moving to orgasm.

—WOMAN, 28

Along with the primary genital muscle contractions of orgasm, both men and women may have rhythmic contractions of the muscles around the rectum and lower abdomen. The intensity and duration of muscle contractions can range from mild, brief contractions localized in the genital area to powerful, spasmodic contractions involving muscles of the lower abdomen, thighs, and extremities as well. Orgasm intensity varies greatly, and may be related to individual differences, the level of sexual tension, and the duration of the preceding excitement and plateau phases. Masters and Johnson found that most people experience stronger muscle contractions and more intense orgasms with masturbation stimulation than with intercourse. The strength and intensity of orgasm contractions, however, are not necessarily related to the person's perception of satisfaction.

In addition to the physical events that Masters and Johnson were able to document with recording instruments, there are many other responses to orgasm that men and women report. Whole novels have been written about them. These responses include a total absorption that blocks awareness of the environment, or a flood of pleasant warmth. Men often report an impetus to push for the deepest possible vaginal penetration and a tremendously satisfying release of pressure as ejaculation occurs. Responses after orgasm may include a sense of release, total relaxation, and serenity; often there is a sense of physical exhaustion similar to that after sustained, exhilarating physical exertion. Muscles throughout the body may feel heavy, warm, and weak. The rapid breathing (hyperventilation) of the late plateau phase and orgasm may cause a tingling sensation in the extremities, cramping of muscles in the hands and feet, and flashes of light (stars) in the visual field. Many people report a sense of well-being and affection toward their partner.

Sometimes orgasm is a purely physical thing for me, pleasant and satisfying but not profound—just a good way for me to deal with a certain kind of tension. Other times, especially with my partner, it can be
overwhelmingly wonderful, and the physical part seems almost incidental.

—WOMAN, 36

The intensity of orgasm may vary on different occasions and in different circumstances. The physical responses, however, appear to follow a uniform, predictable pattern. Similar muscular contractions occur with orgasm whether sexual stimulation has involved vaginal intercourse or other forms of stimulation such as masturbation or breast stimulation. Many women are able to reach orgasm with vaginal intercourse, but many find that more direct clitoral stimulation is necessary as well as, or instead of, intercourse. Masters and Johnson's research **does not** support the concept that two different types of orgasm—vaginal and clitoral—exist for women.

Although orgasm and the immediate release of sexual tension are usually obvious to the man or woman himself or herself, orgasm may **not** be recognizable to a partner. The general high level of muscle tension during the plateau phase may make it impossible for a partner to identify with certainty the specific contractions of orgasm.

Resolution.   Immediately after orgasm, both men and women often notice an interval of genital hypersensitivity. The glans of the clitoris and the tip (glans) of the penis may be so exquisitely sensitive that any form of stimulation is irritating or intolerable. Both men and women may notice the sudden appearance of perspiration on the face, trunk, and extremities within seconds after orgasm. As the resolution phase is established, there is a rapid decrease in blood vessel engorgement. Penis erection subsides by about 50%, and the clitoris returns to its normal unretracted position within seconds after orgasm. The thickened walls of the outer vagina and the engorged testicles gradually return to normal.

During the resolution phase, most men rapidly return to a low level of physical sexual tension, comparable to the early excitement phase. Some women, on the other hand, have a slower resolution in their physical level of sexual tension, more comparable to the plateau phase, and are able to resume sexual responsiveness and experience several orgasms within a short period of time. Most men, however, are not responsive to further sexual stimulation during the resolution phase and can return to the orgasm phase only after resuming sexual activity that reestablishes both the excitement phase and plateau phase physical events. Typical time patterns for sexual response phases are shown in Illustration 43-1.

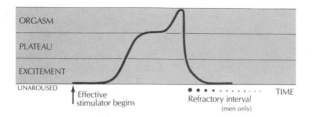

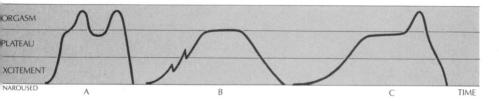

ILLUSTRATION 43-1 A typical arousal response pattern. Men and women have similar patterns, but there are substantial individual variations, and your own pattern is likely to vary from one experience to another. For example, arousal and orgasm may occur very quickly (A), or ups and downs may occur during the excitation phase (B). Arousal may be slow and gradual (C) with a prolonged plateau phase (B). This is particularly common for older men. Renewed stimulation after an initial orgasm may be effective after the refractory interval so that a second orgasm occurs without full resolution in between (A). Sometimes orgasm doesn't occur at all (B). (Adapted from Masters WH, Johnson VE: *Human Sexual Response.* Boston: Little, Brown, 1966.)

A refractory time interval, during which stimulation is not effective in producing increased excitation, occurs only for men, and varies from individual to individual. It may also be influenced by age. For young men, the refractory period may be as short as 10 to 15 minutes; for men over 60 it may be many hours.

THE G (GRÄFENBERG) SPOT

The organs and physical structures involved in sexual responsiveness that were so carefully studied by Masters and Johnson are all well-known human body parts. Anatomists, however, do not agree about the controversial G spot described in 1944 by Ernest Gräfenberg, a famous German gynecologist who also developed one of the first IUDs (intrauterine devices). Gräfenberg, and some other researchers since, describe this area as a collection of erectile and possibly glandular tissue located alongside the urethra where it joins the base of the bladder. This tissue becomes engorged with sexual arousal, and swells to form a ¾-inch to 1 ½-inch structure large enough to feel with an examining finger, located just under the vaginal lining at the back of the vaginal roof. At other times it is too small to be noticeable (2). Direct pressure or stimulation in the area of the G spot is intensely pleasurable and effective in increasing sexual excitation. Gräfenberg also believed that orgasmic contractions of this tissue can expel secretions into and through a woman's urethra, in effect a female ejaculation that occurs with effective stimulation of the G spot. And subsequent researchers, in two small studies, were able to collect samples of a clear colorless urethral ejaculate and found that its chemical composition was quite different from urine (2).

Many women do notice leakage of clear fluid with orgasm, and may assume that it is involuntary urine loss. Urine loss can occur as a result of stress incontinence, with a cough or sneeze for example, and could be a source of embarrassment for a woman who experiences this problem with intercourse as well. It may be that urethral secretions instead are the entirely normal cause of leakage for some women.

CONTROL OF HUMAN SEXUAL RESPONSES

Physical events in the human sexual response cycle are controlled by the automatic (autonomic) nervous system, as are many other body functions, such as heart rate, blood pressure, and digestion. The autonomic nerve pathways, for example, cause the smooth muscle walls in the vessels (arteries) of the penis and vagina to dilate; thus, the rate of blood flow to these organs increases and blood vessels become engorged. You do not have direct voluntary control over your physical sexual responses.

There are two distinct parts of the autonomic nervous system—the sympathetic and the parasympathetic systems—and each seems to have a distinct role in sexual responsiveness. The parasympathetic system plays the primary role in the physical events of the excitation and plateau phases, and the sympathetic system is responsible for orgasm (3). This division of responsibility may explain why a person might have no problem with arousal but be unable to have an orgasm, or (in rarer cases) experience orgasm without prior arousal.

The conscious mind and the voluntary muscles nevertheless hold **ultimate** control over sexuality. Physical sexual changes occur in response to adequate sexual stimulation. Allowing an opportunity for and being receptive to effective sexual stimulation are, for the most part, **voluntary** factors. Stimuli may include conscious thoughts and emotions as well as physical sensations.

For many people, the initiation of sexual tension and the physical events of the early excitation phase typically occur in response to voluntary, conscious thoughts or fantasies. Some people are even able to achieve plateau phase physical changes solely by responding to thoughts and fantasies. Most people, however, require direct physical sensations to achieve plateau responses. For some, nongenital physical sensations are sufficient, but more typically, effective stimulation specifically involving the breast, clitoris, or penis is necessary for plateau phase arousal and orgasm.

There is no simple universal formula for effective physical stimulation. Attention, and the feeling of being loved, are important as well as physical stimuli; this is especially true for many women. In general, gentle, repetitive, rhythmic, caressing stimulation is likely to be pleasurable. Most women respond to direct pressure, such as stroking or moving the shaft of the clitoris within the clitoral hood; some prefer firm pressure, while others find that all but the gentlest direct manipulation of the clitoris itself is unpleasantly sensitive. Most men respond to direct pressure, such as stroking along the bottom side of the shaft of the penis or the glans; for some, direct stimulation of the tip of the penis is too intense to be pleasurable. The range of individual responses is very wide and the same person may find one form of touching pleasurable on one occasion and irritating on another. One of the important tasks in improving sexual functioning is to learn through experimentation what is pleasurable and effective for you and for your partner.

SEX AND AGING

Sexuality, including intercourse, continues to be a pleasurable and important part of life for many people into very old age. A survey of 4,000 U.S. adults conducted by Consumers Union found that 65% of women and 79% of men age 70 and over were sexually active, including about half of the people in the age 80 and over group (4).

Aging does, however, bring noticeable change in sexual functioning for most people, and may add problems related to medical illness. For women, menopause is a fairly clear transition point. Menopause occurs at about age 51, and brings abrupt hormone changes that are likely to impact physical responses to sexual stimulation. For men, the transition is less precisely defined, but gradual alterations in sexual responses for men are also likely to begin at about age 50.

Men are likely to notice a longer refractory time after orgasm (reported by 65% of men over 50 in the Consumers' survey), a longer time for erection to occur (50%), lessened stiffness with full erection (44%), and more frequent loss of erection during sex (32%). Precisely how or why these changes occur is not known; they may reflect normal aging changes in the nervous system or vascular system. The net effect for some couples is quite positive. More time and more direct physical stimulation may be necessary for intercourse and orgasm, and problems with rapid ejaculation may be diminished.

For women, hormone production by the ovaries drops significantly after menopause. Estrogen levels remain low unless the woman is taking hormone medication, and physical changes in the vulva and vagina are likely to result (see Chapter 34). Without estrogen, the tissues of the vaginal lips and vaginal lining become thinner and more delicate, and the woman's lubrication response may be less profuse and/or slower. The vagina may shrink somewhat in overall size, and its elasticity may be diminished. These changes may make intercourse less comfortable, or necessitate use of supplementary lubrication (see the "Inadequate Vaginal Lubrication" section near the end of this chapter). Hormones may also affect sex drive for some women, although the links are not precisely known. About one third of women report a diminished interest in sex after menopause, and this is also a fairly common complaint (25% to 45% in various studies) after hysterectomy surgery, especially when the ovaries have been removed as well as the uterus (5).

Normal ovaries produce the female hormones estrogen and progesterone, and small amounts of male hormones (androgens) as well. Hormone production continues to some extent even after menopause, and the male hormone component actually increases slightly. One effect of male hormones is to increase sex drive for both men and women, and this may explain why some women experience an increase in sexual desire after menopause rather than a decrease.

Partner problems are also likely to affect both women and men as they age. Medical problems for one partner cannot help but impact the other partner, and sexual changes as well impact both.

Common Sexual Problems

You are a very unusual person if you have never experienced a sex problem of any kind: problems are quite universal. Many of the problems described below are temporary and resolve spontaneously. You may already have a good idea about the cause of a problem yourself. Success in overcoming even simple sexual problems will probably require recognition of the problems and their likely causes, discussion with your partner, and mutual commitment to making the changes necessary. If you are suffering, or are having difficulty making changes, then by all means ask for help. Talking to your clinician is entirely appropriate; she/he may be able to help you directly or may refer you to a qualified counselor or sex therapist. This is especially important if you are concerned or feel uncertain about possible medical causes for a sexual problem.

Successful treatment of persistent problems usually involves education about the physical aspects of sexual functioning, development of sexual skills, and help with communication between partners, as well as some reassessment of reasonable expectations, of personal attitudes, and of the emotional environment of sexual functioning.

This discussion is intended only as a brief overview of common problems; the causes and cures for persistent sexual disorders are not as simple and clear-cut as these brief descriptions might imply. Often there are multiple causes, and problems often occur in combination. Relationship conflicts and psychological issues may be involved as well; therefore, your therapist must be able to recognize and deal at least to some extent with emotional and interpersonal factors, as well as the specific sexual problem.

DIMINISHED SEXUAL DESIRE

Many people worry about having too little interest in sex. Since people vary so greatly in what is for them an ideal amount of sexual activity, it is not hard to understand why so many couples feel that they are mismatched. Compromise is necessary in almost every partner relationship.

Diminished interest in sexual expression may simply reflect a stressful personal time in general. Unresolved relationship conflict, serious personal problems, fatigue, intense involvement in school or work, illness or surgery, and fear of pregnancy are common underlying factors. Pain during intercourse or repeatedly frustrating sexual experiences may also result in diminished sexual interest. In some cases, medications are a factor; for example, birth control Pills, tranquilizers, antihypertensive agents, and sedatives may directly alter sexual interest for some people.

If diminished sex drive is the result of an unrelated problem or a side effect of medicines, then initial treatment efforts should start with the underlying problem itself. If unresolved relationship conflict is a factor, you may need professional help to learn to improve communication and resolve conflict.

For most people, sexual interest is also strongly influenced by factors within the realm of voluntary, conscious control: sex requires time, energy, and an appropriate physical and emotional setting. Sexuality is not something that can be taken for granted. Like everything else, it requires planning and attention. If a busy lifestyle allows no opportunity for thinking about satisfying sexual experiences in the past, sexual fantasies, and the emotionally positive aspects of your relationship with your partner, then your interest in sexual expression may be diminished. You may find, for example, that your sexual functioning improves dramatically while you are on vacation.

To overcome this problem, and other sexual problems as well, you will probably need to change your normal life routine to allow for more privacy, more relaxed time with your partner, and less physical fatigue. Mental fatigue as well may be an important factor. You may need to find a better balance between work and the other essential ingredients in life such as vigorous physical exercise and activities that emphasize the creative and spiritual parts of yourself.

Remember too that making changes is a very difficult and slow process. Start with something specific, realistic, and small. For example, you might decide on an exercise class twice a week for two months, or two Tuesday nights each month set aside for "date" time alone with your partner. You may be amazed to see how much difference one small change can make.

Fatigue and Preoccupation. Fatigue and preoccupation are very common causes of sexual problems. Sexual functioning requires physical and mental energy. Fatigue blunts your ability to be receptive to stimulation. You may feel numb, and find that strong, prolonged stimulation is necessary to achieve a level of sexual arousal that seems effortless at other times. Fatigue may also interfere with your ability to be receptive to sexual thoughts, and may therefore diminish the likelihood of establishing even an initial level of sexual tension. You may perceive this as a decrease in sex drive or interest in sex.

I really love my husband, and I like to have sex with him, but somehow it's just not like it used to be. I'm tired a lot of the time, and I
worry a lot about the children, bills, and my work. . . . And me—I don't
think I'm as sexy as I used to be. When we start to make love, my
mind often wanders off on a hundred different things, and Bob just gets
discouraged and says he is tired of trying to make me turn on.

—WOMAN, 27

Occasional fatigue is a normal and inevitable part of a busy human life. Constant
fatigue, however, can be a danger sign that changes are needed. Overcoming fatigue is
likely to necessitate some reassessments:

• Are the priorities in your life for work, family, and personal growth receiving their
  fair shares of your time?
• Are you able to include vigorous exercise as a routine part of life at least three or
  four times each week?
• Do you need to change your expectations for yourself or for your partner?
• Do you need to find ways to reduce your workload? Could other members of the
  family help? Could you hire someone to help? Would you and your family be better
  off with a little more dust but more personal energy?

Preoccupation with problems or other nonsexual thoughts may block receptivity to
initial sexual stimuli, reducing both your interest in sex and your ability to respond to
sexual stimulation.

Sometimes preoccupation is a symptom of other problems altogether. A serious
relationship strain, for example, or unresolved conflicts may make it impossible for one
or both partners to focus attention on positive sexual thoughts. Another common
problem is time. For some people, transition from normal daily activities to a focus on
sexuality is much easier with an hour or two of relaxed time to unwind and let go of
distracting thoughts.

Relationship Problems.   Strains or imbalances in the relationship between partners
are among the most common causes of diminished sexual desire and/or responsiveness. Emotions like anger, fear, resentment, hostility, and disappointment are quite
likely to block receptivity to the idea of sexual interaction, and may block responses to
stimulation that would lead to sexual excitation in other circumstances. Refusing to be
open to sexual response may be a sign that one partner feels less valued or powerful in
the relationship and has no other effective tools to regain equality (6). Counseling in
this situation is most likely to be helpful if underlying relationship issues can be
identified, and communication skills improved. Work on sexual techniques is not likely
to be effective.

Differences between partners in the meaning sexuality has for them may also be a source of strain. Differences are inevitable, at least at some times. One partner, for example, may desire sexual expression most at times of tension and insecurity, to gain reassurance and comfort from intimacy. If sexuality for the other partner is most desirable when the relationship feels strong and loving, their needs may not jibe. Timing and the overall emotional atmosphere will be off for one partner or the other much of the time, and one or both partners may find that interest in sexuality is diminished.

Pregnancy and Childrearing. Many couples find that sexual function is at least temporarily altered by pregnancy and childbirth. Profound physical and hormone changes during pregnancy, as well as psychological changes in preparation for parenthood, may necessitate adjustments in sexual functioning as well. In the first weeks after delivery, estrogen and progesterone levels are low, and vaginal lubrication is diminished because of the low hormone levels. Many women find intercourse uncomfortable in the first weeks or months after childbirth. An episiotomy incision (requiring stitches at the bottom of the vagina) heals in about two or three weeks, but the area may remain sensitive to stretching or pressure for many weeks or months after that. Also, your genital structure itself (the size and length of your vagina, your genital muscle tone, and the position of your cervix) can be permanently altered to some degree by full term pregnancy. Time, experimentation, and patience may be required for you and your partner to find intercourse positions and patterns that give you effective stimulation without discomfort.

In addition, life for both mother and father is dramatically altered by the presence of a newborn infant. Caring for a baby requires countless hours of work and involves a great deal of intimate physical contact. The new mother's need for rest, personal privacy, and time for herself alone may be more pressing than her sexual needs, and this is entirely normal. Many couples find that their previous sexual patterns are not compatible with the baby's sleeping and waking schedule, and many are acutely aware of their loss of privacy as a couple. **Time away from the responsibilities of parenthood is essential.** Many mothers are reluctant to leave a 3-week-old baby with a sitter, even for short periods, but experienced mothers almost always recall the decision to have a sitter as an essential first step back to normal life. And returning to patterns of sexual activity more like their prepregnancy life is likely to require a conscious decision by the couple and intentional steps to achieve it. Nursing mothers find that allowing for one or two bottle feedings each week, to give them time away from the baby, does not interfere with nursing once breast milk flow is well established during the first two or three weeks.

Raising young children, too, is an emotionally draining and often exhausting enterprise. Mothers, and fathers as well, may find that sexual activity takes a lower priority in their lives, so the issues of diminished sexual desire may persist long after the infancy stage of childrearing.

Any woman who is pregnant or has preschool children at home should be presumed to have chronic fatigue until proven otherwise.

—SEX THERAPIST

Fertility Issues.   Sexual problems often arise when couples are anxious to conceive, especially if they suspect that they have a fertility problem or if fertility treatment is already under way. Both partners may find that the pressure to have intercourse at specific scheduled times blocks their normal sexual responsiveness and interferes with arousal, orgasm, or both.

Some couples find that a joint decision to take a vacation from trying to conceive is helpful. One or two months with no calendar records, no temperature charts, and no medical visits may help, but fertility stresses are often very severe. A chance to talk about fears, frustrations, and personal hurt is also important, so support from friends or a couples' group may be good choices. Counseling, too, is a reasonable idea, especially if fertility problems are adding to resentments or conflicts between partners.

Fear of unplanned pregnancy may also cause sexual problems for both men and women. Confidence in the high level of birth control protection afforded by birth control Pills may be one reason that many women and/or their partners experience increased sexual interest and responsiveness when they use this method of contraception. Similarly, some couples report increased sex drive and responsiveness after vasectomy or tubal ligation, procedures that do not alter hormone patterns but do provide extremely effective, permanent protection from pregnancy.

Aversion to Sexual Activity.   Aversion or distaste for any form of genital exploration is an uncommon but distressing problem. Some women and men feel unable even to touch their external genital structures, and a woman may have prolonged spasm contraction of all the genital muscles (vaginismus) when any form of vaginal penetration is attempted. As extreme as this condition seems, treatment is often dramatically effective. Treatment for the problem includes careful education and conditioning exercises that help the woman or man acclimate gradually to genital touching and to vaginal penetration.

Less dramatic forms of aversion may also occur as a result of intense anger or hostility originating from relationship problems or from negative conditioning. Sexual experiences that are physically or emotionally painful can lead to avoidance or even aversion.

INABILITY TO ACHIEVE ORGASM

Preorgasmia is very common among women and much less common among men. Women with this problem often are able to experience arousal and may achieve the physical responses of the excitement phase or even the plateau phase, but they do not have orgasm. Sex experts use the term **preorgasmia** because treatment is successful for more than 90% of women who seek treatment. Often only a few weeks of therapy are required. It is such a common problem that relatively inexpensive group treatment is available in many parts of the country. Often women undertake therapy alone without involving their partners, at least during the initial phases of treatment.

In most cases, the treatment needed for preorgasmia is education. Many women simply never have had an opportunity to learn what kinds of emotional, mental, and physical sensations are sexually pleasurable and effective for them. Treatment includes thorough education about female reproductive organs and physical sexual responses. Women learn through self-exploration about their own responses to a range of physical sensations, and they learn to develop **patterns** for effective stimulation.

In some cases, a woman who has been successful in achieving orgasm through masturbation finds that the transition to orgasm with a partner is no problem. Many times, however, this transition involves education for the partner as well, and joint therapy may be needed to improve communication between partners.

It's really funny. For years I've been faking orgasms, and Harry never knew. Now I know how to have orgasms, and I know our techniques are all wrong. I can't decide whether to tell him it's all been fake, and how I really need to be handled, or just forget the whole thing. He may be hurt, whichever I do.

—WOMAN, 34

A woman who has been orgasmic on only rare occasions or who has been orgasmic in the past but then develops lingering problems with orgasm may benefit from the education and training in skills that have been designed for preorgasmic women. Her problems, however, may be more similar to the vicious cycle of **performance anxiety** that is characteristic of a man's inability to achieve or maintain an erection.

INABILITY TO ACHIEVE OR MAINTAIN ERECTION

For men, difficulty in achieving erection is much more common than difficulty in achieving orgasm. Erection is the first physical event in the excitement phase for men.

Erection is a nonvoluntary response. When sexual activity begins, a man cannot help but notice whether erection is occurring. If it is not, then **anxiety** is an almost universal reaction. Performance anxiety itself and the distraction it causes can create an unrelenting vicious cycle.

A man or woman who is worrying about sexual failure is unable to focus attention on sexual stimuli, and he or she is therefore unable to be receptive to stimulation that might otherwise be extremely pleasurable and effective. Treatment for this problem involves exercises designed to help the person **interrupt** the performance anxiety cycle. The man or woman needs an opportunity to learn to enjoy and lose himself or herself in sensory experiences. This may be possible only when performance is out of the picture and the person is free to be a participant, rather than a spectator who is watching and evaluating performance. The term Masters and Johnson use for sensory enjoyment that is free of the need to perform is **sensate focus**. With agreement in advance that intercourse is not a goal, nor is orgasm, a leisurely backrub or foot massage would be examples of sensate focus activities. In many cases, men (and women) find that their own, natural, automatic physical arousal responses resume when they are able to be receptive to sensory experiences through sensate focus.

Erection problems may also occur because of medical problems (see below), medications, and drugs. Alcohol in small doses may enhance **interest** in sexual activity, but is also a common cause of impaired responsiveness. Its effects are not unlike the effects of fatigue: overall sensitivity to effective stimulation may be reduced so that more intense and prolonged stimulus is required for arousal, or arousal is blocked altogether. Illicit drugs, too, may profoundly reduce sexual responsiveness. Marijuana reduces testosterone (male hormone) production with chronic use, and testosterone influences both sex drive and responsiveness.

For some men, erection problems occur as the most obvious sign of more subtle issues like diminished sexual desire or relationship difficulties. The couple may not be aware of the underlying strains, but absence of erection is unmistakable. Depression and fatigue are very common culprits, as well as unrecognized anger or resentment.

It is entirely normal for a man to have occasional times when erection is difficult or impossible; this is a universal problem and it is also normal to find these occasions anxiety-provoking. Some anxiety is likely to carry over to the next sexual encounter as well. Taking extra time and effort to be sure that factors like distraction, fatigue, and alcohol are minimized is a good first step. If erection problems persist more than a month or two, or are causing suffering, however, it makes sense to seek help early. Repeated frustrating experiences may add to the problem.

RAPID (PREMATURE) EJACULATION

There is no clear-cut definition of rapid ejaculation. In rare cases, control is so limited that ejaculation occurs as soon as 30 to 60 seconds after erection or immediately after the penis enters the vagina. More commonly, men have some ejaculatory control but ejaculate long before they are ready to and have difficulty delaying ejaculation long enough for their partner to achieve orgasm during intercourse. Ejaculatory control can almost always be improved by simple approaches such as the pause technique or the squeeze technique. With the pause, or stop–start, technique the couple simply pauses for a little while when the man feels excitation building toward orgasm. The squeeze technique utilizes firm pressure on the tip of the man's penis to reduce the sexual tension level. The man signals to his partner when a squeeze is needed, but after a brief period of time most men are able to control ejaculation themselves, and only need to rely on this maneuver from time to time in special situations.

Trying harder on your own is unlikely to be successful with this problem, and learning to use the techniques described above is not as simple as it might sound. It makes sense to get help. Success rates for short-term treatment specifically designed to improve control are very high.

MEDICAL AND GYNECOLOGIC PROBLEMS

It is especially important to discuss sex with your clinician when you or your partner has had a serious illness or surgery that temporarily interrupts sexual activity. You will need to learn from your clinician what is an appropriate convalescent period, when it is safe to resume normal sexual activity, and whether there are any particular precautions you need to observe. Your clinician may also be able to suggest specific sexual techniques to minimize discomfort or stress during the recovery period.

Medical problems and surgery can cause sexual problems, or aggravate problems already existing. In some cases specific medical treatment, or a change in medications, may be of help. In other cases the couple may need to make changes in their own sexual patterns to help accommodate to changes caused by the problem situation.

Sexual problems are common after surgery or after illness that affects the reproductive organs. A woman who has had breast surgery or hysterectomy may need to adjust psychologically to illness, to the change in her body image, and also to the physical changes in her sensory perceptions. Similarly, some kinds of prostate surgery can damage nerve pathways essential for a man's sexual responsiveness and can have a psychological impact as well.

Medical problems unrelated to the reproductive organs can sometimes cause sexual problems. Pain, fatigue, worry, or just preoccupation with a serious medical illness or impending surgery can alter sexual interest and responsiveness. Diabetes may cause sexual problems, possibly through alteration in sensory nerve responses. Men and women recovering from major surgery or heart attack may be fearful of the stress of sexual activity. Nervous system disabilities or other chronic physical disabilities may pose unique problems and you may need specialized help to understand the limits of the problem and techniques possible for dealing with it.

Medical problems, however, do not need to mean an end to sexuality. Even severe problems, such as erection impairment caused by circulatory disease or the nerve damage of diabetes, can often be ameliorated or even corrected by treatment. Medical causes of erection difficulty, sometimes called "organic" causes, are now recognized as a quite common reason for erection problems; treatment with medication, or a change in the drugs needed for your medical problem, may help, and sophisticated surgical techniques that utilize controllable erection implants may be a possibility.

Sexual functioning does not necessarily require physically strenuous activity, and it is very unlikely that sex would lead to a heart attack or stroke even if the person did have heart disease or a serious medical problem like high blood pressure. It is entirely appropriate to talk with your clinician about sexual activity if you or your partner has such a problem. Your clinician should give you specific, detailed guidelines including precautions or warning signs and when and what kind of sexual activity would be safe. In general, sexual intercourse requires about the same physical reserve as walking up one flight of stairs. In some cases it may even be possible to adjust the timing of drug treatment, such as medication for chest pain, so that you have the benefit of maximum drug effect at the time you anticipate intercourse.

Birth Control. Birth control methods may have a direct effect on sexual functioning, or an indirect effect through increased or diminished fear of pregnancy. Women using birth control Pills may have diminished sexual interest and responsiveness, probably a direct hormone effect in some cases, or they may have heightened sexual functioning, possibly because of a hormone effect and possibly because of diminished fear of pregnancy. If diminished desire is a problem, changing to a different Pill brand may be helpful (see Chapter 13). An IUD may result in improved sexual functioning for some women, and for others cause problems; the IUD provides continuous protection with no need for paraphernalia or interruptions in lovemaking, but it can also cause prolonged vaginal bleeding and/or discomfort during intercourse. Some couples have no difficulty integrating a diaphragm, contraceptive foam, or condoms into comfortable sexual patterns, but others find them intrusive. Couples who use natural family planning may find that sexual responsiveness is heightened by the long periods of abstinence required, or they may develop problems with **performance pressure**, similar to those experienced by couples who are trying to conceive.

Inadequate Vaginal Lubrication. Inadequate vaginal lubrication is a very common problem among women. Often the problem is simply a result of beginning intercourse before the physical changes of the excitement phase have had a chance to occur. A little more time devoted to sexual arousal and some attention to improving techniques for effective stimulation may solve the problem. Inadequate lubrication is also very likely to be a problem if intercourse is attempted despite lack of desire or arousal on the woman's part.

Some women notice that their lubrication response varies during the normal hormone cycle, and many find that using a water-soluble lubricant such as K-Y Jelly is helpful the first few days after a menstrual period when hormone levels are low and vaginal moisture tends to be scant. Vaginal dryness may be particularly troublesome if you have intercourse immediately after removing a vaginal tampon. A woman using decongestant cold medications may notice diminished vaginal lubrication along with the dryness in her nose and mouth.

Persistent problems with vaginal dryness are also common after menopause. When estrogen hormone levels are low, the vaginal lining becomes thinner and less resilient, and its ability to produce lubrication may be diminished. Treatment with hormones by mouth or in vaginal cream and/or use of vaginal lubricants are usually quite helpful (see Chapter 34).

Pain During or After Intercourse.　　Discomfort or pain during or after intercourse often leads to diminished interest in sexual activity and to problems with sexual performance. Inadequate vaginal lubrication can result in genital and vaginal irritation, and painful symptoms of vaginal infection are often greatly aggravated by intercourse. Abdominal or pelvic pain during or after intercourse has many causes. These problems are discussed in Chapter 40.

Finding the cause of pain is an essential first step; in most cases the cause is an identifiable gynecologic problem. Treatment therefore depends on the problem. Understanding the source of pain, though, may also help and in some cases a change in intercourse position or use of extra lubrication may reduce pain. When pain has been a problem, it may help to have the woman take responsibility for timing insertion of the penis, and also the depth of thrusting.

Some women experience genital and lower abdominal discomfort when they are sexually aroused but do not have orgasm; if orgasm does not occur, the blood vessel engorgement of the inner and outer lips, vaginal walls, and uterus may be maintained for several hours. Discomfort caused by prolonged congestion can be immediately relieved by orgasm, either through intercourse or masturbation. Prolonged sexual arousal without ejaculation can cause similar discomfort for men.

Clitoral Adhesions.　　Clitoral adhesions, strands of scar tissue between the clitoris and its hood, can cause pain during intercourse. Also, some experts believe that full mobility of the clitoral hood is important for optimal stimulation of the clitoris. Clitoral adhesions, however, are uncommon, and many women who have them have no problem with sexual responsiveness.

Finding Help for a Sexual Problem

Your clinician may be a good person to see when you decide to tackle a sexual problem. Some gynecologists and family physicians have special interest and training in this area and can provide sex therapy themselves. Many clinicians, however, choose to refer their patients to a specialist in sexual problems if it appears that more than brief counseling will be required. If you do not feel comfortable about discussing a sexual problem with your clinician or if your clinician is uncomfortable or unable to recommend a resource for therapy, then you might get in touch with a local family service agency, Planned Parenthood, or community mental health center for the names of reputable, experienced sex therapists.

Professionals working in the field have varied backgrounds, and professional degrees may include psychology, psychiatry, social work, and others. You may not find it easy to select a therapist, but the effort to ascertain her or his professional reputation in your community is important. You will want to work with someone who is competent.

Sex therapy involves learning and personal change, but it does not mean abandoning your moral principles or becoming sexually indiscriminate. **Reputable sex therapy does not include the therapist as a sex partner or sex object.** If you think your therapist may be taking advantage of you or that therapy techniques are inappropriate, then respect your own instincts. You are probably right.

Your therapy will begin with a thorough sexual history. You will be asked to describe the problems you are experiencing, and your therapist will also need to understand your past sexual functioning and any medical and social factors that might be related to the problem. You and your therapist can decide whether both partners should participate in all your sessions, some of the sessions, or not at all. Many therapists prefer to have both partners involved from the beginning, with individual sessions for each of the partners perhaps once or twice during the entire treatment. Therapy sessions consist of discussion and education. Sexual activity is reserved for "homework" assignments. Some therapy programs involve whole blocks of time, such as the two-week, full-time program that Masters and Johnson have developed. Most, however, require only weekly sessions of an hour or two.

SUGGESTED READING

Barbach, Lonnie: *For Each Other*. New York: New American Library, 1984. Comprehensive, wise, and clear guidelines for assessing both relationship problems and technique problems that may affect sexual response. Exercises to help overcome common problems are also described.

Barbach, Lonnie: *For Yourself*. Garden City, N.Y.: Anchor Press, 1976. This easy-to-understand book is an excellent starting place for preorgasmic women.

Bing, Elisabeth, and Colman, Libby: *Making Love During Pregnancy*. New York: Bantam Books, 1977. A reassuring and helpful book for couples adjusting to pregnancy.

Brecher, Edward M., and the Editors of Consumer Reports Books: *Love, Sex and Aging.* Mount Vernon: Consumers Union, 1984. A fascinating and inspiring survey of sexuality among fully adult adults.

Heiman, Julie, LoPiccolo, Joseph, LoPiccolo, Leslie: *Becoming Orgasmic—A Sexual Growth Program for Women.* New York: Prentice Hall, 1976. Another excellent book for preorgasmic women, written in a slightly more technical style.

Offit, Avodah K.: *The Sexual Self* (revised edition). New York: Congdon & Weed, 1983. Sexual issues in the context of human personality. A sensitive and truly insightful book.

REFERENCES

1. Masters WH, Johnson VE: *Human Sexual Response.* Boston: Little, Brown, 1966.
2. Weisberg M: Physiology of female sexual function. *Clinical Obstetrics and Gynecology* 27:697–705, 1984.
3. Kaplan HS: *The New Sex Therapy.* New York: Brunner/Mazel, 1974.
4. Brecher EM, Editors of Consumer Reports Books: *Love, Sex and Aging.* Mount Vernon: Consumers Union, 1984.
5. Cutler WB, Garcia C-R, Edwards DA: *Menopause. A Guide for Women and the Men Who Love Them.* New York: W.W. Norton & Co., 1983.
6. LaFerla JJ: Inhibited sexual desire and orgasmic dysfunction in women. *Clinical Obstetrics and Gynecology* 27:738–749, 1984.

44

❖

Rape

Rape is a violent crime of aggression that happens to resemble a sexual act. It is an assault on a person's whole being and leaves most people feeling vulnerable, naked, and powerless.

Being careful helps, of course, but careful behavior won't always prevent rape. As long as people express violent aggression in a sexual mode, we will be coping with the aftermath of rape.

The aftermath of rape is much like the grieving period after any profound experience of loss; the victim's sense of inviolable personhood may literally die. Most victims experience typical grieving emotions, such as denial, anger, and depression. With time, with good emotional support, and with access to competent counseling when it is needed, most victims can resolve rape and leave the experience in the past. "It took two years, but now I think I can stop being a rape victim," one woman said.

In this chapter, we refer to rape victims as women and to rapists as men because that is by far the most common situation. In prison settings, men frequently express dominance by raping other men, and women rapists are not unheard of. There is no intention to slight male victims, whose problems and needs are much the same as those female victims experience.

Most rape victims aren't seriously injured, because most rapists (about 85%) (1) are either armed or threaten to use physical force if the victim doesn't cooperate. Most women realize that arguing with a gun, a knife, or a person who outweighs her by 30 pounds or more is folly, so they submit, bargaining with rape in return for staying alive. Most victims feel lucky to be alive; it is common to feel numb and shocked, as you would after a brush with death of any kind.

If you don't know where to find help after rape, look in your telephone book or ask an operator for a 24-hour crisis line. In some cities, rape crisis centers have 24-hour telephone counselors of their own, and most cities have crisis lines operated by a community center, health department, or mental health association. Crisis line counselors can advise you about getting medical care and about the police procedures for reporting rape. They can discuss the pros and cons of prosecuting your attacker and help you through the court process if you decide to prosecute. Perhaps most important, they can talk with you about your emotional needs.

Medical Care for Rape Victims

It didn't hurt, and it didn't feel any different from any other pelvic exam. Maybe it took a couple of minutes longer. I was really tense about it, though. I was *afraid* it would hurt, and I really didn't want *another* strange man looking at me naked, you know? That already happened once tonight.

—WOMAN, 35

The medical examination for rape is essentially the same as a routine pelvic exam (see Chapter 3), with several additional procedures specifically relating to rape. **Make sure that you are examined by a clinician who is trained to handle rape evidence properly.** All potential physical evidence must be dealt with in a rigorous chain-of-custody procedure, signed into the safekeeping of a physician or police officer, and stored under lock and key.

Remember that rape is a legal term, not a medical diagnosis. If you notice that your clinician writes "alleged" or "possible" rape or sexual assault on your chart, it doesn't necessarily mean she/he doesn't believe you, only that she/he is paying careful attention to legal language.

If you have been **beaten or injured** in any way, your clinician will care for your injuries first. She/he will carefully record all injuries, including minor ones, in your medical record.

During your examination your clinician will collect a routine Pap smear specimen and ask the pathologist to examine the slide for **sperm cells.** She/he will also wash your cervix and vaginal walls with about a tablespoon of saline solution and then draw the fluid back up into a syringe. Part of the fluid sample can be tested for acid phosphatase, a chemical produced by the male prostate gland, and the remainder will be used for microscopic examination to detect sperm cells. Your clinician will record on your chart the number of sperm found and whether the sperm were moving.

These routine tests do not distinguish between an attacker's sperm and your partner's sperm, and they may show no sperm at all, although in fact you have been raped. Your attacker may not have ejaculated, or could possibly have used a condom or even be sterile. One important reason for having your exam promptly is that **evidence of sperm may disappear in eight to ten hours.**

Tests performed immediately after rape will not reveal whether you caught a sexually transmitted infection from your attacker. Your clinician will test you for infection anyway, and you must have your tests repeated in a week's time. The national Centers for Disease Control (CDC) recommends these procedures for detecting sexually transmitted infection that may be acquired from rape (2):

- Test for gonorrhea (cervical secretions)
- Test for chlamydia (cervical secretions)
- Microscope check for trichomonas (vaginal fluid)
- Test for syphilis (blood)
- Serum sample to be frozen and saved for future testing (blood)

Remember to have all these tests repeated in one week, with the exception of your blood test for syphilis. Wait six weeks before that test is repeated. Testing two to three months later for evidence of AIDS (acquired immunodeficiency syndrome) may be reasonable if your attacker was an intravenous drug user (3). The stored serum sample may be needed for testing later if there is any question of hepatitis exposure in your case. Tell the clinician who performs your initial and repeat exams if you were orally or anally raped; if so, she/he can collect specimens from your throat and/or rectum for testing and examine you carefully for evidence of other signs of infection. (The symptoms of and treatment for sexually transmitted infections are described in Chapters 22 to 29.)

According to the CDC, although the risk of infection after rape is unknown, it is thought to be low. If you and your clinician believe a course of antibiotics makes sense in your case, the treatment options recommended by the CDC are (2):

- Tetracycline, 500 mg four times a day for seven days **or**
- Doxycycline, 100 mg two times a day for seven days **or**
- Amoxicillin, 3.0 grams, or Ampicillin, 3.5 grams, given with 1.0 gram of probenecid as a single oral dose, for women who are **pregnant or allergic to tetracycline**

COLLECTION OF EVIDENCE

A thorough medical exam for rape includes a careful check for any substances on your body or your clothing that might be used as evidence. Some examples are:

- Dirt, blood, or grass stains on clothing
- Scrapings from under your fingernails, especially if you struggled with your attacker
- Pubic or scalp hair that looks different from your own, with samples of your hair for comparison
- Anything clinging to your hair or clothing that might be matched with the scene of your attack. You may be asked to leave your clothing with your clinician if she/he thinks it might be needed as evidence.
- Photographs of your body or clothing
- Scraped or blotted secretions from your skin that could be semen, saliva, blood, or other evidence

Douching, bathing, and tampons can all remove evidence of rape, so avoid them if possible until after you see a clinician. Samples should be collected during your exam in any case, however, and your clinician will take special precautions in labeling and storing them for possible future use as evidence (4).

ASSESSING YOUR PREGNANCY RISK

Most women who are raped are eager to be sure that pregnancy does not result from the attack, and a short regimen of emergency, "morning-after" birth control Pills is extremely effective for preventing pregnancy in such circumstances. The likelihood of conception after a single act of intercourse and your morning-after options are discussed in detail in Chapter 15. Your clinician can help you weigh the pros and cons in your case. **If you decide to use morning-after birth control, you must begin taking it within 72 hours after the rape, and the sooner the better.** You must not use morning-after Pills if you have a breast lump or unexplained vaginal bleeding, or if there is any chance you could already be pregnant.

Reporting Rape to the Police

In addition to arranging for medical care, you may also want to report your rape to the police. You can report the rape immediately and decide later whether you want to prosecute. If you do decide to prosecute, you'll have a stronger case if you have reported the rape promptly. Reporting rape only means giving the police a full account of what happened, what your attacker looked like, and all other details you can remember. Most rape specialists believe that it is advisable at least to report your rape. Prosecuting your attacker means that the police will try to arrest him so that he can be tried on your charges. **Whether or not you bring charges against your attacker is completely up to you.**

Recovering from Rape

Emotional reactions to rape can be profound, and many women find that professional counseling is extremely helpful, whether rape occurred three hours or three years ago.

Counselors who work with rape victims report that it is common for a woman to work through times of denial, anger, and/or depression before she can resolve the rape experience and put it to rest. Generally, rape triggers a disorganized, confused state in the beginning, followed by a lengthy, more organized period of emotional recovery (5).

> I went to work the next morning as usual and didn't tell *anybody* what happened. After three months I had broken up with my boyfriend and was practically becoming an alcoholic. I called the rape crisis center. I talked to them on the phone three or four times and finally figured out that it was never going to *go away* until I could admit it was *there*.
>
> —WOMAN, 23

It can be hard to admit you need help getting through a crisis, especially if you are an independent person. If you don't feel like talking to a friend, partner, or family member, try a rape crisis center, mental health clinic, psychologist, or psychiatrist.

> I started crying in class, and I couldn't stop. It was about two weeks after I was raped. I was so *tired* of being brave and strong and picking up the pieces and all that crap. I felt *sorry* for myself, by God, and I think I had a right to!
>
> —WOMAN, 19

Depression, fears, nightmares, and feelings of alienation and helplessness are common after a few days, or even months later—whenever the full impact of what has happened really hits you. Most women are acutely aware of a loss of control, and it is a terrifying feeling.

> About six weeks after they raped me, I started getting really mad at the whole world. I yelled at my secretary, my husband, and everybody else. My husband said, "Why don't you get mad at those punks who did it? I'm on your side, remember?"
>
> —WOMAN, 40

Counselors say that anger can often be a very good sign of healing, especially when it is directed—appropriately—at the rapist. Anger means that your internalized feelings are finding a way out. Try to channel your anger where it belongs; misdirected anger won't help you in the long run.

The day eventually comes, sooner or later, when you can stop being a rape victim. Emotional wounds do heal in time for most women. You can help yourself by relying on trusted family and friends and competent counselors to help you clarify your feelings. **Don't hesitate to get professional help** if your feelings are more than you can handle, even if it means long distance calls to a rape crisis center a hundred miles away.

It took me a long time to admit I couldn't get over it by myself. *Everybody* knew I needed help before I could admit to it myself! I started seeing a psychologist once a week, and I read some things she recommended. It was a relief to learn it was *normal* to check every closet twice a night, and *normal* to worry that he'd find me, even though we'd moved to a different apartment. I'll never forget it, that's for sure. But it no longer haunts me.

—WOMAN, 50

How Family and Friends Can Help

When someone you care about has been raped, you will want to help and support her. She will probably have a lot of powerful feelings she needs to express, so make sure she knows you are willing to listen. You can help her best if you know the facts about rape in general. There are many myths about rape ("no woman can be raped against her will," for example), and if you aren't certain about your own perceptions of rape, do some reading or get in touch with a rape crisis center for advice.

Rape affects you too, and you may have very distressing feelings of your own to sort out. You could feel angry or even guilty, as though her rape were somehow your fault. You may be uncertain about how to handle your own relationship with her, especially if the two of you are sexual partners. Make sure she knows you are willing to put her needs first during this difficult time. She could want and need sexual intimacy with you very much, or she may not be interested in sex at all. Talk with her and ask her what will help her most. No one expects you to be a professional therapist, so don't hesitate to seek help from a rape crisis center or a mental health center when you need it.

SUGGESTED READING

Grossman, Rochel; and Sutherland, Joan (eds.); *Surviving Sexual Assault.* New York: Congdon & Weed, 1983.

REFERENCES

1. Brownmiller S: *Against Our Will: Men, Women and Rape.* New York: Simon & Schuster, 1975.
2. Centers for Disease Control: 1985 STD treatment guidelines. *Morbidity and Mortality Weekly Report, Supplement.* Vol 34, No 4S, October 18, 1985.
3. Glaser JB, Hammerschlag MR, McCormack WM: Correspondence: Sexually transmitted disease in victims of sexual assault. *New England Journal of Medicine* 316:1023–1025, 1987.
4. Sexual assault. *ACOG Technical Bulletin,* No 101, February 1987.
5. Burgess AW: Rape trauma syndrome: A nursing diagnosis. *Occupational Health Nursing* 33:405–406, 1985.

45

❖

Basic Facts About Surgery

Don't be surprised if you feel anxious or even fearful when your clinician recommends surgery. These feelings are common and normal. Most people find that a detailed understanding of their particular health problem, and of the treatment possibilities involved, helps relieve anxiety. It is usually easier to cope with specific fears based on clear information about possible risks and complications than it is to ease the fear of something unknown. You may feel genuinely relieved after your clinician has reviewed the worst possibilities with you in detail.

Before you make a decision about surgery, it is essential for you to know what all your options are, both surgical and nonsurgical. You need to know enough about each option so that you can weigh all of them rationally. Be sure you understand, for each option, the likely benefits that you can expect, the precise procedure or treatment proposed, the possible complications that might occur immediately or later on, and what follow-up treatment, if any, you will need.

Once your decision is made, you will probably find the whole surgery process easier if you understand in advance exactly what will happen. Even pain is easier to bear if you know what is causing it, how it can be treated, and how long it will last.

A clear understanding of your problem and of your treatment is also important for your future medical care. You may want to write down the details of your surgery so you will be able to report them accurately to clinicians caring for you in the future. It may be hard to remember ten years after surgery whether your right or your left ovary was the problem, exactly what was removed, or what the technical name for your cyst was. Your surgeon should be able to give you a copy of your surgical record and the pathologist's report to keep in your personal health files.

Deciding About
Surgery—Informed Consent

As soon as she said "I think your uterus should come out," this wave of fear washed over me, even though I half expected her to say that. Now, 48 hours later, I'm a little less afraid and I am getting used to the idea of surgery, but I do feel scared and depressed. I feel . . . old. But I know she's right. I said yes without any hesitation.

—WOMAN, 43

Deciding whether or not to have surgery is your decision, and no one else's. Your clinician will help you evaluate your options and will probably give you her/his clear recommendations, but you yourself are the one who must make the decision. No matter what kind of surgery your clinician has recommended, you will probably have many questions, not only about your specific medical problem and the surgery you are considering, but also about hospital procedures, anesthesia, and how to plan for your recovery after surgery. You will give proof of your understanding and of your decision to have surgery by signing your surgical consent form. It is your right to have a full explanation and to have all your questions answered before you give your consent. It is your surgeon's responsibility to be sure you have the information you need in order to give informed consent. The components of informed consent are:

- A detailed understanding of the recommended surgery. You need to know what the goal of surgery is and exactly what will be removed or done.
- An understanding of all other treatment options (if any) in your situation, and what would happen if you did not have surgery
- An understanding of possible complications with surgery and with any other possible treatment options. You need to know about serious risks even if they are very rare, and about all common minor risks.
- An understanding of the benefits you can reasonably expect with surgery and with other treatment options as well

Your responsibility in assuring that your consent to surgery is truly informed is to ask questions. Your clinician can't read your mind! You must ask—and keep asking— until you understand the answers, no matter how busy your clinician seems to be.

(And by all means ask about costs if you want to know.) Remember that you have the right to change your mind any time before surgery.

It is entirely appropriate to ask about success rates for the surgery proposed, and your surgeon's experience with the procedure. Percentage figures may be helpful. For people with your diagnosis how often does surgery succeed? How often does it fail? How many patients experience minor or serious complications with the procedure? What is the risk of death, and is your risk lower or higher than average?

Complication rates and risks are likely to be lowest if your surgeon has experience with the specific surgical procedure planned, and performs it frequently. You can ask how many times she/he has performed this operation, and how many times in the last year. If the answer is less than 10 or 20, then finding a more experienced surgeon may be wise.

Surgery is the best alternative for many problems discussed in this book, either to confirm a diagnosis or to treat your problem. Nevertheless, any surgery, and especially major surgery, has the potential for serious complications and even death. You will certainly want to make your decision carefully.

The following suggestions on how to **avoid unnecessary surgery** are summarized and adapted from Herbert S. Dennenberg's "A Shopper's Guide to Surgery: Fourteen Rules on How to Avoid Unnecessary Surgery"(1).

1. **Go first to your primary care clinician; ideally, your internist or family doctor.** Your own doctor may be able to treat you without surgery in many cases.

2. **Make sure that your surgeon is board certified and a Fellow of the American College of Surgeons or the American College of Obstetricians and Gynecologists.** These organizations certify your physician's competence as a surgeon by oral, written, and clinical examinations. An appointment on the faculty of a medical school may also be an indication of competence. You can check at a large public library or a medical library in the *Directory of Medical Specialists* for information on where your surgeon went to medical school and had specialty training. When you are selecting a surgeon, ask for at least two names from your primary care physician. Friends, other doctors or nurses (possibly an operating room nurse), or organizations such as the National Organization for Women or Planned Parenthood may also be able to recommend specific surgeons. **Talk to your surgeon.** You must have confidence in her or him. If you do not, find another surgeon.

3. **Get a second opinion from another clinician or surgeon before you agree to major surgery.** A second opinion from an independent source (rather than your surgeon's office partner, for example) may reveal other treatment options or clarify questions for you. Reputable, competent surgeons are always comfortable about a second opinion. If your surgeon seems unwilling for you to seek a second opinion, you may want to consider finding another surgeon. Be sure that you have a clear idea from

your first surgeon about the urgency of the proposed surgery; you need to know how much time you have to get a second opinion.

4. **Make sure that your surgery is performed in an accredited hospital.** A list of accredited hospitals in your area is available from the Joint Commission on Accreditation of Hospitals, 645 North Michigan Avenue, Chicago, Illinois 60611.

5. **Don't push a doctor to perform surgery.** If you insist on a surgical solution to your problem, you are quite likely to find a surgeon willing to go along with you, even if surgery is not needed.

6. **Make sure that you understand your consent forms completely before you sign them.**

7. **Make sure that your surgeon knows and is willing to work with your primary care clinician.** If you are over age 60, you may need an internist as well as a surgeon or gynecologist involved in your postoperative care. If your surgeon belongs to a medical group that includes an internist, it may be easier to involve other specialists in your postoperative care if needed. Make sure that you know any other physicians your surgeon works with for night coverage.

8. **Select a surgeon who is not too busy to give you enough time and attention.** Good surgeons are busy, but they should answer all your questions and take the time to oversee your care before and after surgery.

9. **Be especially thoughtful if your surgeon recommends hysterectomy, hemorrhoidectomy, or tonsillectomy and adenoidectomy (T&A).** These are often cited as the most common unnecessary operations. Be certain that you understand whether your surgeon believes your operation is **necessary** or whether it is **elective**. Remember that except for cancer, uncontrollable infection, and uncontrollable hemorrhage, surgery is almost always elective rather than medically essential. Elective surgery may be desirable and in your best interest (hernia repair, for example); but unjustifiable, unnecessary surgery does occur. Be wary of a surgeon who seems to be pressuring you into elective surgery. Take the time to think it over, talk with your family and friends, obtain another opinion, and do some reading.

10. **You are entitled to make the final decision about surgery.** Don't let anyone else make the decision for you.

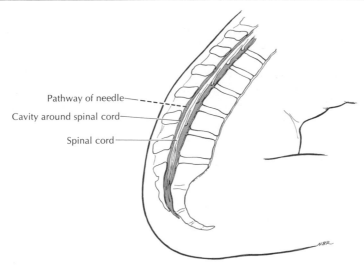

ILLUSTRATION 45-1 Pathway of spinal anesthesia injection. Anesthetic enters the space that surrounds the spinal cord.

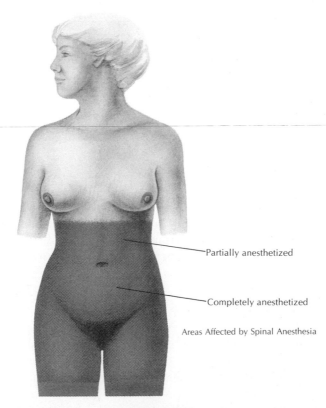

ILLUSTRATION 45-2 Areas anesthetized by spinal injection.

Anesthesia

Local anesthesia is often sufficient for minor surgical procedures that are short and technically simple. An anesthetic drug (similar to dental Novocain) injected into the surgical site blocks pain nerves in the area for about 30 to 60 minutes. Adverse reactions to local anesthesia are rare. Rash, hives, swelling, or asthma symptoms can occur because of allergy, and fatal allergic reactions are possible but are extremely rare. Local anesthetics can also cause heart rhythm changes, seizures, stroke, or even heart arrest if large or repeated doses are used. Local anesthesia is not recommended for long procedures that would require repeated injections of anesthetic drug, or when anesthesia of an extensive body area is needed.

General anesthesia is a term that includes both the many different techniques that produce sleep and regional anesthesia that produces a complete nerve block in large areas of the body.

Regional techniques such as **spinal, epidural, or caudal block** anesthesia are commonly used for full term delivery and for relatively minor surgical procedures. An anesthetic is injected into space surrounding the spinal cord (see Illustration 45-1) or in the area of a major nerve. The anesthetic drug blocks all nerve messages from the area supplied by that nerve, making a large portion of the body numb. If you have spinal anesthesia, for example, the entire lower half of your body, including your legs and feet, will be temporarily numb and paralyzed (see Illustration 45-2). You will be fully conscious and alert during regional anesthesia surgery. You may be given a sedative so that you won't be anxious or bothered by any discomfort that does occur. Regional anesthesia is most effective for blocking pain from superficial tissues such as skin and muscle, and to some degree it also diminishes pain sensations from pelvic organs inside the abdomen.

Headache is the most common side effect with spinal anesthesia. It is less likely to occur if anesthesia is administered by an experienced anesthesiologist who uses a small needle to inject the drug, but headaches can be severe enough to delay discharge from the hospital and may persist for as long as two weeks. Injury or infection that damages the spinal cord could cause permanent paralysis, but is extremely rare. It is important that your anesthesiologist watch you carefully until the regional anesthesia effects have worn off, for muscle relaxation in the anesthetized area can cause a sudden drop in blood pressure. Your blood pressure and heart rate will be checked frequently, and your anesthesiologist will use drugs to raise your blood pressure if it drops to a dangerous level.

General anesthesia to induce **anesthetic sleep** is usually recommended for major operations such as hysterectomy and can also be used for minor procedures such as D&C or abortion. Your anesthesiologist will use a combination of anesthesia drugs and gases to induce sleep and block pain sensations. An intravenous tube will be placed in your arm before surgery so that drugs can be administered. You may be given a mild sedative prior to surgery, along with a drug such as atropine to dry up mucus and saliva production. After you are in the operating room and lying on the operating table, your anesthesiologist will begin by recording your blood pressure and pulse, and connecting the monitoring equipment that will be used during surgery to detect any changes in your heart rhythm or pulse rate. To begin anesthesia, the anesthesiologist will probably inject a rapid-acting barbiturate such as Pentothal to induce sleep. Pentothal takes effect within seconds and produces sound sleep almost immediately. You will not be able to say more than one or two words before you fall asleep. After you are asleep, a tube will be placed through your mouth into your windpipe to insure a clear pathway for breathing. Anesthetic gas that you breathe along with oxygen will block pain sensations. The anesthesiologist may use muscle-paralyzing drugs to insure complete muscle relaxation, in which case the anesthesiologist will breathe **for you** by pumping oxygen and anesthesia gas from the anesthesia machine into your lungs. As your surgery is nearing completion, the anesthesiologist will stop the anesthetic gas, and you will be awake before you leave the operating room. You probably will not remember the operating room, however, and are more likely to remember waking up in the recovery room, where you will be under close observation for about two hours after surgery.

If anesthesia sleep is brief, as for a tubal ligation or D&C, for example, you will recover quickly from the anesthesia. Most women are fully awake, able to walk comfortably, and fairly alert within four hours after a tubal ligation or D&C. Anesthesia drugs do slow reflexes and impair coordination, however, so it is essential that you avoid driving or operating dangerous machinery for at least 24 hours after any general anesthesia.

Anesthesia sleep is less risky than you might imagine, but complications are possible. The overall death rate for complications of anesthesia is about 1 or 2 per 10,000 procedures (2). The risk of serious problems that could lead to permanent damage or death, such as stroke, heart arrest, or breathing arrest, is very low for young, healthy women and higher for older women or women with serious medical problems such as heart disease or emphysema.

Anesthesiologists use a standard classification system to evaluate risk for each patient. Table 45-1 shows definitions for each of the five anesthesia classes. The overall risk of death with surgery (including anesthesia) correlates with class and is about 5 times higher for a class 2 patient than it is for a class 1 patient, about 50 times higher for a class 3 patient, and 100 or more times higher for a class 4 or 5 patient.

If you are in risk class 1 your own personal risk for surgery is significantly lower than the **overall** risks reported for that procedure. Most of the serious problems that make up the overall total actually occur among the high-risk patients. If your medical problems put you in risk class 3 or higher, however, you need to weigh the pros and cons of any surgery very carefully.

Before surgery the anesthesiologist will review your medical history, answer your questions, and discuss the type of anesthesia she/he plans in your case. **Be sure to tell**

TABLE 45-1
RISK CLASSIFICATION
(AMERICAN SOCIETY OF ANESTHESIOLOGISTS)

CLASS	DEFINITION
1	Healthy
2	Mild systemic disease[a] with no impairment of body function
3	Severe systemic disease [a] with definite impairment of body function
4	Severe systemic disease[a] that is a constant threat to life
5	Near death; unlikely to survive 24 hours with or without surgery

[a]Systemic disease means any significant ongoing medical condition such as high blood pressure, diabetes, asthma, or kidney disease.

SOURCE: Adapted from Miller RD (ed): *Anesthesia* (ed 2). New York: Churchill Livingstone, 1986.

her/him about any drug allergies or adverse reactions you have had, and answer all questions honestly and completely. Your anesthesiologist needs to know about (2):

• Significant medical problems now or in the past
• Previous surgery
• Orthopedic problems
• Any possibility that you might be pregnant
• Any evidence of abnormal bleeding (abnormal vaginal bleeding, blood in your urine, or bloody or dark black bowel movements)
• Any possibility of hepatitis or recent hepatitis exposure
• Recent weight loss of 10 pounds or more
• Recent fever, cough, or symptoms of flu or a cold
• All recent or current medications including aspirin

Be sure to discuss any medications you take routinely with your surgeon ahead of time. You may be advised to continue them as usual until the night before surgery, or in some cases it may be better to stop them beforehand. Aspirin and birth control Pills, for example, can affect blood clotting, so allowing several weeks for your blood to return to normal may be desirable.

Some drugs can interact with agents used for anesthesia, including glaucoma eye drops, some tranquilizers, and narcotics such as heroin, marijuana, and cocaine (3). Exposure to the insecticide parathion may also affect anesthesia. Your anesthesiologist needs a **complete** list of current and recent medications and drugs.

Just before surgery, the anesthesiologist will ask you if you have had anything to eat or drink in the last eight hours. Be sure that your answer is accurate. Anesthesia risk is greatly increased if you have anything in your stomach, for you could vomit and inhale stomach fluid into your lungs. If your surgery is not an emergency, your anesthesiologist will recommend that surgery be rescheduled or delayed to allow time for your stomach to empty.

Preparing for Surgery

It is very important for you to understand and follow preoperative instructions precisely. If you are late arriving at the hospital or have not had the proper lab tests in advance, for example, hospital rules may force your surgeon to cancel your surgery appointment.

A blood count and urinalysis are usually required before general anesthesia. If you are having a hysterectomy or other major surgery, additional tests to determine your blood-clotting time and blood type and a blood crossmatch for transfusion may also be required. Your surgeon or anesthesiologist may recommend more thorough evaluation including a cardiogram and a chest x-ray if you have had previous medical problems or are over age 40.

Thorough cleansing of the planned incision area, and in some cases shaving, is the next step in surgery after anesthesia. If you will be having an abdominal incision, your entire abdomen including any pubic hair on your lower abdomen may be shaved. Vaginal surgery preparation will require shaving all your pubic hair and your upper thighs as well. Shaving is not usually necessary for D&C or laparoscopic tubal sterilization. Your surgeon may order an enema the evening before major surgery.

Just before major surgery, a narrow rubber tube called a catheter will be inserted through your urinary opening (urethra) into your bladder. The catheter insures that your bladder will remain empty throughout surgery and therefore will be less vulnerable to injury. Insertion of the catheter is quick, but if you are not already under anesthesia, you may have a slight stinging sensation for a second or two.

COMMON SURGERY PROCEDURES

There are many aspects of the surgical experience that vary depending on the type of procedure you are having, so you will need to look elsewhere in this book to read about your own surgery. Table 45-2 lists common types of gynecologic surgery and the chapter in which each is described.

ADVANCE PLANNING

If you know about surgery ahead of time, it makes sense to do whatever you can to be sure you are in the best physical condition possible when your surgery is done. This is an ideal time to stop smoking, for example. Even a few days of cigarette-free living can

TABLE 45-2
COMMON SURGERY PROCEDURES

PROCEDURE	CHAPTER
Abortion	18
Bartholin's gland removal	39
Biopsy (skin, cervix, endometrium)	4
Breast biopsy	37
Conization of the cervix	35
D&C (dilation and curettage)	47
Ectopic pregnancy	8, 10
Hysterectomy	49
Hysteroscopy	46
Laparoscopy	48
Laparotomy	48
Lysis of adhesions	10
Oophorectomy	49
Ovarian cystectomy	48
Pelvic repair	49
Tuboplasty (salpingoplasty)	10
Tubal sterilization	20
Vasectomy	21

make a significant difference to your lungs and may reduce your risk for lung problems after surgery. The week before surgery is also a good time to avoid drugs such as marijuana, cocaine, and alcohol.

You may also be able to reduce the likelihood that you would need a blood transfusion. Careful blood screening for hepatitis A and B, and AIDS (acquired immunodeficiency syndrome), are routine in all U.S. blood banks, so risks for acquiring these diseases with transfusion are small. Non-A non-B hepatitis, however, is a significant threat because it cannot be detected in screening, and blood sensitivity reactions do occur occasionally. Also, there is a remote risk that you could be exposed to AIDS from blood donated by a person who was infected with the AIDS virus within the preceding three months, so she/he has not yet formed detectable AIDS antibodies.

If possible, have a blood count to check for anemia several months in advance of surgery, and be faithful about iron supplements or any other anemia treatment your clinician recommends. Your blood count may improve within just a few weeks. It may be possible to donate your own blood ahead of time for banking in case blood is needed during your surgery.

Overall nutrition is also a reasonable concern. Being overweight increases surgical risk and the likelihood of problems such as incision infections and postoperative pneumonia. If you have sufficient advance warning, then exercise and diet to bring your weight closer to the normal range is a very good idea. A drastic weight loss diet during the last few weeks before surgery, however, is not likely to help and may even be unwise. Make sure your nutrition quality is excellent before surgery, including plenty of fresh foods that are the source of dietary vitamins. Vitamin C in particular may play a direct role in healing (4).

What to Expect After Surgery

The major effects of general anesthesia subside gradually over the first two to six hours, but you may have fatigue, mild nausea, drowsiness, and impaired reflexes for 24 to 48 hours. The length of time you need to allow for recovery from surgery depends on what kind of surgery you have had and on the specific medical problem(s) that necessitated your surgery. Recovery is rapid after minor procedures such as D&C or tubal ligation, and you can safely plan to resume normal activities within the first week; many women are fully recovered within two or three days after such surgery.

Major surgery such as hysterectomy will require about six weeks for full recovery, assuming that you do not have any serious complications. During the first two days after surgery, you will probably have narcotic pain shots, and you may not remember this time clearly. You will be getting out of bed to urinate as soon as your catheter is removed, usually the morning after surgery. During the first three or four days your pain will subside so that pain injections can be replaced with milder pain pills, and your intestines will gradually resume normal functioning. You will first be given clear liquids to drink and can have normal foods once you begin to have bowel contractions, rectal gas, and bowel movements. You will not feel hungry until your stomach and intestines have resumed normal contractions, and if you do eat solid food too soon, you will probably have bloating and nausea. Once your bowel function is normal, perhaps with the aid of an enema, you are ready to go home. Most women go home about five days after major surgery.

SURVIVING IN THE HOSPITAL

With a little planning and good information, you can make any hospital stay less unpleasant. You may be surprised to find that your hospital is able and quite willing to cooperate in arranging to meet your needs or desires. A smoke-free room, for example, is a very normal request. Competition and consumer pressure have made hospitals more accommodating and flexible, and many offer previously unheard of services and amenities. Some suggestions for making your hospital stay as pleasant as possible are:

- **Have a clear idea of what is going to happen.** If you know beforehand what kind of incision you will have, whether or not a catheter will be used, how long you will need intravenous tubes, and what medications you will be given, you can minimize surprises once you are in the hospital.
- **Remember that your surgeon must write all orders.** If something doesn't happen when you want it to, it is probably because there is no order in your chart. Nurses can only carry out your surgeon's orders and provide routine nursing care. If you need something, be sure that your surgeon knows about it, including simple things such as taking a shower or having your hair washed.
- **Gain the support of the nursing staff.** Thoughtfulness and courtesy do pay off. Ask for what you need, but let your surgeon be the one to make demands or settle any problems. If you are labeled a "difficult" patient, your hospital stay can be miserable.
- **Have your surgeon talk to an appointed family member or friend after your surgery.** When you wake up, your family member or friend can tell you how your surgery went and how you are doing. Your surgeon probably won't see you until that evening or even the next morning.
- **Order the food you want.** If you are a vegetarian or have special dietary needs, talk to the dietary department before you enter the hospital. If your hospital has a reputation for bad food, you might try the vegetarian meals; often they are of higher quality than regular meals.
- **Bring something simple you like to do.** You will probably be able to rent a television set for your hospital room, but you will also enjoy having several good books or a portable hobby.

HOME RECOVERY

Before you leave the hospital, your surgeon will remove the clips or stitches from your incision and will give you instructions on caring for your incision, taking medications, bathing, eating, exercising, and other activities. In some cases absorbable stitches are used on the skin, and these do not have to be removed. Your incision will seal closed within about three to four days, and after it seals you can safely bathe or shower. Your incision will be prominent, a deeper red than the normal skin, and will have a firm lump or cord of fibrous tissue just underneath. The fibrous lump and deep color of the incision gradually subside, and your incision will be much less conspicuous within a year or so after surgery. If you are particularly concerned about the appearance of your scar, let your surgeon know. Careful plastic surgery techniques to close your incision may be possible to minimize scar formation. Numbness in the incision area is also common and may persist for several months.

Think of your home recovery time after major surgery as three separate two-week periods. During the first two weeks you will need complete rest; do not plan any activities outside the house, and do *no* cleaning, cooking, lifting, or housework. Take your temperature with a thermometer three times each day (at 2, 6, and 10 P.M.)

45:3   DANGER SIGNS AFTER SURGERY

Fever (temperature over 100.4 degrees F.)
Pain not relieved by the medication your surgeon has given you
Pain, swelling, tenderness, or redness in your leg (calf or thigh)
Chest pain, cough, difficulty breathing, or coughing blood
Fainting or dizziness that persists more than a few seconds
Red or tender skin near your incision
Bleeding or oozing from your incision
Persistent bladder discomfort, burning with urination, blood in your
    urine, or inability to urinate
More than 3 days without a normal bowel movement
Bright red or heavy vaginal bleeding that is not a normal menstrual
    period

Contact your surgeon at once or go to a hospital emergency room
if you develop any of these symptoms after surgery.

and any time you feel feverish or have chills; drink plenty of fluids, and plan a mild, bland diet. Do not put *anything* in your vagina if your surgery involved a vaginal incision or dilation of your cervical canal.

During the first few weeks at home you will also need to watch for danger signs of possible surgery complications. Illustration 45-3 lists danger signs common to most surgical procedures; be sure you also understand any additional warning signs your surgeon wants you to report for your specific surgery. Possible surgical complications for common gynecologic procedures are discussed along with each surgery elsewhere in this book (see Table 45-2).

During the second two weeks at home (three to four weeks after surgery), you can begin limited activity. Short walks in your yard, a short ride (do not drive yourself), or a trip out to dinner would be reasonable. Wait until your incision discomfort has subsided and you no longer are taking pain pills before you resume driving. Medication and pain could slow your reflexes. You may begin to resume limited household activities, but avoid heavy lifting or prolonged standing. Rest if you feel tired, and take your temperature at least once a day or any time you feel feverish.

During the last two weeks (five to six weeks after surgery), you can gradually increase all your activities to normal. Your postoperative checkup will probably be scheduled during this interval.

In other words, **someone else** must do the cooking, cleaning, and shopping, and take over any child care responsibilities you have for **at least four to five weeks after surgery**. During the first two weeks or so you will need someone available to **help take care of you** during at least part of the day and in the evening. Unless you have unusual medical problems or complications, however, you will not need professional nursing care at home.

SUGGESTED READING

Gots, Ronald; Kaufman, Arthur: *The People's Hospital Book.* New York: Avon, 1978. Thoughtful and helpful advice on how to evaluate and choose an appropriate hospital and how to cope with hospital life.

Annas, George J.: *The Rights of Hospital Patients: The Basic ACLU Guide to a Hospital Patient's Rights.* New York: American Civil Liberties Union and Avon, 1975. Clear information on your rights when health care problems or disputes occur.

Directory of Medical Specialists. Chicago: Marquis' Who's Who, 1983.

ABMS Compendium of Certified Medical Specialists. Evanston, Il: American Board of Medical Specialists, 1986.

REFERENCES

1. Dennenberg HS: A shopper's guide to surgery: Fourteen rules on how to avoid unnecessary surgery. Unpublished paper.
2. Miller RD (ed): *Anesthesia* (ed 2). New York: Churchill Livingstone, 1986.
3. Orkin FK, Cooperman LH (eds): *Complications in Anesthesiology.* Philadelphia: J.B. Lippincott Co., 1983.
4. Brody JE: *Jane Brody's Nutrition Book.* New York: W.W. Norton & Co., 1981.

46

Hysteroscopy

Hysteroscopy permits your surgeon to see the inside of your cervical canal and uterus without an incision. This feat is possible with the help of a hysteroscope, a metal tube narrow enough to slip through the cervical canal into the uterine cavity. Hysteroscopy is not a common procedure, but is becoming more widely available in the mid 1980s. It may be helpful in evaluating and treating problems such as (1):

- Suspected abnormality in the shape of the uterine cavity when repeated, spontaneous pregnancy loss or abnormal hysterosalpingogram results (x-ray dye test) suggest that an abnormality may be present
- Possible uterine cavity abnormality when unexplained infertility persists, and results of other fertility studies are normal
- An IUD that is lost, or embedded in the uterine wall so that simpler procedures cannot retrieve it
- Suspected scar tissue (adhesions) blocking all or part of the uterine cavity (a condition called Asherman's syndrome, which can cause scant or absent periods; see Chapter 33)
- Suspected uterine septum, a thin sheet of uterine tissue extending downward from the top of the uterus, which can interfere with conception and pregnancy success
- Abnormal uterine bleeding or bleeding after menopause whose cause needs to be determined
- Suspected uterine polyps
- Suspected fibroid tumors located just under the surface of the uterine cavity lining (called submucous myoma, or leiomyoma) that are causing impaired fertility or excessive bleeding

Hysteroscopy also may be helpful in evaluating precancerous cervical abnormalities that extend up inside the cervical canal.

The main goal of hysteroscopy simply may be to inspect the cervical canal and uterine cavity. Your surgeon also may be able to obtain tiny tissue samples for microscopic evaluation by a pathologist, or actually carry out treatment; a lost IUD, for example, may be removed, or a thin septum snipped away with narrow surgical instruments inserted through the hysteroscope tube.

Hysteroscopy Procedure

I'd never even *heard* of hysteroscopy, and at first I wasn't too thrilled about the idea. See, I'm the type who buys a new car when the big innovations have been tried out for at *least* two years.

My alternative was a 5-inch scar and several weeks of missing work. All of a sudden hysteroscopy looked pretty good.

—WOMAN, 26

Before scheduling hysteroscopy, your surgeon will want to be certain you are not pregnant, and that you do not have active infection involving the uterus or tubes. Hysteroscopy during pregnancy could be dangerous for the fetus and also for the woman because her enlarged uterus may be softer and more susceptible to damage. If possible, it may be preferable to schedule hysteroscopy during the first half of your menstrual cycle just after you have finished a menstrual period, to be certain you are not pregnant. In some situations, such as evaluation for abnormal bleeding, this delay may not be feasible. In the case of infection, hysteroscopy might result in further spread of infection upward into the fallopian tubes or abdominal cavity.

Hysteroscopy can sometimes be performed as an office procedure with local anesthesia only. In some cases, however, general anesthesia is recommended, especially if surgical manipulation is anticipated. Also, equipment for hysteroscopy is not commonly available, and a hospital in your community may be the only facility equipped to perform the procedure.

Hysteroscopy can be performed in conjunction with laparoscopy (see Chapter 48), a surgical procedure that allows your surgeon to inspect the outer surface of your uterus, tubes, and ovaries through an illuminated tube inserted into the abdominal cavity. It is a common part of fertility evaluation. Hysteroscopy, if indicated for evaluation of impaired fertility in your case, can be done while you are under anesthesia for your laparoscopy procedure.

For hysteroscopy you will be positioned on the exam table with your legs in stirrups just as for a pelvic exam. If general anesthesia is used, you will be asleep during the following steps in hysteroscopy procedure. With local anesthesia, however, you will remain awake and quite aware of what is happening. It is helpful to know in advance what you can expect.

Before beginning hysteroscopy, your surgeon will perform a bimanual exam, with two fingers inside your vagina and the other hand on your abdomen, to confirm the position and size of your uterus. Next, a speculum will be placed in your vagina so your cervix can be seen easily (see Chapter 3 for more details on bimanual exam and vaginal specula). After washing your cervix and vagina with antiseptic your surgeon will begin by administering local anesthetic solution. By injecting the anesthetic on each side of your cervix (a technique called paracervical block) the main nerves to the uterus can be temporarily deadened. You may have some crampy discomfort during the injection or because of the cervical clamp (tenaculum) that is used to steady your cervix. You may, however, feel little or no pain with the anesthesia process.

Paracervical block is quite effective in eliminating pain, but it does not make your vagina or abdomen numb. You will be able to feel movements as your surgeon inserts and manipulates instruments, and you may have some cramping as well if the surgery stimulates uterine contractions.

If your surgeon is using a small hysteroscope, it may be possible to insert it through the cervical canal with no dilation. If not, the first step in the procedure will be dilation, using tapered metal rods, to stretch the cervical canal gradually until its diameter is about 8 or 9 mm (a little less than one half inch). Following dilation your surgeon will insert the hysteroscope through your cervical canal. The hysteroscope in place, along with the view of your uterine cavity your surgeon will see, is shown in Illustration 46-1.

The small, "contact" hysteroscope is designed to inspect one tiny area at a time, with the tip of the instrument in direct contact against the wall of the cervical canal or uterine cavity. If your surgeon is using this instrument, she/he will proceed immediately to systematic evaluation of each part of the canal and cavity.

If your surgeon is using a larger hysteroscope, designed for treatment as well as inspection, then it will be necessary to expand your uterine cavity slightly with carbon dioxide gas or a liquid solution prepared for this purpose. The gas or liquid will be flushed through the hysteroscope equipment under gentle pressure into your uterine cavity. It holds the walls of the uterine cavity apart to give your surgeon a better view. The irrigating fluid or gas flow is maintained throughout the rest of the procedure as your surgeon inspects the cavity and performs any biopsy or surgery that is necessary. Then the instruments are removed, and the procedure is over.

Afterward, you should be able to resume normal activities within a few minutes if you have had local anesthesia. Recovery from general anesthesia is a little slower (see Chapter 45), but most women feel well within eight to ten hours, and entirely back to normal within one or two days.

Irrigating fluid or gas may pass upward from the uterus into the fallopian tubes and out into the abdominal cavity, and irritation of the abdominal cavity lining may

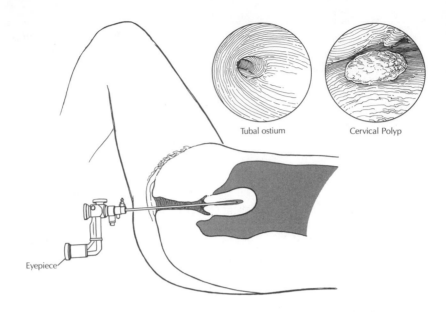

Tubal ostium   Cervical Polyp

Eyepiece

ILLUSTRATION 46-1   For hysteroscopy, a slender tube is inserted through the cervix into the uterine cavity, as shown above. Looking through the hysteroscope, the surgeon can see inside the cervical canal and uterine cavity, in one small area at a time. By moving the hysteroscope, abnormalities such as a polyp or uterine leiomyoma (benign fibroid tumor) may be located and identified.

cause shoulder and abdominal pain. The fluid or gas is absorbed within a day or two, however, pain subsides, and there is no evidence that these substances cause any persisting effects.

After hysteroscopy, you may have light bleeding or spotting for a few days, or possibly none at all. You will need to watch for the danger signs of possible complications shown in Illustration 46-2, especially during the first week or so after hysteroscopy. Also, your surgeon may advise you to avoid putting anything into your vagina for the first two weeks, until your dilated cervical canal has a chance to return to normal size. That means no intercourse, no douching, and no tampons. These precautions are intended to reduce the risk of introducing bacteria into your cervical canal at a time when your defenses against spread of infection upward to your uterus may be diminished.

Risks and Complications

Hysteroscopy is a fairly simple procedure, not unlike endometrial biopsy or insertion of an IUD, and serious complications are rare. It is classified as minor surgery, not major surgery, because instruments do not enter your abdominal cavity.

46:2   DANGER SIGNS AFTER HYSTEROSCOPY

Fever (temperature over 100.4 degrees F.)
Persistent abdominal pain or severe cramps
Heavy bleeding that lasts more than 6 to 12 hours, or requires
    5 pads or more in 1 hour
Faintness or dizziness that persists more than a few seconds
Abnormal or foul-smelling vaginal discharge

Contact your surgeon at once or go to a hospital emergency room
if you develop any of these symptoms after surgery.

ANESTHESIA COMPLICATIONS

Local anesthesia has few risks, but severe allergic reactions or overdosing problems can occur. General anesthesia, too, has overall risks that are low for a young, healthy person. Fatal complications are possible with both local and general anesthesia, but are exceedingly rare. Anesthesia risks are described in detail in Chapter 45.

INFECTION

Any procedure that involves instruments traversing the cervical canal into the uterus carries with it a risk of infection. Usually, the bacteria responsible for an infection after surgery originate from your own cervix, vagina, or bowel. The surgery serves to transport them upward into the uterus, and also may facilitate their growth because of bleeding that provides a good growth medium for bacteria, or because of trauma to the lining of the cervical canal and uterus. Infection risk is greatly increased if you already have a sexually transmitted infection such as gonorrhea or chlamydia, have recently been exposed to one, or if you have had pelvic infections in the past. If you have cervicitis, inflammation of the cervix often caused by bacterial infection, you should be treated with antibiotics first to clear up the problem before having hysteroscopy.

DAMAGE TO THE CERVIX,
UTERUS, OR OTHER PELVIC ORGANS

Serious damage is rare. The clamp used to position the cervix and uterus could cause a tear in the cervix that might require repair with stitches. Puncture of the cervical canal or uterus is also possible. A puncture (perforation) is likely to close and heal without treatment, but further surgery for repair is a possibility. If nearby structures such as the bladder, bowel, or blood vessels were to be injured at the time of perforation, emergency abdominal surgery to evaluate and repair the damage would be necessary. Perforation probably occurs in no more than 1 out of 500 hysteroscopy procedures (2). The risk may be somewhat higher for a woman who has a very narrow and tight cervical canal (cervical stenosis), and hysteroscopy for inspection and diagnosis has a lower risk than hysteroscopy surgical procedures.

The gas or liquid solution used to distend the uterus is another potential hazard. If an excessive amount of gas or liquid is infused, serious complications including impaired lung or heart function could occur. Similarly, accidental infusion of the gas or liquid into a blood vessel could cause serious problems. Either of these problems could potentially be fatal. Distention with fluid or gas could also cause rupture of a fallopian tube whose end was blocked by scar tissue from previous infection. All of these potential problems are extremely rare, and specialized equipment developed for this procedure is designed specifically to avoid these problems.

Bleeding can occur after hysteroscopy surgery, and repeat hysteroscopy to locate and cauterize a bleeding area might be necessary.

In some cases hysteroscopy is unsuccessful for technical reasons. It may not be possible for your surgeon to insert the hysteroscope if your cervical canal is very narrow and cannot be dilated. And problems with bubbles or heavy bleeding may interfere with a clear view.

Contraindications

A contraindication is a medical condition that renders a course of treatment inadvisable or unsafe that might otherwise be recommended. Contraindications for hysteroscopy include:

• Pregnancy
• Current or recent infection involving the uterus or fallopian tubes (pelvic infection)
• Cervical cancer

Several additional conditions are relative contraindications. Hysteroscopy should be delayed if possible, or performed only if the anticipated benefits warrant the additional risk these situations may impose:

• Current menstrual flow
• Cervicitis (cervical inflammation that may be caused by bacterial infection)
• Possible gonorrhea or chlamydia infection of the cervix, or recent possible exposure to infection
• Cervical stenosis (a narrow and tight cervical canal)
• Recent full term pregnancy or recent abortion

Benefits

Hysteroscopy is an elective procedure; there are no situations in which this surgery is a medical necessity. However, hysteroscopy is frequently the simplest and least risky way to obtain helpful information, and in some cases solve a problem. Alternatives for removing a uterine septum, or a lost or embedded IUD, for example, may involve major abdominal surgery (laparotomy; see Chapter 48).

As hysteroscopy equipment and surgeons trained in its use become more widely available, this procedure will, no doubt, become more common. New applications are also likely as other uses are explored.

As with any surgical procedure, safety and success are most often attained in the hands of an experienced and well-trained surgeon. Before deciding on hysteroscopy, be sure that your surgeon has had special training and is experienced in this procedure. You might ask, for example, how many times she/he has performed hysteroscopies in the last year. An answer of 20 or more means this is a fairly common surgical technique in her/his repertoire.

New developments in hysteroscopy, already being used in some centers, allow the surgeon to use magnification to study the surface of the cervical canal and uterine cavity. The magnified view is similar to the detail that is visible under a microscope, and may help in assessing the extent and severity of precancerous cervical or uterine abnormalities.

Research is also under way to utilize hysteroscopy for placement of chemicals or inert plugs inside the fallopian tubes for the purpose of contraceptive sterilization. It may be possible to develop a temporary tubal plug that will effectively block conception, but can be removed in case pregnancy is desired later.

Hysteroscopy equipment is being adapted for a technique called embryoscopy; this procedure, still at the experimental stage, may allow the surgeon to inspect a living fetus through the amniotic membrane.

REFERENCES

1. Gomel V, Taylor PJ, Yuzpe AA, et al: *Laparoscopy and Hysteroscopy in Gynecologic Practice.* Chicago: Year Book Medical Publishers, 1986.
2. Taylor PJ, Hamou J: Hysteroscopy. *Journal of Reproductive Medicine* 28:359–388, 1983.

47

❖

Dilation and Curettage
(D&C, Uterine Scraping)

Dilation and curettage (D&C) is one of the most frequently performed of all surgical procedures. One out of every 200 U.S. women undergoes D&C each year, and it is quite likely that D&C may be recommended for you at some time in your life (1). The primary purpose of D&C is to **diagnose and/or treat abnormal uterine bleeding.**

The D&C procedure allows your surgeon to scrape away part of your uterine lining (endometrium). Shreds of tissue from the lining are submitted to a pathologist, who prepares microscope slides. By examining the size, shape, and arrangement of cell layers from the lining on these slides, the pathologist can determine whether or not cancer is present. Precancerous abnormalities should be apparent, and the pathologist may also be able to identify problems such as abnormal hormone patterns or polyps that can cause abnormal bleeding.

D&C removes only part of the uterine lining (see Illustration 47-1), and the continuous growth of lining cells means that the missing parts should be replaced within a few weeks. Also, it is entirely possible that a small area of abnormal tissue in the lining might be missed with D&C. Even the most thorough scraping probably removes no more than 50% or 60% of the surface, so if problems persist after a D&C, it may be necessary to repeat the D&C, or your surgeon may recommend hysteroscopy as an alternative. Hysteroscopy allows the surgeon to look inside the uterus through a slender tube (see Chapter 46), and it may be possible with this procedure to identify abnormal areas that were previously missed.

Abnormal bleeding from the uterus can be an early sign of uterine cancer or precancerous abnormalities in the uterine lining. Thorough evaluation to find the cause and correct it is especially important for a woman over 35 who has abnormal bleeding patterns, since uterine cancer risks are higher after age 35. **After menopause**

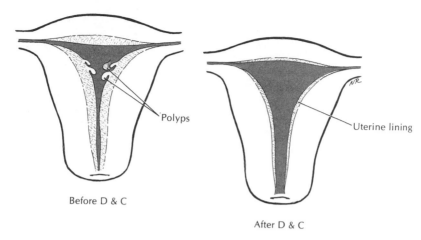

Before D & C

After D & C

ILLUSTRATION 47-1   The D&C procedure removes most of the uterine lining and any polyps that arise from the lining.

any bleeding at all requires investigation unless you are taking hormone medication; a few days of bleeding in conjunction with each monthly medication cycle is normal.

Office procedures such as endometrial biopsy or vacuum scraping (described in the last section of this chapter) may provide the information you and your clinician need in evaluating abnormal bleeding, but if the results are inconclusive, D&C probably will be recommended.

In some cases D&C provides effective treatment as well as diagnostic information. It is sometimes needed as an emergency measure to treat heavy bleeding or hemorrhage. Uterine bleeding is likely to be reduced or stopped at least temporarily after D&C unless the bleeding is caused by traumatic injury to the uterus or benign uterine fibroids (leiomyomas). Bleeding from uterine polyps is also likely to be cured by D&C if your surgeon is able to locate and remove all the polyps that are present.

D&C may also be recommended if your clinician suspects that you have fragments of placental tissue or fetal tissue remaining in your uterus after a miscarriage, abortion, or full term delivery. In this situation a vacuum aspiration procedure similar to the technique used for elective abortion will be used.

In the past, D&C was commonly recommended as a routine procedure just prior to hysterectomy, and performed in the operating room after general anesthesia had been administered. Its purpose was to detect unsuspected uterine cancer, in which case hysterectomy surgery would be delayed to allow for further evaluation. Studies have shown that this approach is not accurate in detecting early cancer (2), and that treatment for early cancer is not compromised after hysterectomy that was performed for other reasons. If cancer is suspected, then endometrial biopsy or D&C should be scheduled well before hysterectomy to allow time for preparation and reading of accurate, permanent microscope slides and any further evaluation that may be needed.

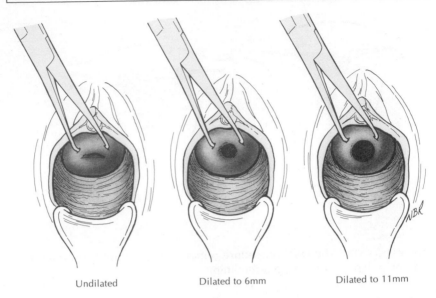

Undilated   Dilated to 6mm   Dilated to 11mm

ILLUSTRATION 47-2   The first step of a D&C is dilation of the cervical canal. Graduated metal rods are used to widen the cervical opening.

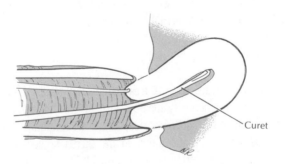

Curet

ILLUSTRATION 47-3   The surgeon scrapes away uterine lining with a sharp, spoon-shaped curet.

The D&C Procedure

General anesthesia (anesthesia sleep) or spinal anesthesia is usually recommended for a D&C. Local anesthesia similar to that for abortion can be used for D&C (see Chapter 18), but local anesthesia does not fully eliminate pain. Since the goal of D&C is careful, thorough exploration of the entire uterine cavity, it is important that patient discomfort not be an obstacle to performing the procedure properly.

Once anesthesia is complete, you are placed in the standard pelvic examination position. Your vulva, inner thighs, and vagina are thoroughly cleansed, and the entire area is covered with sterile towels to leave just your vagina exposed.

47:4   DANGER SIGNS AFTER D&C

Fever (temperature over 100.4 degrees F.)
Persistent abdominal pain or severe cramps
Heavy bleeding that lasts more than 6 to 12 hours, or requires
    5 pads or more in 1 hour
Faintness or dizziness that persists more than a few seconds
Abnormal or foul-smelling vaginal discharge

Contact your surgeon at once or go to a hospital emergency room
if you develop any of these symptoms after surgery.

The first step is pelvic examination. Your abdominal and pelvic muscles are completely relaxed under anesthesia, and your surgeon can use this opportunity to examine your uterus, tubes, and ovaries very carefully.

Next, a speculum is placed in your vagina so that your surgeon can see your cervix. The cervix is held steady with a clamp (tenaculum), and the angle of your cervical canal and depth of your uterus are determined by inserting a thin metal rod called a uterine sound through the canal and up to the top of your uterus.

At this point, your surgeon may obtain some tissue specimens from your cervical canal lining itself. A very narrow curet that has a sharp, spoon-shaped tip is used for the scraping.

Next your surgeon will widen or dilate your cervical canal by inserting tapered rods (dilators) in graduated sizes until the canal is about 1/2 inch in diameter (see Illustration 47-2).

After dilation, your surgeon locates and removes any polyps that you may have on the uterine lining, and then uses a slightly larger curet to scrape each area of your entire uterine lining (see Illustration 47-3). All the shreds of tissue that are removed are carefully collected so that they can be microscopically examined. When scraping is completed, the curet, clamp, and speculum are removed.

The entire D&C procedure takes about 10 to 15 minutes. Once you are fully awake, you will be ready to return to your regular hospital room or to be discharged to return home. If you plan to leave immediately after surgery, be sure to arrange for someone to accompany you. Don't try to drive a car until at least 24 hours after having anesthesia.

It is common to have light bleeding or spotting for a few days after a D&C, although some women have no bleeding at all. **Get in touch with your surgeon immediately if you develop any of the danger signs listed in Illustration 47-4.**

Most surgeons advise women to avoid intercourse, douching, and tampons for the first two weeks after D&C until the cervical canal has had a chance to shrink back to normal size. These precautions may help avoid contaminating the uterus with bacteria that might cause infection.

Be sure to see your surgeon for your postoperative checkup about two weeks after surgery. This visit is almost always included in her/his surgical fee, and it is very important. Your surgeon will check for tenderness in your uterus or tubes that might indicate infection, and will check to be certain that your cervical canal has returned to normal size. The pathologist's report on your D&C specimen will be completed about one week after your surgery. Your clinician may call you to give you the results by phone or may discuss them with you at your checkup visit.

Risks and Complications

I had a D&C in 1980 and another one this year. Nothing is scary except being put to sleep, and I do find that truly frightening. Afterward I was fine.

—WOMAN, 35

D&C is a simple procedure, and complications are rare. The overall death rate for healthy women under 50 years of age undergoing D&C is probably less than 2 deaths per 10,000 procedures (3). The following sections discuss possible problems you should be aware of, other than complications of anesthesia (see Chapter 45).

INFECTION

Infection inside the uterus and tubes is the most common serious problem following D&C. Infection can occur any time instruments are inserted into your uterine cavity and is usually caused by bacteria carried into your uterus from your own cervix, vagina, or bowel. The risk of infection is greatly increased if you have gonorrhea or chlamydia, have recently been exposed to gonorrhea or chlamydia, or have had pelvic infections in the past. Infections usually resolve quickly with antibiotic treatment, but they may be serious enough to require further surgery, including total hysterectomy, and can even cause death. Approximately 1 woman in 200 experiences an infection after D&C (4).

HEMORRHAGE

Heavy bleeding during or after a D&C is possible if your uterine walls are injured during scraping, if a polyp or fibroid tumor is only partially removed, if your cervix is injured by the clamp, or if you have abnormal bleeding tendencies. Hemorrhage is rare; more often, D&C will decrease or stop abnormal bleeding.

DAMAGE TO THE UTERUS OR OTHER PELVIC ORGANS

Puncture (perforation) of the uterus by a surgical instrument is a possible complication of D&C, although it is uncommon. If the puncture damages only the uterus, chances are good that the defect will close and heal spontaneously without further treatment. Damage to nearby blood vessels, the bladder, or bowel is possible, and immediate surgery to repair the injury could be necessary. If your surgeon suspects that you have a perforation, she/he may want you to stay in the hospital for observation, and may recommend laparoscopy (see Chapter 48) to assess whether there is any damage to your uterus or internal organs that needs surgical repair. Reported rates for perforation are about 1 in every 160 cases; the risk is highest for a woman who has a very tight cervical canal, a condition called cervical stenosis (4). In some cases, insertion of slender dilating rods or laminaria prior to surgery may be recommended. Laminaria are slender strips of seaweed prepared for medical use. The dilating rods or laminaria absorb water and swell over several hours, so they produce gentle and gradual cervical dilation when they are inserted in the cervical canal.

SCAR TISSUE FORMATION IN THE UTERINE CAVITY

An uncommon complication of a D&C is formation of scar tissue that partially or completely covers the uterine lining, obliterating the uterine cavity. This problem, called **Asherman's syndrome**, can cause infertility and the absence of menstrual periods; it most commonly occurs among women who have a D&C at the time they have an infected uterus, but can occur after a routine D&C or uncomplicated vacuum abortion procedure as well.

Contraindications

A contraindication is a medical condition that renders inadvisable or unsafe a course of treatment that might otherwise be recommended. Because D&C is a procedure of great importance for detecting uterine cancer as early as possible, **there are no absolute contraindications to D&C.** There are several medical conditions, however, that may mean that D&C should not be performed unless it is absolutely necessary:

• Uterine infection, tubal infection, or cervicitis. It is highly desirable to treat and cure infection before surgery.
• Pregnancy. D&C must be avoided if you wish to continue your pregnancy. D&C is an abortion technique, but the vacuum technique is safer and more effective when abortion is your goal (see Chapter 18).

• Serious medical problems such as heart or kidney disease that increase anesthesia risk
• Blood disorders that impair blood clotting or cause excessive bleeding

Alternative Office Procedures

Depending on the reason D&C is being considered, an endometrial biopsy or a vacuum scraping procedure may be reasonable options.

Endometrial biopsy is commonly used in evaluating fertility problems or bleeding problems experienced by young women when the main goal is to assess the hormone response of the uterine lining. Endometrial biopsy is like a miniature D&C. Little or no cervical dilation is required and the curet or scraper that is used is very narrow so it can pass through the undilated cervical canal. It is possible in most cases to obtain a few shreds of uterine lining satisfactory for microscopic evaluation using this technique.

A local anesthetic to temporarily block nerves in the cervix and the base of the uterus is commonly used for endometrial biopsy. The anesthetic, however, does not completely eliminate pain, and fairly intense cramping during each scrape is likely. Extensive or thorough scraping, therefore, may not be possible.

Vacuum scraping with a local anesthetic is also feasible as an office procedure. Instead of a metal curet, a slender plastic tube attached to a vacuum is inserted through the cervical canal and scraped along the uterine lining to obtain the strands of lining tissue needed. Several types of vacuum equipment are available for this purpose; some use vacuum created by an electric vacuum pump and some use a large, hand-held syringe as a vacuum source. Vacuum probably permits a more thorough scraping of the lining surface with less discomfort than endometrial biopsy, and is more comparable to D&C in its goals. Studies of vacuum scraping accuracy show that it is comparable to D&C in its ability to detect uterine cancer, but may not be as useful in detecting and removing uterine lining polyps (5).

The choice between endometrial biopsy, vacuum scraping, and D&C with anesthesia depends on your feelings about possible discomfort and anesthesia risk, as well as financial and medical considerations. D&C is essentially painless with general anesthesia, but may cost as much as $1,000 more than office procedure options. General anesthesia also involves greater risk than local anesthesia, and complication rates after D&C from bleeding, infection, and perforation are somewhat higher than rates after an office vacuum procedure or endometrial biopsy (5). In comparing risks, however, it is important to remember that the vacuum scraping patients studied were probably younger and healthier overall than D&C patients; the D&C may have been chosen because of extremely heavy bleeding, a very tight cervical canal, or a strong suspicion of cancer.

Neither D&C nor vacuum scraping can provide absolute assurance that uterine cancer is not present. They are among the best techniques available, but small areas of abnormal lining could be missed. If bleeding problems persist after an initial D&C or vacuum procedure, follow-up and further evaluation will be essential. The procedure may need to be repeated periodically until your problems are resolved.

REFERENCES

1. National Center for Health Statistics, Graves EJ: Utilization of short-stay hospitals, United States, 1983 Annual Summary. *Vital and Health Statistics,* Ser 13, No 83, DHHS Publication Number (PHS) 85–1744, Public Health Service. Washington, D.C.: U.S. Government Printing Office, 1985.
2. Lerner HM: Lack of efficacy of prehysterectomy curettage as a diagnostic procedure. *American Journal of Obstetrics and Gynecology* 148:1055–1056, 1984.
3. Moses L: Comparison of crude and standardized anesthetic death rates, in Bunker JP, Forest WH, Mosteller F, et al (eds): *The National Halothane Study: Report of the Subcommittee on the National Halothane Study.* Washington, D.C.: U.S. Government Printing Office, 1969.
4. Mattingly RF, Thompson JD: *Te Linde's Operative Gynecology* (ed 6). Philadelphia: J.B. Lippincott Co., 1985.
5. Grimes DA: Diagnostic dilation and curettage: A reappraisal. *American Journal of Obstetrics and Gynecology* 142:1–6, 1982.

48

Laparoscopy and Exploratory Laparotomy

"Laparo" is the Greek word for flank. In medicine the prefix "laparo" is used incorrectly to mean abdomen, so laparotomy means surgery that involves an incision into the abdominal cavity. Laparoscopy means examination of the inside of the abdomen through a lighted tube (scope).

Both laparoscopy and laparotomy are classified as major surgery, but they are quite different from the patient's point of view. Laparoscopy involves only a brief anesthesia and surgery time and very small incisions, so recovery is rapid. You can expect to feel entirely back to normal within just a few days. Laparotomy, on the other hand, is full abdominal surgery, much like hysterectomy. Several days in the hospital and convalescence at home for at least four to six weeks will be necessary.

Laparoscopy is commonly used for performing tubal ligation (see Chapter 20); in other situations the main goal often is diagnosis. Your surgeon can see the pelvic organs clearly with laparoscopy and can identify abnormalities such as an ectopic (tubal) pregnancy, patches of endometriosis, an ovarian cyst, or scarring from infection. Your surgeon's laparoscopy view is usually clear enough that she/he can also be certain that a possible abnormality such as ectopic pregnancy or endometriosis is **not** present because, if it were, it would probably be visible. Laparoscopy is an invaluable procedure for confirming a suspected diagnosis. Treatment during laparoscopy, however, is limited. It may be possible for your surgeon to remove ovarian cyst fluid, obtain a small biopsy specimen, or use cautery to eradicate small patches of endometriosis or scar tissue strands. New laparoscopy techniques that exploit laser surgery equipment and specialized laparoscopy instruments are being developed. As these are perfected, laparoscopy may become the preferred approach for more complex surgical tasks as well. For extensive surgery laparotomy will be needed.

Laparotomy surgery provides your surgeon with a clear view of your pelvic organs and the opportunity to make needed surgical repairs at the same time. In some situations laparoscopy is combined with laparotomy. When ectopic pregnancy is suspected, for example, a laparoscopy procedure may be done first to determine whether or not a tubal pregnancy is present. If none is seen, then your surgery will be stopped. If an ectopic pregnancy is present, your surgeon will proceed directly to laparotomy to remove the pregnancy, and in some cases the affected fallopian tube as well.

In some situations laparoscopy is not a logical first step. If you have symptoms of severe internal hemorrhage and ectopic pregnancy is suspected, for example, the delay involved in initial laparoscopy would not be wise. Your surgeon is also unlikely to recommend laparoscopy if she/he is fairly certain that laparotomy surgery will be necessary anyway. A large mass in an ovary will probably need to be removed regardless of what it looks like with laparoscopy. Thorough microscopic evaluation of tissue from the mass will be necessary for a precise diagnosis.

If you are having laparoscopy or laparotomy because of a medical problem, and you have been considering permanent sterilization for birth control, discuss sterilization with your surgeon ahead of time. In most situations, the additional surgery steps for tubal sterilization can be done easily and safely during either laparoscopy or laparotomy.

Laparoscopy

With my laparoscopy the goal was to find out once and for all if my horrible cramps were from endometriosis. (Yes.) I was scared about anesthesia, and scared I'd be wiped out for days, but I wasn't. I felt sore and tired, but well enough to watch a VCR movie that evening at home. My roommate rented *The Young Interns*. Cute.

I wouldn't want to have one a week, but it was okay. I've felt worse with flu.

—WOMAN, 26

Laparoscopy is usually performed in a hospital or outpatient surgical center with general anesthesia. In some cases local anesthesia and sedatives or tranquilizers may be an option. Local anesthesia does avoid possible risks of general anesthesia and

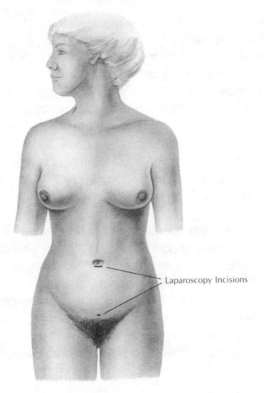

ILLUSTRATION 48-1   For laparoscopy a small incision just below your navel will be needed; a second tiny incision near your pubic hairline may be needed for other instruments.

reduces surgery cost. Some discomfort is likely with local anesthesia, however, because of the gas used to inflate the abdominal cavity during laparoscopy. Since it is essential that the patient remain absolutely motionless during surgery, especially if cautery instruments are being used, local anesthesia may not be advisable (1).

Once anesthesia is complete, you will be positioned on the operating table with your feet in stirrups and your hips elevated. Your abdomen, thighs, and vagina will be washed with antiseptic solution and covered with sterile drapes leaving only your vagina and a small area of your abdomen exposed. Your bladder may be drained with a catheter to be sure it is completely empty, and your surgeon will perform a pelvic exam. Next, your surgeon will position an instrument to move your uterus later during surgery. She/he may simply insert the instrument into your vagina and attach it by vacuum to your cervix, or a vaginal speculum may be necessary so your surgeon can place a clamp on your cervix. Your surgeon may also use a uterine elevator—a blunt rod inserted through your cervix and into the uterus—to provide better mobility of the

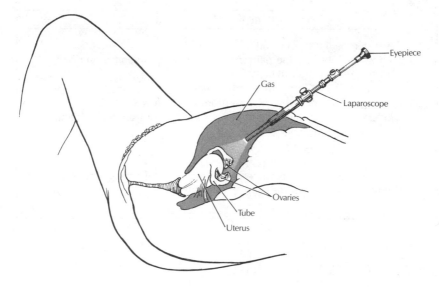

ILLUSTRATION 48-2   The laparoscope light illuminates the abdomen. Looking through the laparoscope your surgeon should be able to see your uterus, tubes, and ovaries quite clearly.

uterus and tubes during surgery. If dye injection is planned to assess your fallopian tubes, the equipment needed will be fitted to your cervix at this time. If you are having a D&C (see Chapter 47) at the same time as your laparoscopy, it will also be done at this stage.

The next step in laparoscopy is inflation of the abdominal cavity with a gas. Your surgeon will insert a needle into your abdomen through which gas gradually flows until it lifts up the abdominal wall. Next your surgeon makes a 1-inch incision just below your navel and inserts the laparoscope tube (see Illustration 48-1). By moving the laparoscope your surgeon can inspect each area in your pelvis. Your uterus, tubes, and ovaries should be clearly visible (see Illustration 48-2) as well as other abdominal organs unless you have dense scar tissue that blocks the view or makes it impossible for your surgeon to move the laparoscope into position.

With your pelvic organs in view, your surgeon may use cautery to remove strands of scar tissue or endometriosis patches if they are not too extensive. Dye may be used to check for blockage inside your fallopian tubes. Dye injected through your cervix should travel through your uterus and tubes and spill out freely into the abdominal cavity, where it is visible through the laparoscope.

When your surgeon is finished with the procedure, the inflation gas is allowed to escape from your abdomen, and the laparoscope and instruments are removed. Your surgeon will use one or two dissolving stitches to close your incision(s) and will cover them with one or two Band-Aids.

48:3   DANGER SIGNS AFTER LAPAROSCOPY

Fever (temperature over 100.4 degrees F.)
Pain not relieved by the pain medication your surgeon prescribed,
     or persisting longer than 12 hours
Chest pain, cough, or shortness of breath
Fainting or dizziness that persists more than a few seconds
Moderate or heavy bleeding from your incision or from your vagina
Red or tender skin near your incision(s)
Bleeding or oozing from an incision

Contact your surgeon at once or go to a hospital emergency room
if you develop any of these symptoms after surgery.

WHAT TO EXPECT AFTER SURGERY

Recovery after laparoscopy mainly involves recovery from anesthesia. The procedure is likely to take 15 to 45 minutes, and you will probably be ready to return home within two to six hours after surgery. By then you will be fully alert, and able to walk without difficulty. You will need to have someone to take you home, however, because anesthesia effects may slow your reflexes. You should not drive for at least 24 hours after surgery.

Your incisions are not likely to be painful. You may notice generalized muscle soreness as a result of muscle relaxant drugs used during surgery and a mild sore throat from the windpipe tube used for anesthesia. You may also have temporary shoulder pain because the gas used to inflate your abdomen during surgery is irritating to the lining of the abdominal cavity. It may collect at the top of your abdomen just under the diaphragm, the structure that separates your abdomen from your lungs. Nerves to the diaphragm are in the same nerve trunk as your shoulder nerves, so the pain message feels like shoulder pain. The gas is gradually absorbed within the first 24 to 36 hours, so pain should stop and any sense of abdomen bloating will also subside.

Pain and discomfort after surgery should not be severe; aspirin, aspirin substitute, or pain medication prescribed by your surgeon and rest should relieve it. Be sure to maintain good fluid intake during the first 24 hours and urinate regularly, because a full bladder may aggravate discomfort. Vaginal bleeding or spotting may also occur after surgery and last for a few days, but you should feel quite normal within two or three days.

You will need to **watch for the danger signs of possible laparoscopy complications during the first week** or so after surgery. If you have any of the problems shown in Illustration 48-3, you must see your surgeon right away for evaluation.

Your incisions should heal quickly. If your stitches need to be removed, your surgeon will tell you to schedule a postoperative visit about a week after surgery;

otherwise you can assume that absorbable stitches were used. Keep your incision(s) clean and dry, and covered with a Band-Aid for the first week. Unless your surgeon advises otherwise, it should be safe to shower or bathe any time after surgery. As your incision heals you may notice a firm, painless lump just under the skin. This is a normal phase in connective tissue regrowth. The lump will gradually disappear over several months, and your incision scar probably will be almost invisible when it is fully healed.

Your follow-up exam will be scheduled for one or two weeks after surgery, and is almost certain to be included in the fee for your surgery. Your surgeon will check to be sure your incisions are healing properly and you will have an opportunity to discuss your laparoscopy results and make plans for any further treatment needed.

PROBLEMS AND RISKS

Serious complications and deaths with laparoscopy are rare: approximately 1 death occurs in every 20,000 laparoscopies performed for diagnosis (1). Anesthesia complications, bleeding, and infection are the leading causes of serious problems.

Overall, about 1 woman in 120 will experience a significant complication (2). Rates have been thoroughly studied for the various possible problems after laparoscopy for tubal sterilization. Statistics on complications after **diagnostic** laparoscopy are not as extensive, but rates are probably no higher than for sterilization and may be lower. Complication risks are lower for women whose surgeons perform laparoscopy 100 or more times each year, and for young, healthy women. Personal medical factors such as diabetes, obesity, and lung problems caused by asthma, bronchitis, or emphysema increase risks (3). Previous pelvic surgery or pelvic infection history also may increase laparoscopy risks (2).

Anesthesia Problems. If general anesthesia is used, severe complications including cardiac arrest and even death are possible. Local anesthesia can also cause serious problems if too much of the anesthetic drug reaches the bloodstream.

Damage to Abdominal Organs. Accidental damage to the stomach, intestine, or bladder, or to large blood vessels in the abdomen is possible as laparoscopy instruments are inserted into the abdominal cavity, or later as they are moved or cautery is used. The risk for damage is higher than average for a woman who already has extensive scarring from previous surgery or infection. Scar tissue may hold abdominal organs to the abdominal wall, so they are not able to float out of the way as they normally would with abdominal inflation. Severe damage is rare, but if it occurs, it would usually require immediate laparotomy surgery (described later in this chapter) to repair the problem. Approximately 1 woman in 500 requires further surgery because of laparoscopy complications (2).

Problems with Gas Inflation. If the gas inflation needle is not correctly positioned inside the abdominal cavity initially or later slips out of place, gas may be inadvertently pumped into the wrong structure, and might cause damage if it stretched the stomach or bowel wall, for example. Gas pressure inside the abdominal cavity might also cause problems for a woman who has a hernia.

Abdomen inflation may also trigger heart rhythm problems because of abdominal stretching or interference with the lungs' ability to maintain normal blood oxygen and carbon dioxide levels. Gas inflation problems can be serious in rare cases, but are usually minor and subside without further treatment.

Infection. Urinary tract infection, wound infection, and infection involving the uterus and tubes or pelvic organs are possible after laparoscopy. Injury to the bowel may be a cause of infection, or bacteria from the vagina and cervix may be introduced into the uterus by instruments placed for uterine manipulation. Severe infection could spread to the lining of the abdominal cavity and cause peritonitis, or form a pocket of pus (abscess) that might require surgical drainage. Infection can also cause permanent damage to the uterus and fallopian tubes.

I had a pelvic infection and got admitted to the hospital four days after my laparoscopy. They weren't sure whether the infection started before or after surgery. I stayed in three days, and started feeling like myself in a couple of weeks. My doctor kept saying he'd never had this happen before. Well neither had I.

—WOMAN, 27

Infection problems are not common. Significant infection occurs in about 1 case in 500 and approximately 1 woman in 1,000 may require hospitalization because of infection problems (2). Most infections are minor, such as superficial infection in an incision, and will resolve with incision cleansing or antibiotic treatment at home.

Bleeding. Internal bleeding could occur as a result of accidental damage to a pelvic organ or blood vessel. Internal bleeding is likely to be evident during surgery, but later bleeding can occur, so watching for signs of bleeding after surgery is important (see Illustration 48-3). With internal blood loss, there would be no vaginal bleeding; bleeding might cause abdominal pain and faintness or weakness, especially when standing up.

External vaginal bleeding can also occur if instruments used in the cervix or uterus cause a tear or injury. Light bleeding or spotting for a few days after surgery is common, but heavy bleeding requires immediate evaluation.

Other Surgical Problems.   After any major surgery, risks for problems such as pneumonia, bronchitis, and abnormal blood clot formation (thrombophlebitis) in leg veins or pelvic veins are temporarily increased. Clots, particularly, can cause serious problems if part or all of a clot dislodges and travels to the lungs (embolism) These problems are very rare in healthy young women.

Unsuccessful Laparoscopy.   Laparoscopy may turn out to be impossible for a woman who is very obese or has extensive abdominal scar tissue. Your surgeon could encounter technical difficulties when she/he attempts abdominal inflation or first tries to insert the laparoscope. Scar tissue may block your surgeon's view even with equipment properly positioned. Such problems may occur in as many as 1 case in 100 (2). If laparoscopy cannot be completed, your surgeon can either discontinue surgery or proceed immediately with a routine abdominal incision and laparotomy.

It makes sense to discuss this possibility ahead of time so you and your surgeon can agree on what would be best. If you are having laparoscopy as an entirely elective procedure (to evaluate fertility, for example), you may not wish to have any further surgery. On the other hand, if your laparoscopy is needed for emergency evaluation of possible ectopic pregnancy, then further surgery may be the only reasonable option.

Open laparoscopy is a term used for a modified laparoscopy technique. With open laparoscopy, the instruments are inserted through a surgical incision slightly larger than the standard laparoscopy incision so that your surgeon can identify each layer in the abdominal wall. This technique may help your surgeon avoid puncturing areas where scar tissue may be in the way, or where bowel may be adhering to the abdominal lining. Open laparoscopy is somewhat more time-consuming, but may be recommended if your surgeon suspects that you have extensive scar tissue.

CONTRAINDICATIONS

A contraindication is a medical condition that renders unsafe or inadvisable a treatment or procedure that otherwise might be recommended. You and your surgeon must consider possible contraindications carefully in deciding about laparoscopy. In some situations, laparotomy surgery may be your only other option, so laparoscopy risks must be weighed against laparotomy risks. **Laparoscopy must not be attempted when intestinal obstruction is known or suspected.** The medical conditions listed below are relative contraindications: possible benefits and laparoscopy alternatives must be weighed carefully against risks on an individual basis (4).

• Intestinal obstruction
• Peritonitis (inflammation or infection involving the abdominal lining)
• Severe heart or lung disease
• Abdominal or diaphragm hernia
• Uterine pregnancy (especially advanced pregnancy)
• A large abdominal mass

• Previous abdominal surgery
• Previous pelvic infection or abdominal infection
• Body weight substantially below or above the normal range

ADVANTAGES OF LAPAROSCOPY

Laparoscopy can provide valuable information that otherwise would be unavailable except with laparotomy surgery. Compared with laparotomy, surgical risks with laparoscopy are low and recovery is rapid; and limited surgical treatment can be undertaken with laparoscopy. Situations for which laparoscopy is commonly recommended include (5):

• Suspected ectopic pregnancy
• Suspected endometriosis
• Suspected pelvic infection
• Pelvic pain evaluation
• Fertility evaluation when (1) an x-ray dye test (hysterosalpingogram) shows possible uterine or tubal abnormalities, (2) endometriosis or tubal damage from infection is suspected, (3) rapid evaluation is advisable because of the woman's age, or (4) pregnancy has not occurred despite four to six months of effective treatment for any other problems present
• Assessing advisability of tubal repair surgery for fertility treatment
• As part of in vitro fertilization treatment for fertility problems
• To remove an IUD lost in the abdominal cavity
• To assess treatment success after initial endometriosis treatment, ovarian cancer treatment, or tubal repair surgery

More extensive surgical tasks are also possible with laparoscopy, and new techniques are being developed actively. Specialized instruments for laparoscopic surgery and use of laser surgery equipment may allow the surgeon to treat more extensive endometriosis or scar tissue than is possible with standard laparoscopy. Surgical removal of ovarian tumors, an entire ovary, or early ectopic pregnancy through laparoscopy is also being performed in some medical centers (6).

Laparotomy

When I had it, it used to be called an "exploratory," going in for a look, and for treatment if they found anything. Of course, I suspected the worst, because I had a mass. It turned out to be a benign cyst on my ovary. I'll tell you, though, my soul felt well long before my body did! It was quite a jolt!

—WOMAN, 66

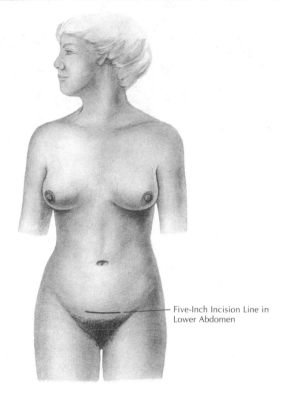

Five-Inch Incision Line in Lower Abdomen

ILLUSTRATION 48-4   Laparotomy may be performed with a horizontal (Pfannenstiel) abdominal incision (shown here) or an up-and-down incision beginning a few inches below your navel and extending down to your pubic hairline.

Laparotomy is almost always performed in a hospital operating room, and requires a hospital stay of several days. General anesthesia is usual for laparotomy, although regional anesthesia such as a spinal or epidural block may be possible.

For surgery you will be positioned lying on your back on the operating table. After anesthesia is complete, your abdomen will be washed with antiseptic solution and sterile drapes will be placed over your body and legs leaving only a small area of your abdomen exposed. Your bladder will be drained with a catheter tube, and the catheter may be left in place for some time after surgery.

Surgery begins with an incision about 5 inches long. Unless serious problems are anticipated, your surgeon will probably use a horizontal incision line across the middle of your lower abdomen just above the pubic hairline (see Illustration 48-4). If you have had previous surgery, your surgeon may follow the old incision line so that the old scar tissue can be removed, leaving you with only one scar when healing is complete. If cancer is suspected or extensive surgery needed, then an up-and-down incision will be necessary so your surgeon will be able to enlarge the incision if necessary.

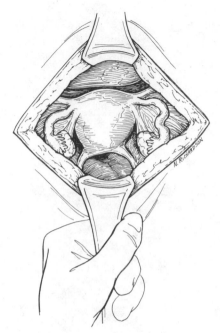

ILLUSTRATION 48-5   Your surgeon can see your pelvic organs clearly during laparotomy surgery.

The incision opening is next extended through the muscle and connective tissue layers of the abdominal wall and through the peritoneum, the thin membrane that lines your abdominal cavity. Loops of intestine are visible and your surgeon can reach other organs in the abdomen including your liver, gallbladder, and kidneys with her/his fingers to check for abnormalities. Your surgeon uses instruments to hold the edges of the incision apart, and move your intestines out of the way so that your uterus, tubes, and ovaries can be seen clearly (see Illustration 48-5).

The middle part of your surgery depends on the reason for your laparotomy and what is found. Your surgeon will have discussed these possibilities with you beforehand and any surgical procedures anticipated will have been listed on your surgical consent form. With ectopic pregnancy, for example, your surgeon may be able to make an incision in the fallopian tube and remove just the pregnancy, leaving the tube in place to heal; or it may be necessary to remove part or all of the involved tube. On occasion, unexpected findings may require additional surgery steps.

If your laparotomy was needed for repair of tube damage, your surgeon will remove scar tissue or endometriosis patches to free your tubes. If an ovary mass was the reason for surgery, the mass will be removed and given to the pathologist for microscopic evaluation.

When surgery is completed, your surgeon will make a final inspection to be sure

48:6   DANGER SIGNS AFTER SURGERY

Fever (temperature over 100.4 degrees F.)
Pain not relieved by the medication your surgeon has given you
Pain, swelling, tenderness, or redness in your leg (calf or thigh)
Chest pain, cough, difficulty breathing, or coughing blood
Fainting or dizziness that persists more than a few seconds
Red or tender skin near your incision
Bleeding or oozing from your incision
Persistent bladder discomfort, burning with urination, blood in your
    urine, or inability to urinate
More than 3 days without a normal bowel movement
Bright red or heavy vaginal bleeding that is not a normal menstrual
    period

Contact your surgeon at once or go to a hospital emergency room
if you develop any of these symptoms after surgery.

there are no areas of bleeding, and will allow the intestines to shift back into normal position. Then each abdominal layer will be repaired with stitches that are permanent or absorbable. Absorbable stitches may also be used for your skin incision, or your surgeon may prefer clips or temporary stitches that are removed after several days.

WHAT TO EXPECT AFTER SURGERY

You will remain in the surgery recovery room for an hour or so until you are fully awake, and then move to a regular hospital room. You are likely to have pain in the area of your incision and abdomen during the first few days, but pain shots will be available until you are able to swallow and absorb pills. Intestinal activity stops temporarily after any abdominal surgery, so you will not be able to eat or drink for a few days, and intravenous fluids will be needed instead. As your intestines resume normal function, you will feel hungry again and bowel gas will return—clues that you are ready for food.

You should plan for a hospital stay of five to seven days. You may be able to return home a day or two earlier, but a longer stay is also possible if you have had extensive surgery or if complications occur.

At home, about four to six weeks will be needed for convalescence. You will need lots of rest and help with household tasks such as cooking for the first week or two, and you should not plan to return to work any sooner than five or six weeks after surgery. Also, you should not plan to drive until you no longer need pain pills and your incision discomfort is entirely gone. Your reflexes may be slowed if your body resists sudden motion that might cause pain in the area of your incision.

Your incision should be kept clean and dry for the first four days after surgery; after that no special precautions with showering or bathing will be necessary. The incision may form a firm, nontender cord just under the skin as it first heals; this cord will subside gradually over the next 6 to 12 months. The incision itself may appear bright pink initially, but the color will gradually fade. Numbness in the incision area is also common and usually subsides over several months.

Most surgery problems occur within the first few days, while you are still in the hospital. When you return home, however, you do need to watch for the danger signs of possible surgery complications shown in Illustration 48-6.

PROBLEMS AND RISKS

Laparotomy is major surgery and its risks and complications are similar to those for abdominal hysterectomy. Your age and general health status are important factors in risk, as are the reason for surgery and the competence of your surgeon. Overall, the risk of death for a young healthy woman who undergoes laparotomy is low, probably less than the 1 in 1,000 risk for hysterectomy (4). Severe complications are also rare, but less serious problems are common.

Infection. Treatment for minor infection problems is necessary for as many as 25% of hysterectomy patients (4), and rates are similar for laparotomy. Bladder infections and superficial incision infections are by far the most common. Severe infections can occur, and may necessitate further surgery to drain an abscess or even remove your uterus or tubes. Infection risk is highest for a woman who has had previous pelvic infection.

Bleeding. Excessive blood loss during surgery may necessitate blood transfusion, and internal bleeding after surgery might require another operation to find and stop the bleeding. Hemorrhage problems are most common with ectopic pregnancy because internal bleeding may have already begun before surgery. Later bleeding is much less common.

Bladder and Bowel Problems. Bladder problems are quite common, especially bladder infection, and several days or even longer of catheter drainage may be required after surgery for return of normal bladder function if surgical manipulations in the area of the bladder have been necessary.

Accidental damage to bowel or urinary tract structures can also occur with laparotomy. Bladder injury or perforation is possible, and so is damage to the ureters, the tubes that carry urine from the kidneys to the bladder. If injury is recognized during surgery, additional surgical steps to repair the damage will be done immediately. A second surgery might be necessary for repair if problems are discovered after surgery.

Other Surgical Complications. Thrombophlebitis, abnormal blood clot formation in leg veins or pelvic veins, is a possible risk with any major surgery. Inactivity and bed rest, as well as infection, contribute to thrombophlebitis risk. It is a serious problem because part or all of an abnormal clot could break loose (embolize) and travel to the lung, and lead to severe breathing problems, a stroke, or even death.

Cautery used to eradicate endometriosis patches confers a risk of possible bowel or bladder burn injury. Conservative surgery for ectopic pregnancy, with your fallopian tube left in place to heal, means that your future risk for another ectopic pregnancy is higher than average. Your surgeon can explain any extra risks that are specific to the surgery planned in your case.

CONTRAINDICATIONS

A contraindication is a medical condition that renders unsafe or inadvisable a treatment or procedure that otherwise might be recommended. Laparotomy may be an essential, life-saving procedure so **there are no absolute contraindications** to this surgery. In some situations, however, laparotomy surgery may be inadvisable because of high-risk factors such as:

• Severe heart or lung disease
• Uterine pregnancy
• Serious medical problems such as diabetes, high blood pressure, or a blood clotting disorder that may increase surgery risks

ADVANTAGES OF LAPAROTOMY

Laparotomy allows your surgeon to confirm a diagnosis and treat the problem in one step. When your symptoms, exam, and laboratory studies suggest that internal hemorrhage or overwhelming infection are present, immediate laparotomy may be the only reasonable option.

For me there was no careful decision making or reviewing pros and cons for surgery. By the time I got to the emergency room, I could hardly stand up. The emergency room doctors thought it must be a ruptured tubal pregnancy, but there wasn't even time to wait for a pregnancy test result. My gynecologist did the surgery within two hours after I arrived. It turned out to be a cyst on my ovary that was bleeding. Luckily, I didn't have to have the ovary removed, though, just repaired—and I was able to get along without a blood transfusion. I was able to go home four days after surgery, but the combination of anemia and surgery left me exhausted for a full two months.

—WOMAN, 23

Laparotomy may also be the most appropriate choice in the case of an enlarged ovary. Your surgeon will be able to remove the abnormal tissue for full evaluation by a pathologist.

Laparotomy may also be needed if you decide on elective surgery for fertility. With laparotomy, your surgeon can repair previous damage to the fallopian tubes, correct a structural abnormality in your uterus, or remove benign uterine fibroid tumors (leiomyoma) that may be interfering with pregnancy success (see Chapter 10).

In the case of elective fertility surgery, initial laparoscopy is likely to be recommended. Laparoscopy will allow your surgeon to assess the feasibility of repair surgery and give you an estimated success rate as you decide whether or not repair is reasonable in your situation.

REFERENCES

1. Ohlgisser M, Sorokin Y, Heifetz M: Gynecologic laparoscopy. A review article. *Obstetrical and Gynecological Survey* 40:385–396, 1985.
2. DeStefano F, Greenspan JR, Dicker RC: Complications of interval laparoscopic tubal sterilization. *Obstetrics and Gynecology* 61:153–158, 1983.
3. Liskin L, Rinehart W: Female sterilization. *Population Reports* Ser C, No 9, May 1985. Baltimore: Johns Hopkins University.
4. Mattingly RF, Thompson JD: *Te Linde's Operative Gynecology* (ed 6). Philadelphia: J.B. Lippincott & Co., 1985.
5. Gomel V, Taylor PJ, Yuzpe AA, et al: *Laparoscopy and Hysteroscopy in Gynecologic Practice.* Chicago: Year Book Medical Publishers, 1986.
6. Martin DC, Diamond MP: Operative laparoscopy: Comparison of lasers with other techniques. *Current Problems in Obstetrics, Gynecology and Fertility* 9:568–601, 1986.

49

❖

Hysterectomy

Hysterectomy is major surgery, and deserves careful decision making. ("Hyster" means uterus; "ectomy" means surgical removal.) It is such a common operation that you no doubt have friends and relatives who have had hysterectomies, most likely with no problems whatsoever. If you face the decision yourself, be sure that you take time to weigh the pros and cons in your own situation. As with any major surgery, serious complications are possible with anesthesia or with the surgery itself. Serious problems are rare, but postoperative complications are common and risks are indeed real, so avoid surgery that is done as a convenience only. Because it isn't always clear whether hysterectomy is your best option, you will need lots of facts and all your wits and instincts about you as you decide.

The five situations in which hysterectomy is necessary to preserve or save a woman's life are:

- To remove cancer originating in the vagina, cervix, uterus, fallopian tubes, or ovaries
- To treat precancerous abnormalities of the uterus or cervix when other treatments have not been effective or are not preferable
- To stop severe, uncontrollable hemorrhage
- To stop severe, uncontrollable infection
- As part of surgery for life-threatening problems affecting the intestine or bladder when it is technically impossible to correct the primary problem without removing the uterus as well

Hysterectomy in any other situation is elective. Elective surgery may be an entirely appropriate choice when the problem is serious and other treatment is not available or has been ineffective. Surgery may also be justified for problems that are likely to become more severe at some future time, because surgery that is delayed until a simple problem becomes a severe problem or until emergency surgery is necessary incurs a higher overall surgery risk than does elective surgery. Some of the non-life-threatening problems that may justify hysterectomy are:

- Recurrent attacks of pelvic infection; infection accompanied by severe, persistent pain or continuing pain with intercourse
- Endometriosis that is causing severe symptoms, or is a threat to other organs such as the bladder or bowel
- Fibroid tumors (benign leiomyoma) that are causing bladder pressure or disabling symptoms or have grown rapidly
- Loss of pelvic muscle support from childbirth injury that is severe enough to interfere with bladder or bowel function or cause the uterus to descend so far that the cervix protrudes through the vaginal opening
- Vaginal bleeding that is excessive enough to cause anemia and cannot be controlled with hormones

Hysterectomy may be a wise choice in other situations as well, but when medical reasons for surgery are vague and other treatment alternatives with lower risks are available, it is especially important to consider surgery cautiously. Most clinicians believe, for example, that **hysterectomy is not appropriate when the main goal of surgery is sterilization;** tubal ligation and vasectomy are safer alternatives. Problems such as pelvic pain, backache, pelvic pressure, menstrual cramps, and heavy discharge often can be managed effectively without surgery.

Unless you have a life-threatening problem such as cancer, hemorrhage, or infection, **you have time to think about hysterectomy before you make a final decision.** You may find it helpful to do some reading and see a second clinician for an independent assessment of your treatment options.

Assessing personal pros and cons may not be easy, particularly when a problem such as endometriosis or uncontrollable, flooding periods from benign fibroid tumors is the reason surgery is being considered. Even if your current symptoms are severe, there may be other factors to consider. With uterine fibroids, for example, many surgeons would recommend surgery if your uterus is the size of a 12- to 14-week pregnancy or larger, particularly if you are having symptoms. The assessment is not clear-cut, however, especially if you are within a few years of menopause: fibroid problems are likely to resolve on their own after menopause and so are endometriosis problems. Also, an unrelated medical problem that increases your risk with surgery may make surgery a less desirable option.

Large fibroids are not necessarily dangerous. If you do not have uncontrollable bleeding or pain, and your fibroids are not growing rapidly, you may be able to coexist with them peacefully until menopause. The likelihood of malignancy in a fibroid is so

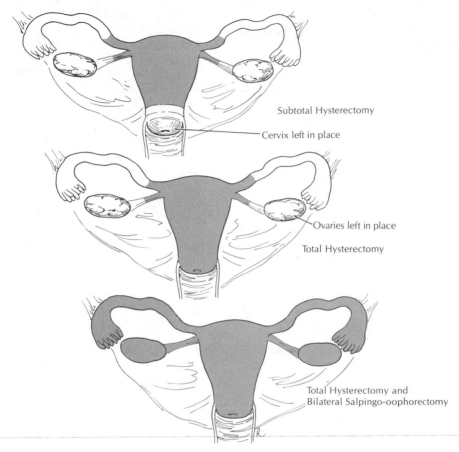

Subtotal Hysterectomy

Cervix left in place

Ovaries left in place

Total Hysterectomy

Total Hysterectomy and
Bilateral Salpingo-oophorectomy

ILLUSTRATION 49-1   Subtotal hysterectomy leaves the cervix in place. Total hysterectomy means that all of the uterus (including the cervix) is removed. The operation for removal of the uterus, tubes, and ovaries is called total hysterectomy and bilateral salpingo-oophorectomy.

low that surgery should not be recommended solely because of cancer fear. Surgery may be needed, however, if your surgeon cannot be certain that your tumors are fibroids. Endometriosis, too, may remain stable and does not necessarily require medical intervention unless it is causing troublesome symptoms.

Your own feelings about how your symptoms are affecting your life are very significant, and entirely appropriate considerations. If your symptoms are not really bothering you, and you do not have cancer or a life-threatening problem, then it is safe to decide against surgery or to delay your decision. On the other hand, if your symptoms are interfering with your ability to do the things you want to do, then surgery may be entirely reasonable and its risks worth taking, even though there is no medical necessity involved.

Hysterectomy Choices

There are several different hysterectomy techniques (see Illustration 49-1), so be sure that you understand exactly which procedure your surgeon plans to use and why.

Total abdominal hysterectomy (TAH): Removal of the uterus and cervix through an incision in the lower abdomen. The fallopian tubes and ovaries are not removed.

Total abdominal hysterectomy and bilateral salpingo-oophorectomy (TAH and BSO): Removal of the ovaries (oophorectomy) and fallopian tubes (salpingectomy) along with the uterus and cervix through an incision in the lower abdomen.

"Complete hysterectomy": A lay term sometimes used for removal of the ovaries in addition to the uterus, fallopian tubes, and cervix. "Complete hysterectomy" is the same as TAH and BSO.

Vaginal hysterectomy: Removal of the uterus and cervix through an incision inside the vagina. The fallopian tubes and ovaries are usually not removed.

Subtotal hysterectomy: Removal of the uterus but not the cervix. The fallopian tubes and ovaries are not removed. This procedure is rarely used today except in emergency situations when the additional time and surgery steps needed for removal of the cervix are inadvisable because the woman's medical condition is so poor. Under normal circumstances most surgeons recommend total hysterectomy because they feel the cervix has no essential functions when the uterus is not present, and does pose a future risk of cervical cancer. However, this operation may become more popular in the future. In some situations, removal of the cervix is not an essential goal and Pap testing can provide good protection against future cervical cancer risk. The cervix plays a role in female sexuality, and its removal in "total" hysterectomy also involves some shortening of the vagina that may make intercourse uncomfortable for some women.

Pelvic repair (vaginal repair): Surgery to improve muscle and fibrous tissue support for the bladder and/or rectum. Pelvic repair may correct the vaginal bulges, cystocele and/or rectocele that are caused by lax support of the bladder and/or rectum adjacent to the vaginal walls. Depending on the structural abnormalities that need correction, pelvic repair may involve abdominal and/or vaginal incisions that allow the surgeon to carry out one of the many surgical techniques developed for this purpose. The uterus is often removed at the time of repair, and in some cases the tubes and ovaries as well.

DECIDING ON THE MOST APPROPRIATE PROCEDURE

Any form of hysterectomy is major surgery and requires general anesthesia. You can expect to stay in the hospital for about four to six days, and should plan for a recuperation period at home of about four to six weeks. Complete recovery is likely to take several months. Read Chapter 45 carefully to review preoperative procedures for major surgery, anesthesia, and what to expect after surgery.

Your choice among hysterectomy options involves several factors:

• The reason hysterectomy is needed
• Whether vaginal surgery or abdominal surgery is more appropriate
• Whether or not your ovaries will be preserved

In some situations your choice may be quite limited. With surgery for cancer or severe infection, an abdominal incision is necessary, and it may not be reasonable, or technically possible, to leave your ovaries in place.

Vaginal hysterectomy is popular because the incision scar is inside your vagina, out of sight, and because recovery after surgery is often quicker and less painful than with abdominal surgery. This operation is not likely to be recommended if your ovaries will be removed along with your uterus. Vaginal surgery also may not be advisable if your uterus is very large or if you have extensive scarring from infection or endometriosis, or have had previous pelvic surgery such as cesarean section delivery.

In many cases, however, the decision about hysterectomy options is not clear-cut. Your surgeon should be willing to discuss and consider your own preferences, and often it is appropriate to make the choice jointly. Most crucial—and controversial—is your decision about whether or not your ovaries should be removed at the time of surgery.

PRESERVING THE OVARIES: PROS AND CONS

Without a doubt, the most confusing part of the whole hysterectomy decision for me was what to do about ovaries, in or out?

—WOMAN, 39

Policies and guidelines for deciding about ovary removal have never been universal so they vary from surgeon to surgeon, and, of course, depend as well on the specific medical needs of the individual woman.

Traditional teaching in the past was that ovaries after menopause are completely inactive and serve no useful purpose. Postmenopausal ovaries do appear inactive—shrunken in size, with none of the outward signs of follicle development so easily visible during the reproductive years. Because surgeons believed that postmenopausal ovaries had no value, and might later become a cancer site, it is easy to understand why routine ovary removal at the time of hysterectomy has been a common policy. Research evidence now shows, however, that the ovaries do continue to produce some hormones after menopause (1). The possible importance of this hormonal role in later life is under investigation, and policies regarding ovary removal are being reevaluated (2).

A woman's ovaries are her counterpart of the testicles in a man; the technical term for both is gonads, and the term for their removal, castration. Gonads are the primary source of reproductive hormones for both men and women. For men, hormone production is essential for sexual functioning as well as reproduction and normally persists throughout life, although the amount of hormone produced does decline somewhat in older age. For women, hormone function is essential for reproduction but not for intercourse. Hormones, however, do play a role in the physical aspects of sexual response and also in sex drive.

Hormone production by the ovaries is altered dramatically during the menopausal years. Production of estrogen declines about 90%, ovulation stops, and, without ovulation, there is little or no progesterone production. These changes are responsible for cessation of menstrual periods, or menopause, at about age 51. After menopause the ovaries continue to produce only low levels of estrogen, but **increase** their production of male hormones (androgens) somewhat, and also produce hormone precursors. Androgens and precursors are **converted to estrogen** in body fat cells, and a woman's resulting total estrogen level may be fairly substantial. Approximately 10% of women have sufficient natural estrogen after menopause that symptoms of estrogen deficiency such as vaginal dryness do not occur (1). Whether or not androgens and hormone precursors have other direct functions for women after menopause is not known. Androgens may, however, affect a woman's sex drive as well as her energy and muscle strength.

Effects of Ovary Removal Before and After Menopause. Removing a woman's ovaries before menopause causes immediate and dramatic hormone changes. This procedure is often called surgical menopause, although the term is not technically accurate since removal means that *post*menopausal hormone production is lost as well. After surgery the woman is no longer fertile, and the abrupt drop in estrogen is almost certain to cause severe menopause symptoms such as hot flashes within just a few days. Treatment with hormone replacement medication will be started immediately if at all possible. Premature loss of estrogen without hormone replacement treatment increases risks for the bone mineral loss of osteoporosis and for cardiovascular diseases such as heart attack as well (3). Continued hormone treatment will be needed until at least age 50 to protect against these risks.

A woman whose ovaries are removed after menopause is unlikely to notice any immediate changes, and may not notice long-term effects of hormone alterations either. Hormone changes that occur as a result of ovary removal after menopause are subtle, and possible symptoms and consequences are not precisely known.

Reasons for Removing Ovaries. In some situations ovary removal is an unavoidable or essential part of hysterectomy surgery. Surgery for cancer of the uterus or ovaries is an example. Success in treating the cancer might be compromised by continuing ovarian hormone production, because some types of cancer grow faster

TABLE 49-1
OVARIAN CANCER IN RETAINED OVARIES

STUDY (YEAR)	NUMBER OF HYSTERECTOMIES	CANCER IN RETAINED OVARIES	PERCENT
Randall (1963)	915	2	0.2
Gevaerts (1962)	300	0	0.0
Reycraft (1955)	4,500	9	0.2
Funck-Brentano (1958)	580	1	0.2
Whitelaw (1959)	1,215	0	0.0
Ranney (1977)	2,136	4	0.2
Funt (1977)	992	0	0.0
Total	10,638	16	0.1

SOURCE: Mattingly RF, Thompson JD: *Te Linde's Operative Gynecology* (ed 6). Philadelphia: J.B. Lippincott Co., 1985. Used with permission.

in the presence of estrogen. In some cases it is technically impossible to preserve the ovaries and still fulfill the purpose of surgery. Extensive scar tissue from infection or severe endometriosis, for example, may involve the ovaries directly so that they cannot be left in place, or they may be so diseased that leaving them would make continuing problems likely.

In many cases ovary removal is optional and the reason it is recommended is as a precaution against ovarian cancer later in life. Approximately 1 woman in 100 can expect to develop ovarian cancer sometime during her life. Ovarian cancer is a devastating disease because it does not have early warning signs that might allow early detection. Advocates of routine ovary removal feel that the hormone-producing role of ovaries after menopause is not important enough to justify any future risk for ovarian cancer, and that treatment with estrogen hormone medication is a satisfactory alternative.

Research data to document future benefits of routine ovary removal are limited. Summarizing available data, one expert concludes that approximately 1% to 2% of women who have ovaries left in place will subsequently need surgery again because of an ovary or tube problem (3). Follow-up studies after hysterectomy for women with ovaries left in place, however, have shown very low ovarian cancer rates: about 1 in 1,000 (see Table 49-1). Why ovarian cancer rates might be so much lower than expected in women after hysterectomy, or even whether rates truly are lower, is not known. Age may be one factor. Women in the studies were followed for as long as 20 years, and during that time the rate for ovarian cancer would normally be expected to decline. Future ovarian cancer risk is highest (about 1%) with surgery at age 45; thereafter it drops gradually so that a woman who is 70 years old has only a 0.3% (one third of 1%) risk for developing ovarian cancer sometime in the future (3). It is also possible that removing the uterus might in some way protect against later cancer in the ovary, or that women in these studies had lower than average risk factors.

In addition to age, risk for ovarian cancer is influenced by other factors as well. Your own risk may be lower than average if you have had several full term pregnancies or used birth control Pills in the past. The most important high-risk factors are:

• Strong family history of ovarian cancer: mother, sister(s)
• Previous cancer of the colon or rectum, hereditary intestinal polyps, or family history of colon or rectal cancer
• Previous breast cancer or family history of hereditary-pattern breast or uterine cancer

If you have one or more high-risk factors for ovarian cancer, it is logical to consider ovary removal when surgery is necessary for some other reason. In rare cases, when risk is very high because of hereditary patterns for ovary, breast, and colon cancer in the family, surgery specifically to remove the ovaries may even be recommended. If you are concerned about this issue, you may need genetic counseling to map your family medical history and determine whether or not your family has a high-risk pattern. Unfortunately, even removing both ovaries may not be sufficient to protect against the disease. Out of 28 women in one study who had preventive ovary removal because of very high family risk for ovarian cancer, 3 women nevertheless later developed cancer in the abdomen that was microscopically identical to ovarian cancer (3).

Removing just one ovary, a seemingly logical middle-ground approach, may not be a good idea. Ovarian cancer rates in one study were higher for women who had only one ovary preserved at the time of hysterectomy than they were for women with both ovaries preserved (4).

Reasons for Leaving Ovaries in Place.   Ovary removal is not likely to be recommended for a woman who is 40 or younger at the time of hysterectomy unless her surgery is for cancer or it is technically impossible to preserve her ovaries.

For a woman nearing or already at menopause, the ovaries' small but persisting contribution to hormone production is the main reason for considering ovary preservation. Artificial replacement of hormones through medication is not always satisfactory. Most women tolerate estrogen treatment well, but side effects can occur, and a woman who develops a problem such as diabetes, serious high blood pressure, or gallbladder disease may have to stop using hormones. Treatment with hormone medication may also be unwise for a woman who has severe heart disease or liver disease or has had problems with blood clots or a previous stroke.

Hormone treatment cannot fully duplicate the ovaries' role. Estrogen medication is a good substitute for ovarian estrogen, but replacing hormone precursors and androgen is not usually attempted. Treatment to replace androgens is possible, but undesirable side effects such as hair growth are common. Prolonged use of androgen drugs can cause serious liver problems and may be a cause of liver cancer (5).

Androgen hormones influence sex drive for women both before and after menopause. Loss of ovary androgen production may be one of the reasons that some women report a decreased desire for sexual activity after hysterectomy (4). Estrogen also affects sexual function, and a woman who is unable to take hormone medications may have significant problems with intercourse as a result of estrogen deficiency. (Hormonal and surgical effects of hysterectomy on sexual function are discussed in detail later in this chapter.)

For a woman who cannot take estrogen medication, loss of ovary hormone production may involve medical risks. **Heart disease risk is higher than average for a woman who loses estrogen hormone production before age 40** whether through premature menopause or surgery. There is some evidence that estrogen hormone levels after age 40 and even after menopause provide significant protection against heart disease for older women. Ovary removal means that the small but continuing ovarian source of estrogen for a woman after menopause is not available. This issue is of special concern for any woman who cannot take estrogen medication and is at high risk for heart disease because of such factors as:

• Diabetes
• High blood pressure
• High blood fat levels (cholesterol, triglycerides) or hereditary blood lipid problems
• Smoking cigarettes
• Strong family history of heart disease (parent, brother, or sister had heart attack before age 50)

Osteoporosis risk, too, may be affected for a woman who is unable to take hormone medication. Estrogen loss before age 40 is known to be a significant risk factor for bone density loss, and the level of continuing estrogen after menopause is also significant. Research evidence to show what role ovarian hormones play after menopause is lacking, but it is reasonable to assume that **continuing hormone production by the ovaries would be desirable for bone protection,** especially for a woman unable to take hormone medication. For some women, osteoporosis risk is low. It is not a common problem for black women because of a hereditary disposition for thicker, stronger bones. Common risk factors other than estrogen hormone deficiency that increase osteoporosis risk include:

• Inactivity
• Family history of osteoporosis (loss of height, dowager's hump, hip fracture)
• Slender body build
• Low calcium intake, milk intolerance

- Diet high in protein, caffeine, salt
- Excessive vitamin A or vitamin D
- Medications including thyroid (3 grains or more daily), cortisone, Dilantin, aluminum antacids, and some diuretics
- Medical problems including kidney disease, diabetes, alcoholism, and bowel diseases such as colitis

Breast Cancer Risk.   Available research evidence does not show whether breast cancer risk is increased, decreased, or unaffected by ovary removal. Breast cancer is definitely influenced by hormone patterns, however, and is also one of the most common reasons that a woman might be unable to take hormone medications later in life.

Approximately 9% of women develop breast cancer, usually after age 40. Estrogen hormone stimulates tumor growth for some breast cancers, and despite sophisticated laboratory studies that can detect tumor cell receptors for estrogen, there is no way to be certain whether estrogen medication would be safe. For this reason, a woman who has had breast cancer will be advised to **avoid** estrogen medication, at least for the first few years after her cancer diagnosis, even if she has osteoporosis or symptoms of estrogen deficiency.

Ovary removal before age 40 is statistically linked to a **lower than average** future risk for breast cancer. Whether, or how, ovary removal after age 40 may affect risk is not clearly documented. It is possible that reduced exposure to estrogen between age 40 and 50 and even after menopause might be protective. In general, known breast cancer risk factors involve exposure to natural estrogen production that is longer or higher than average. On the other hand, extensive research on women who take estrogen medication after menopause has not found any significant overall risk increase for breast cancer. It may be that hormone levels during and after the menopause years are not important, and that breast cancer risk depends instead on hormone patterns earlier in life.

This is obviously an important issue for all women, and especially for women who have had previous breast cancer or a strong family history of breast cancer. Unfortunately, medical knowledge cannot yet provide clear guidelines for assessing whether ovary removal might be beneficial or whether ovary removal may be harmful overall. A woman who develops breast cancer may be unable to take hormone medication and may therefore have higher risks for heart disease and osteoporosis.

Summary: Weighing Pros and Cons.   If ovary removal is recommended, your surgeon will be able to tell you whether it is necessary in your case, or whether future cancer risk is the main reason for the removal recommendation. **If future cancer risk is the reason, then your own feelings and opinions are an appropriate part of the decision-making process.**

Ovary removal is **medically necessary** if you are having surgery because of:

• Uterine or ovarian cancer
• Severe infection that involves the ovaries as well as the uterus and/or fallopian tubes

Ovary removal may also be a **wise choice, or an unavoidable** part of surgery if:

• Scar tissue and/or technical difficulties in performing surgery make it impossible for your surgeon to leave them in place
• Endometriosis is the reason for surgery, and your ovaries contain endometriosis tissue that is likely to cause further problems in the future
• Your ovaries are abnormal, because of benign tumor growth, for example, and further problems in the future are likely

You may also want to **consider ovary removal** if your personal medical history involves:

• High risk for future ovarian cancer

Otherwise it is entirely reasonable to decide in favor of preserving your ovaries even if you have already completed menopause. Continuing ovary function may be especially important if your personal medical history includes:

• High risk factors for osteoporosis
• High risk factors for heart disease
• Problems with sex drive or sexual function
• Medical problems that may make future treatment with hormone medication impossible or unwise

Hysterectomy Procedures

ABDOMINAL HYSTERECTOMY

Surgical procedures are very similar for both TAH (total abdominal hysterectomy) and TAH with BSO (bilateral salpingo-oophorectomy added).

After surgical preparations and anesthesia are complete, your surgeon makes a horizontal 5-inch incision across the middle of your lower abdomen (see Illustration 49-2). (If you have had previous surgery with a vertical incision, your surgeon may follow your old incision line in order to remove the original scar tissue and leave you with just one vertical scar; a vertical incision may also be needed if there is a possibility you have an ovarian tumor.) The incision is extended through the connective tissue layers of your abdomen and through the thin, translucent membrane (peritoneum) that lines your abdominal cavity, and the abdominal muscles are separated (usually not cut) and spread apart temporarily. Once the abdominal cavity is

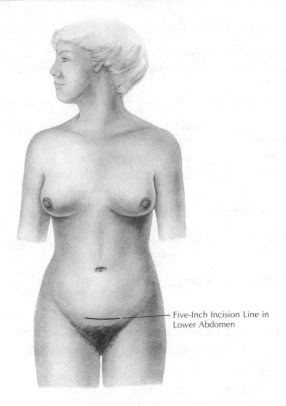

Five-Inch Incision Line in
Lower Abdomen

ILLUSTRATION 49-2   Hysterectomy is often performed with a horizontal
(Pfannenstiel) abdominal incision.

open, your surgeon inspects your pelvic organs, intestines, and bladder, and checks
your kidneys, liver, and gallbladder with her/his fingers to detect any abnormalities.
Then instruments are used to hold your incision open and hold your intestines out of
the way so that your uterus, tubes, and ovaries can be seen clearly (see Illustration
49-3). Your surgeon removes your uterus (or uterus, tubes, and ovaries) by first
placing clamps across the ligaments and blood vessels that attach these organs to the
rest of your pelvis. Each clamp site is then carefully cut and stitched to prevent
bleeding. The juncture of the cervix with the back of the vagina can be stitched closed,
or in some cases left partially open to allow fluid from the surgery site to drain out
during healing; in that case, the vaginal incision site will close on its own within four
to six weeks.

    After your uterus and cervix (and sometimes ovaries and tubes) are removed, your
surgeon repairs each layer—the peritoneum, connective tissue, muscle, and skin—to
close your incision.

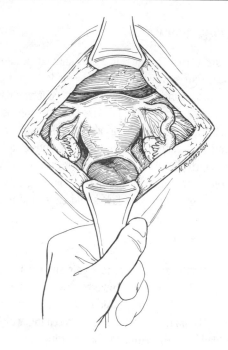

ILLUSTRATION 49-3   Your surgeon can see all your pelvic organs clearly during abdominal hysterectomy.

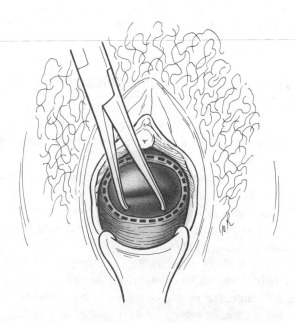

ILLUSTRATION 49-4   Incision for vaginal hysterectomy.

VAGINAL HYSTERECTOMY

After anesthesia, you are placed in the pelvic examination position and your vagina and thighs are cleansed. Your surgeon uses instruments to hold open the walls of your vagina and makes an incision through the inside of your vagina where the vaginal walls meet the cervix (see Illustration 49-4). The incision is extended through connective tissue and peritoneum into your abdominal cavity. Your surgeon uses a clamp to pull down on your cervix in order to locate, suture, and cut the ligaments and blood vessels that attach the uterus to other pelvic structures. As your uterus is cut free, the uterus and cervix are removed through the opening in your vagina. Finally, your surgeon repairs each of the incision layers and closes the incision.

PELVIC REPAIR

From your point of view as a patient, pelvic repair surgery is very similar to either abdominal hysterectomy or to vaginal hysterectomy, depending on which repair technique is needed in your particular situation. An abdominal incision is needed for techniques such as the Marshall-Marchetti-Krantz procedure, which is used to reposition the base of the bladder and urethra to correct urine control problems. "Anterior and posterior repair," techniques commonly used to correct cystocele and rectocele, involve vaginal surgery. An incision through the vaginal lining is used to expose the bladder bulge (cystocele) or bulging rectal tissue (rectocele) and reposition the fibrous and muscle tissue layer to prevent future bulging. Stitches are used to hold the supporting tissue firmly in place, and the vaginal incision(s) is stitched closed.

Hysterectomy Complications and Risks

After you leave the hospital, it will be up to you to watch for signs of possible problems. If you have any of the danger signs shown in Illustration 49-5, prompt evaluation is essential.

Also, be sure that you understand clearly any instructions that your surgeon has for your care after you leave the hospital. You will need to allow several weeks for the incision inside your vagina to heal. You should not have vaginal intercourse or put anything inside your vagina until after your postoperative checkup, when your surgeon determines that your healing is satisfactory.

The overall risk of death for a healthy woman undergoing elective hysterectomy is less than 1 in 1,000. Your risk with hysterectomy depends on your age and general health status, the competence of your surgeon and anesthesiologist, the quality of hospital care, and the specific reasons for the procedure in your case. About 1 or 2 deaths occur for every 1,000 hysterectomies performed (6). As with any surgery, the

49:5   DANGER SIGNS AFTER HYSTERECTOMY

Fever (temperature over 100.4 degrees F.)
Pain not relieved by the medication your surgeon has given you
Pain, swelling, tenderness, or redness in your leg (calf or thigh)
Chest pain, cough, difficulty breathing, or coughing blood
Fainting or dizziness that persists more than a few seconds
Red or tender skin near your incision
Bleeding or oozing from your incision
Persistent bladder discomfort, burning with urination, blood in
   your urine, or inability to urinate
More than 3 days without a normal bowel movement
Bright red or heavy vaginal bleeding that is not a normal menstrual
   period
Pain or bleeding during or after intercourse

Contact your surgeon at once or go to a hospital emergency room
if you develop any of these symptoms after surgery.

death risk is substantially higher for a woman 55 or older at the time of surgery, or a woman who has one or more anesthesia or surgery risk factors such as high blood pressure. The reason for hysterectomy is also a crucial factor (see Table 49-2). About 60% of hysterectomy deaths occur in the small group of women (8% of total) who undergo medically necessary hysterectomy because of cancer or severe complications associated with pregnancy.

Deaths are quite rare, but serious complications are not rare. **At least 25%, and as many as 50%, of patients in reported studies have one or more complications following hysterectomy** (7).

INFECTION

Infection is the most common hysterectomy complication. About 30% of women who have abdominal hysterectomy and 15% of women who have vaginal hysterectomy require treatment for infection (7). In most cases, infection is mild and involves only the bladder or the surface of the incision, so it responds readily to antibiotic treatment. Infection problems can be severe, however. An abscess might require further surgery, and infection is a major cause of the few deaths that do occur with hysterectomy.

In older studies, infection risk was higher after vaginal hysterectomy than after abdominal hysterectomy. Antibiotics immediately before and after vaginal surgery are now used routinely, and a 1982 study of hysterectomy complications showed that **overall** complication rates after vaginal hysterectomy were lower (25%) than the rates after abdominal surgery (48%). Infection problems accounted for the largest share of

TABLE 49-2
DEATH RISK WITH HYSTERECTOMY[a]

| | APPROXIMATE RISK OF DEATH | |
AGE	VAGINAL HYSTERECTOMY	ABDOMINAL HYSTERECTOMY (NONMALIGNANT DISEASE)
35–44	1 in 20,000	1 in 3,600
45–54	1 in 3,700	1 in 2,200
55–64	1 in 5,300	1 in 530
65–74	1 in 550	1 in 220

[a]Age is an important factor in surgery risk and so is the *reason for surgery*. Abdominal and vaginal hysterectomies are often done for different reasons, and the abdominal surgery statistics include almost all women who required surgery for serious medical problems.

SOURCE: Adapted from Wingo PA, Huezo CM, Rubin GL, et al: The mortality risk associated with hysterectomy. *American Journal of Obstetrics and Gynecology* 152:803–808, 1985.

complications in both groups: 17% of vaginal surgery patients compared to 38% of abdominal surgery patients (8). In comparing these rates it is important to remember that the abdominal surgery group included patients who had more serious problems before surgery, and therefore **required** abdominal surgery rather than vaginal surgery.

HEMORRHAGE

Bleeding can occur during surgery, and 10% of women who have hysterectomy require blood transfusion (7). Heavy bleeding can also occur after you go home, and is most common about 7 to 14 days after surgery, when your internal stitches begin to dissolve. Less than 1% of women require hospitalization or transfusion because of late bleeding, however.

URINARY AND BOWEL PROBLEMS

Problems with urination are quite common during the first few weeks after hysterectomy, but usually are not serious. Bladder infection is extremely common, especially when a urine catheter through the urethra is needed for more than a few hours after surgery. If prolonged bladder drainage is anticipated, a drainage tube temporarily inserted through the abdominal wall may be used instead of a urethral catheter because infection rates are lower (3). Bladder muscles are likely to require several days to regain the normal contraction strength that empties the bladder effectively, and in some cases the inability to urinate persists as long as several weeks. This can result in longer hospitalization than expected, or continued catheter drainage at home after discharge.

Injury to urinary tract structures is a fairly common complication with hysterectomy. Approximately 1 woman in 200 will have a bladder injury and 1 woman in 300 an injury to the ureters, the tubes that drain urine from the kidney to the bladder (7). Additional surgical steps during hysterectomy may be necessary to repair damage if it is recognized immediately. In some cases, the injury is not evident until after surgery and a second operation may be needed later for repair. Bladder fistula, an abnormal opening from the bladder into the vagina, is one example of possible bladder injuries. In the past, childbirth injury was the most frequent cause of fistula; now accidental injury during surgery is its most common cause. A fistula results in continuous leakage of urine from the vagina, and surgery is usually necessary for repair.

Bowel problems are rare, but could occur if your intestines are damaged during surgery or if scar tissue interferes with intestinal contractions. Later surgery to remove scar tissue might be necessary in rare cases, or even colostomy if a persistent rectal–vaginal fistula forms or severe injury to the intestine occurs during surgery.

THROMBOPHLEBITIS AND LUNG BLOOD CLOTS

Problems with abnormal blood clot formation, called thrombophlebitis, are uncommon but potentially very serious. Thrombophlebitis in a leg vein is a risk with any kind of major surgery because of bed rest and inactivity; risk is also higher after pelvic surgery, especially when infection occurs, because large veins there can be a site for clot formation. The danger of thrombophlebitis is that part or all of an abnormal clot could break loose from its origin in a leg vein or pelvic vein and travel to the lungs (embolize) and seriously or fatally impair breathing. A block in blood circulation caused by a large clot could cause a stroke, with permanent brain damage or even death.

VAGINAL PROBLEMS

The most common vaginal problem after hysterectomy is slow healing of the incision at the back of the vagina. As the normal healing process occurs, dark pink, lush tissue called granulation tissue may form along the incision line. It is more fragile than normal vaginal lining tissue and may bleed slightly with trauma such as penile thrusting during intercourse; it may also cause excessive watery vaginal discharge. Granulation tissue that persists can be treated in the office with a chemical cautery stick to encourage complete healing.

Vaginal shortening is another possible complication. A portion of the vagina must be removed with hysterectomy in order to cut the cervix free from its attachment to the vagina. If excessive vaginal tissue is removed, the final vaginal depth may be shortened enough that intercourse becomes uncomfortable or even impossible. Also, scar tissue along the back of the vagina will be less elastic than the normal lining and may add to the problem of shortness.

OVARIAN PROBLEMS

If the ovaries are left in place at the time of hysterectomy, common ovarian problems such as benign cysts can occur later, just as they might for any woman. In addition, the hysterectomy surgery itself may be a cause of later ovarian problems. Scar tissue formation or surgical damage to the blood vessels that supply the ovary may be responsible for later pain or tenderness during intercourse. In rare cases, later ovarian problems such as these occur even when the ovaries have been removed at the time of hysterectomy. A tiny shred of remaining ovary tissue may be the culprit.

Damage to ovarian blood vessels during hysterectomy surgery can also cause premature loss of ovary function, even though the ovaries are left in place. There is some evidence that this problem occurs more frequently than is commonly believed. Researchers have found that as many as 40% to 50% of premenopause-age women who have had hysterectomies report symptoms of insufficient ovarian hormone production. Lower than average estrogen and progesterone levels were documented in one study of premenopausal women whose ovaries were left in place at hysterectomy (9).

A retained fallopian tube may also cause problems if the tube becomes swollen with trapped secretions. A swollen tube may be painful, and would be evident as an abnormal mass in the pelvis. Further surgery would be necessary in this situation to be certain that the mass is not a tumor.

EFFECTS ON SEXUAL FUNCTION

It is entirely reasonable to be concerned about possible sexual problems in relation to hysterectomy. Unfortunately, there are no precise research data to show how frequently new sexual problems might occur after surgery, or how hysterectomy may effect problems that are already present.

Often, gynecologic problems that make hysterectomy appropriate also interfere with sexual function. Pain caused by pelvic infection or endometriosis, or prolonged and excessive bleeding, may make intercourse unpleasant or impossible, for example. In these situations, improvement in sexual enjoyment and function is likely following hysterectomy.

Temporary vaginal discomfort during intercourse is very common for the first few months after surgery. Permanent and serious sexual problems can also occur as a result of hysterectomy for a woman who has surgery complications. Severe vaginal shortening or scarring, for example, could make intercourse difficult or even impossible. These problems are very rare, however, and sexual problems that are more commonly reported are more subtle; evaluating the role of hysterectomy surgery in causing or contributing to such problems is a thorny research task. Researchers in 1950 and 1961 concluded that 10% to 15% of women experience sexual problems after hysterectomy; subsequent studies in 1967, 1974, and 1977 found higher rates: 28%, 38%, and 37%, respectively (3). It is hard to interpret these findings, however, because sexual problems are very common for all women. It is quite possible that 40% of comparable women who did not undergo hysterectomy might report similar problems.

Approaching this issue from a different direction, a questionnaire survey conducted by Consumers Union found that hysterectomy did not have a major impact on the reported frequency of sexual intercourse or on sexual enjoyment among older people. Overall, 70% of the women surveyed reported high levels of enjoyment of sex, and 68% of women who had had hysterectomy also reported high enjoyment; ovary removal had no significant impact in this study (10).

Nevertheless, hysterectomy with or without ovary removal does affect sexual function. Some women notice only minor alterations. For some women, the changes may cause problems; for others, sexual function may be improved.

Hormone Patterns and Physical Aspects of Sexual Response.   The uterus, cervix, and the ovaries are not necessary for sexual arousal or orgasm. All these organs do play roles in the normal sexual response, however, so even if you do not experience any difficulty or problems with sexual function, you will probably be able to identify some differences in your own response patterns and sensations after surgery.

The ovaries provide estrogen hormone, which stimulates cervical mucus production and also maintains a vaginal lining that is lush, resilient, and able to produce lubricating fluid as the sexual arousal response begins. Loss of estrogen commonly causes vaginal dryness problems, with markedly reduced lubricating fluid. Low estrogen also is responsible for a gradual loss of vulvar tissue. If the vaginal lips shrink in size and substance, their ability to swell during arousal and transmit sensations of penile thrusting to the clitoris may also be reduced.

Ovarian hormones may also affect sex drive. Small amounts of androgen (male hormones) are normally produced by the ovaries, and this role persists after menopause. (Androgens are also manufactured by the adrenal glands.) Increased interest in sex is one effect of androgens. Many other factors affect sex drive and the precise role of hormones is not known, but ovarian androgen production may be significant.

The cervix and uterus both participate in the physical changes of sexual arousal, and in muscular contractions during orgasm. Movements of the penis striking the cervix are transmitted to the uterus. The uterus responds to sexual arousal with engorgement, and as it moves with thrusting, the sensations can be perceived deep in the pelvis. During orgasm, the muscular wall of the uterus undergoes rhythmic contractions along with the muscles in the vulvar area. When the cervix and uterus are absent, the physical structure of the pelvis, and its physical adaptations in response to arousal, are undeniably altered.

If the ovaries are left in place, problems caused by hormone changes should not occur, except when hormone loss is a result of damage to the blood supply of preserved ovaries. If hormone deficiency is causing problems, then treatment with hormone medication is very likely to be helpful.

Physical changes may prompt you to explore or revise your lovemaking techniques. You may find that your optimal intercourse position, for example, is altered. And because emotions are so important in sexual functioning, it is also possible that your feelings about surgery and loss of fertility may have an impact, negative or positive, on sexual functioning for you, and possibly for your partner as well.

I didn't have any trouble having orgasms after my hysterectomy, but I certainly was *afraid* I would. My orgasms do feel a little bit different now. There is definitely something *missing* that I used to feel—a kind of muscle contraction deep inside during orgasm. It doesn't really bother me, but I do notice it.

—WOMAN, 37

PSYCHOLOGICAL PROBLEMS

Surgery of any kind is a significant stress. In the case of hysterectomy, it also means loss of a body part, and one that has substantial meaning because of its role in fertility. Grief is an entirely normal reaction to loss, and is likely to be more intense with hysterectomy than it would be with removal of the gallbladder, for example. Grief typically begins with a phase of denial, a temporary optimistic interval that occurs during the initial days or weeks after loss before the reality of what has happened is really incorporated. Periods of guilt, depression, and anger are also quite likely, followed finally by acceptance and readiness to move on to other issues in life. These are all entirely normal and healthy human responses that help us deal with loss, but may be tough to live through, especially when you are also recovering from surgery. During the first weeks and months after surgery you are likely to feel especially vulnerable and tired. The physical fatigue of the recovery period may also intensify feelings of depression.

The psychological impact of hysterectomy is likely to be especially intense for a woman who desires future pregnancy but must nevertheless undergo surgery, or when hysterectomy is an unexpected emergency procedure (11).

Severe or prolonged postoperative psychological problems are not normal, and are not common among women who have been in good psychological health prior to surgery. Hysterectomy can be a major setback, however, for a woman who already has depression problems. **Possible psychological impact deserves careful consideration just as any other surgery risk factor when the pros and cons of elective surgery are being weighed.**

WEIGHT GAIN

Many women fear weight gain after hysterectomy, and there are indeed several ways in which weight might be affected. If surgery is necessary because of a problem such as prolonged infection, then appetite may increase along with overall well-being after the problem is eliminated. Surgery also necessitates a period of reduced physical activity; if calorie intake is not similarly reduced, then weight gain during convalescence is quite likely. Alternatively, a woman who has had pain or problems with bladder control severe enough to interfere with exercise may find that maintaining ideal weight is easier after surgery with a more active lifestyle.

Weight gain is not among the reported short-term or long-term complications of hysterectomy, with or without ovary removal. Research to determine the precise effects of hysterectomy and hormones on weight, however, is lacking.

LONG-TERM EFFECTS

Research on possible long-term effects of hysterectomy in the past focused specifically on the impact of hormone loss when ovary removal was performed at the same time. The uterus itself was presumed to be inert, hormonally speaking, and therefore of no significance to other body functions. It is now clear that uterine lining cells can and do manufacture certain hormones that enter the bloodstream and thus affect other organs. Prostaglandin hormones are one example, and researchers suspect that the uterus may be a significant source of other hormones that influence blood vessel dilation and clotting (7). These discoveries are significant because of the potential impact on heart disease risk. Heart disease risk might also be affected by premature loss of ovary function that occurs because of damage to the ovary's blood supply during hysterectomy surgery. Hysterectomy with ovary removal prior to menopause has long been known to increase a woman's risk for heart disease; studies show that premenopausal **hysterectomy alone (with ovaries preserved) may also increase heart attack risk** for the remaining premenopause years (12). If further research substantiates and clarifies this risk, heart disease impact may become one of the most important issues in considering elective hysterectomy.

Long-term effects also include **beneficial health consequences** for many women. After hysterectomy menstrual bleeding and cramps are eliminated, and the likelihood of anemia is reduced. Pregnancy risks are eliminated, along with cervical and uterine cancer risks, and pelvic infection is extremely unlikely.

TABLE 49-3

VARIATIONS IN HYSTERECTOMY RATES

NUMBER OF HYSTERECTOMIES PERFORMED IN 1982
FOR EVERY 100,000 WOMEN AGE 15 TO 44

Overall in the United States	750
White women	770
Black women	670
Women in northeastern states	420
Women in western states	690
Women in north central states	700
Women in southern states	1,050

SOURCE: Irwin KL, Peterson HB, Hughes JM, et al: Hysterectomy among women of reproductive age, United States, update for 1981–1982. *CDC Surveillance Summaries* Vol 35, No 1SS, 1986.

What About
Unnecessary Surgery?

Hysterectomy is one of the most common of all surgical procedures and it is often cited as an example of unnecessary surgery.

Hysterectomy was first performed in 1843 (3). It reached maximum popularity in the United States in about 1975, a year when more than 900 hysterectomies were performed for every 100,000 women between 15 and 44 years of age. By 1980, the rate had declined to 750 per 100,000, and thereafter remained fairly stable at least through 1982 (13).

As might be expected, rates are highest for women during their reproductive years; these are the years that gynecologic problems are common. There are, however, significant variations in hysterectomy rates that are hard to explain logically. For example, rates are higher in some geographic areas than others (see Table 49-3).

Significant differences in gynecologic health may explain part of the variation in hysterectomy rates, but the wide range of rates probably means that differences also exist in the likelihood that hysterectomy will be recommended by a surgeon, and in the willingness of women to agree to surgery. If hysterectomy is commonplace in your geographic and social environment, then you may not be as surprised to hear surgery recommended, and may be more likely to decide in favor of surgery. Your surgeon, too, is almost certain to be influenced to some extent by the philosophy and practice of her/his colleagues.

Financial issues may also influence surgery decisions. A liberal policy in making recommendations for surgery certainly can impact the income of a surgeon. Also, availability of insurance reimbursement might influence a woman in making her decision, or encourage her to have surgery sooner rather than delaying in the hope that surgery may be avoided. At some later time she might not have favorable coverage.

None of these are intellectually satisfying reasons to decide for or against major surgery. In an ideal world, medical and personal factors would be weighed in a vacuum, free of financial pressure or community trends. It is disquieting, but not surprising, to see the effects of "reality" in our health statistics.

I read a short research report on surgery rates for male gynecologists compared to female gynecologists, and it made me really question my own policies. *The women surgeons just didn't do nearly as many hysterectomies.* Am I underestimating the meaning of hysterectomy to a woman? Should I be more conservative? These are tough questions for anyone in this field today. No answers, of course.

—GYNECOLOGIST, 45 (Male)

As you assess the issues of hysterectomy and unnecessary surgery, however, it is important to remember that in most cases the woman undergoing surgery is doing so voluntarily, is probably fairly well informed about her risks, and is sometimes very eager to have the surgery. There are many situations in which hysterectomy, although not necessary to preserve or save a woman's life, does add greatly to the quality of life. A woman who has incapacitating menstrual cramps for seven days each month because of endometriosis may feel that the risks and expense of surgery are justified, even though hysterectomy is not medically necessary in her case.

REFERENCES

1. Scott JZ, Cumming DC: The menopause. *Current Problems in Obstetrics, Gynecology and Fertility* 8:4–58, 1985.
2. Garcia C-R, Cutler WB: Preservation of the ovary: A reevaluation. *Fertility and Sterility* 42:510–514, 1984.
3. Mattingly RF, Thompson JD: *Te Linde's Operative Gynecology* (ed 6). Philadelphia: J.B. Lippincott Co., 1985.
4. Cutler WB, Garcia C-R: *The Medical Management of Menopause and Premenopause.* Philadelphia: J.B. Lippincott Co., 1984.
5. *Physicians' Desk Reference* (ed 40). Oradell, N.J.: Medical Economics Co., 1986.
6. Wingo PA, Huezo CM, Rubin GL, et al: The mortality risk associated with hysterectomy. *American Journal of Obstetrics and Gynecology* 152:803–808, 1985.

7. Easterday CL, Grimes DA, Riggs JA: Hysterectomy in the United States. *Obstetrics and Gynecology* 62:203–212, 1983.

8. Dicker RC, Greenspan JR, Strauss LT, et al: Complications of abdominal and vaginal hysterectomy among women of reproductive age in the United States. The Collaborative Review of Sterilization. *American Journal of Obstetrics and Gynecology* 144:841–848, 1982.

9. Riedel H-H, Lehmann-Willenbrock E, Semm K: Ovarian failure phenomena after hysterectomy. *Journal of Reproductive Medicine* 31:597–599, 1986.

10. Brecher EM, editors of Consumer Reports Books: *Love, Sex, and Aging. A Consumers Union Report.* Mount Vernon, N.Y.: Consumers Union, 1984.

11. Tang GWK: Reactions to emergency hysterectomy. *Obstetrics and Gynecology* 65:206–210, 1985.

12. Punnonen R, Ikalainen M, Seppala E: Premenopausal hysterectomy and risk of cardiovascular disease. *Lancet* 1:1139, 1987.

13. Irwin KL, Peterson HB, Hughes JM, et al: Hysterectomy among women of reproductive age, United States, update for 1981–1982. *CDC Surveillance Summaries* Vol 35, No 1SS, 1986.

I N D E X